T0383259

Sleep Disorders

Editor

BRADLEY V. VAUGHN

NEUROLOGIC CLINICS

www.neurologic.theclinics.com

Consulting Editor
RANDOLPH W. EVANS

November 2012 • Volume 30 • Number 4

ELSEVIER

1600 John F. Kennedy Boulevard • Suite 1800 • Philadelphia, Pennsylvania 19103-2899

http://www.theclinics.com

NEUROLOGIC CLINICS Volume 30, Number 4
November 2012 ISSN 0733-8619, ISBN-13: 978-1-4557-4951-5

Editor: Donald Mumford

Neurologic Clinics (ISSN 0733-8619) is published quarterly by Elsevier Inc., 360 Park Avenue South, New York, NY 10010–1710. Months of issue are February, May, August, and November. Periodicals postage paid at New York, NY, and additional mailing offices. Subscription prices are $285.00 per year for US individuals, $470.00 per year for US institutions, $140.00 per year for US students, $359.00 per year for Canadian individuals, $564.00 per year for Canadian institutions, $397.00 per year for international individuals, $564.00 per year for international institutions, and $199.00 for Canadian and foreign students/residents. To receive student/ resident rate, orders must be accompanied by name of affiliated institution, date of term, and the *signature* of program/residency coordinator on institution letterhead. Orders will be billed at individual rate until proof of status is received. Foreign air speed delivery is included in all *Clinics* subscription prices. All prices are subject to change without notice. **POSTMASTER:** Send address changes to *Neurologic Clinics*, Elsevier Health Sciences Division, Subscription Customer Service, 3251 Riverport Lane, Maryland Heights, MO 63043. **Customer Service: Telephone: 1-800-654-2452 (U.S. and Canada); 314-447-8871 (outside U.S. and Canada). Fax: 314-447-8029. E-mail: journalscustomerservice-usa@elsevier.com (for print support); journalsonlinesupport-usa@elsevier.com (for online support).**

Reprints. For copies of 100 or more of articles in this publication, please contact the Commercial Reprints Department, Elsevier Inc., 360 Park Avenue South, New York, New York, 10010-1710; Tel.: (+1) 212-633-3812; Fax: (+1) 212-462-1935, and E-mail: reprints@elsevier.com.

Neurologic Clinics is also published in Spanish by Nueva Editorial Interamericana S.A., Mexico City, Mexico.

Neurologic Clinics is covered in *Current Contents/Clinical Medicine, MEDLINE/PubMed (Index Medicus), EMBASE/Excerpta Medica, and PsycINFO, and ISI/BIOMED.*

Printed and bound by CPI Group (UK) Ltd, Croydon, CR0 4YY

Transferred to digital print 2012

Contributors

CONSULTING EDITOR

RANDOLPH W. EVANS, MD
Clinical Professor, Department of Neurology, Baylor College of Medicine, Houston, Texas

GUEST EDITOR

BRADLEY V. VAUGHN, MD
Chief of the Division of Sleep and Epilepsy, Vice Chair, Department of Neurology; and Professor of Neurology and Biomedical Engineering, Department of Neurology, University of North Carolina School of Medicine, Chapel Hill, North Carolina

AUTHORS

CHARLES H. ADLER, MD, PhD
Professor, Movement Disorders Division, Department of Neurology, Mayo Clinic, Scottsdale, Arizona

IMRAN ALI, MD
Professor of Neurology, Associate Dean for Clinical Undergraduate Medical Education, Professionalism and Diversity; Director, Comprehensive Epilepsy Program, Department of Neurology, University of Toledo, College of Medicine and Life Sciences, Toledo, Ohio

ALON Y. AVIDAN, MD, MPH
Department of Neurology, Professor of Neurology, Director, UCLA Sleep Disorders Center, Los Angeles, California

SUSHANTH BHAT, MD
NJ Neuroscience Institute at JFK Medical Center, Seton Hall University, Edison, New Jersey

SUDHANSU CHOKROVERTY, MD
NJ Neuroscience Institute at JFK Medical Center, Seton Hall University, Edison, New Jersey

AMIT CHOPRA, MD
The Center for Sleep Medicine, Mayo Clinic, Rochester, Minnesota

NANCY A. COLLOP, MD
Woodruff Health Sciences Center, Emory University, Atlanta, Georgia

ANTONIO CULEBRAS, MD, FAAN, FAHA, FAASM
Professor of Neurology, Department of Neurology, Upstate Medical University, Syracuse, New York

MARYANN C. DEAK, MD
Clinical Instructor, Division of Sleep Medicine, Harvard Medical School, Sleep Health Centers, Brigham and Women's Hospital, Brighton, Massachusetts

ERIKA D. DRIVER-DUNCKLEY, MD
Associate Professor, Movement Disorders Division, Department of Neurology, Mayo Clinic, Scottsdale, Arizona

CHARLENE E. GAMALDO, MD, FAASM
Assistant Professor, Neurology, Assistant Professor, Pulmonary and Critical Care Medicine, Director, Johns Hopkins Sleep Disorders Center, Baltimore, Maryland

DIVYA GUPTA, MD
NJ Neuroscience Institute at JFK Medical Center, Seton Hall University, Edison, New Jersey

SHELBY F. HARRIS, PsyD
Sleep-Wake Disorders Center, Montefiore Medical Center, Bronx, New York

SARA K. INATI, MD
EEG Section, National Institute of Neurologic Disorders and Stroke, National Institutes of Health, Bethesda, Maryland

OCTAVIAN C. IOACHIMESCU, MD, PhD
Atlanta Veterans Affairs Medical Center, Emory University School of Medicine, Decatur, Georgia

DOUGLAS B. KIRSCH, MD
Regional Medical Director, Division of Sleep Medicine, Department of Medicine, Brigham and Women's Hospital, Sleep HealthCenters; Clinical Instructor, Harvard Medical School, Brighton, Massachusetts

SURESH KOTAGAL, MD
The Center for Sleep Medicine; Departments of Neurology and Pediatrics, Mayo Clinic, Rochester, Minnesota

ANDREW D. KRYSTAL, MD, MS
Director, Sleep Research Laboratory and Insomnia Program, Professor of Psychiatry and Behavioral Science, Department of Psychiatry, Duke University Medical Center, Durham, North Carolina

RAMAN K. MALHOTRA, MD
Assistant Professor of Neurology, Co-Director, SLUCare Sleep Disorders Center, Director, Department of Neurology and Psychiatry, Saint Louis University School of Medicine, St Louis, Missouri

JUSTIN C. MCARTHUR, MBBS, MPH, FAAN
Professor of Neurology, Pathology, Medicine, and Epidemiology, Director, Department of Neurology, Neurologist-in-chief, The Johns Hopkins Hospital, Johns Hopkins University School of Medicine, Baltimore, Maryland

RENEE S. MONDERER, MD
Sleep-Wake Disorders Center, Montefiore Medical Center, Bronx, New York

ALEX MOSZCZYNSKI
University of Toronto, Toronto, Ontario, Canada

BRIAN JAMES MURRAY, MD, FRCPC, DABSM
Department of Medicine, Director of Integrated Medical Education, University of Toronto;
Associate Professor, Neurology and Sleep Medicine, Sunnybrook Health Sciences
Center, Toronto, Ontario, Canada

J. STEVEN POCETA, MD
Division of Neurology, Sleep Center, Scripps Clinic, La Jolla, California

JEANETTA C. RAINS, PhD
Center for Sleep Evaluation, Manchester, New Hampshire

MARC RAPHAELSON, MD
Leesburg, Virginia

HEIDI L. ROTH, MD
Associate Professor, Department of Neurology, Cognitive Neurology and Sleep Medicine,
University of North Carolina, Chapel Hill, North Carolina

DAVID B. RYE, MD, PhD
Professor of Neurology, Program in Sleep, Department of Neurology, Emory University
School of Medicine, Atlanta, Georgia

ANNUM K. SHAIKH, BS
MPH Candidate, Emory University Rollins School of Public Health, NE Atlanta, Georgia

MICHAEL THORPY, MD
Director, Sleep-Wake Disorders Center, Montefiore Medical Center, Bronx, New York

LYNN MARIE TROTTI, MD, MSc
Assistant Professor of Neurology, Program in Sleep, Department of Neurology, Emory
University School of Medicine, Atlanta, Georgia

BRADLEY V. VAUGHN, MD
Chief of the Division of Sleep and Epilepsy, Vice Chair, Department of Neurology; and
Professor of Neurology and Biomedical Engineering, University of North Carolina School
of Medicine, Chapel Hill, North Carolina

MARI VIOLA-SALTZMAN, DO
Clinician Educator, Department of Neurology, Pritzker School of Medicine, NorthShore
University HealthSystem, Evanston, Illinois

NATHANIEL F. WATSON, MD, MSc
Associate Professor of Neurology, University of Washington (UW) School of Medicine;
Co-director, UW Medicine Sleep Center, Seattle, Washington

JOHN W. WINKELMAN, MD, PhD
Associate Professor, Harvard Medical School, Sleep Health Centers, Brigham and
Women's Hospital, Brighton, Massachusetts

PHYLLIS C. ZEE, MD, PhD
Professor of Neurology, Director Sleep Disorders Centers, Department of Neurology,
Circadian Rhythms and Sleep Research Lab, Northwestern University, Chicago, Illinois

LIRONG ZHU, MD, PhD
Department of Neurology, Circadian Rhythms and Sleep Research Lab, Northwestern
University, Chicago, Illinois

Contents

Sleep is characterized by changes in neural firing and chemistry compared with wakefulness. Many neurologic diseases affect pathways that regulate control of sleep state and some primary sleep disorders have abnormalities of this circuitry. Nonrapid eye movement (NREM) and rapid eye movement (REM) sleep alternate in an approximately 90-minute cycle. Recent findings have expanded understanding of the control of sleep state, and will facilitate development of novel therapeutics to assist patients with a variety of disorders of sleep and wakefulness. Treatment of sleep and wake disorders can assist patients with a variety of neurologic problems.

Sleep medicine has been evolving over the past few decades and methods of patient evaluation have changed. Given the strong overlap between neurologic disorders and sleep disorders, neurologists should be familiar with currently available tools in sleep medicine to best care for their patients. This article lists some of the most common assessments that a neurologist might use in clinical practice to evaluate patients with sleep complaints. Both subjective and objective tools have important roles in a complete sleep evaluation; however, knowing when and how to use these assessments is also essential.

Neurologists treat many people with unrecognized sleep disorders. This review recommends that new and established patients routinely complete standard sleep questionnaires as an aid to clinical history. Because there is high prevalence of treatable primary sleep disorders among neurologic patients, routine diagnostic sleep testing is indicated for patients with stroke, neuromuscular disease, dementia, REM behavioral disorder, atypical or treatment-refractory insomnia, and chronic and unexplained fatigue or sleepiness. As local and national regulatory momentum favors increasing care coordination and integration, neurologists should develop a clinical pathway to diagnose and treat sleep disorders within the practice or through a collegial expert network.

networks. Insufficient mobilizable iron stores increase expressivity in some individuals. The sensorimotor features are relieved by dopamine, especially dopamine agonists, gabapentin and its derivatives, and opioids. A diagnosis relies on recognition of key primary and supportive features, and treatments are generally well tolerated, efficacious, and life-changing.

There have been remarkable advances in our understanding of the molecular, cellular, and physiologic mechanisms underlying the regulation of circadian rhythms, and of the impact of circadian dysfunction on health and disease. This information has transformed our understanding of the effect of circadian rhythm sleep disorders (CRSD) on health, performance, and safety. CRSDs are caused by alterations of the central circadian timekeeping system, or a misalignment of the endogenous circadian rhythm and the external environment. This article reviews circadian biology and discusses the pathophysiology, clinical features, diagnosis, and treatment of the most commonly encountered CRSDs in clinical practice.

Sleep-wake problems are common during childhood and adolescence. They are of diverse cause, and can contribute significantly to alterations in behavior, cognition, and learning. Obstructive sleep apnea, central hypoventilation syndrome, narcolepsy, periodic hypersomnia, delayed sleep phase syndrome, restless legs syndrome, parasomnias, and sleep disruption consequent to psychiatric disorders are some of the commonly encountered conditions. Some aspects of sleep architecture and its organization change with age and maturation. Diagnostic criteria and sleep laboratory techniques and findings for some childhood sleep disorders differ from those of adults. Most pharmacologic agents used to treat pediatric sleep disorders are off-label.

Sleep in Neurological Disorders

Sleep evaluation can be essential in the treatment of dementia because sleep-related issues are common in dementia, often treatable, affect patient function, and are a major cause of caregiver distress. This article provides a practical approach to treatment of sleep in patients with dementia. Certain specific sleep disorders can be associated with certain underlying disorders and greater knowledge of these relationships is leading to more refined treatment approaches. Whether a sleep-related disorder such as obstructive sleep apnea, or limited sleep time, predisposes to the development of dementia is an active area of research.

Sleep and epilepsy have a dynamic interaction that presents the clinician opportunities for diagnosis and treatment. Sleep complaints are very common in patients with epilepsy and these complaints may be related to the underlying epilepsy, the treatment of epilepsy or other sleep related issues. Appropriate treatment of epilepsy may improve sleep, and treatment of sleep disorders may reduce the frequency of recurrent seizures. Sleep and sleep deprivation may provoke seizures and can provide further diagnostic information about the seizure type and location. For the clinician, understanding the relationship of sleep and epilepsy expands the diagnostic and therapeutic armamentarium.

There is abundant and still evolving scientific clinical evidence linking sleep apnea with stroke risk factors, cardiovascular disease, and stroke. Sleep apnea is a modifiable risk factor and efforts to control this condition should be pursued vigorously, particularly in patients at risk of vascular disease. Emerging evidence has also linked other sleep disorders, such as periodic limb movements of sleep and restless legs syndrome, with vascular risk.

Irrespective of diagnosis, chronic daily, morning, or "awakening" headache patterns are soft signs of a sleep disorder. Sleep apnea headache may emerge de novo or may present as an exacerbation of cluster, migraine, tension-type, or other headache. Insomnia is the most prevalent sleep disorder in chronic migraine and tension-type headache, and increases risk for depression and anxiety. Sleep disturbance (eg, sleep loss, oversleeping, schedule shift) is an acute headache trigger for migraine and tension-type headache. Snoring and sleep disturbance are independent risk factors for progression from episodic to chronic headache.

Sleep disturbance is common after traumatic brain injury (TBI). Insomnia, fatigue, and sleepiness are the most frequent post-TBI sleep complaints with narcolepsy (with or without cataplexy), sleep apnea (obstructive or central), periodic limb movement disorder, and parasomnias occurring less commonly. In addition, depression, anxiety, and pain are common TBI comorbidities with substantial influence on sleep quality. Diagnosis of sleep disorders after TBI may involve polysomnography, multiple sleep latency testing, or actigraphy. Treatment is disorder-specific and includes the use of medications, continuous positive airway pressure, or behavioral modifications. Unfortunately, treatment of sleep disorders associated with TBI often does not improve sleepiness or neuropsychologic function.

Research models show a strong interrelationship between sleep quality and immune function. The proinflammatory cytokines, interleukin-1, interleukin-6, and tumor necrosis factor α are classified as official sleep-regulatory substances. However, sleep-promoting properties are also possessed by several other immune and proinflammatory cellular classes. This article reviews the current physiologic evidence for the prominent somnogenic and sleep-regulatory properties inherent to these immune substances. Clinical examples of this relationship are discussed from the perspective of infectious and primarily immune-related conditions associated with significant sleep disruption and from the perspective of immune dysregulation associated with several primary sleep disorders.

This article summarizes what is currently known about sleep disturbances in several movement disorders including Parkinson disease, essential tremor, parkinsonism, dystonia, Huntington disease, myoclonus, and ataxias. There is an association between movement disorders and sleep. In some cases the prevalence of sleep disorders is much higher in patients with movement disorder, such as rapid eye movement sleep behavior disorder in Parkinson disease. In other cases, sleep difficulties worsen the involuntary movements. In many cases the medications used to treat patients with movement disorder disturb sleep or cause daytime sleepiness. The importance of discussing sleep issues in patients with movement disorders cannot be underestimated.

Sleep disorders are common in patients with neuromuscular diseases, but are often overlooked. Recognizing and treating issues relating to sleep disturbances improves the quality of life for these patients. This article provides an overview of the sleep dysfunction that occurs in neuromuscular diseases, of which the most common is sleep-disordered breathing. In addition, the current literature is reviewed to provide primary care physicians, sleep specialists, neurologists, and neuromuscular specialists with information on available diagnostic and treatment modalities.

There is growing experimental evidence that the relationship between psychiatric disorders and sleep is complex and includes bidirectional causation. This article provides the evidence that supports this point of view, reviewing data on sleep disturbances seen in patients with psychiatric disorders as well as data on the impact of sleep disturbances on psychiatric conditions. Although much has been learned about the psychiatric disorders–sleep relationship, additional research is needed to better understand the relationship. Such work promises to improve comprehension of these phenomena and lead to better treatment for the many patients with sleep disorders and psychiatric disorders.

NEUROLOGIC CLINICS

RELATED INTEREST

Sleep Medicine Clinics, March 2012
Sleep-Related Epilepsy and Electroencephalography
Madeleine Grigg-Damberger, MD and Nancy Foldvary-Schaefer, DO, MS, *Guest Editors*

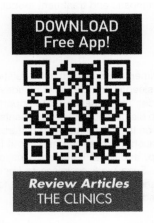

DOWNLOAD
Free App!

Review Articles
THE CLINICS

NOW AVAILABLE FOR YOUR iPhone and iPad

Preface

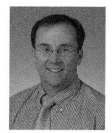

Bradley V. Vaughn, MD
Guest Editor

Sleep is a function of the brain. We have discovered that sleep is an active state with a variety of physiological processes that improve our abilities during wakefulness. These states provide benefit to brain function and can be a benchmark for health and neurologic function. Disruption of sleep can lead to negative effects for both brain and body health. Approximately 1 in 3 individuals in the general population have a sleep complaint and the prevalence of sleep issues is much higher in patients with neurologic disorders. Sleep disruption can cause an enhancement of these neurologic symptoms and lower quality of life. Several studies also indicate that improvement in sleep may decrease the severity of symptoms associated with some neurologic disorders. In addition, some neurologic disorders may present initially with sleep issues. This is most well demonstrated by REM sleep behavior disorder, which can present decades prior to the other symptoms of synucleinopathies. Despite this rich dynamic relationship of sleep and neurologic disorders, many neurologists have little training regarding the physiology of sleep or dealing with sleep issues. The articles in this issue of *Neurologic Clinics* are specifically written to elucidate these important areas for neurologists who may be unfamiliar with sleep medicine. These articles also emphasize many clinical approaches and pearls and include cases to highlight these key points.

A thorough clinical approach to sleep issues requires understanding the basic neurologic components and principles of sleep. The authors have reflected this in their articles. This edition has 3 major sections: Basics of Sleep, Approach to Sleep Issues, and Sleep in Neurological Disorders. The first article is written to provide a general understanding of the physiological basis of sleep and how the brain incorporates 2 major components, circadian rhythm and the drive to sleep, into determination of sleep–wake state. From there, the next article maps out the tools a neurologist may use to understand and define sleep disorders. This article reviews practical tools that apply to the general population and some tools that are more specific for patients with neurologic conditions. The third article discusses how sleep medicine fits into a neurologic practice and is written specifically by a private practitioner who blended sleep and neurology specialties into 1 practice. The author's inclusion of real-life experience demonstrates the practicalities of using sleep medicine to enhance the care of patients with neurologic issues.

Neurol Clin 30 (2012) xiii–xiv
http://dx.doi.org/10.1016/j.ncl.2012.08.020
neurologic.theclinics.com
0733-8619/12/$ – see front matter © 2012 Elsevier Inc. All rights reserved.

Approximately 1 in 3 people note intermittent insomnia and 12% of our population complain about excessive sleepiness. The second section of this edition is designed to give the practicing neurologist an understanding of the approach to common sleep problems. Articles on insomnia, hypersomnia, and parasomnias give an approach to these typical complaints. In addition, articles on specific sleep disorders, such as sleep apnea, circadian rhythm disorders, and restless legs syndrome, enhance the reader's understanding of these diagnoses and enhance the opportunities of treating patients with these conditions successfully. Sleep disorders are not limited to our adult population. As such, this section concludes with an insightful article regarding the approach of sleep issues in children.

The third section concentrates on the interaction of sleep and sleep disorders in neurologic disease. The major categories of neurologic disorders seen in clinical practice are addressed. This section highlights the opportunities available for neurologists to utilize sleep as a benchmark of brain health and treatment of sleep issues as an opportunity to benefit patients with neurologic disease. Areas such as dementia, stroke, epilepsy, headache, traumatic brain injury, immunologic and infectious disorders, movement disorders, neuromuscular disorders, and psychiatric disorders give a full breadth for the practicing neurologist. These articles deliver practical approaches and treatments for sleep issues with many clinical pearls. For neurologists who are perplexed or feel limited in their abilities in addressing these often "by the way" complaints, this series of articles can give a new array of options for the treatment of sleep and neurologic issues.

I would like thank all of the authors who contributed to this issue of *Neurologic Clinics*. I am very honored to work with these distinguished, enthusiastic, and insightful authors. I also would like to give special thanks to Donald Mumford, editor of *Neurologic Clinics*, who was instrumental in seeing this publication to fruition. His sage advice and understanding made this publication possible. Last, I would like to dedicate this issue to all of the patients, whom we, as health care providers, have learned from. We each entered medicine to help others, but without patients from whom we learn, we could not improve our practice and expertise. I hope you enjoy and benefit from this edition as much as I have.

Bradley V. Vaughn, MD
Department of Neurology
University of North Carolina School of Medicine
CB #7025, 2122 Physician Office Building
Chapel Hill, NC 27599-7025, USA

E-mail address:
vaughnb@neurology.unc.edu

Basics of Sleep

Neurobiological Aspects of Sleep Physiology

Alex Moszczynski[a], Brian James Murray, MD, FRCPC, DABSM[b,c],*

KEYWORDS

• Sleep • Sleep physiology • Sleep disorders • Alertness • Wakefulness

KEY POINTS

- A simple model for understanding the physiology of sleep is to consider rhythm-generating thalamocortical circuits that are modulated by external neuronal influences.
- Alertness is derived from ascending cholinergic and monoaminergic projecting systems that facilitate cortical activity.
- Orexin/hypocretin is helpful in stabilizing states to prevent rapid changes.
- Sleep is composed of nonrapid eye movement (NREM) and rapid eye movement (REM) sleep, which alternate in an approximately 90-minute cycle.
- NREM is characterized by a decreased in aminergic function, and marked decrease in cholinergic activity.
- REM sleep is notable for a return of cholinergic activity and a sustained decrease in aminergic activity.
- Narcolepsy is associated with rapid and incomplete state transitions and is associated with blockade of the orexin system.
- REM sleep behavior disorder is a condition marked by loss of skeletal muscle atonia and subsequent dream enactment that helps predict incipient Parkinson disease, thereby potentially identifying patients for neuroprotective strategies.
- Homeostatic sleep pressures as well as circadian factors contribute to alertness at any given point in time.
- Clock genes are rhythmically transcribed in all cells in the body and can influence physiology.
- Polysomnography collects a wealth of physiologic information that can be explored for further understanding of a variety of neurologic conditions.
- Simple treatments for common sleep disorders can benefit patients with a variety of neurologic problems.

Disclosure: Dr Murray received unrestricted educational funds and consulting fees from UCB Pharma, and Valeant in the last year but has no ongoing relationship with these or any other companies.
[a] University of Toronto, Toronto, Ontario, Canada; [b] Department of Medicine, University of Toronto, Toronto, Ontario, Canada; [c] Neurology and Sleep Medicine, Sunnybrook Health Sciences Center, Room M1-600, 2075 Bayview Avenue, Toronto, Ontario M4N 3M5, Canada
* Corresponding author. Neurology and Sleep Medicine, Sunnybrook Health Sciences Center, Room M1-600, 2075 Bayview Avenue, Toronto, Ontario M4N 3M5, Canada.
E-mail address: brian.murray@utoronto.ca

INTRODUCTION

Most humans spend roughly a third of their lives asleep, but physiologists and physicians frequently overlook this time. Sleep is an important and complex physiologic process requiring proper function of multiple diverse brain regions. These structures must work together electrically and chemically in a network to facilitate sleep, and if neurologic diseases compromise these regions the process can be disrupted with significant consequences.

Sleep is fundamental for optimal brain function and represents a novel therapeutic target for many neurologic disorders. In modern society there is a tendency to decrease sleep time and increase daytime sleepiness as a consequence. Fatigue is observed in many neurologic disorders. The problem with the term fatigue is that it encompasses several factors, including sleepiness as well as mood, reduced neuromuscular function, pain, and other features. Patients with stroke,[1] multiple sclerosis,[2,3] neuromuscular disorders,[4] and mood disorders[5] have been shown to exhibit fatigue, which may at least in part be caused by underlying sleep disturbances that are common in these disorders. Neurodegeneration of orexin and dopamine neurons may contribute to the sleepiness observed in many patients with Parkinson disease.[6–8] There are many common sleep disorders[9] with sleep apnea representing at least 3% of the population[10] and restless legs syndrome being present in at least 6%.[11] Decreased sleep, as well as decreased quality of sleep, has been associated with diminished health, increased incidence of injury, decreased quality of life, and increased mortality.[12,13] Sleep disorders have important implications for vascular disorders, which can manifest neurologically in stroke. For example, untreated sleep apnea is a contributing factor in the metabolic syndrome[14] and is an established risk factor for hypertension[15] and stroke.[16] However, many sleep disorders are amenable to simple therapies that can reduce risk, improve neurologic function, and improve quality of life. For example, risk of future stroke may be reduced by treatment of sleep disordered breathing,[17] and stroke recovery seems to be enhanced with treatment of sleep disordered breathing via continuous positive airway pressure (CPAP).[18] Treatment of sleep disordered breathing may improve health in patients with neuromuscular disorders[19] and epilepsy,[20] among other neurologic conditions. Treatment of other sleep disorders represents further opportunities for improving neurologic function.

Many complex physiologic changes accompany sleep. Some examples include differences in behavioral state, motor control, autonomic, and endocrine function. Because many physiologic systems change in sleep, problems with specific brain structures may present themselves during sleep. Therefore, sleep may be a useful diagnostic indicator for some neurologic disorders. A routine polysomnogram contains a wealth of physiologic information. Physiologic variables of interest in typical sleep studies include electroencephalography (EEG), electrooculography (EOG), surface electromyography, respiratory activity, cardiac rhythm, and oxygen saturation.[21] Sleep physiology can assist in the diagnosis of various neuropsychiatric conditions. One particularly important instance in which sleep can be a predictive indicator is in the rapid eye movement (REM) sleep behavior disorder (RBD), in which there is a loss of the normal skeletal muscle atonia of REM sleep, which can precede Parkinson disease by many years.[22,23] As another example, a reduced latency to REM sleep is typically observed in depressed individuals.[24] Therefore objective physiology may help establish physiologic endophenotypes that may suggest better response to various specific neurotherapeutics. A neurologist can readily appreciate the significance of identifying a primary generalized epilepsy pattern on an EEG, because this helps direct appropriate anticonvulsant choice. Advanced engineering and computer science techniques should yield more information from this complex physiology aside from what can be appreciated on casual visual inspection.

Understanding of the control of sleep and wake state has increased greatly in the last few decades. The discovery of orexin/hypocretin and its disruption in narcolepsy has opened up a new understanding of the control of state in recent years.[25,26] This article focuses on the current understanding of the fundamental physiologic processes regulating sleep state. It will be useful for the reader to conceptualize sleep as the neurochemical modulation of a set of intrinsically rhythmical thalamocortical circuits. Although many fundamental questions remain, there have been large advances in understanding of the control of state in the last several years.

SLEEP DEFINITION

Sleep may be defined as a rapidly reversible state of reduced mobility and sensory awareness[27] that is not simply an absence of consciousness, but an actively generated state.

Sleep seems to serve an important function. Animal studies suggest that, after long periods of sleep deprivation, health is impaired and mortality may be increased.[28] Sleep is homeostatically regulated but is also influenced by circadian rhythms.[29,30] When deprived of sleep for a certain amount of time, humans experience a sleep rebound characterized by proportionally increased slow wave sleep as well as increased δ EEG power.[31] Symptomatic sleep loss from the prion disease fatal familial insomnia is associated with premature mortality, although the underlying condition may contribute rather than sleep loss itself.[32] However, sleep loss may have a role in neurodegeneration.[33] Related to its apparent vital function, sleep has been proposed to be particularly important for energy conservation during restorative processes in non-REM (NREM) sleep.[34]

BASIC CONTROL OF SLEEP/WAKE STATE

The drive for sleep may be theoretically modeled to be driven by 2 independent processes, known commonly as process C and process S. Process C[35] is the circadian time-of-day fluctuation in arousal, which follows a nearly 24-hour cycle[36] and is entrained by light. All cells in the body exhibit a 24-hour rhythm in genetic transcription and translation of clock genes.[37] The suprachiasmatic nucleus (SCN) is the master pacemaker in the brain with direct input from the retina via the retinohypothalamic tract. The SCN coordinates rhythms throughout the body. In the absence of light input, other factors can entrain circadian rhythms, such as social cues or timing of feeding. However, process S accumulates with longer periods of wakefulness and represents homeostatic sleep drive. Process S decreases exponentially during sleep. A greater proportion of slow wave sleep (SWS) tends to be observed in this recovery state, indicating that SWS may be responsible for decreasing this particular sleep debt.[38]

Sleep is not a passive process, but it is an actively produced state generated by activity of specific brain structures and networks, with the active inhibition of others. With the epidemic of encephalitis lethargica during World War I, Constantin von Economo observed patients who exhibited 2 different conditions. One group was unable to remain awake, and was in a constant lethargic state, whereas the other was unable to sleep, and experienced severe insomnia that led to death.[39] Through careful observation, von Economo realized that lesions of 2 distinct areas of the brain caused these 2 conditions, providing the first evidence of separate sleep-promoting and wake-promoting centers in the brain. Patients with insomnia showed lesions in the preoptic area of the hypothalamus, whereas those with hypersomnolence presented with lesions in the posterior hypothalamus/rostral midbrain. In experiments, lesions of the posterior region of the hypothalamus lead to reduced wakefulness[40] and lesions of the anterior hypothalamus lead to insomnia. Electrical stimulation of the anterior hypothalamus can also promote sleep.

NEUROANATOMY AND NEUROPHYSIOLOGY OF THE BASIC RHYTHM GENERATORS

External neuromodulation by chemical factors in remote brain regions influence the basic rhythmical thalamocortical circuits. A full description of the basis of cortical EEG rhythms is beyond the scope of this article. In summary, the anatomy of thalamocortical circuits and the thalamic reticular core lead to an intrinsic rhythmicity (**Fig. 1**).[41] This circuitry consists of 3 fundamental components:

1. Corticothalamic projections: from cortex to thalamocortical and reticular nuclei of the thalamus
2. Thalamocortical (TC) relay nuclei: these nuclei send signals about sensation to the cortex for perception of stimuli
3. Thalamic reticular (RE) nucleus: these γ-aminobutyric acid (GABA)–ergic neurons form a covering around the dorsal and lateral thalamus and provide intrinsic feedback to the thalamus

The cortex projects to the thalamus and excites TC and RE cells. Cortex to thalamocortical projections have weak direct glutamatergic excitation and strong indirect polysynaptic inhibition. Cortex to reticular projections are glutamatergic. TC cells project to cortex and give collaterals to RE cells. RE cells project back to TC cells (not cortex) leading to an intrathalamic inhibitory circuit. This reticular feedback leads to a modulation of the signal between thalamus and cortex. Reticular core to thalamocortical projections are GABAergic and high-frequency spike bursts lead to potent inhibition in NREM. A reduction in reticular spike burst activity leads to less inhibition

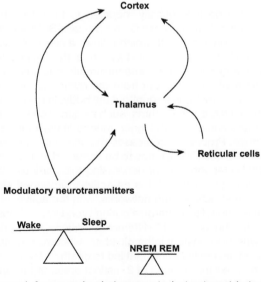

Fig. 1. Basic conceptual framework: thalamocortical circuits with intrinsic and extrinsic modulation.

in REM and wakefulness. The connections between the thalamic reticular cells and thalamocortical cells set up robust oscillations in NREM sleep. NREM sleep represents rhythmical inhibitory postsynaptic potentials with rebound excitation.

All sensory information except for the sense of smell reaches the cortex through the thalamus. In this way, the thalamus is a gatekeeper for the transmission of sensory stimuli to the cortex. During sleep, the brain has a pattern of activity whereby the transmission of sensory stimuli to the cortex is reduced. Sleep can therefore be considered a cortical disconnect from the outside world. However, the sensory responsiveness observed in sleep may be specific to the stimulus involved. Arousal in lighter NREM sleep may be more easily evoked by more significant stimuli such as hearing one's own name.[42] The lateral dorsal tegmental nucleus and pedunculopontine nucleus are cholinergic nuclei that project to the thalamus and are active in desynchronized brain states and fire less during NREM sleep, which contributes significantly to the gating of sensory information.

Neuronal membranes are polarized at rest. Action potentials are accompanied by sodium influx and depolarization. Outward flowing current (anions in or cations out) lead to a local positivity. Active sources and current sinks are accompanied by passive sinks and sources at remote locations, which are recorded in clinical EEG as the summation of electrical signal at radially arranged apical dendrites. Transient EEG activity leads most prominently to surface negative discharges representing the most visually obvious electrical events in cortical EEG. The standard convention is to represent the EEG with negativity polarity upwards; therefore, most transients in sleep are upward on visual inspection.

Spindle rhythms can be recorded in the thalamus after decortication and high brainstem transection. This manifestation therefore relies on network interactions between reticular and thalamocortical cells. The cortex synchronizes spindles and facilitates sensory blockade. Sleep spindles occur when the cortex enters a depolarized state in which cortical firing excites GABAergic neurons in the reticular nucleus of the thalamus leading to inhibition of thalamocortical neurons triggering intrinsic currents that produce a burst of action potentials.

The cortical oscillation is a periodic rhythm of 1 to 5 seconds seen in sleep that entrains spindles and K-complexes that can be triggered by sensory events.[43] The term K-complex was derived from the observation that technologists could knock on the door of the room of a sleeping patient and elicit this response. It has been proposed that K-complexes may be a mechanism of preventing arousal from sleep while still allowing some cortical processing of sensory input, allowing sleep to be consolidated into 1 period of time, but still being potentially alerted by meaningful stimuli.[44,45] The slow cortical rhythm continues in thalamectomy models. The slow cortical oscillations entrain spindle oscillations in the thalamus. In NREM sleep, with hyperpolarization of cells by the removal of acetylcholine and consequent opening of potassium leak channels, a set of slow oscillations occur with a hyperpolarization phase called the down-state, which lasts a few hundred milliseconds, and a slightly longer up-state. During the down-state there is a near cessation of synaptic activity in the cortex, whereas during the up-state the cortex fires rapidly.[46]

δ Rhythms can be intrinsically generated in the thalamus even after decortication. The cortex prevents thalamic δ oscillations in wakefulness. δ Oscillations are entrained by the slow cortical oscillation. In NREM sleep, there is a spread of the oscillatory activity as synchronized waves through the brain. The high voltage is related to the high degree of synchronization caused by extensive lateral connections. Given prominent cortical-cortical connections, and thalamocortical connections, a series of slow waves progress over the cortex, most prominently from anterior to posterior regions.[47]

The thalamus is modified by state-dependent neurotransmitters. The thalamus generates δ activity and spindles only at hyperpolarized resting membrane potentials. Hyperpolarization of thalamic neurons is accomplished by removal of depolarizing cholinergic and adrenergic input. All of the brain regions that produce neurotransmitters associated with arousal (**Table 1**) that project to the cortex also have projections to the thalamus and modulate thalamic rhythms as well. In this way they act as a source of drive for wakefulness that is withdrawn during sleep.

Fast rhythms of wakefulness can be generated by cortical neurons. Intracortical circuits contribute to the synchronization of the fast rhythm. Cholinergic nuclei such as the laterodorsal tegmental nucleus and the pedunculopontine nucleus depolarize thalamocortical cells and hyperpolarize reticular cells. Cholinergic nuclei thereby potentiate higher frequency rhythms associated with alertness and block δ oscillations associated with sleep.

The heavy connections within the brain regions that allow synchronization to occur can be problematic if there is an abnormal source of oscillation, as in epilepsy, which can take over the normal rhythm and contributes to the increased frequency of seizures in sleep.[48]

AN OVERVIEW OF SLEEP STATE PROGRESSION

The stages of sleep occur repeatedly throughout the night in a recurring NREM-REM cycle of approximately 90 minutes' duration. The general progression from wakefulness is a short time in N1, followed by a greater period of time in N2, N3, and then REM. The proportional amount of time spent in each phase changes through the sleep period. In the first hours of the night, more N3 sleep is observed, consistent with a homeostatic role in lowering the accrued sleep debt. As the night progresses, longer REM bouts are seen in each cycle. REM sleep timing is influenced by permissive circadian factors. Therefore, if a person is awake through the early hours of their normal sleep period, they may have proportionally increased REM sleep.

Sleep stage is characterized by specific EEG, EOG, and electromyography (EMG) findings. The traditional scoring system[49] has been replaced by new quantification

Table 1
Key structures and neurotransmitter activity in major states of sleep and alertness

Locus	Neurotransmitter	Wake Activity	NREM Activity	REM Activity
Laterodorsal tegmental nucleus	Acetylcholine	+	−	+
Pedunculopontine nucleus	Acetylcholine	+	−	+
Dorsal raphe	Serotonin	+	−	−
Locus coeruleus	Norepinephrine	+	−	−
Substantia nigra	Dopamine	+	−	+
Tuberomammillary nucleus	Histamine	+	−	−
Ventrolateral preoptic nucleus	γ-Amino butyric acid	−	+	+ (extended VLPO)
Posterolateral hypothalamus	Orexin	+	−	−

methods that were published by the American Academy of Sleep Medicine in 2007.[21] The critical physiology of each stage is summarized in **Table 2**.

NEUROANATOMY OF STATE MODULATION

The control of state is modulated by regions that promote sleep, and others that promote arousal (see **Table 1**). These centers are mutually inhibitory, and therefore only 1 state can normally exist at a time. It has long been recognized that stimulation of the brainstem reticular formation increases arousal.[50] Specific arousal centers include the tuberomammillary nucleus (TMN), locus coeruleus (LC), dorsal raphe nuclei, substantia nigra (SN), pedunculopontine (PPN), and laterodorsal tegmental nucleus (LDT). These interact with one another and send diffuse projections to cortex and thalamus to promote wakefulness while inhibiting the activity of sleep-promoting centers. Sleep-promoting centers include the ventrolateral preoptic nucleus (VLPO) and the median preoptic nucleus (MnPO), which are less well understood.

WAKE-PROMOTING SYSTEMS

The main alerting stimuli come from the cholinergic basal forebrain and a group of cholinergic and predominantly monoaminergic neurons running along the central brain stem typically referred to as the reticular activating system. **Fig. 2** shows some of the major wake-promoting centers and a prototypical ascending projecting system of wakefulness: projections from the LC. The main mechanism by which cortical activation is achieved by these neurotransmitters is by closing leakage potassium channels in cortical and thalamic neurons, leading the cells to depolarize and thus becoming more prone to fire. Stimulation of the reticular activating system results in EEG activation and the cortical desynchronization characteristic of wakefulness.[50,51] Lesions of this area lead to slow waves in the cortex and coma. Sensory afferents send branches to the ascending reticular activation system such that sensory stimulation can be directly responsible for promoting wakefulness. It is therefore important that, for sleep to occur, sensory stimulation must be minimized and there must be some active inhibition, thereby disconnecting sensation from the cortex.

However, not all wakefulness is the same. A variety of factors may differentially be responsible for components of alertness. For example, fight-or-flight responses may more directly involve norepinephrine, whereas rewarding behaviors may be more directly reinforced by dopamine.

Acetylcholine

Basal forebrain lesions lead to slowing of cortical activity and loss of vigilance.[52] These cholinergic neurons are most active in wakefulness and, to a lesser degree, in REM sleep.[53] They are least active in SWS. Neurons in the LDT and PPN have also been shown to be active during waking. These neurons project to the basal forebrain, thalamus, and the posterior hypothalamus. Studies using acetylcholine (ACh) antagonists have shown SWS-like activity, and have implicated ACh as an important contributor to mediation of conscious arousal.[54] Increased cortical levels of ACh are also found in REM sleep.[53]

Norepinephrine

Norepinephrine (NE) is produced in the LC and has been shown to promote arousal, particularly in times of stress in which increased alertness would benefit survival. Cooling of the LC leads to sleep and lesions can lead to coma.[55] LC neurons are most active in wake[56] and depolarize thalamic neurons.[57]

Table 2
Key physiologic features of adult human sleep stages

Stage	EEG	EOG	EMG	% Total Sleep Time (Adult)	Comments
Wake	8–13 Hz α activity for >50% of 30-s epoch	Blinking Rapid eye movements	High tone	—	—
N1	α Rhythm <50% of an epoch Low-amplitude mixed-frequency activity Vertex sharp waves	Slow roving eye movement	Tone reduced from wakefulness (readily appreciated as head nodding in lecture halls)	~5%	Transitional sleep: a marker of sleep disruption Increased in sleep disorders with sleep fragmentation
N2	K-complexes Sleep spindles	Eyes normally are still	—	~50%	—
N3 (SWS; δ sleep; previously stages 3 and 4)	High-amplitude, low-frequency (0.5–2 Hz) activity for >20% of epoch	—	Further decreases in motor tone	~20%	Homeostatic sleep
REM	Low-voltage, fast activity slightly slower than wakefulness Sawtooth waves	Rapid eye movements	Skeletal muscle atonia	~25%	Reduction in primary sensory cortex activation, but increases in associative cortical areas and limbic systems Dreaming state

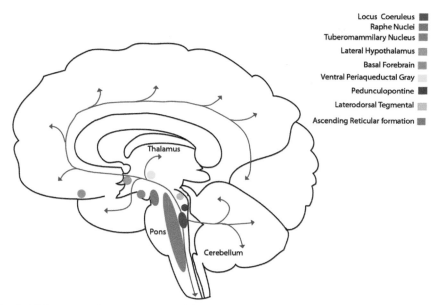

Locus Coeruleus
Raphe Nuclei
Tuberomammilary Nucleus
Lateral Hypothalamus
Basal Forebrain
Ventral Periaqueductal Gray
Pedunculopontine
Laterodorsal Tegmental
Ascending Reticular formation

Fig. 2. Wake promotion systems: LC with major projections.

Another important part of LC activity is that, in addition to mediating cortical arousal, descending projections from this nucleus also promote muscle tone.[58] Optogenetic studies have recently shown that increasing LC activity can awaken an animal from sleep,[59] and unexpectedly produces a behavioral state in animals similar to cataplexy (the loss of motor tone with emotional stimuli). It had been previously noted that LC neuron activity ceases during cataplexy in narcoleptic dogs[60] but that the activity of serotonin neurons does not,[61] implying that lack of LC activity is conducive to producing the atonia observed in cataplexy. Ongoing studies of the interaction of various neurotransmitter systems may help in understanding the issues around motor control in cataplexy.

Serotonin

Serotonin (5-hydroxytryptamine [5-HT]) is produced in the dorsal raphe nuclei (DRN) and is another important mediator of arousal and muscle tone. These cells are suppressed during REM sleep. The removal of serotonin-mediated muscle activation in REM sleep may contribute to obstructive sleep apnea.[62] In addition, suppression of 5-HT release specifically increases REM sleep, indicating that these neurons play some role in suppressing the neural activity responsible for REM sleep.[63] These neurons fire rapidly when awake, less in NREM sleep, and are almost inactive during REM sleep. These neurons also affect mood, behavior, motor control, feeding, and thermoregulation.

Histamine

Histamine (HA) produced in the TMN of the hypothalamus is associated with promotion of arousal.[64] Intraventricular administration of histamine leads to arousal[65] and lesions of this region are associated with somnolence.[40] Histamine neurons are wake active.[66]

Dopamine

Dopamine (DA) also seems to promote cortical arousal in wake and REM. Dopaminergic neurons in the caudal hypothalamus seem to express increased amounts of the immediate early gene c-fos while awake, indicating a role in alertness.[67] The wake-promoting effects of the drug modafinil seem to occur through a dopamine receptor–dependent mechanism and, when dopamine receptor activity was blocked by the antagonist quinpirole, the wake-promoting effects were abolished.[68]

Orexin/Hypocretin

Orexin has recently been identified as a novel neuropeptide; blockade of this system can induce narcolepsy.[25,26] There are 2 forms of orexin (also known as hypocretin). Orexin-A and orexin-B target OX1 and OX2 receptors, which are both excitatory G-protein–coupled receptors. Orexin cells have diffuse projections to cortex and other activating nuclei.[69,70] Orexin neurons are active in wake, particularly with novelty[71] and inactive in SWS.[72] It is thought that orexin neurons are particularly important in the maintenance of wakefulness, and prevention of sudden transitions between wake and sleep. Orexin neurons have been shown to be absent or reduced in human narcolepsy,[73] in which patients experience excessive daytime sleepiness, hypnagogic hallucinations, sleep paralysis, and cataplexy. Orexin is thought to be a stabilizing input that reinforces activation of the arousal-promoting neurons. When orexin is lost, frequent incomplete transitions of state occur more rapidly. Optogenetic studies have recently shown that silencing these neurons can induce sleep in mice, further indicating their importance in maintaining arousal.[74] These neurons have different modes of firing in different types of wakefulness. In dogs, the orexin neurons fire at a higher frequency during active exploration than while running on a treadmill. It is therefore unlikely to be the increased physical activity that is responsible for the increased firing of these neurons, but rather the increased stimulation that goes along with novelty, which may explain how motivated behavior can promote arousal.

SLEEP-PROMOTING SYSTEMS

Although arousal-promoting centers have been well studied, sleep is an active process requiring the proper function of sleep-promoting centers, which are less understood. The ventrolateral preoptic area (VLPO) in the hypothalamus has been a leading player in this story. This center seems to be influenced by both the circadian rhythm and the homeostatic drive (**Fig. 3**). The VLPO expresses the immediate early gene c-fos during sleep[75] and, when the VLPO is lesioned, insomnia results.[76] Most neurons in this area fire most actively during sleep[77] and have inhibitory influences on arousal systems.[78,79] This region is thought to be particularly important in sustaining sleep and shows activity in NREM and REM sleep. GABAergic and galaninergic projections from the VLPO inhibit arousal-promoting centers. An extended VLPO has been described that contains REM-on neurons and may play a role in REM sleep control. Other areas such as the median preoptic nucleus (MnPO) also seem to play a role in initiating NREM through GABAergic mechanisms.[80]

Adenosine

Adenosine is a known somnogen, acting on A_1 and A_2 receptors to promote sleep as levels increase with prolonged wakefulness. Therefore, this may represent the substance that best marks the theoretic process S.[81] Blocking adenosine receptors with agents such as caffeine reduces the drive for sleep. Adenosine has been shown

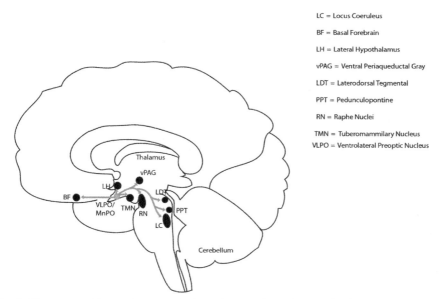

LC = Locus Coeruleus

BF = Basal Forebrain

LH = Lateral Hypothalamus

vPAG = Ventral Periaqueductal Gray

LDT = Laterodorsal Tegmental

PPT = Pedunculopontine

RN = Raphe Nuclei

TMN = Tuberomammilary Nucleus

VLPO = Ventrolateral Preoptic Nucleus

Fig. 3. Sleep promotion systems: ventrolateral preoptic nucleus projections.

to act on A_1 receptors in wake-promoting centers in which it inhibits activity and decreases arousal.[82]

Other somnogens are known, including prostaglandin D2, which has similar properties to adenosine, galanin, δ sleep–inducing peptide, and other inflammatory factors such as interleukin-1 and tumor necrosis factor, which can even induce local sleep when applied on animal cortex.[83]

INTERACTIONS BETWEEN SLEEP-PROMOTING CENTERS AND WAKE-PROMOTING CENTERS DETERMINES STATE OF AROUSAL

The mutually inhibitory flip-flop model of state control[84] is widely accepted as a plausible explanation for the observed rapid state changes between wake and sleep. The VLPO inhibits arousal centers such as TMN, LC, DRN, and lateral hypothalamus. In contrast, arousal centers inhibit the VLPO.[85,86] The wake-promoting and sleep-promoting systems form mutually inhibitory connections. In doing so, they create a binary oscillator, normally allowing only 1 state of arousal to occur at a time. This switch is thought to be responsible for the sudden and complete shift from wake to sleep and vice versa under normal circumstances. As the activity of 1 set of systems decreases, the other increases, which further drives the other down, acting as a positive feedback for itself, and a negative feedback for the opposing systems. At some critical point, there is a change in the dominantly active systems that manifests itself as a change in state. Orexin is thought to represent an important factor in state stability, which would explain the rapid state transitions seen in disorders such as narcolepsy in which orexin signaling is lost.[87] Lesions of the VLPO similarly lead to increased state transitions.[76]

INTERACTIONS WITH CIRCADIAN AND INFRARADIAN RHYTHMS

An extension of this model includes the influence of circadian factors that primarily influence the VLPO/MnPO as well as basal forebrain.

The key circadian pacemaker in the brain is the suprachiasmatic nucleus. The SCN is a paired structure in the anterior hypothalamus that is the basic anatomic clock in the brain. There is a core and shell. The core contains rhythmical neurons and the shell consists of light-responsive cells. Neurons in the SCN fire in a 24-hour cycle driven by an intrinsic transcriptional-translational loop.[37] All cells in the body have this rhythmical expression, and cells in culture maintain this rhythm for some time before the entraining influence of light is removed. Clock genes are rhythmically transcribed in a 24-hour cycle and entrained by the retinohypothalamic tract projections to the suprachiasmatic nucleus. In absence of photic input, such as in blindness, the rhythm can be entrained by other factors such as exogenous melatonin,[88] strict feeding times, or behavioral factors such as social interactions.

Four main proteins PERIOD (PER), CRYPTOCHROME (CRY), and translational factors CLOCK and BMAL1 are involved in the basic molecular clock (**Fig. 4**). The transcription factors combine and activate Cry and Per to increase production of their respective proteins. CRY and PER dimerize and inhibit activity of CLOCK/BMAL1. Phosphorylation leads PER and CRY levels to drop. Kinases such as casein kinase I ε further modulate this cycle.[35] The role of several other factors influencing this basic cycle are being clarified and are beyond the scope of this article.

Mutations in clock genes can lead to altered phase lengths of the circadian rhythm in humans.[89] A complex behavior such as being a night owl or morning lark might be influenced by a single codon mutation.

The ventral subparaventricular zone has particular circadian influence on sleep with lesions in this zone disrupting circadian rhythms.[90] The major projection is to the dorsomedial nucleus of the hypothalamus. This area has GABAergic projections to the VLPO[91] and glutamatergic projections to the lateral hypothalamus.

Other longer rhythms are less well understood, although endocrine influences of the monthly cycle are significant in influencing sleep in women.[92,93] Seasonal rhythms are also profound in sleep-wake behaviors and influence conditions such as seasonal affective disorder and cluster headache.[94] There is significant plasticity in the SCN system, with significant changes in cell counts noted over the course of seasons.[95]

CONTROL OF REM SLEEP

Although there have been significant recent advances in understanding of the mechanisms of REM/NREM regulation, some questions remain. The cholinergic REM-on and monoaminergic REM-off antagonistic model has been a major model of REM

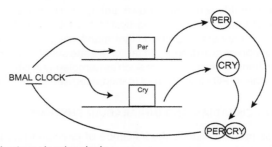

Fig. 4. Simplified basic molecular clock.

control. More recently, GABAergic and glutamatergic mechanisms have been suggested to be particularly important for the control of REM/NREM cycling.

Anatomic transection studies have pointed to an important influence of the pons in generating REM sleep. The LDT and PPN are cholinergic nuclei that seem to be particularly important.[96] Activity in the PPN is most striking in REM sleep and wakefulness.[97] Electrical stimulation of the PPN region may even increase REM sleep in humans.[98]

The subcoeruleus region or sublateral dorsal region (SLD) seems to be a key area for REM generation. Lesions to the SLD result in disrupted, fragmented REM sleep periods in rats.[99] The ventrolateral periaqueductal gray (vlPAG) and lateral pontine tegmentum (LPT) represent novel REM-off regions. When these regions are lesioned, REM sleep is increased.

A REM flip-flop model has been proposed whereby the SLD sends GABAergic projections to the vlPAG/LPT and vice versa, which would lead to similar properties of state control to those discussed earlier. The extended VLPO, with melanin-concentrating hormone and orexinergic neurons, modulates this REM flip-flop switch. The extended VLPO region also seems to be active in REM,[100] whereas the lateral hypothalamus in which orexin is found is inactive during REM.[72] The eVLPO seems to inhibit the REM-off machinery found in the LPT and vlPAG. Melanin-concentrating hormone activity in the lateral hypothalamus has also been noted to be increased in REM sleep, with reduced amounts in NREM and even less in wakefulness. This activity seems to be inhibitory to arousal centers. This pathway requires further clarification.

The mechanisms of REM sleep atonia represent important descending manifestations of REM sleep. Traditional models suggest that SLD glutamatergic projections to the spinal cord lead to a hyperpolarization of the α motor neurons and causes the sleep paralysis characteristic of normal REM sleep.

It has been proposed that, because the nuclei responsible for the different aspects of REM sleep are located in separate loci that seem to be under independent regulation, these cells may enter a state of dyscontrol if stabilizing orexinergic inputs are removed, as is the case with narcolepsy.[84]

PHYSIOLOGIC CHANGES IN SLEEP

Although the effects of sleep on systemic physiology are significant and beyond the scope of this article, a few features are particularly important and are highlighted.

Respiratory drive occurs through multiple mechanisms.[101] There is an underlying pattern that results from activity of central pattern generators in the brainstem, such as the pre-Botzinger complex (PreBotC), which act as a constant input to the muscles of respiration. There is also an arousal-mediated drive to breathe that is reduced during sleep. Chemoreceptor-based responses to hypercapnia are also reduced in sleep, requiring further increases in blood CO_2 levels before responses are elicited. All of these factors result in reduced respiratory activity during sleep marked by a decreased tidal volume and respiratory rate.

The decrease in respiration is further exacerbated in REM sleep, because of the lower aminergic input to the respiratory centers and active inhibition of the muscles of the upper airway. REM sleep is associated with further reduced responsiveness to increased CO_2 levels and low oxygen levels. In addition, the muscle relaxation results in decreased upper airway diameter and increased upper airway resistance leading to reduced airflow. In extreme cases, this reduction of upper airway muscle activation can result in complete collapse of the upper airway, contributing to obstructive sleep apnea.

Endocrine

Because of the hypothalamic modulation of sleep, endocrine activity changes according to different states of arousal. Hormone release can be coupled to sleep, can follow a circadian influence that is independent of sleep, or follow an ultradian pulsatile pattern of release depending on the hormone in question.[102]

Growth hormone is released largely in SWS, especially in the early hours of the sleep period. Sleep deprivation results in reduced growth hormone release, which may contribute to short stature in children with poor-quality sleep.

With decreased cortical and muscular activity in sleep, the body's need for high levels of glucose decreases and, as such, the level of insulin required to control the glucose is also reduced.

Thyroid stimulating hormone (TSH) typically peaks in a circadian fashion at night but sleep inhibits TSH secretion. Therefore TSH is maximal before sleep onset, and further release seems to be inhibited by sleep because measured TSH levels are increased significantly during sleep deprivation and in disturbed sleep.

Cortisol follows a circadian rhythm, and is not generally affected by sleep or wake state, but higher levels of circulating cortisol may affect sleep onset, or reduce the amount of SWS achieved. Cortisol levels in the blood normally reach a peak in the early morning and are linked to the circadian cycle.

Melatonin is secreted at night in the absence of light. The production of melatonin is entrained by light. Photoreceptors in the retina signal the SCN in the thalamus, which then regulates hormonal, temperature, and behavioral activity accordingly. Neurons from the SCN signal the pineal gland where melatonin is produced from 5-HT (ultimately from the amino acid tryptophan). There are 2 melatonin receptor types: MT1 and MT2. The MT1 receptor may reduce the SCN alertness message, although this is a small effect. The phase-changing properties of melatonin are largely mediated by the MT2 receptor.

SOME IMPORTANT PHYSIOLOGIC CHANGES IN REM SLEEP

REM sleep is characterized by low-voltage fast activity in the EEG and a decrease in muscle tone. In REM sleep there is an active inhibition of motor neurons. This decrease is partly mediated by inhibition of the LC.[103] Obstructive sleep apnea worsens because of muscular impairment of airway patency. This impairment is an important contributor to the sleep apnea syndrome, which leads to poor sleep quality and quality of life in many patients.[104]

REM sleep also normally suppresses behaviors that may otherwise be elicited by the increased cortical activity accompanying REM sleep. In the RBD this suppression is not sufficient to prevent motor activation from eliciting movements, and so dream-enacting behaviors are observed, accompanied by a high muscle tone uncharacteristic of normal REM sleep. Injurious dream-enacting behavior can follow.

REM sleep can be divided into 2 types, each with different physiologic markers. Tonic REM sleep is constant throughout the REM state and includes decreased responsiveness to temperature changes. This phase is accompanied by a reduction of activity in the EMG. In addition to the more severe respiratory suppression, phasic REM is associated with bursts of sympathetic activity, and is marked by an irregular heart rate, rapid eye movements, and bursts in the EMG that may appear as twitching. This increased muscle tone can also result in irregular respiratory activity.

SOME NEUROLOGIC STATE CONTROL PROBLEMS

The breadth of sleep disorders are discussed elsewhere in this issue, but it is useful for the reader to consider a few important examples in the context of understanding the fundamental physiology of sleep.

Orexin and State Dyscontrol

The discovery of orexin and its subsequent implication in narcolepsy has provided a significant development in the understanding of sleep physiology and its disorders. Orexin can be conceptualized as glue that maintains state and stabilizes the flip-flop switch. Maintaining 1 state helps prevent problems that are evident in a variety of sleep disorders in which incomplete state transitions occur. For example, intrusion of sleep into wakefulness may have catastrophic implications while driving for a patient with narcolepsy. Intrusion of the atonia of REM sleep into wakefulness could similarly contribute to cataplexy. Hallucinations at sleep onset represent an unusually early expression of REM sleep in the sleep cycle. In the RBD, patients lose the normal atonia of REM sleep and this represents a component of wake physiology that manifests itself during REM sleep.

SWS Arousals

Somnambulism (sleepwalking) may manifest itself in varying degrees of activity including complex behaviors. Somnambulism occurs when there is an incomplete arousal from SWS, triggered by an external arousal[105] or intrinsic sleep disorders such as sleep apnea or periodic limb movements. δ Oscillatory activity is seen in the EEG in the early parts of the behavior, suggesting that it takes some time for sleep to be overcome and for the cortex to be fully reactivated. This disorder tends to be in the first third of the night, when NREM sleep is more likely to occur. Patients may have no recollection of the events, consistent with the reduced amount of acetylcholine in the brain to facilitate memory formation.[106]

DRUGS/PHARMACOLOGIC INFLUENCES ON SLEEP

It is possible to manipulate controlling systems pharmacologically at many points to promote wakefulness or sleep. Because of the diversity of neurotransmitters and receptors involved in sleep/wake processes, it is possible to inadvertently disturb bystanding pathways and have unwanted side effects. Sleep achieved by pharmacologic means is generally not the same as sleep achieved naturally, and can be detected through different profiles in the EEG and underlying physiology.[107]

Catecholaminergic drugs such as amphetamines and cocaine promote wakefulness. In contrast, catecholamine-depleting drugs such as reserpine produce somnolence. Administration of common pharmacologic agents affecting these systems may affect normal sleep activity. Antihistamines are notorious for causing sedation. Antidepressants, including tricyclic antidepressants as well as selective serotonin reuptake inhibitors,[108] increase 5-HT and antagonize REM sleep. A prolonged REM latency is typically seen in most patients on antidepressants.

Cholinergic systems contribute to arousal. Agonists such as neostigmine lead to enhanced vigilance, whereas drugs that block cholinergic nuclei, such as atropine, lead to reduced vigilance.

Many of the drugs commonly used to reduce consciousness or promote sleep, such as sedatives, hypnotic, and anesthetics, target the $GABA_A$ receptor. This receptor is ubiquitously expressed throughout the central nervous system (CNS), and is thought to be largely responsible for the changes in neural activity during sleep. Many sleep-promoting drugs, including ethanol[109] and benzodiazepines,[110] are known to act on these receptors.

Along with the sleep-promoting effects of GABAergic drugs are other less desirable effects. For example, zolpidem, a sedative drug that is known to interact with the benzodiazepine-binding site of the $GABA_A$ receptor, has been associated with somnambulism.[111] In contrast, benzodiazepines such as clonazepam are among the most commonly used drugs for the treatment of somnambulism[112] because they markedly suppress restorative homeostatic SWS. This difference in effect has been proposed to be the result of a difference in the half-life of the drugs,[113] because zolpidem has a much shorter half-life than clonazepam. Memory impairment and falls are a particular concern in the elderly on benzodiazepines and should be avoided.[114]

Additional side effects of GABA agonists include the potentiation of obstructive sleep apnea, as observed with ethanol ingestion.[115] Alcohol acts on $GABA_A$ receptors, which are ubiquitously expressed throughout the CNS. It is thought that the sleep-promoting effects of alcohol are produced through this mechanism. A major issue with sleep induced by alcohol is that the upper airway is prone to collapse. $GABA_A$ receptors are found in the hypoglossal motor nucleus (HMN), which is responsible for maintaining genioglossal tone. With alcohol's inhibition of motor activity,[116] the upper airway is prone to collapse and obstructive sleep apnea occurs more frequently, leading to fragmented sleep and early morning awakening.

In addition to their effects on the $GABA_A$ receptor, many anesthetic drugs are known to act on potassium ion channels promoting inhibitory activity and preventing neuronal firing in a similar fashion to GABAergic drugs.[117] Although there are similarities in the behavior as well as the EEG pattern of sleep and anesthesia,[118] there are marked differences between the 2 states. Sleep is rapidly reversible, whereas anesthesia is not. This difference is important as an indicator of sleep as an active process, and not simply an inhibitory process. General anesthesia more closely resembles coma than sleep in its EEG profile and its lack of responsiveness to vigorous stimulation caused by brain stem inhibition.[119]

Caffeine is in common use as an adenosine receptor antagonist. Through recent knockout studies in rats, it has been proposed that its arousal effect is caused by an inhibition of the adenosine A2A receptors in the shell of the nucleus accumbens.[120] Other antagonists of the adenosine receptor include theophylline, which has been shown to delay sleep onset and increase wakefulness during the sleep period.[121] That adenosine receptor antagonists promote arousal or inhibit sleep onset supports the hypothesis that adenosine is a key mediator of the homeostatic sleep drive.[81]

Another new, commonly prescribed wake-promoting drug is modafinil. Modafinil acts to enhance the activity of arousal systems including dopamine,[122] histamine, and orexin[123] while decreasing GABAergic activity[124] through poorly understood mechanisms[125] but most likely through the dopamine system. Modafinil has been used to successfully treat excessive daytime sleepiness associated with narcolepsy.[126]

The small molecule sodium oxybate/γ-hydroxybutyrate has also been used to treat narcolepsy, for the cataplexy seen this condition,[127] and is a particularly interesting agent in that SWS and REM sleep are preserved, with intense sedation.

Orexin agonists for promotion of alertness and orexin antagonists for the treatment of insomnia are currently in development.

SUMMARY

Sleep is a complex physiologic process requiring the synchronized activity of many different brain regions. As such, it results in many physiologic changes in the body.

A simple model to consider for understanding sleep and wakefulness is to conceptualize that rhythmical circuits exist in the intrinsic wiring of thalamocortical circuits and that these are modulated by external chemical factors that change over time. Intrinsic thalamocortical rhythms are influenced by wakefulness-promoting cholinergic/monoaminergic systems and sleep-promoting GABAergic systems. Orexin/hypocretin is important in sustaining wakefulness and preventing rapid state changes. Sleep is composed of NREM and REM sleep that alternate in an approximately 90-minute cycle. NREM is characterized by a decrease in aminergic function and a marked decrease in cholinergic activity. REM sleep is notable for a return of cholinergic activity. Circadian factors influence the timing of sleep and physiology of all cells in the human body. Abnormalities in brain regions involved in sleep can result in characteristic changes to sleep architecture or cause deviations from the normally occurring series of events. These changes may be of use in diagnosing or predicting outcomes in different neurologic disorders. Treating common sleep disorders in many cases can help to mitigate neurologic impairment and improve recovery. A rapidly expanding understanding of this neurophysiology should further improve current treatment options.

REFERENCES

1. Staub F, Bogousslavsky J. Fatigue after stroke: a major but neglected issue. Cerebrovasc Dis 2001;12:75–81.
2. Cantor F. Central and peripheral fatigue: exemplified by multiple sclerosis and myasthenia gravis. PM R 2010;2:399–405.
3. Rotstein D, O'Connor P, Lee L, et al. Multiple sclerosis fatigue is associated with reduced psychomotor vigilance. Can J Neurol Sci 2012;39:180–4.
4. McElhiney MC, Rabkin JG, Gordon PH, et al. Prevalence of fatigue and depression in ALS patients and change over time. J Neurol Neurosurg Psychiatry 2009; 80:1146–9.
5. Gerber PD, Barrett JE, Barrett JA, et al. The relationship of presenting physical complaints to depressive symptoms in primary care patients. J Gen Intern Med 1992;7:170–3.
6. Thannickal TC, Lai YY, Siegel JM. Hypocretin (orexin) cell loss in Parkinson's disease. Brain 2007;130:1586–95.
7. Knie B, Mitra MT, Logishetty K, et al. Excessive daytime sleepiness in patients with Parkinson's disease. CNS Drugs 2011;25:203–12.
8. Drouot X, Moutereau S, Lefaucheur JP, et al. Low level of ventricular CSF orexin-A is not associated with objective sleepiness in PD. Sleep Medicine 2011;12:936–7.
9. American Academy of Sleep Medicine. The international classification of sleep disorders: diagnostic and coding manual. 2nd edition. Westchester (IL): American Academy of Sleep Medicine; 2005.
10. Lurie A. Obstructive sleep apnea in adults: epidemiology, clinical presentation, and treatment options. Adv Cardiol 2011;46:1–42.
11. Winkelman JW, Shahar E, Sharief I, et al. Association of restless legs syndrome and cardiovascular disease in the Sleep Heart Health Study. Neurology 2008; 70:35–42.
12. Doi Y, Minowa M, Tango T. Impact and correlates of poor sleep quality in Japanese white-collar employees. Sleep 2003;26:467–71.
13. Martin JL, Fiorentino L, Jouldjian S, et al. Sleep quality in residents of assisted living facilities: effect on quality of life, functional status, and depression. J Am Geriatr Soc 2010;58:829–36.

14. Sharma SK, Agrawal S, Damodaran D, et al. CPAP for the metabolic syndrome in patients with obstructive sleep apnea. N Engl J Med 2011;365:2277–86.

15. Peppard PE, Young T, Palta M, et al. Prospective study of the association between sleep-disordered breathing and hypertension. N Engl J Med 2000; 342:1378–84.

16. Marin JM, Carrizo SJ, Vicente E, et al. Long-term cardiovascular outcomes in men with obstructive sleep apnoea-hypopnoea with or without treatment with continuous positive airway pressure: an observational study. Lancet 2005;365: 1046–53.

17. Chan W, Coutts SB, Hanly P. Sleep apnea in patients with transient ischemic attack and minor stroke: opportunity for risk reduction of recurrent stroke? Stroke 2010;41:2973–5.

18. Ryan CM, Bayley M, Green R, et al. Influence of continuous positive airway pressure on outcomes of rehabilitation in stroke patients with obstructive sleep apnea. Stroke 2011;42:1062–7.

19. Perrin C, D'Ambrosio C, White A, et al. Sleep in restrictive and neuromuscular respiratory disorders. Semin Respir Crit Care Med 2005;26:117–30.

20. Malow BA, Foldvary-Schaefer N, Vaughn BV, et al. Treating obstructive sleep apnea in adults with epilepsy: a randomized pilot trial. Neurology 2008;71: 572–7.

21. Iber C, American Academy of Sleep Medicine. The AASM manual for the scoring of sleep and associated events: rules, terminology, and technical specifications. Westchester (IL): American Academy of Sleep Medicine; 2007.

22. Schenck CH, Mahowald MW. REM sleep behavior disorder: clinical, developmental, and neuroscience perspectives 16 years after its formal identification in SLEEP. Sleep 2002;25:120–38.

23. Postuma RB, Gagnon JF, Vendette M, et al. Quantifying the risk of neurodegenerative disease in idiopathic REM sleep behavior disorder. Neurology 2009;72: 1296–300.

24. Kupfer DJ, Foster FG. Interval between onset of sleep and rapid-eye-movement sleep as an indicator of depression. Lancet 1972;2:684–6.

25. Chemelli RM, Willie JT, Sinton CM, et al. Narcolepsy in orexin knockout mice: molecular genetics of sleep regulation. Cell 1999;98:437–51.

26. Lin L, Faraco J, Li R, et al. The sleep disorder canine narcolepsy is caused by a mutation in the hypocretin (orexin) receptor 2 gene. Cell 1999;98:365–76.

27. Siegel JM. Do all animals sleep? Trends Neurosci 2008;31:208–13.

28. Everson CA, Bergmann BM, Rechtschaffen A. Sleep deprivation in the rat: III. Total sleep deprivation. Sleep 1989;12:13–21.

29. Borbely AA, Achermann P. Sleep homeostasis and models of sleep regulation. J Biol Rhythms 1999;14:557–68.

30. Dijk DJ, Czeisler CA. Contribution of the circadian pacemaker and the sleep homeostat to sleep propensity, sleep structure, electroencephalographic slow waves, and sleep spindle activity in humans. J Neurosci 1995;15:3526–38.

31. Borbely AA, Baumann F, Brandeis D, et al. Sleep deprivation: effect on sleep stages and EEG power density in man. Electroencephalogr Clin Neurophysiol 1981;51:483–95.

32. Medori R, Tritschler HJ, LeBlanc A, et al. Fatal familial insomnia, a prion disease with a mutation at codon 178 of the prion protein gene. N Engl J Med 1992;326: 444–9.

33. Kang JE, Lim MM, Bateman RJ, et al. Amyloid-beta dynamics are regulated by orexin and the sleep-wake cycle. Science 2009;326:1005–7.

34. Tononi G, Cirelli C. Sleep function and synaptic homeostasis. Sleep Med Rev 2006;10:49–62.
35. Manthena P, Zee PC. Neurobiology of circadian rhythm sleep disorders. Curr Neurol Neurosci Rep 2006;6:163–8.
36. Czeisler CA, Duffy JF, Shanahan TL, et al. Stability, precision, and near-24-hour period of the human circadian pacemaker. Science 1999;284:2177–81.
37. Reppert SM, Weaver DR. Coordination of circadian timing in mammals. Nature 2002;418:935–41.
38. Dijk DJ, Beersma DG, Daan S. EEG power density during nap sleep: reflection of an hourglass measuring the duration of prior wakefulness. J Biol Rhythms 1987;2:207–19.
39. Triarhou LC. The percipient observations of Constantin von Economo on encephalitis lethargica and sleep disruption and their lasting impact on contemporary sleep research. Brain Res Bull 2006;69:244–58.
40. Sallanon M, Sakai K, Buda C, et al. Increase of paradoxical sleep induced by microinjections of ibotenic acid into the ventrolateral part of the posterior hypothalamus in the cat. Arch Ital Biol 1988;126:87–97.
41. Steriade M. The corticothalamic system in sleep. Front Biosci 2003;8:d878–99.
42. Langford GW, Meddis R, Pearson AJ. Awakening latency from sleep for meaningful and non-meaningful stimuli. Psychophysiology 1974;11:1–5.
43. Amzica F, Steriade M. The K-complex: its slow (<1-Hz) rhythmicity and relation to delta waves. Neurology 1997;49:952–9.
44. Jahnke K, von Wegner F, Morzelewski A, et al. To wake or not to wake? The two-sided nature of the human K-complex. Neuroimage 2012;59:1631–8.
45. Caporro M, Haneef Z, Yeh HJ, et al. Functional MRI of sleep spindles and K-complexes. Clin Neurophysiol 2012;123:303–9.
46. Steriade M, Timofeev I, Grenier F. Natural waking and sleep states: a view from inside neocortical neurons. J Neurophysiol 2001;85:1969–85.
47. Massimini M, Huber R, Ferrarelli F, et al. The sleep slow oscillation as a traveling wave. J Neurosci 2004;24:6862–70.
48. Vaughn BV, D'Cruz OF. Sleep and epilepsy. In: Carney PR, Berry RB, Geyer JD, editors. Clinical sleep disorders. Philadelphia: Ovid Technologies, Lippincott Williams & Wilkins; 2005. p. 403–19.
49. Rechtschaffen A, Kales A. A manual of standardized terminology, techniques and scoring system for sleep stages in human subjects. Los Angeles: US Government Printing Office; 1968.
50. Moruzzi G, Magoun HW. Brain stem reticular formation and activation of the EEG. Electroencephalogr Clin Neurophysiol 1949;1:455–73.
51. Steriade M, Oakson G, Ropert N. Firing rates and patterns of midbrain reticular neurons during steady and transitional states of the sleep-waking cycle. Exp Brain Res 1982;46:37–51.
52. Stewart DJ, MacFabe DF, Vanderwolf CH. Cholinergic activation of the electrocorticogram: role of the substantia innominata and effects of atropine and quinuclidinyl benzilate. Brain Res 1984;322:219–32.
53. Jasper HH, Tessier J. Acetylcholine liberation from cerebral cortex during paradoxical (REM) sleep. Science 1971;172:601–2.
54. Montplaisir JY. Cholinergic mechanisms involved in cortical activation during arousal. Electroencephalogr Clin Neurophysiol 1975;38:263–72.
55. Schott B, Michel D, Mouret J, et al. Monoamines and the regulation of wakefulness. II. Lesional syndromes of the central nervous system. Rev Neurol (Paris) 1972;127:157–71 [in French].

56. Hobson JA, McCarley RW, Wyzinski PW. Sleep cycle oscillation: reciprocal discharge by two brainstem neuronal groups. Science 1975;189:55–8.

57. McCormick DA, Bal T. Sleep and arousal: thalamocortical mechanisms. Annu Rev Neurosci 1997;20:185–215.

58. Jones BE. Modulation of cortical activation and behavioral arousal by cholinergic and orexinergic systems. Ann N Y Acad Sci 2008;1129:26–34.

59. Carter ME, Yizhar O, Chikahisa S, et al. Tuning arousal with optogenetic modulation of locus coeruleus neurons. Nat Neurosci 2010;13:1526–33.

60. Wu MF, Gulyani SA, Yau E, et al. Locus coeruleus neurons: cessation of activity during cataplexy. Neuroscience 1999;91:1389–99.

61. Wu MF, John J, Boehmer LN, et al. Activity of dorsal raphe cells across the sleep-waking cycle and during cataplexy in narcoleptic dogs. J Physiol 2004; 554:202–15.

62. Cui L, Wang JH, Wang M, et al. Injection of L: -glutamate into the insular cortex produces sleep apnea and serotonin reduction in rats. Sleep Breath 2011. [Epub ahead of print].

63. Portas CM, Thakkar M, Rainnie D, et al. Microdialysis perfusion of 8-hydroxy-2-(di-n-propylamino)tetralin (8-OH-DPAT) in the dorsal raphe nucleus decreases serotonin release and increases rapid eye movement sleep in the freely moving cat. J Neurosci 1996;16:2820–8.

64. Steininger TL, Alam MN, Gong H, et al. Sleep-waking discharge of neurons in the posterior lateral hypothalamus of the albino rat. Brain Res 1999;840:138–47.

65. Monnier M, Sauer R, Hatt AM. The activating effect of histamine on the central nervous system. Int Rev Neurobiol 1970;12:265–305.

66. Vanni-Mercier G, Sakai K, Jouvet M. Specific neurons for wakefulness in the posterior hypothalamus in the cat. C R Acad Sci III 1984;298:195–200 [in French].

67. Leger L, Sapin E, Goutagny R, et al. Dopaminergic neurons expressing Fos during waking and paradoxical sleep in the rat. J Chem Neuroanat 2010;39:262–71.

68. Wisor JP, Eriksson KS. Dopaminergic-adrenergic interactions in the wake promoting mechanism of modafinil. Neuroscience 2005;132:1027–34.

69. Peyron C, Tighe DK, van den Pol AN, et al. Neurons containing hypocretin (orexin) project to multiple neuronal systems. J Neurosci 1998;18:9996–10015.

70. Takahashi K, Koyama Y, Kayama Y, et al. Effects of orexin on the laterodorsal tegmental neurones. Psychiatry Clin Neurosci 2002;56:335–6.

71. Mileykovskiy BY, Kiyashchenko LI, Siegel JM. Behavioral correlates of activity in identified hypocretin/orexin neurons. Neuron 2005;46:787–98.

72. Lee MG, Hassani OK, Jones BE. Discharge of identified orexin/hypocretin neurons across the sleep-waking cycle. J Neurosci 2005;25:6716–20.

73. Thannickal TC, Moore RY, Nienhuis R, et al. Reduced number of hypocretin neurons in human narcolepsy. Neuron 2000;27:469–74.

74. Tsunematsu T, Kilduff TS, Boyden ES, et al. Acute optogenetic silencing of orexin/hypocretin neurons induces slow-wave sleep in mice. J Neurosci 2011;31: 10529–39.

75. Sherin JE, Shiromani PJ, McCarley RW, et al. Activation of ventrolateral preoptic neurons during sleep. Science 1996;271:216–9.

76. Lu J, Greco MA, Shiromani P, et al. Effect of lesions of the ventrolateral preoptic nucleus on NREM and REM sleep. J Neurosci 2000;20:3830–42.

77. Szymusiak R, Alam N, Steininger TL, et al. Sleep-waking discharge patterns of ventrolateral preoptic/anterior hypothalamic neurons in rats. Brain Res 1998; 803:178–88.

78. Sherin JE, Elmquist JK, Torrealba F, et al. Innervation of histaminergic tubero-mammillary neurons by GABAergic and galaninergic neurons in the ventrolateral preoptic nucleus of the rat. J Neurosci 1998;18:4705–21.

79. Steininger TL, Gong H, McGinty D, et al. Subregional organization of preoptic area/anterior hypothalamic projections to arousal-related monoaminergic cell groups. J Comp Neurol 2001;429:638–53.

80. Benedetto L, Chase MH, Torterolo P. GABAergic processes within the median preoptic nucleus promote NREM sleep. Behav Brain Res 2012;232:60–5.

81. Porkka-Heiskanen T, Strecker RE, Thakkar M, et al. Adenosine: a mediator of the sleep-inducing effects of prolonged wakefulness. Science 1997;276:1265–8.

82. Portas CM, Thakkar M, Rainnie DG, et al. Role of adenosine in behavioral state modulation: a microdialysis study in the freely moving cat. Neuroscience 1997; 79:225–35.

83. Krueger JM. The role of cytokines in sleep regulation. Curr Pharm Des 2008;14: 3408–16.

84. Saper CB, Fuller PM, Pedersen NP, et al. Sleep state switching. Neuron 2010;68: 1023–42.

85. Chou TC, Bjorkum AA, Gaus SE, et al. Afferents to the ventrolateral preoptic nucleus. J Neurosci 2002;22:977–90.

86. Gallopin T, Fort P, Eggermann E, et al. Identification of sleep-promoting neurons in vitro. Nature 2000;404:992–5.

87. Mochizuki T, Crocker A, McCormack S, et al. Behavioral state instability in orexin knock-out mice. J Neurosci 2004;24:6291–300.

88. Sack RL, Brandes RW, Kendall AR, et al. Entrainment of free-running circadian rhythms by melatonin in blind people. N Engl J Med 2000;343:1070–7.

89. Toh KL, Jones CR, He Y, et al. An hPer2 phosphorylation site mutation in familial advanced sleep phase syndrome. Science 2001;291:1040–3.

90. Lu J, Zhang YH, Chou TC, et al. Contrasting effects of ibotenate lesions of the paraventricular nucleus and subparaventricular zone on sleep-wake cycle and temperature regulation. J Neurosci 2001;21:4864–74.

91. Chou TC, Scammell TE, Gooley JJ, et al. Critical role of dorsomedial hypothalamic nucleus in a wide range of behavioral circadian rhythms. J Neurosci 2003;23:10691–702.

92. Herzog AG. Neuroactive properties of reproductive steroids. Headache 2007; 47(Suppl 2):S68–78.

93. Mong JA, Baker FC, Mahoney MM, et al. Sleep, rhythms, and the endocrine brain: influence of sex and gonadal hormones. J Neurosci 2011;31:16107–16.

94. Pringsheim T. Cluster headache: evidence for a disorder of circadian rhythm and hypothalamic function. Can J Neurol Sci 2002;29:33–40.

95. Hofman MA, Swaab DF. Seasonal changes in the suprachiasmatic nucleus of man. Neurosci Lett 1992;139:257–60.

96. Shouse MN, Siegel JM. Pontine regulation of REM sleep components in cats: integrity of the pedunculopontine tegmentum (PPT) is important for phasic events but unnecessary for atonia during REM sleep. Brain Res 1992;571: 50–63.

97. Steriade M, Pare D, Datta S, et al. Different cellular types in mesopontine cholinergic nuclei related to ponto-geniculo-occipital waves. J Neurosci 1990;10: 2560–79.

98. Lim AS, Moro E, Lozano AM, et al. Selective enhancement of rapid eye movement sleep by deep brain stimulation of the human pons. Ann Neurol 2009; 66:110–4.

99. Lu J, Sherman D, Devor M, et al. A putative flip-flop switch for control of REM sleep. Nature 2006;441:589–94.

100. Lu J, Bjorkum AA, Xu M, et al. Selective activation of the extended ventrolateral preoptic nucleus during rapid eye movement sleep. J Neurosci 2002;22: 4568–76.

101. Horner RL. Emerging principles and neural substrates underlying tonic sleep-state-dependent influences on respiratory motor activity. Philos Trans R Soc Lond B Biol Sci 2009;364:2553–64.

102. Morris CJ, Aeschbach D, Scheer FA. Circadian system, sleep and endocrinology. Mol Cell Endocrinol 2012;349:91–104.

103. McGregor R, Siegel JM. Illuminating the locus coeruleus: control of posture and arousal. Nat Neurosci 2010;13:1448–9.

104. Baldwin CM, Ervin AM, Mays MZ, et al. Sleep disturbances, quality of life, and ethnicity: the Sleep Heart Health Study. J Clin Sleep Med 2010;6:176–83.

105. Broughton RJ. Sleep disorders: disorders of arousal? Enuresis, somnambulism, and nightmares occur in confusional states of arousal, not in "dreaming sleep". Science 1968;159:1070–8.

106. Stickgold R. Sleep: off-line memory reprocessing. Trends Cogn Sci 1998;2: 484–92.

107. Staner L. Sleep-wake mechanisms and drug discovery: sleep EEG as a tool for the development of CNS-acting drugs. Dialogues Clin Neurosci 2002;4:342–50.

108. Armitage R. The effects of antidepressants on sleep in patients with depression. Can J Psychiatry 2000;45:803–9.

109. Jia F, Chandra D, Homanics GE, et al. Ethanol modulates synaptic and extrasynaptic GABAA receptors in the thalamus. J Pharmacol Exp Ther 2008;326: 475–82.

110. Sigel E. Mapping of the benzodiazepine recognition site on GABA(A) receptors. Curr Top Med Chem 2002;2:833–9.

111. Poceta JS. Zolpidem ingestion, automatisms, and sleep driving: a clinical and legal case series. J Clin Sleep Med 2011;7:632–8.

112. Kavey NB, Whyte J, Resor SR Jr, et al. Somnambulism in adults. Neurology 1990;40:749–52.

113. Juszczak GR. Desensitization of GABAergic receptors as a mechanism of zolpidem-induced somnambulism. Med Hypotheses 2011;77:230–3.

114. Madhusoodanan S, Bogunovic OJ. Safety of benzodiazepines in the geriatric population. Expert Opin Drug Saf 2004;3:485–93.

115. Issa FG, Sullivan CE. Alcohol, snoring and sleep apnea. J Neurol Neurosurg Psychiatry 1982;45:353–9.

116. Horner RL. The tongue and its control by sleep state-dependent modulators. Arch Ital Biol 2011;149:406–25.

117. Franks NP. General anaesthesia: from molecular targets to neuronal pathways of sleep and arousal. Nat Rev Neurosci 2008;9:370–86.

118. Franks NP, Zecharia AY. Sleep and general anesthesia. Can J Anaesth 2011;58: 139–48.

119. Brown EN, Lydic R, Schiff ND. General anesthesia, sleep, and coma. N Engl J Med 2010;363:2638–50.

120. Lazarus M, Shen HY, Cherasse Y, et al. Arousal effect of caffeine depends on adenosine A2A receptors in the shell of the nucleus accumbens. J Neurosci 2011;31:10067–75.

121. Roehrs T, Merlotti L, Halpin D, et al. Effects of theophylline on nocturnal sleep and daytime sleepiness/alertness. Chest 1995;108:382–7.

122. Volkow ND, Fowler JS, Logan J, et al. Effects of modafinil on dopamine and dopamine transporters in the male human brain: clinical implications. JAMA 2009;301:1148–54.
123. Ishizuka T, Murotani T, Yamatodani A. Modanifil activates the histaminergic system through the orexinergic neurons. Neurosci Lett 2010;483:193–6.
124. Huang Q, Zhang L, Tang H, et al. Modafinil modulates GABA-activated currents in rat hippocampal pyramidal neurons. Brain Res 2008;1208:74–8.
125. Gerrard P, Malcolm R. Mechanisms of modafinil: a review of current research. Neuropsychiatr Dis Treat 2007;3:349–64.
126. Broughton RJ, Fleming JA, George CF, et al. Randomized, double-blind, placebo-controlled crossover trial of modafinil in the treatment of excessive daytime sleepiness in narcolepsy. Neurology 1997;49:444–51.
127. Houghton WC, Scammell TE, Thorpy M. Pharmacotherapy for cataplexy. Sleep Med Rev 2004;8:355–66.

A Neurologist's Guide to Common Subjective and Objective Sleep Assessments

Douglas B. Kirsch, MD

KEYWORDS

- Polysomnography • MSLT • MWT • Assessment tools • Sleep questionnaires
- Sleep assessments • Polysomnography • Epworth sleepiness scale

KEY POINTS

- Appropriate use of both subjective and objective tools is necessary to balance medical costs with patient results.
- Subjective questionnaires are available for broad evaluation of sleep disorders, as well as long-term assessment and tracking of specific sleeping problems.
- Objective testing is considered the gold standard for evaluation of certain sleep disorders, removing the possibility of reporting bias and allowing an improved assessment of the patient's symptom severity.

INTRODUCTION

Sleep medicine has grown over the last several decades; however, interest in sleep, from both the public and the medical community has been particularly strong in the last several years. Neurologists have played key roles in understanding the relationship between sleep and the brain, as well as improving the understanding of many sleep disorders.

The field of sleep medicine is currently comprised of physicians of several primary specialties, including neurologists, pulmonologists, psychiatrists, and internal medicine. However, practitioners of family medicine, pediatrics, otolaryngology, and anesthesiology are also eligible to be board certified in sleep medicine. Being an expert sleep physician requires time and dedication and, as of 2011, requires a sleep medicine fellowship for most specialties. However, even neurologists who are not sleep-specialized are likely to see patients with sleep disorders as part of their practice and, therefore, should be familiar with several aspects of the sleep evaluation. There are known links between sleep-disordered breathing and stroke, epilepsy, and neuromuscular conditions; between restless legs syndrome (RLS) and neuropathies; and

Division of Sleep Medicine, Department of Medicine, Brigham and Women's Hospital, 1505 Commonwealth Ave., 5th Floor, Sleep Health Centers, Brighton, Brookline, MA 02135, USA
E-mail address: Doug_Kirsch@Sleephealth.com

Neurol Clin 30 (2012) 987–1006
http://dx.doi.org/10.1016/j.ncl.2012.08.009
0733-8619/12/$ – see front matter © 2012 Elsevier Inc. All rights reserved.

between rapid eye movement (REM) sleep behavior disorder and neurodegenerative conditions—just to name a few.

This article reviews common assessment tools, both subjective and objective, that are used in clinical practice. Some measures are brief and easily available via the Internet, whereas others require a nearly 24-hour stay in a sleep laboratory. Regardless of cost and complexity, each test has an important role in screening, diagnosis, or treatment of a patient with a sleep disorder, which can have a significant impact on a patient's morbidity and quality of life.

An essential tool for the practice of sleep medicine is the International Classification of Sleep Disorders (ICSD). The ICSD was compiled by the American Academy of Sleep Medicine (AASM) to categorize the variety of sleep disorders as they are currently understood based on scientific and clinical evidence and to present clear diagnostic criteria for those disorders. The second edition of this manual was updated in 2005 by a task force of more than 100 members of the sleep medicine community from around the world; the process for a third edition is currently underway.

Subjective Tools

There are many questionnaires that are used to assess for the presence of sleep disorders; this section will cover several of the most common ones. Selection of the most appropriate questionnaire will depend on the patient's presenting symptom and age group. Therefore, this section will be segmented into six parts: general sleep, excessive daytime sleepiness (EDS), insomnia, obstructive sleep apnea (OSA), RLS, and pediatrics. The tools discussed are listed in **Table 1** and Internet locations for some of these tools are located in **Table 2**.

General sleep assessments

Patients are often referred to sleep disorder centers with a suspicion of a rare sleep disorder, such as narcolepsy. Before considering a complex or rare sleep disorder, physicians should obtain a clinical sleep history. As part of the information-gathering phase after an initial visit, patients complaining of insomnia or hypersomnia

Table 1 Discussed sleep questionnaires by category	
General Sleep Assessments	Sleep diary (See **Fig. 1** for example) Short Form-12, Short Form-36 Sleep Disorders Questionnaire[3] PROMIS Questionnaires[4]
Excessive Daytime Sleepiness	Epworth Sleepiness Scale[45] Stanford Sleepiness Scale[46] Functional Outcomes of Sleep Questionnaire[12]
OSA	Berlin Questionnaire[27] STOP-BANG Questionnaire[47]
Insomnia	Pittsburgh Sleep Quality Index[21] Insomnia Severity Index[22]
RLS	International Restless Legs Syndrome Scale[33] RLS Single Question Screen[32]
Pediatrics	Pediatric Sleep Questionnaire Children's Sleep Habits Questionnaire Pediatric Daytime Sleepiness Scale Modified Epworth Sleepiness Scale for children

Abbreviations: OSA, Obstructive Sleep Apnea; RLS, Restless Legs Syndrome.

Table 2	
Internet-based locations of some sleep disorder scales (links active as of spring 2012)	
Epworth Sleepiness Scale	http://epworthsleepinessscale.com/
Stanford Sleepiness Scale	http://www.stanford.edu/~dement/sss.html
Berlin Questionnaire	http://www.aafp.org/afp/2000/0315/p1825.html
STOP-BANG Questionnaire	sleepapnea.org/assets/files/pdf/STOP-BANG%20 Questionnaire.pdf
Pittsburgh Sleep Quality Index	http://www.sleep.pitt.edu/content.asp?id=1484&subid= 2316
Insomnia Severity Index	https://www.myhealth.va.gov/mhv-portal-web/resources/ jsp/help.jsp?helpDirectRequest=sleep_insomnia_index print.htm
International RLS Scale	http://www.medicine.ox.ac.uk/bandolier/booth/RLS/ RLSratingscale.pdf
Sleep Diary	yoursleep.aasmnet.org/pdf/sleepdiary.pdf
The Sleep Disorders Questionnaire	http://stanfordhospital.org/clinicsmedServices/clinics/ sleep/documents/SDQ_version_2.03%20_English_.pdf

should be given a sleep diary to complete. The sleep diary is an instrument in which the patient typically tracks their sleep patterns on a daily basis. Information may include medications taken, bed time, time to sleep onset, number of awakenings, time of waking, time out of bed, and any naps taken. Typically, a sleep diary is kept for at least a week, but it may also be used as a long-term method of assessing a patient's sleep.

In the case of the patient with daytime sleepiness, the diary is most useful for assessing an estimate of total sleep time. One of the most common reasons for daytime sleepiness is insufficient daytime sleep. It is worth remembering that insufficient sleep may be subtle; chronic mild sleep deprivation may still cause daytime symptoms.

In cases of patients with insomnia, a sleep diary may help ascertain too much time in the bed or excessive daytime napping. A sample sleep diary is provided in **Fig. 1**; another example is from the AASM is available on the Internet, referenced in **Table 2**.

A nonspecific assessment of the effect of sleep disorders on patients may be performed by the Short Form Health Survey (SF). The SF-36 is a 36-question survey with "an 8-scale profile of functional health and well-being scores as well as psychometrically-based physical and mental health summary measures and a preference-based health utility index."[1] This survey has been used in assessment of many medical disorders, including many sleep disorders. A shorter, one-page, 2-minute form, the SF-12, is also available and has been used in sleep research.[2]

The Sleep Disorders Questionnaire was developed in 1986 based primarily on Stanford University's Sleep Questionnaire and Assessment of Wakefulness. The 175 item, eighth-grade reading level instrument was developed as a comprehensive clinical tool, with hope it would be used to develop a research database.[3] The strength of this questionnaire is its all-inclusiveness, but that same trait may also limit its use in a typical clinical practice.

The Patient-Reported Outcomes Information System, a National Institutes of Health project analyzing a framework of physical, mental, and social health domains, had a sleep questions as a portion of the larger initiative. One hundred and twenty eight questions were initially evaluated for sleep disorders, with two smaller question sets developed out of the larger set. The sleep-disturbance item bank is a 27-question

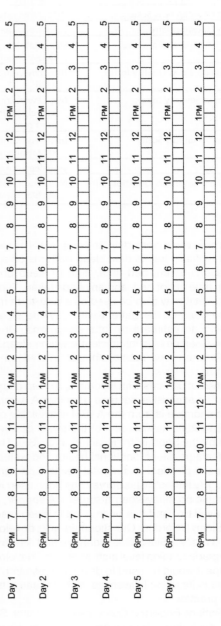

Fig. 1. A sample sleep diary. (Courtesy of Sleep HealthCenters, Brighton, MA; with permission.)

set and the sleep-related impairment set is a 16-question set. Based on sensitivity analysis, a few questions may show promise as potential screening tools for daytime impairment (eg, "I felt tired," "I was sleepy during the daytime") and for sleep disturbance (eg, "My sleep quality was [very poor to very good]," "I was satisfied with my sleep").[4] These questions have been validated in a general population, but their utility in a population with neurologic disorders is unclear at this time.

Excessive daytime sleepiness (EDS)

Hypersomnia, or EDS, is defined as "the inability to stay awake and alert during the major waking episodes of the day, resulting in unintended lapses into drowsiness or sleep." It is a common symptom of insufficient sleep, intrinsic sleep disorders, medication-related side effects, and many medical conditions. Many neurologic patients may suffer from EDS, including patients with movement disorders, neuromuscular diseases, multiple sclerosis, dementia, cerebrovascular diseases, head trauma, and epilepsy.[5]

The most widely used questionnaire specific for daytime sleepiness is the Epworth Sleepiness Scale (ESS). Developed in Australia by Murray Johns in 1991, the ESS has been consistent when testing and retesting individuals over time. The ESS evaluates a patient's self-report of sleepiness by asking about the likelihood of a patient dozing in eight situations. The Likert-response scale ranges from 0 ("would never doze") to 3 ("high chance of dozing"). The sum of the eight responses quantifies subjective sleep propensity "in recent times." High ESS scores (>16) were observed in patients with narcolepsy, idiopathic hypersomnolence, or moderate-to-severe OSA.[6] Many studies have been performed on the ESS because of its ease of use. However, conflicting results exist regarding how well the ESS predicts objective measures of daytime sleepiness.[7,8] When initial evaluation of the ESS was performed comparing the results of ESS with objective data from a patient's multiple sleep latency test (MSLT) results, the findings demonstrated low-to-moderate statistical significance. Some of the discrepancies in the research may arise from patient underestimation of sleep propensity. These results suggest that, in practice, the ESS is best used to assess subjective sleepiness in a standardized manner, although it is unlikely to replace objective testing. Tracking ESS scores longitudinally for individual patients does seem useful in assessing change or treatment response over weeks to months. Medicare adopted the ESS in 2008 as a standard in the evaluation of all patients with suspected sleep apnea and as a requirement for some forms of treatment.[9]

The Stanford Sleepiness Scale provides a validated, subjective measure of instantaneous sleepiness as a single question on a seven-point scale.[10,11] The scale ranges from 1 ("Feeling active, vital, alert, or wide awake") to 7 ("No longer fighting sleep, sleep onset soon; having dream-like thoughts"). This scale, in contrast to the ESS, can be used by the same patient many times in a day. However, that makes this scale less meaningful when used over longer time periods (weeks to months) because many factors (particularly circadian ones) may have a strong effect on the result.

The impact of daytime sleepiness on activities of daily living can be assessed by the Functional Outcomes of Sleep Questionnaire (FOSQ). The FOSQ was designed at a fifth-grade reading level, is designed to take 15 minutes to complete, and contains 74 questions over six domains (orientation, physical independence, mobility, occupation, social integration, and economic self-sufficiency), as well as assessment of several additional daily endeavors potentially affected by daytime sleepiness. Initially, this questionnaire was validated to discriminate between normal subjects and those seeking medical attention for a sleep problem.[12] It has since been shown to change with positive pressure therapy for OSA,[13] treatment with modafinil,[14] and with other treatments of OSA.[15] A modified short form of the FOSQ, the FOSQ-10, has also been validated and may be easier for clinical use in following patients over time.[16]

Insomnia

The ISCD, edition 2, specifies criteria for insomnia: (1) a complaint of difficulty initiating sleep, difficulty maintaining sleep, or waking up too early, or sleep that is chronically nonrestorative or poor in quality with duration of at least 1 month; (2) the sleep difficulty occurs despite adequate opportunity and circumstances for sleep; and (3) at least one of the following forms of daytime impairment (fatigue, attention or memory impairment, mood disturbance, daytime sleepiness) related to the night-time sleep difficulty is reported by the patient.[17] In a 772-person community population, 7.3% of patients with chronic insomnia reported neurologic disorders compared with 1.2% of patients without insomnia.[18] An adequate tool for insomnia should review common contributors to the insomnia. In a recent review of 26 questionnaires for insomnia, Vernon and colleagues[19] surmised that no adequate questionnaire existed for insomnia. Neurologic diseases associated with insomnia include: Parkinson disease, multiple sclerosis, dementia, stroke, traumatic brain injury, and epilepsy.[20] In some cases, insomnia may present as another symptoms that the patient cannot describe well—such as misinterpretation of sundowning or acting out in the evening.

The Pittsburgh Sleep Quality Index (PSQI) was developed in 1988 as a method of assessing sleep quality in clinical psychiatric populations. It is a self-rated questionnaire that assesses sleep quality and disturbances over 1-month. There are 19 questions that generate seven "component" scores: subjective sleep quality, sleep latency, sleep duration, habitual sleep efficiency, sleep disturbances, use of sleeping medication, and daytime dysfunction.[21] An cumulative global score up to 21 is obtained; the lower the score the better the perception of sleep. Global scores on the PSQI greater than 5 provided a sensitive and specific measure of poor sleep quality, relative to clinical and laboratory measures. Furthermore, a PSQI score greater than 5 also indicates that a subject is having severe difficulties in at least two areas, or moderate difficulties in more than three areas. This assessment has been frequently used, cited in hundreds of research studies since its creation.

In 2001, Morin and colleagues[22] developed the Insomnia Severity Index as a brief method of screening for difficulty with sleep and as a measure of treatment outcome. The questionnaire is a seven-question assessment, with each question having an answer range from 0 to 4. As the score increases, the severity of the insomnia increases. The scale queries about the severity of each type of sleeping difficulty (falling asleep, staying asleep, and waking up too early), then has four more questions about the subject's perception of their insomnia. The total score is interpreted as follows: absence of insomnia (0–7), subthreshold insomnia (8–14), moderate insomnia (15–21), and severe insomnia (22–28). It has been reliable in detection of insomnia within populations and changes over time with treatment.[23]

Obstructive sleep apnea (OSA)

OSA is a disorder that affects 4% of middle-aged men and 2% of middle-aged women.[24] This disorder of repetitive collapse of the upper airway causing oxygen desaturation and electroencephalographic arousals increases risk of hypertension, heart disease, and cardiovascular disease.[25] Sleep apnea has been associated with stroke, dementia, and encephalitis, particularly when central respiratory centers are injured.[26]

Many of the sleep disorders have specific questionnaires designed to screen for them or assess the severity of the patient's symptoms. The Berlin Questionnaire may be the most commonly used clinical screening tool for assessment of OSA: "The Berlin

Questionnaire was an outcome of the Conference on Sleep in Primary Care, which involved 120 U.S. and German pulmonary and primary care physicians and was held in April 1996 in Berlin, Germany. Questions were selected from the literature to elicit factors or behaviors that, across studies, consistently predicted the presence of sleep-disordered breathing."[27] The questionnaire has three sections. The first section assesses symptoms such as snoring and witnessed apneas, the second section evaluates effects of OSA such as daytime sleepiness, and the third section asks about the presence of hypertension and calculates a body mass index (BMI). In category 1, high-risk was defined as persistent symptoms (3–4 times per week) in two or more questions about their snoring. In category 2, high-risk was defined as persistent (3–4 times per week) wake-time sleepiness, drowsy driving, or both. In category 3, high-risk was defined as a history of high blood pressure or a body BMI more than 30 kg/m^2. If two of the three sections are considered high-risk, the patient is considered to be at high risk for OSA.[27] Although many questionnaires require only written patient input based on symptoms, this instrument requires a BMI calculation and knowledge of blood pressure status.

The STOP-BANG questionnaire was developed as a short pre- or peri-operative screen for OSA for use by anesthesiologists. It contains eight questions, covering similar material to that of the Berlin questionnaire. The question content matches the questionnaire acronym: **S**noring, **T**iredness, **O**bserved apneas, blood **P**ressure, **B**MI, **A**ge, **N**eck circumference, and **G**ender. Although the questions on snoring, tiredness, apneas, high blood pressure, age (>50 years), and gender are straightforward (eg, presence or absence, male or female), questions on BMI (>35 kg/m^2) and neck circumference (>40 cm) may require clinician measurement. A positive answer to three or more questions gives a high probability of OSA.[28] Thus, this questionnaire is easier to score than the Berlin questionnaire, but also may require some clinical measurements.

Restless legs syndrome (RLS)

The first modern description of RLS in a scientific article came from Ekbom[29] in the 1940s, although it was only recently that the disorder was recognized to be more common (approximately 4.4% of the population).[30] The disorder has been described to have four components, listed below with the acronym URGE[31]:

U = urge to move the legs, usually associated with unpleasant leg sensations
R = rest induces symptoms;
G = getting active (physically and mentally) brings relief
E = evening and night make symptoms worse

A one-question screen has been tested to help gauge the prevalence of restless legs syndrome, "When you try to relax in the evening or sleep at night, do you ever have unpleasant, restless feelings in your legs that can be relieved by walking or movement?"

The single question had 100% sensitivity and 96.8% specificity for the diagnosis of RLS in the more than 500 screened patients when referenced against clinician evaluation in the study. This question has the advantage of being quick to finish and an easy tool for screening of patients, but does not evaluate severity of symptoms or change over time.[32]

The International Restless Legs Syndrome rating scale is a 10-question tool and is probably the most widely applied tool to evaluate and track RLS symptoms over time. Twenty centers in six countries participated in the validation of this instrument. Generally, the questionnaire reviews the severity of the symptoms, the effect of those symptoms on daytime function, and the frequency of the symptoms. Scoring categories for the RLS scale are: mild (score 1–10), moderate (score 11–20), severe (score 21–30), and very severe (score 31–40). "This scale meets performance criteria for a brief, patient completed instrument that can be used to assess RLS severity for purposes of clinical assessment, research, or therapeutic trials. It supports a finding that RLS is a relatively uniform disorder in which the severity of the basic symptoms is strongly related to their impact on the patient's life."[33]

Pediatrics

Adult questionnaires are unlikely to be optimal for use with children and adolescents. For these age groups, one of the first parental EDS assessments to be validated is contained within the Pediatric Sleep Questionnaire (PSQ). The PSQ contains more than 70 close-ended questions that parents answer "yes," "no," or "don't know," and several open-ended questions that obtain a medical history. The PSQ and four-item sleepiness subscale have proved useful in research conducted in general pediatric waiting rooms.[34]

Another instrument also used primarily for research is the Children's Sleep Habits Questionnaire (CSHQ), which screens children between ages 4 and 19 for sleep problems and includes a subscale on daytime sleepiness.[35] The CSHQ includes items relating to the major presenting clinical sleep complaints in this age group: bedtime behavior and sleep onset, sleep duration, anxiety around sleep, behavior occurring during sleep and night waking, sleep-disordered breathing, parasomnias, and morning waking or daytime sleepiness. Parents rate the sleep behaviors occurring during a recent typical week. Items are rated on a three-point scale; usually whether the sleep behavior occurred five to seven times per week, sometimes for two to four times per week, and rarely for zero to one time per week. Higher scores on this scale indicate more sleep disturbance.

The Pediatric Daytime Sleepiness Scale is a 13-question survey suitable for assessment of EDS in middle-school-age children. All questions were presented in a Likert-scale format (eg, never, seldom, sometimes, frequently, always); the higher the score, the more sleepy the subject.[36]

Finally, the ESS also has been modified and used with children for research purposes. The ESS was modified slightly in this study to be more applicable to children. The mention of alcohol was deleted and another question was changed to indicate that the subject was a passenger in the car.[37]

Objective Testing

Although subjective testing has the advantages of being quick and inexpensive, for many sleep disorders, objective testing is considered the gold standard. Objective testing removes the possibility of any reporting biases and allows an improved assessment of the patient's symptom severity. In sleep medicine, objective testing may include an overnight polysomnography, out-of-center sleep test, MSLT, maintenance of wakefulness test (MWT), and actigraphy.

Overnight polysomnography

The polysomnogram is considered the gold standard for objective testing of sleep, evaluating electroencephalography (EEG), respiratory parameters, and muscle activity during sleep. Current guidelines from the AASM recommend that polysomnography assess the following parameters: EEG, eye movements (electro-olfactogram), chin and leg motor activity (electromyogram [EMG]), airflow parameters (typically nasal pressure transducer and nasal-oral thermistor), respiratory effort parameters (thoracic and abdominal), oxygen saturation, and body position (**Fig. 2**).[38] Laboratories performing sleep studies should be accredited by one of several agencies (eg, the Joint Commission of Accreditation of Healthcare Organizations, AASM) to ensure that quality metrics are being upheld. A technologist places all of the appropriate probes

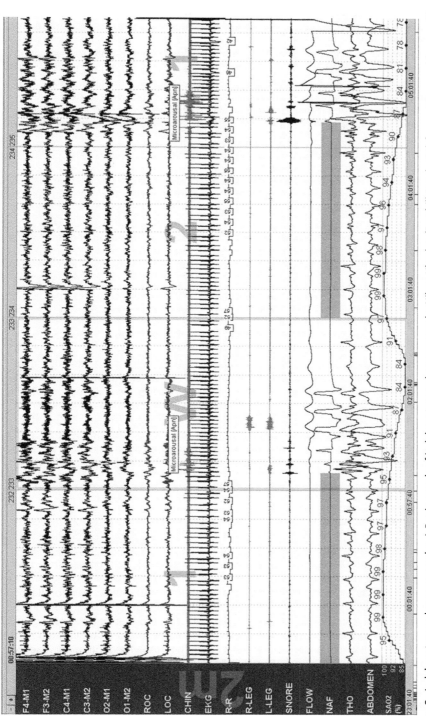

Fig. 2. In-laboratory polysomnography. A 2-min epoch of in-laboratory polysomnography Nihon Khoden (Foothill Ranch, CA) from a 55-year-old man with OSA. The top six leads are EEG (right and left frontal, central, and occipital), followed by two eye leads (ROC and LOC), the chin lead (CHIN), EKG with heart rate below (R-R), two leg leads (R-LEG, L-LEG), snore channel (SNORE), oronasal thermistor (FLOW), nasal pressure transducer (NAF), effort bands (THO [thorax] and ABDOMEN), and oxygen saturation (SAO2). Two obstructive apneas are observed at the boxes in the NAF signal with absent nasal-oral airflow and continued respiratory effort. The respiratory events are associated with increased frequency signal (arousals) in the EEG signals and oxygen desaturations.

and wires on the patient before the study initiation and observes the patient throughout the night, ensuring that the patient is medically stable and that the recorded data are accurately obtained.

Most commonly, patients are sent for in-laboratory polysomnography for evaluation of OSA, treatment of OSA with positive pressure therapy, or evaluation of treatment of OSA, such as weight loss, oral appliances, or surgical intervention. Other reasons for polysomnography may include evaluation for periodic limb movements during sleep, assessment of dangerous parasomnias, and differentiation of seizures and parasomnias. Patients with insomnia are not typically evaluated with polysomnography, unless clinical evaluation suggests a comorbid sleep disorder. A full list of reasons to obtain (or not to obtain) an in-laboratory sleep study from the AASM practice parameters for polysomnography is supplied in **Box 1**.

The advantages of the in-laboratory polysomnogram include the assessment of sleep stage changes over the course of the night and the effect of sleep stage on sleep-disordered breathing, observer reporting and video recording for evaluation of patient behavior, and scoring of EEG-based arousals from sleep. Based on Medicare criteria, an apnea-hypopnea index (AHI) of 5 events per hour in association with a symptom (EDS, impaired cognition, mood disorders, insomnia, hypertension, ischemic heart disease, or history of stroke) or an AHI of 15 events per hour without associated symptoms is considered diagnostic of OSA.[9,17] However, because there are multiple standards for the scoring of respiratory events, AHI values may have inter-laboratory variability. Some standard terminology and definitions on sleep study reports are summarized in **Table 3**.

In most cases, the diagnostic test will last a minimum of 6 hours. However, many sleep centers have opted to perform "split-night" studies. The first half of the study (2–3 hours) is diagnostic and the second half is a positive pressure treatment trial to minimize health care costs in cases of patients with a high likelihood of OSA. Overnight testing may also be in the form of an all-night positive airway pressure (PAP) titration study because the technologist adjusts the PAP pressures to eliminate or minimize sleep-disordered breathing. Polysomnography with 16-lead EEG and/or extra EMG leads may be considered in specific circumstances, particularly with patients who have epilepsy and who may be having seizures during sleep, or patients who have parasomnias requiring more thorough evaluation for potential underlying seizures.

Out-of-center sleep testing

Monitoring of sleep-related breathing at home was reviewed at a national level by Medicare in 2007to 2008. Many portable monitors measure a subset of the measures of a typical polysomnogram (eg, airflow, respiratory effort, heart rate, and snoring).[39] AASM guidelines (2007) suggest that a home sleep test (HST) may be performed on patients who have moderate-to-high likelihood of OSA in the absence of comorbid conditions, such as significant intrinsic lung disease or neuromuscular conditions that may cause hypoventilation. Although the AASM also suggests limiting these tests on patients who have comorbid sleep or medical disorders, current insurance regulations may guide patients who have risk for OSA and another sleep disorder to an HST instead of than allowing an in-laboratory study. The AASM algorithm for use of portable monitoring is provided in **Fig. 3**. A limitation for most HST monitors is the lack of EEG leads because absence of brain wave measurement limits accurate sleep staging and identification of cortical arousals.[40] In some instance, overnight oximetry may also be used to diagnose cases of severe sleep apnea or to assess the efficacy of treatment of OSA; however, oximetry will likely fail to detect mild OSA.

Box 1
Practice parameters for polysomnography, 2005

Polysomnography is routinely indicated for:

1. The diagnosis of sleep-related breathing disorders (SRBD) (standard)

2. Positive airway pressure (PAP) titration in patients with SRBDs (standard)

3. A preoperative clinical evaluation to evaluate for the presence of OSA in patients before they undergo upper airway surgery for snoring or OSA (standard)

4. The assessment of treatment results in the following circumstances (standard):

    a. After good clinical response to oral appliance treatment in patients with moderate to severe OSA

    b. After surgical treatment of patients with moderate-to-severe OSA

    c. After surgical or dental treatment of patients with SRBD whose symptoms return

5. For the assessment of treatment results in the following circumstances (standard):

    a. After substantial weight loss or gain (eg, 10% of body weight) has occurred in patients on continuous PAS (CPAP) for treatment of SRBDs for potential adjustment of PAP pressures

    b. When clinical response is insufficient or when symptoms return; in these circumstances, testing should be devised with consideration that a concurrent sleep disorder may be present (eg, OSA and narcolepsy)

6. Patients with heart failure, if they have nocturnal symptoms suggestive of SRBD (disturbed sleep, nocturnal dyspnea, snoring) or if they remain symptomatic despite optimal medical management (standard)

7. Patients with coronary artery disease, if there is suspicion of sleep apnea (guideline)

8. Patients with history of stroke or transient ischemic attacks, if there is suspicion of sleep apnea (guideline)

9. Patients with significant tachyarrhythmias or bradyarrhythmias, if there is suspicion of sleep apnea (guideline)

10. Patients with neuromuscular disorders and sleep-related symptoms for evaluation of symptoms of sleep disorders beyond the sleep history (standard)

11. Patients with suspected narcolepsy in combination with a multiple sleep latency test (standard)

12. Diagnosis of paroxysmal arousals or other sleep disruptions that are thought to be seizure related when the initial clinical evaluation and results of a standard EEG are inconclusive; with additional EEG derivations in an extended bilateral montage, and video recording, recommended in addition to standard leads (optional)

13. For evaluating sleep-related behaviors that are violent or otherwise potentially injurious to the patient or others in combination with additional EEG derivations and video recording (optional)

14. When evaluating patients with unusual or atypical parasomnias (age at onset; the time, duration, and frequency of behavior; and the specifics of the motor behavior, including stereotypical, repetitive, or focal) (guideline)

15. Situations with forensic considerations, (eg, if onset follows trauma or if the events themselves have been associated with personal injury) (optional)

16. When the presumed parasomnia or sleep-related seizure disorder does not respond to conventional therapy (optional)

17. When a diagnosis of periodic limb movement disorder is considered because of complaints by the patient or an observer of repetitive limb movements during sleep and frequent awakenings, fragmented sleep, difficulty maintaining sleep, or EDS (standard).

Polysomnography is NOT routinely indicated for:

1. Patients treated with CPAP whose symptoms continue to be resolved with CPAP treatment (optional)

2. A multiple sleep latency test is not routinely indicated for most patients with SRBD (standard)

3. Diagnosis of chronic lung disease (standard)

4. In cases of typical, uncomplicated, and noninjurious parasomnias when the diagnosis is clearly delineated (optional)

5. Patients with a seizure disorder who have no specific complaints consistent with a sleep disorder (optional)

6. Diagnosis or treatment of RLS, except where uncertainty exists in the diagnosis (standard)

7. Establishing the diagnosis of depression (standard)

8. Diagnosis of circadian rhythm sleep disorders (standard).

Adapted from Kushida CA, Littner MR, Morgenthaler T, et al. Practice parameters for the indications for polysomnography and related procedures: an update for 2005. Sleep 2005;28(4): 499–521; with permission.

Out-of center-testing is a growing area of sleep medicine given the large number of patients with likely OSA, the limited number of sleep laboratories across the country, and the cost savings to insurance programs of doing HST compared with an in-laboratory test. These tests tend to underestimate OSA severity. The numerator in

Table 3
A brief glossary of sleep study terms

Stage N1	The lightest stage of sleep; represented by theta activity on EEG
Stage N2	The stage of sleep in which most adults spend most of their time; represented by K-complexes and spindles on EEG
Stage N3	Slow-wave sleep; at least 20% of the epoch being slow waves (0.5–2 Hz, peak-to-peak amplitude >75 μV) on EEG
Stage R	REM sleep; often the state where dreaming is most vigorous. Sleep-disordered breathing is often at its worst in this stage. Motor activity is generally minimal and EEG is mixed frequency
Hypopnea	A reduction in airflow for more than 10 s is associated with an oxygen desaturation or an arousal from sleep. These are often obstructive, but at times may have more central characteristics
Obstructive apnea	Cessation of airflow related to upper airway closure for more than 10 s with continued thorax and abdominal muscle movement
Central apnea	Cessation of airflow for more than 10 s with reduction in movement of thorax and abdomen; may be related to changing from wake to sleep, cardiac problems, neurologic problems or medications like narcotics
Mixed apnea	Cessation of airflow for more than 10 s that starts as a central apnea then develops obstructive characteristics
AHI/RDI	Apnea-Hypopnea Index/Respiratory Disturbance Index: the number of respiratory events/h of sleep; generally considered the primary marker of sleep apnea severity
PLM	Periodic Limb Movement of Sleep; a polysomnographic finding of leg movements occurring in a specific pattern with unclear clinical significance

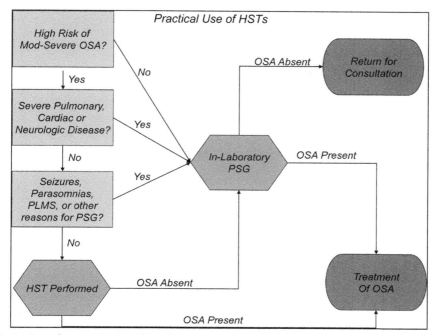

Fig. 3. Out-of-center testing algorithm. PLMS, periodic limb movement syndrome; PSG, polysomnography. (*Adapted from* Collop NA, Anderson WM, Boehlecke B, et al. Clinical guidelines for the use of unattended portable monitors in the diagnosis of OSA in adult patients. Portable monitoring task force of the American Academy of Sleep Medicine. J Clin Sleep Med 2007;3(7):737–47; with permission.)

the AHI (respiratory events) is lower than an in-laboratory test because subtle breathing events may not be scored and the denominator in the AHI is elevated because recording time is assessed instead of sleep time as in an in-laboratory polysomnogram (no EEG signal-to-score sleep occurs in most HSTs). Also, the failure rate of a HST is significantly higher than an in-laboratory test, owing to the absence of a sleep technologist fixing electrical leads during the testing night and the limitations of the technology of current HST devices.

Not all portable testing devices measure the same parameters. Most of the devices will measure airflow, respiratory effort, and oximetry via standard signals (ie, oral-nasal thermistor or nasal pressure, oximetry or pulse rate, respiratory effort belt) (**Fig. 4**). However, some devices have used alternative signals, such as peripheral artery tonometry in the WatchPAT (Itamar Medical, Ltd., Franklin, MA) device as a substitute for airflow and respiratory effort, or venous pulsation as a surrogate for respiratory effort in some versions of the ARES (Advanced Brain Monitoring, Inc, Carlsbad, CA) device. When selecting an HST device for a practice, it is wise to trial a few devices to understand the pros and cons of each device.

MSLT and MWT

The MSLT remains the gold standard test for objective assessment of EDS. This test measures the physiologic tendency of a patient to fall asleep in a quiet environment. The recommendations for the MSLT protocol are described in detail in the January 2005 practice parameters published by the AASM.[41] Although this test has only

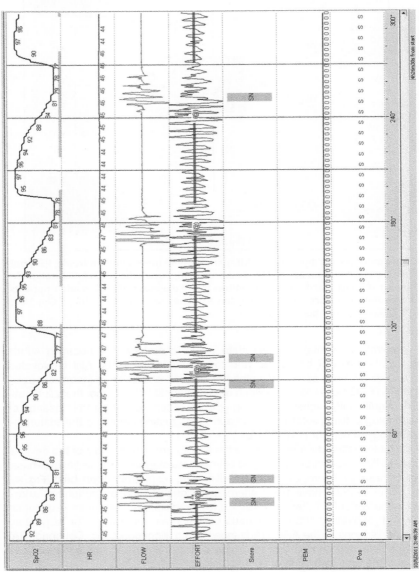

Fig. 4. A 2-minute epoch of home sleep testing (HST). This is a 5-minute epoch from a Stardust (Philips HealthCare, Andover, MA) HST device of a 64-year-old woman with OSA. The top channel is oximetry (SpO2), followed by heart rate (HR), nasal pressure (FLOW), respiratory effort (EFFORT), snoring (Snore), patient event marker (PEM), and position (Pos), in this case, supine. The epoch demonstrates repetitive apneas with absent nasal pressure and continuous respiratory effort.

been validated for the diagnosis of narcolepsy, it has been applied by many practitioners as a tool for the assessment of sleepiness of all causes.

Preparation is essential before a patient undergoes the MSLT. It is recommended that the patient obtain 2 weeks of regular sleep before the test; use of actigraphy and/or sleep diaries may help track the patient's sleep patterns. Stimulants, stimulant-like medications, and REM-suppressing medications (eg, many antidepressants) should be discontinued, if safe to do so, at least 15 days or five half-lives before the patient undergoes testing. Urine drug screening is often performed the morning of the MSLT to ensure that findings of the MSLT are not altered pharmacologically. Caffeine and alcohol may alter sleep time and sleep architecture; these substances should not be used immediately before or during the test. Withdrawal from these agents may also change test results.[42] The night before the MSLT, an in-laboratory polysomnogram should be performed to document quality and duration of sleep. At least 6 hours of documented sleep should occur before administration of the MSLT to ensure an accurate daytime test. Patients with abnormalities of circadian phase should consider an altered test schedule, although this may be difficult in typical sleep practices.

A standard MSLT montage includes a referential EEG from frontal, central, and occipital locations, two electrooculograms (left and right) at the outer canthi, a mental or submental EMG, and an ECG (**Fig. 5**). These leads will allow determination of sleep onset, sleep stage, and the patient's heart rhythm. The nap attempts should take place in a bedroom that is dark, quiet, and at a comfortable temperature setting. Five nap opportunities begin 1.5 to 3 hours after the end of the overnight polysomnogram and continue every 2 hours. No sleeping should be allowed between the nap tests, nicotine use should be avoided 30 minutes before each test, and vigorous activity should be suspended 15 minutes before each trial. Before each attempt, the patient is told to "please lie quietly, assume a comfortable position, keep your eyes closed, and try to fall asleep."[41] The results of the test demonstrate two things: the mean sleep latency, which is the arithmetic average of how quickly the patient had an epoch scored as sleep in each nap, and the number of sleep-onset REM periods, which is the number of naps in which the patient had at least one epoch scored as REM sleep. Based on the ICSD, 2nd edition, a diagnosis of narcolepsy requires

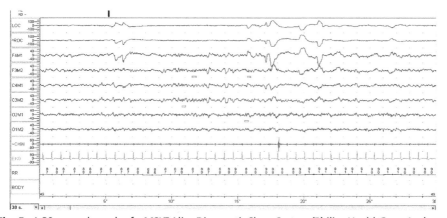

Fig. 5. A 30-second epoch of a MSLT Alice Diagnostic Sleep System (Philips HealthCare, Andover, MA). The layout is more limited than a full polysomnogram and demonstrates from top to bottom: left and right eye leads (LOC, ROC), six EEG leads (right and left frontal, central, and occipital), chin EMG lead (CHIN), EKG lead, and heart rate (R-R). This image demonstrates REMs in the eye leads, mixed frequency EEG signal, and low chin EMG tone, all of which suggest stage R sleep.

Table 4
40-min MWT normative data

Sleep onset definition	Mean (min)	Standard Deviation	2 Standard Deviation Below (min)
First epoch any stage	32.6	9.9	12.9
Three epochs stage 1 or one epoch any other stage	35.2	7.9	19.4

Data from Doghramji K, Mitler MM, Sangal RB, et al. A normative study of the maintenance of wakefulness test (MWT). Electroencephalogr Clin Neurophysiol 1997;103(5):554–62.

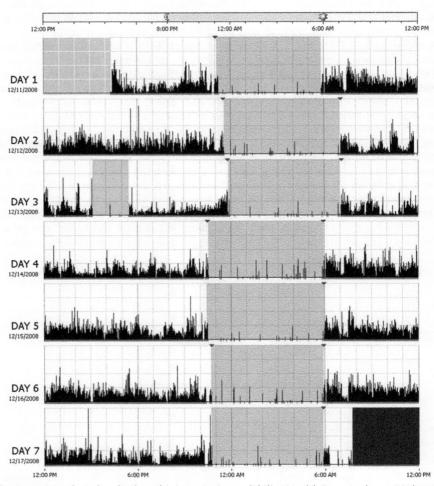

Fig. 6. Actigraph, 7-day display. This is an Actiware (Philips HealthCare, Andover, MA) actigraphy report. The shaded areas are scored as rest time. This patient has an approximate bedtime from 11 PM to 12 midnight to a wake time of about 6 AM. One nap is observed on day 3 in the middle of the afternoon.

a mean sleep latency of less than 8 minutes and two sleep-onset REMs.[17] However, physicians should recognize that other sleep disorders (eg, OSA, behaviorally induced insufficient sleep, and circadian rhythm disturbances) may cause similar findings; therefore, assessment of the results from an MSLT should always be performed within a clinical context.

The MWT is effectively the inverse of the MSLT. Though similar in that the patient is tested four times over the course of a day for 40 minutes per nap episode in a dim room while reclining, the subtle, but important, difference in the instructions is that the patient should attempt to "remain awake as long as possible."[41] The MWT has been used by the Federal Aviation Administration to test pilots who have been diagnosed with OSA and treated, assessing if they are alert enough to return to work safely.[43] Although this test evaluates the ability of patients to stay awake in a circumscribed set of conditions, it has not been clearly demonstrated to be predictive of motor vehicle accidents or other activities in which reduced alertness may impact safety. It is also a difficult test to interpret because the meaning of the result is unclear when the test does not demonstrate either no sleep or clearly alert or clearly abnormally sleepy. **Table 4** demonstrates the normative data from the MWT to aid in result interpretation.

Actigraphy

Actigraphy is a method of tracking activity over time via an accelerometer and has been demonstrated to be a reasonably accurate reflection of states of activity and rest.[44] Care should be taken when analyzing data from this device because rest times do not always reflect sleep time (sitting quietly with minimal movement is often scored as rest). Sleep diaries should be used simultaneously to compare subjective and objective sleep times. This device is most useful in assessing patients for circadian changes and in tracking approximate sleep times in patients with insomnia or hypersomnia **Fig. 6** provides one example of actigraphy data.

SUMMARY

Neurologists' interest in sleep medicine has grown over the years and data has demonstrated the impact of sleep disorders on many neurologic disorders. Understanding the proper use of subjective and objective assessment tools to evaluate for the presence of sleep disorders in clinical neurologic practice may improve patient outcomes, even if the primary symptoms are not sleep-specific. Many subjective assessment tools are brief and can be used to assess a patient's symptoms over time. The objective tests are more expensive and time-consuming but are often necessary for appropriate diagnosis of a suspected sleep disorder.

REFERENCES

1. Available at: http://www.sf-36.org/tools/sf36.shtml. Accessed February 15, 2012.
2. Siccoli MM, Pepperell JC, Kohler M, et al. Effects of continuous positive airway pressure on quality of life in patients with moderate to severe obstructive sleep apnea: data from a randomized controlled trial. Sleep 2008;31(11):1551–8.
3. Douglass AB, Bornstein R, Nino-Murcia G, et al. The sleep disorders questionnaire. I: creation and multivariate structure of SDQ. Sleep 1994;17(2):160–7.
4. Buysse DJ, Yu L, Moul DE, et al. Development and validation of patient-reported outcome measures for sleep disturbance and sleep-related impairments. Sleep 2010;33(6):781–92.
5. Happe S. Excessive daytime sleepiness and sleep disturbances in patients with neurological diseases: epidemiology and management. Drugs 2003;63(24):2725–37.

6. Murray WJ. A new method for measuring daytime sleepiness: the Epworth Sleepiness Scale. Sleep 1991;14(6):540–5.
7. Punjabi NM, Bandeen-Roche K, Young T. Predictors of objective sleep tendency in the general population. Sleep 2003;26(6):678–83.
8. Chervin RD, Aldrich MS. The Epworth sleepiness scale may not reflect objective measures of sleepiness or sleep apnea. Neurology 1999;52(1):125–31.
9. Available at: http://www.medicarenhic.com/dme/medical_review/mr_bulletins/mr_bulletin_current/091808_pap_phys_letter.pdf. Accessed March 12, 2012.
10. Hoddes E, Zarcone V, Smythe H, et al. Quantification of sleepiness: a new approach. Psychophysiology 1973;10(4):431–6.
11. Herscovitch J, Broughton R. Sensitivity of the Stanford sleepiness scale to the effects of cumulative partial sleep deprivation and recovery oversleeping. Sleep 1981;4(1):83–91.
12. Weaver TE, Laizner AM, Evans LK, et al. An instrument to measure functional status outcomes for disorders of excessive sleepiness. Sleep 1997;20(10):835–43.
13. Faccenda JF, Mackay TW, Boon NA, et al. Randomized placebo-controlled trial of continuous positive airway pressure on blood pressure in the sleep apnea-hypopnea syndrome. Am J Respir Crit Care Med 2001;163(2):344–8.
14. Schwartz JR, Hirshkowitz M, Erman MK, et al. Modafinil as adjunct therapy for daytime sleepiness in obstructive sleep apnea: a 12-week, open-label study. Chest 2003;124(6):2192–9.
15. Lye KW, Waite PD, Meara D, et al. Quality of life evaluation of maxillomandibular advancement surgery for treatment of obstructive sleep apnea. J Oral Maxillofac Surg 2008;66(5):968–72.
16. Chasens ER, Ratcliffe SJ, Weaver TE. Development of the FOSQ-10: a short version of the Functional Outcomes of Sleep Questionnaire. Sleep 2009;32(7):915–9.
17. American Academy of Sleep Medicine. The international classification of sleep disorders: diagnostic and coding manual. 2nd edition. Westchester (IL): American Academy of Sleep Medicine; 2005. p. 79.
18. Taylor DJ, Mallory LJ, Lichstein KL, et al. Co-morbidity of chronic insomnia with medical problems. Sleep 2007;30(2):213e8.
19. Vernon MK, Dugar A, Revicki D, et al. Measurement of non-restorative sleep in insomnia: a review of the literature. Sleep Med Rev 2010;14(3):205–12.
20. Mayer G, Jennum P, Riemann D, et al. Insomnia in central neurologic diseases–occurrence and management. Sleep Med Rev 2011;15(6):369–78.
21. Buysse DJ, Reynolds CF 3rd, Monk TH, et al. The Pittsburgh sleep quality index: a new instrument for psychiatric practice and research. Psychiatry Res 1989;28(2):193–213.
22. Bastien CH, Vallières A, Morin CM. Validation of the insomnia severity index as an outcome measure for insomnia research. Sleep Med 2001;2(4):297–307.
23. Morin CM, Belleville G, Bélanger L, et al. The insomnia severity index: psychometric indicators to detect insomnia cases and evaluate treatment response. Sleep 2011;34(5):601–8.
24. Young T, Palta M, Dempsey J, et al. The occurrence of sleep-disordered breathing among middle-aged adults. N Engl J Med 1993;328(17):1230–5.
25. Park JG, Ramar K, Olson EJ. Updates on definition, consequences, and management of obstructive sleep apnea. Mayo Clin Proc 2011;86(6):549–54.
26. Dyken ME, Afifi AK, Lin-Dyken DC. Sleep-related problems in neurologic diseases. Chest 2012;141(2):528–44.

27. Netzer NC, Stoohs RA, Netzer CM, et al. Using the Berlin questionnaire to identify patients at risk for the sleep apnea syndrome. Ann Intern Med 1999;131(7): 485–91.

28. Chung F, Yegneswaran B, Liao P, et al. STOP questionnaire: a tool to screen patients for obstructive sleep apnea. Anesthesiology 2008;108(5):812–21.

29. Ekbom KA. Restless legs. Acta Med Scand 1945;158:1–123.

30. Allen RP, Stillman P, Myers AJ. Physician-diagnosed restless legs syndrome in a large sample of primary medical care patients in Western Europe: prevalence and characteristics. Sleep Med 2010;11:31–7.

31. Available at: http://www.rls.org/Document.Doc?id=1933. Slide 6. Accessed April 1, 2012.

32. Ferri R, Lanuzza B, Cosentino FI, et al. A single question for the rapid screening of restless legs syndrome in the neurological clinical practice. Eur J Neurol 2007; 14(9):1016–21.

33. Walters AS, LeBrocq C, Dhar A, et al, International Restless Legs Syndrome Study Group. Validation of the International Restless Legs Syndrome Study Group rating scale for restless legs syndrome. Sleep Med 2003;4(2):121–32.

34. Archbold KH, Pituch KJ, Panahi P, et al. Symptoms of sleep disturbances among children at two general pediatric clinics. J Pediatr 2002;140(1):97–102.

35. Owens JA, Spirito A, McGuinn M. The Children's Sleep Habits Questionnaire (CSHQ): psychometric properties of a survey instrument for school-aged children. Sleep 2000;23(8):1043–51.

36. Drake C, Nickel C, Burduvali E, et al. The pediatric daytime sleepiness scale (PDSS): sleep habits and school outcomes in middle-school children. Sleep 2003;26(4):455–8.

37. Melendres MC, Lutz JM, Rubin ED, et al. Daytime sleepiness and hyperactivity in children with suspected sleep-disordered breathing. Pediatrics 2004;114(3): 768–75.

38. Iber C, Ancoli-Israel S, Chesson A, et al, American Academy of Sleep Medicine. The AASM manual for the scoring of sleep and associated events: rules, terminology and technical specifications. 1st edition. Westchester (IL): American Acadmey of Sleep Medicine; 2007.

39. Chediak A. Why CMS approved home sleep testing for CPAP coverage. J Clin Sleep Med 2008;4(1):16–8.

40. Collop NA, Anderson WM, Boehlecke B, et al. Clinical guidelines for the use of unattended portable monitors in the diagnosis of obstructive sleep apnea in adult patients. Portable monitoring task force of the American Academy of Sleep Medicine. J Clin Sleep Med 2007;3(7):737–47.

41. Littner MR, Kushida C, Wise M, et al. Practice parameters for clinical use of the multiple sleep latency test and the maintenance of wakefulness test. Sleep 2005;28(1):113–21.

42. Carskadon MA, Dement WC, Mitler MM, et al. Guidelines for the multiple sleep latency test (MSLT): a standard measure of sleepiness. Sleep 1986;9: 519–24.

43. Avialable at: http://www.faa.gov/about/office_org/headquarters_offices/avs/offices/aam/ame/guide/special_iss/all_classes/sleep_apnea/. Accessed January 11, 2011.

44. Morgenthaler T, Alessi C, Friedman L, et al. Practice parameters for the use of actigraphy in the assessment of sleep and sleep disorders: an update for 2007. Sleep 2007;30(4):519–29.

45. Johns MW. A new method for measuring daytime sleepiness: the Epworth sleepiness scale. Sleep 1991;14(6):540–5.

46. Glenville M, Broughton R. Reliability of the Stanford sleepiness scale compared to short duration performance tests and the Wilkinson auditory vigilance task. Adv Biosci 1978;21:235–44.

47. Vasu TS, Doghramji K, Cavallazzi R, et al. Obstructive sleep apnea syndrome and postoperative complications: clinical use of the stop-bang questionnaire. Arch Otolaryngol Head Neck Surg 2010;136(10):1020–4.

Treating Sleep Disorders in Neurology Practice

Marc Raphaelson, MD[a],*, Sara K. Inati, MD[b]

KEYWORDS

- Sleep disorders • Neurology • Practice • Diagnosis • Treatment • Integrate

KEY POINTS

- Most patients in a neurology practice have sleep complaints, and many have comorbid primary sleep disorders.
- A reasoned clinical pathway to diagnose and treat sleep apnea is increasingly important for the long-term health of neurology patients and practices.
- A number of neurology practices now include a comprehensive sleep medicine practice with a board-certified physician and registered and licensed technologists. Facility credentials are evolving and soon may include accreditation in polysomnography testing, out-of-center testing, and providing durable medical equipment.
- The neurologist can play a key role in diagnosing, treating, and managing sleep disorders, helping their patients to improve both their neurologic symptoms and their overall quality of life.

INTRODUCTION

Many neurology patients have sleep disorders. Some have obvious and bothersome symptoms, such as insomnia or loud snoring, but other patients have no symptoms even in the presence of life-threatening sleep apnea or hypoventilation. This article discusses how neurologists might incorporate sleep diagnosis and treatment into their practice. The article also reviews sleep problems in some common neurologic disease categories and recommends routine diagnostic testing in specific clinical circumstances. Case reports illustrate the clinical benefit of sleep testing and treatment in typical patients.

DIAGNOSING SLEEP DISORDERS IN NEUROLOGY PRACTICE

A very high proportion of neurology patients have sleep disorders, but it is often difficult to elicit those symptoms during the face-to-face encounter. In many practices,

This research was supported in part by the Intramural Research Program on the NIH, NINDS.
[a] 224D Cornwall Street, Suite 101B, Leesburg, VA 20176, USA; [b] EEG Section, National Institute of Neurologic Disorders and Stroke, National Institutes of Health, Building 10 CRC, Room 7-5680, Bethesda, MD 20894, USA
* Corresponding author.
E-mail address: raphaels4@aol.com

Neurol Clin 30 (2012) 1007–1025
http://dx.doi.org/10.1016/j.ncl.2012.08.015
0733-8619/12/$ – see front matter © 2012 Elsevier Inc. All rights reserved.

neurologic.theclinics.com

patients complete or update a comprehensive history that includes sleep symptoms before every new or established outpatient visit. This allows patients to provide information as their time and interest permit. With this information, the neurologist may better identify patients with sleep symptoms and those whose neurologic disorders carry a high risk of sleep-disordered breathing. Once high-risk patients have been identified, a practice may then choose how to evaluate and treat them. Options include developing a dedicated sleep medicine practice and laboratory, providing limited testing and treatment, or simply referring patients elsewhere.

One way to evaluate patients for sleep disorders is by establishing an overnight sleep laboratory within the practice. The primary tests performed in a sleep laboratory are the polysomnography (PSG) and multiple sleep latency test (MSLT). When performing a PSG, sleep staging is determined by analysis of the electrical activity of the brain, eye movements, and chin electromyography (EMG). Breathing effort and airflow are recorded using expandable belts, thermistors, nasal pressure transducers, and other technology. Cardiac rhythm, finger oximetry, and end-tidal carbon dioxide partial pressure are also recorded. The MSLT montage is simpler than the PSG montage and is designed mainly to demonstrate sleep stages. Neurologists understand PSG and MSLT technology as extensions of electroencephalography (EEG) technology and service. However, neurologists tend to be less familiar with training, supervising, licensing, and retaining a technologist; providing 24-hour facility access, service, and security; and meeting a rising regulatory burden.

When establishing a sleep laboratory, the practice should expect to hire and retain technologists who have completed standardized training and have passed one of the national standard tests, which have continued to evolve as the field matures. In an increasing number of states the technologist must also meet licensing standards. Salary is similar to that for neurodiagnostic technologists.

Sleep medicine physicians confront an increasing number of regulations. When a laboratory performs PSGs, a physician is required by federal regulations to provide general supervision. "General supervision means the procedure is furnished under the physician's overall direction and control, but the physician's presence is not required during the performance of the procedure... The training of the nonphysician personnel who actually perform the diagnostic procedure and the maintenance of the necessary equipment and supplies are the continuing responsibility of the physician."[1] Medicare requires that the interpreting physician must be board certified or board eligible in sleep medicine if the patient is to qualify for payment for sleep apnea therapy. A 1-year fellowship is now required to sit for this board. Doctors alternatively may qualify to interpret PSG or portable tests if they are affiliated with a sleep center that is accredited by the American Academy of Sleep Medicine, the Joint Commission, or the Accreditation Commission for Health Care. The policies for physician affiliation are specific to each sleep center, and Medicare has not set standards of expertise for affiliation. When establishing an in-practice laboratory, a neurology practice that does not include a board-certified sleep specialist can opt to retrain a member, hire a new member, or contract with a board-certified medical doctor to interpret studies. Business arrangements with outside interpreting physicians are now specifically regulated by Centers for Medicare and Medicaid Services (CMS) "antimarkup" rules that may vary from one locality to another.[2] All financial arrangements between physicians and facilities should pass careful legal review.

Regardless of internal expertise, the practice should also identify a local network of collegial sleep professionals. This includes an otolaryngologist for anatomic evaluation and occasional sleep apnea surgery, a dentist to provide oral appliances for sleep apnea, a pulmonologist to help manage complex sleep apnea and comorbid pulmonary disease, a psychiatrist to evaluate mental health concerns, which are often comorbid with insomnia, a behavioral psychologist for cognitive behavioral therapy of insomnia, a cardiologist to consult on cardiovascular consequences of sleep problems, and a pain specialist to help manage patients with chronic pain and attendant sleep disorders.

The practice also needs to identify one or more providers of durable medical equipment (DME), such as continuous positive airway pressure (CPAP) and related supplies. Federal laws prohibit physicians from dispensing or providing DME to Medicare or other federally insured patients,[3] and state fraud and abuse laws also regulate doctors' economic practices. Some practices do dispense DME to privately insured patients through practice pathways that have passed careful legal review. Information must pass regularly among patients, physicians, and DME companies, and patients should come to follow-up office visits with printouts of CPAP adherence and other data usually supplied by the DME provider. This allows the treating physician to objectively quantify treatment adherence and efficacy, as well as to meet insurer requirements for PAP payment.

Physicians have to guide patients through a changing regulatory maze to get appropriate evaluation and treatment of sleep disorders. Medications commonly used to treat sleep disorders are often dispensed only with prior authorization, and they are subject to frequent utilization reviews. Most Medicare contractors now require that the PSG be performed in an accredited facility by a licensed or registered technologist. They also require that the study be read by a board-certified physician or a physician affiliated with a certified sleep center, whether the test is done in an independent diagnostic testing facility or in the office. If CMS is to approve initial CPAP therapy, further requirements include a physician visit before testing and a documented Epworth Sleepiness Score. Patients are eligible for Medicare payment for sleep apnea therapy if the apnea-hypopnea index (AHI) is greater than or equal to 5 if the patient is symptomatic (specific regulatory language includes daytime hypersomnolence, impaired cognition, mood disorder, insomnia, stroke, hypertension, or ischemic heart disease), or the AHI is greater than or equal to 15 if the patient is not symptomatic.[4] If CMS is to approve ongoing CPAP therapy after an initial 90-day trial, further requirements include a physician visit in months 2 or 3; the visit must document symptomatic improvement and objective evidence of patient adherence to therapy for at least 4 hours, on 70% of nights, during 30 consecutive days. Other conditions limit a practice's ability to provide 1-stop service: the physician cannot dispense DME to governmentally insured patients, and any company that performs home sleep testing also cannot provide DME. In other words, CMS regulations and legal findings by the federal Office of the Inspector General (OIG) increasingly limit relationships among physicians, independent testing facilities, and DME providers. The practice's relationships and procedures should be designed to meet CMS requirements as expressed in your local carrier decisions (LCDs),[5] and they should be reviewed annually, as the LCDs may change without notice. Most private insurers have well-defined policies for sleep testing and for sleep apnea therapy, often posted online. Private payer policies may be more or less exacting than the local CMS policies.

The clinical utility of PSG is limited by its relative inconvenience and cost. As portable EEG expands the reach of neurologic testing beyond the office, so does out-of-center testing (OOCT, also known as portable testing or home sleep testing) extend the availability of sleep testing. After instruction from an office technologist, a patient may put on a simplified set of sensors at bedtime and record a diagnostic test that is not attended by a technologist. The next day, the patient returns to the office, where the stored data are downloaded. The technologist may score the information on site or may upload it to a server for remote analysis. Patients cannot reliably self-apply EEG electrodes, but they can more reliably apply cardiac and respiratory sensors. Devices for OOCT generally use a simplified montage with innovative sensor technology, often with proprietary signal analysis, usually designed specifically to test for sleep apnea.

Current Procedure Terminology (CPT) coding[6] now distinguishes 3 types of limited channel recordings that are in relatively wide use, listed in **Table 1**. The oldest technology, corresponding to code 95806, is unattended cardiopulmonary testing. Two newer codes, 95800 and 95801, refer to measurement of respiratory variables with or without sleep time. Available devices usually measure sleep time indirectly by methods such as actigraphy, and some use limited EEG information.

Commercially available devices differ in their ease of use, in the specific physiologic variables measured, and in the technologies and proprietary algorithms used for event detection. The initial costs of portable sleep monitoring devices differ at least threefold, and the per-patient expenses vary even more. A compact method to classify and evaluate portable monitoring methods was recently proposed.[7] OOCT is technically limited in comparison with PSG. In general, portable devices may underestimate the severity of sleep-disordered breathing, at least in part because the number of events is divided by total recording time, and not necessarily total sleep time. Artifact rates may also be higher than for attended studies, as sensor problems may persist all night when data are not continuously reviewed by an attendant technologist. The physician should assess the raw data for each OOCT study to ensure the integrity of the recording. Because each OOCT method has imperfections, each should be used only as part of a comprehensive sleep evaluation.[8]

Clinically, OOCT is best used to diagnose sleep apnea in patients with a high pretest probability of the disorder.[8,9] Some investigators suggest that for the general population without neurologic disease or contraindications, sleep apnea may be diagnosed with OOCT and treated with auto-adjusting CPAP ("smart PAP"), never sleeping overnight in the laboratory. Some patients would be poor candidates for any type of OOCT technology, and poor candidates most can be excluded from testing based on medical history.[10] The 2007 Clinical Guideline states that OOCT "is not appropriate for the diagnostic evaluation of OSA in patients suspected of having other sleep disorders, including central sleep apnea, periodic limb movement disorder (PLMD), insomnia, parasomnias, circadian rhythm disorders, or narcolepsy."[8] Patients with congestive heart failure or acute stroke may have central apnea; generally they should be studied in a laboratory with a device that measures respiratory effort as well as air flow. Patients with autonomic dysfunction or those on medications that block autonomic output should be tested with technology that does not rely on peripheral arterial tone. Neuromuscular patients at high risk for hypoventilation generally should undergo fully attended PSG to ensure that rapid eye movement

Table 1	
Home sleep testing: CPT codes 2011	
CPT	**Description**
95800	Sleep study, unattended, simultaneous recording; heart rate, oxygen saturation, respiratory analysis (eg, by airflow or peripheral arterial tone), and sleep time
95801	Sleep study, unattended, simultaneous recording minimum of heart rate, oxygen saturation, and respiratory analysis (eg, by airflow or peripheral arterial tone)
95806	Sleep study, simultaneous recording of ventilation, respiratory effort, electrocardiogram or heart rate, and oxygen saturation, unattended by a technologist

(REM) respiration is recorded, as the algorithmic detection of probable REM sleep is not as reliable for OOCT as is formal staging with PSG.

Actigraphy is another commonly used type of outpatient testing. An actigraph uses motion sensors on the wrist or ankle to record movement over a period of 3 to 21 days, and may be repeated. Because there is usually little movement during sleep but frequent movement while awake, a plot of movement over time usually demonstrates high-movement wake periods interspersed with low-movement sleep periods. Procedures to educate the patient, dispense and collect equipment, and to analyze and report data are similar as for other OOCTs. Neurologists can easily incorporate actigraphy into their practice to track sleep-wake patterns for patients with insomnia and non–24-hour rhythms, and to investigate restless legs syndrome and periodic limb movements in sleep.[11]

CMS payments for PSG interpretation dropped by more than 20% in 2010, and technical payments are scheduled to drop by about 20% from 2010 to 2013. Compared with attended PSG, OOCT costs are lower and profit margins are generally slender. Patient education, equipment insurance, and technologist roles are similar for OOCT and for ambulatory EEG testing. If your practice chooses this well-validated clinical pathway, you can serve most of your patients with sleep apnea with a lower investment of time, expertise, and funds than if you open a full-service laboratory.

There are many apparent practice opportunities available to pediatric neurologists with an interest in sleep medicine. There are relatively few pediatric sleep specialists, and many adult sleep specialists are not comfortable interpreting studies on children. A pediatric facility usually is designed to allow parents to stay with minor children, and usually there is a higher technologist-to-patient staffing ratio at children's centers. Technology for pediatric PSG usually includes monitoring of end-tidal or transcutaneous carbon dioxide partial pressure as a measure of ventilation.[12] New CPT codes for pediatric PSG are expected for 2013.

Inpatient sleep medicine is also a burgeoning service. Patients with new cerebral or myocardial infarction, all at high risk for obstructive sleep apnea (OSA), may benefit from immediate diagnosis by OOCT and treatment by auto-adjusting PAP, minimizing disruption to the schedule for attended studies. Other neurology candidates for inpatient sleep consultation include patients with neuromuscular disease, chronic pain, fatigue, or those whose screening questionnaires indicate high risk. Currently Medicare pays most hospitals a fixed fee based on the patient's diagnosis and disease severity, so most hospitals discourage PSG and other elective testing for inpatients. Inpatient testing is likely to increase, however, particularly if evolving hospital quality measures come to include sleep apnea screening before surgery. Newer payment mechanisms may encourage inpatient testing, particularly if accountable care organizations are paid similarly for testing done during or after hospitalization.

Sleep medicine is a relatively new medical specialty. In a 2011 editorial, Pack[13] proposed that sleep medicine should be increasingly focused on scientific and clinical outcomes rather than on processes. Sleep specialists should be prepared to diagnose and treat all sleep disorders, to provide in-laboratory PSG and OOCT, and should offer treatments including positive airway pressure (PAP), dental appliance therapy, surgery, and cognitive behavioral therapy (CBT) for insomnia. He proposed that the sleep practice should include physician and nonphysician providers and often should be embedded with general medicine practices. Neurology practices are well positioned to help increase the application of sleep diagnosis and therapy to a larger patient population.

SLEEP DISORDERS IN NEUROLOGIC DISEASE: WHO NEEDS TO BE TESTED?

Patients in neurologic practice commonly have difficulty falling asleep, and have disrupted sleep, fatigue, excessive daytime sleepiness, poor concentration or memory, irritability, and mood disorders. Primary brain disorders and primary sleep disorders may cause similar symptoms, and many patients have multiple factors contributing to nonspecific symptoms. Additionally, our patients may not express or recognize their sleep-related concerns.

Sleep-disordered breathing (SDB), in particular OSA and central sleep apnea, is common among patients with neurologic disease. The importance of sleep apnea in neurologic disorders is not completely understood, because investigators have used differing test methods and different definitions. Although some studies have diagnosed SDB with attended, overnight PSG, including sleep staging, many others have relied on unattended portable monitoring with limited montages. Although some investigators have required desaturations of 3% to 4% to define hypopnea, others include all episodes of reduced airflow or episodes that are terminated by an arousal. Because clinical symptoms are not adequate to diagnose sleep apnea, PSG testing is a clinical standard in a number of neurologic disorders. **Table 2** summarizes neurologic disorders for which sleep testing should be performed routinely. Treatment is beneficial for most neurologic patients with diagnosed OSA, even when sleep apnea is mild by PSG criteria.

Table 2
Neurologic disorders: Sleep testing is indicated

Disorder	Indicated Test	Rationale
Stroke	PSG Unattended testing may be needed for immediate and acute testing.	High incidence OSA, but also relatively high incidence of central apnea and hypoventilation. Symptoms not reliable as screen
Neuromuscular disease	PSG with end-tidal P_{CO_2}	High incidence OSA and hypoventilation
Dementia	PSG	High incidence OSA CPAP use is feasible.
Nocturnal wandering, parasomnias including REM behavioral disorder, nocturnal seizures	PSG with extra EMG leads, possibly after sleep deprivation	Arousals owing to OSA may be responsible for behavior.
Insomnia (refractory to treatment or atypical)	PSG	High incidence mild OSA; OOCT often insensitive to mild OSA
Refractory morning or nocturnal headache	PSG	Possible sleep apnea, even mild
Refractory epilepsy with OSA symptoms or signs	PSG	Possible sleep apnea, even mild
Fatigue, sleepiness when chronic and unexplained	PSG with MSLT	Possible sleep apnea, narcolepsy, idiopathic hypersomnolence

Abbreviations: CPAP, continuous positive airway pressure; EMG, electromyography; MSLT, multiple sleep latency test; OOCT, out-of-center testing; OSA, obstructive sleep apnea; P_{CO_2}, partial pressure of carbon dioxide; PSG, polysomnography; REM, rapid eye movement.

SLEEP DISORDERS AND STROKE

In a meta-analysis including more than 2000 patients with stroke or transient ischemic attack (TIA), SDB with AHI greater than 5 was found in 72% and AHI greater than 20 was found in 38% of patients; 7% had primarily central apnea or Cheyne Stokes respirations.[14] In this study, neither stroke type (ischemic vs hemorrhagic) nor location (hemispheric vs brainstem) was predictive of sleep apnea. The risk of OSA was higher among patients with snoring, daytime sleepiness, and witnessed apneas, but more than 25% of patients with SDB did not snore. Other studies confirm that clinical symptoms do not accurately predict sleep apnea in stroke.[15]

In the setting of acute stroke, the presence of SDB has been associated with early neurologic worsening[16] and higher acute blood pressure.[17,18] SDB has a negative impact on short-term and long-term neurologic recovery,[19] mortality,[20–22] and stroke recurrence risk.[21,23–25] Early studies indicate that CPAP use in the setting of acute stroke may help reduce recurrent cardiovascular events, improve 5-year mortality,[26,27] and reduce nighttime blood pressure. Low adherence for CPAP therapy is common among stroke patients who are not sleepy or who have dementia, delirium, anosognosia, and pseudobulbar or bulbar palsy.[28]

Fatigue and insomnia are very common following stroke, reported in approximately half of patients in one large study.[24] Sleepiness caused by cerebral damage usually improves over the first few months following stroke, although fatigue may persist.[29,30] Untreated comorbid sleep apnea often contributes to subjective sleepiness in patients who have had stroke. Sleep disruption after stroke may also be related to underlying cardiac failure, anxiety, depression, or pain, and may be exacerbated by noise, light, and intrusive hospital monitoring. Symptomatic therapy of poststroke sleepiness and insomnia may be effective.[31]

Stroke-related cerebral damage can also cause sleep-related movement disorders and parasomnias. New-onset REM sleep behavior disorder has been reported after pontine tegmental strokes.[32] In one study, restless legs syndrome, often with periodic limb movements in sleep, appeared in 12% of patients within 1 week after stroke, most often after pontine, thalamic, basal ganglia, and corona radiata damage.[33]

OSA should be considered in all patients with cerebrovascular disease. A 2005 consensus statement recommended optional PSG when sleep apnea is clinically suspected in patients with stroke or TIA.[34] One emerging clinical pathway is to perform unattended portable testing on all patients who have had a stroke immediately on admission. Another evolving protocol is to use auto-adjusting CPAP empirically on admission to treat patients at clinically high risk of sleep apnea.[35,36] Guidelines in 2007 recommended that portable monitoring "may be indicated for the diagnosis of OSA in patients for whom in-laboratory PSG is not possible by virtue of immobility, safety, or critical illness."[8] PSG may demonstrate the relative importance of obstructive compared with central sleep apnea, informing pulmonary therapy in the acute stoke setting.

Box 1
Case Report

A 64-year-old male suffers a right internal capsule infarction with mild left-sided weakness. His snoring disrupts sleep for his hospital roommate, who complains to the nurses. The patient's wife wears hearing aids during the day and removes them at night, and she is not certain whether her husband snores. The patient's only sleep concern is his need to urinate 2 to 3 times nightly, "because my prostate is old." PSG demonstrates AHI 27/hour with desaturations to a low of 79%. The patient is adherent for CPAP therapy and sleeps through the night. Alertness improves, and the patient is more enthusiastic in therapy.

SLEEP AND NEUROMUSCULAR DISEASE

A variety of mechanisms may contribute to sleep-disordered breathing in patients with neuromuscular disease, including diaphragmatic weakness, chest wall weakness, pharyngeal wall weakness, and restrictive lung disease. Comorbid obesity and cerebral abnormalities may further increase risks of obstructive and central sleep apnea and of sleep hypoventilation. Sleep breathing disorders may be more severe in REM sleep, when the normal reduction in accessory respiratory muscle tone may be exacerbated by weakness. Hypoventilation, with low baseline oxygen saturation and high partial pressure of carbon dioxide, is more common in patients with neuromuscular disease than in the general population with OSA.

Sleep complaints and disorders in neuromuscular patients usually have been reported in small observational series. Excessive daytime sleepiness is common in neuromuscular disorders reported in up to 80% of patients with myotonic dystrophy, for example.[37,38] Painful cramping and spasticity may disrupt sleep and limit movements in bed, and abnormal spontaneous movements may impair sleep onset. Cough and swallow arousals to clear secretions may disrupt sleep. Patients with autonomic disturbances may suffer from incontinence and night sweats. Pain, anxiety, depression, and medication side effects may disrupt sleep as well.[39] SDB was found in 36% to 60% of patients with myasthenia gravis, and was worst during REM sleep.[40,41] Sleep breathing abnormalities have also been reported in 50% of patients with postpolio syndrome,[42] and in patients with hereditary motor and sensory neuropathy[43,44] and diabetic autonomic neuropathy.[45]

Attended PSG is the essential diagnostic test for sleep breathing abnormalities in patients with neuromuscular disease. The study must investigate the effectiveness of REM breathing in these patients, and REM cannot be identified with sufficient reliability by unattended testing with limited montages. End-tidal or transcutaneous carbon dioxide levels usually are the most sensitive indicator of hypoventilation and should be included in the PSG montage when available. One recommended standard in the American Academy of Sleep Medicine (AASM) practice parameters in 2005 was that routine PSG be performed in patients with neuromuscular disorders, who "are not adequately diagnosed by obtaining a sleep history, assessing sleep hygiene, and reviewing sleep diaries."[34]

OSA, when present in patients with neuromuscular diseases, usually is treated with bilevel pressure (BPAP) rather than CPAP. Compared with CPAP therapy, BPAP provides a significant pressure decrease during expiration; the inspiratory boost or "support" pressure seems to be an important treatment component in weak patients. This can improve both quality of life and survival.[46–50] Even with maximal PAP therapy, supplemental oxygen may be needed.[51] Inspiratory muscle training may also be effective.[52] Central components of apnea, when present, usually respond to these treatments, but servo-ventilator PAP, essentially a demand respirator, may be more effective than BPAP in patients with complex sleep apnea owing to neuromuscular disease.

SLEEP AND PARKINSON DISEASE

Sleep disturbances are very common in patients with Parkinson disease (PD). About 60% of patients report insomnia,[53] 30% report excessive daytime sleepiness,[54,55] up to 59% have REM sleep behavior disorder,[56,57] and 12% to 21% report restless legs syndrome.[58,59] In one study, sleep apnea was diagnosed in 20% of patients with PD.[60] In atypical parkinsonism, sleep disorders may be even more prevalent.

REM sleep behavior disorder may be caused by damage to the REM sleep atonia system.[61] PSG in patients with REM behavioral disorder may demonstrate loss of the normal muscle atonia during REM sleep; sensitivity may be improved if PSG includes monitoring of smaller foot muscles as well as the anterior tibialis surface EMG that is commonly monitored during PSG.[62] Diagnostic PSG to investigate possible sleep apnea is essential when parkinsonian patients report parasomnias, because abnormal behaviors in REM may be triggered by apneic arousals and may remit when comorbid OSA is treated.[63] Treatment also consists of ensuring a safe nighttime environment for the patient and bed partner; medical therapy may include clonazepam, melatonin, or other agents.[64]

Excessive daytime sleepiness affects on average one-third of patients with PD, particularly those with advanced disease.[54,55,65,66] The presence or degree of sleepiness often does not correlate with separately diagnosed sleep disorders.[60,67,68] Some patients with PD experience a sudden onset of sleep, without warning or awareness of falling asleep; this was first described in patients taking dopamine agonists, which seem to increase the risk.[65,66,69,70] In one study, almost half of patients with PD fell asleep within a mean of 5 minutes, indicating pathologic sleepiness similar to narcolepsy.[65,66,69,70] Importantly, patients may be unaware of being abnormally sleepy.[71] Thus, patients with PD with severe sleepiness may be best identified by caregiver reports, regular questioning about sudden onset of sleep, and by objective testing with MSLT. Modafinil may improve alertness, but in one report it was effective in fewer than one-third of patients.[72]

Patients with multisystem atrophy (MSA) frequently have sleep disorders and are at risk of developing progressive, life-threatening laryngeal obstruction and stridor during sleep, observed in 42% of patients in one study.[73] CPAP may treat sleep breathing adequately,[74] but tracheotomy may eventually be required.

Patients with PD or MSA need a PSG when parasomnia is suspected, or when there is a high clinical likelihood of sleep apnea. MSLT is needed when sleepiness is unexplained or severe. The Maintenance of Wakefulness Test (MWT), an objective test similar to the MSLT, theoretically measures the patient's ability to stay awake while at rest, whereas the MLST theoretically measures the patient's tendency to fall asleep. The MWT may be a necessary but imperfect tool in evaluating fitness to drive or operate heavy equipment, because severe sleepiness is often asymptomatic in people with PD or related disorders.

Box 2
Case Report

The wife of a patient with PD is distressed because approximately once per week her husband hits her during the night. Episodes usually occur after about 3 hours of sleep; when awakened, the patient recalls dreaming of fighting. He has frequent difficulty initiating sleep and occasional mild snoring. PSG demonstrates an AHI of 14/hour with desaturations to a low of 84%; hypopneas are more frequent and desaturations more severe in REM sleep. On CPAP therapy, parasomnias and insomnia resolve. Three years later, parasomnias return despite good adherence to and efficacy of CPAP therapy. While the patient uses CPAP at the prescribed pressure, PSG demonstrates normal breathing in all stages of sleep, but there is abnormally increased motor activity in the last REM period, noted over the extensor digitorum brevis but not over the anterior tibialis. The parasomnias resolve when the patient takes clonazepam and continues to use CPAP.

SLEEP AND MULTIPLE SCLEROSIS

Sleep disturbances are reported in as many as half of patients with multiple sclerosis.[75,76] Contributing factors include neurologic, endocrine, autoimmune, and psychiatric problems. More than 80% of patients with multiple sclerosis report chronic fatigue, and it is rated as the most disabling symptom by many.[77,78] Fatigue is characterized by a feeling of physical tiredness with lack of energy; it may be independent of a strong desire for sleep, but usually it is difficult to separate fatigue from sleepiness on clinical grounds. Insomnia is also common, and can be caused or worsened by bladder problems, spasticity, muscle spasms, periodic leg movements, depression, anxiety, and brain lesions.[79,80] Medications also contribute; sleepiness may be caused by medications including baclofen, clonazepam, and gabapentin, and insomnia may be caused by others, including amantadine, modafinil, and methylprednisolone. SDB, narcolepsy, RLS, and RBD have been reported as well, although the prevalence is not well studied.[81,82]

PSG with MSLT should be performed when patients with multiple sclerosis have sleepiness or fatigue that is unexplained or not responsive to simple management tools, such as sleep hygiene. Chronic fatigue in patients with multiple sclerosis is often treated with amantadine or modafinil, despite limited evidence of efficacy.[83–85]

Box 3
Case Report

A 42-year-old woman with relapsing-remitting multiple sclerosis complains of fatigue. Treatment with modafinil 400 mg daily improves her Epworth Sleepiness Scale (ESS) score from 20/24 to 16/24, but she still has difficulty staying awake while driving. More complete history reveals that she had difficulty staying awake in high school and college classes, and episodes of sudden weakness have been triggered by hearty laughing. PSG demonstrates fragmented sleep. MSLT is compatible with narcolepsy. More vigorous pharmacologic therapy improves her ESS score to 6/24, and the patient now drives without drowsiness.

SLEEP AND DEMENTIA

Sleep apnea is present with an AHI of 15 or more in 15% to 25% of people older than 55,[86,87] so it is therefore highly prevalent among patients with dementia. Experimental evidence demonstrates that chronic recurrent mild hypoxia may cause neuronal cell death and white matter changes,[88,89] and a prospective study has demonstrated that SDB increases the risk of mild cognitive impairment and dementia in women older than 65 years.[90] Sleep apnea increases morbidity and sleep symptoms in the elderly and specifically in patients with dementia. In a study of patients with mild dementia, AHI of 10 or more, and average age about 78 years, CPAP adherence was acceptable at just over 5 hours per night. Therapy improved objective sleep efficiency and slow-wave sleep, subjective sleepiness, depression, and cognition in patients with sleep apnea and dementia.[91–93]

Insomnia is an early and prominent symptom in the prion disorder fatal familial insomnia, in which thalamic pathology helps to model theories of sleep physiology.[94] Patients with dementia frequently suffer from sleep/wake symptoms including insomnia, sleepiness, and circadian disorders; they usually benefit from sleep hygiene, regular schedules, and review of potential medication side effects.[95] Patients with dementia should be examined with PSG if there is a moderate clinical suspicion of sleep apnea, but it is not recommended routinely.

> **Box 4**
> **Case Report**
>
> A 72-year-old retired scientist has progressive memory loss and depression. He has withdrawn from his family and sleeps much of the day. PSG demonstrates an AHI of 72/hour with desaturations to a low of 82%. The patient is adherent to CPAP therapy and reduces time in bed to 7 hours daily. Daily activities are more numerous and rewarding. Minimal cognitive impairment is diagnosed.

SLEEP AND DEPRESSION, ANXIETY, AND POSTTRAUMATIC STRESS DISORDER

Insomnia is a primary symptom in patients with major depressive disorder, generalized anxiety disorder, panic disorder, and posttraumatic stress disorder. Common complaints also include hypersomnia, fatigue, nonrestorative sleep, and nocturnal panic attacks. Adequate therapy often requires recognizing and treating both psychiatric and sleep disorders.

PSG studies in depressed patients demonstrate reduced slow-wave sleep, shortened REM latency, and disrupted sleep continuity.[96] REM latency often normalizes during effective treatment of depression,[97] Additionally, patients with OSA have an increased risk of developing major depressive disorder,[98] and there is some evidence that treatment of comorbid OSA can result in improvements in depression.[99]

Two sleep symptoms are included in PTSD diagnostic criteria: nightmares and insomnia. Although PSG findings in patients with PTSD are not specific,[100] high rates of SDB[101,102] and parasomnias[103–106] are reported. Patients with PTSD also may have sleep symptoms deriving from comorbid major depression, panic disorder, or substance abuse or dependence.[102] Prazosin may be particularly beneficial for sleep disturbances in patients with PTSD.[107–110]

For chronic insomnia, cognitive behavioral therapy has been more effective than pharmacologic therapy in randomized trials[111] and should be prescribed for all patients with chronic insomnia, particularly with recent evidence of increased morbidity and mortality among patients prescribed hypnotic medications.[112] Medications, including selective serotonin reuptake inhibitors, serotonin-norepinephrin reuptake inhibitors, and bupropion may worsen insomnia in some patients, whereas sedating medications, such as trazodone, nefazodone, and mirtazapine, can improve sleep initiation and maintenance.[113] Thus, attention to sleep symptoms can help to direct the choice of primary treatment for a patient's mood disorder.

Relatively mild sleep apnea is increasingly recognized as a treatable cause of or contributing factor to insomnia, even in the presence of other primary sleep or neurologic disorders.[114–116] Patients with insomnia should undergo PSG when there are atypical features, such as disruptive snoring, or when they fail to respond to usual treatments.[117]

SLEEP, HEADACHE, AND EPILEPSY

The International Classification of Headache Disorders, second edition,[118] introduced diagnostic criteria for sleep apnea headache and hypnic headache. Morning headache occurs in 18% to 74% of patients with OSA, and CPAP therapy often resolves headache as well as sleep apnea.[119,120] Cluster headache often appears at night, both in REM and non-REM sleep.[121] It is common practice to perform diagnostic PSG for patients with unexplained, frequent nocturnal or morning headaches, particularly when they do not respond to treatment.

Epilepsy and sleep are dynamically related; sleep and sleep deprivation can be helpful in diagnosing epilepsy. Seizures can be exacerbated by sleep deprivation, and may occur more often in non-REM than REM sleep.[122,123] Attention to sleep also can improve the treatment of epilepsy. In patients with sleep apnea, good CPAP adherence is associated with improved seizure control in several small series.[124–127] At times, it can also be difficult to distinguish parasomnias from nocturnal seizures. A clinical standard in the 2005 AASM consensus statement recommended PSG for the evaluation of atypical parasomnias, or for seizures or parasomnias that do not respond to usual therapy. Sleep deprivation may increase the number of parasomnias occurring during PSG testing.[128]

SUMMARY

Most patients in a neurology practice have sleep complaints, and many have comorbid primary sleep disorders. As a first step to identify and help them, new and established patients should complete a sleep questionnaire as part of their comprehensive history. Among primary sleep disorders, OSA is highly prevalent among neurologic patients; it increases morbidity and mortality and may worsen neurologic symptoms. Conversely, treating sleep apnea and other sleep disorders can improve neurologic care. A reasoned clinical pathway to diagnose and treat sleep apnea is increasingly important for the long-term health of neurology patients and practices.

As regulatory and practice management momentum builds toward increasing care coordination and integration, most neurology practices can offer actigraphy and out-of-center testing for sleep apnea, using work flow and practice management models similar to those for ambulatory EEG testing. Some practices may choose to offer OOCT testing in selected patients, and some may choose to interpret PSG and MSLT studies performed at another facility to emphasize their neurologic expertise. Finally, a number of neurology practices now include a comprehensive sleep medicine practice with a board-certified physician and registered and licensed technologists. Facility credentials are evolving and soon may include accreditation in PSG testing, OOCT, and providing DME. The neurologist can play a key role in diagnosing, treating, and managing sleep disorders, helping patients to improve both neurologic symptoms and overall quality of life.

REFERENCES

1. Medicare definition of general supervision, from The Code of Federal regulations of the United States of America. 1996. Available at: http://www.cms.hhs.gov/mcd/overview.asp. Accessed March 26, 2012.
2. Cor H, Vegliando K. Medicare claims processing manual. 2008. Chapter 1-General billing requirements. Available at: https://www.cms.gov/manuals/downloads/clm104c01.pdf. Accessed April 3, 2012.
3. Federal Fraud Enforcement and Physician Compliance. Available at: http://www.ama-assn.org/ama/pub/physician-resources/legal-topics/regulatory-compliance-topics/health-care-fraud-abuse/federal-fraud-enforcement-physician-compliance/federal-fraud-abuse-laws.page. Accessed April 3, 2012.
4. National Coverage Determination (NCD) for Continuous Positive Airway Pressure (CPAP) Therapy For Obstructive Sleep Apnea (OSA) (240.4). Available at: http://www.cms.gov/medicare-coverage-database/details/ncd-details.aspx?NCDId=226&ncdver=3&CoverageSelection=Both&ArticleType=All&PolicyType=Final&s=Maryland&KeyWord=CPAP&KeyWordLookUp=Title&KeyWordSearchType=And&bc=gAAAABAAAAAA&. Accessed April 3, 2012.
5. Medicare Coverage Database. Available at: http://www.cms.hhs.gov/mcd/overview.asp. Accessed April 12, 2012.

6. Association AM. CPT Professional 2012 (Spiral bound) (Current Procedural Terminology [CPT] Professional). Spi Ind Th. American Medical Association Press; 2011. p. 700.

7. Collop N, Tracy S, Kapur V, et al. Obstructive sleep apnea devices for out-of-center (OOC) testing: technology evaluation. J Clin Sleep Med 2011;7: 531–48.

8. Collop N, Anderson W, Boehlecke B, et al. Clinical guidelines for the use of unattended portable monitors in the diagnosis of obstructive sleep apnea in adult patients. Portable Monitoring Task Force of the American Academy of Sleep Medicine. J Clin Sleep Med 2007;3:737–47.

9. Trikalinos T, Ip S, Raman G, et al. Home Diagnosis of Obstructive Sleep Apnea-Hypopnea Syndrome. Agency for Healthcare Research and Quality Technology Assessment Program. 2007. Available at: http://www.cms.hhs.gov/determinationprocess/downloads/id48TA.pdf. Accessed April 3, 2012.

10. Kuna S, Gurubhagavatula I, Maislin G, et al. Noninferiority of functional outcome in ambulatory management of obstructive sleep apnea. Am J Respir Crit Care Med 2011;183:1238–44.

11. Morgenthaler T, Lee-Chiong T, Alessi C, et al. Practice parameters for the clinical evaluation and treatment of circadian rhythm sleep disorders. An American Academy of Sleep Medicine report. Sleep 2007;30:1445–59.

12. Wise M, Nichols C, Grigg-Damberger M, et al. Executive summary of respiratory indications for polysomnography in children: an evidence-based review. Sleep 2011;34:389–98.

13. Pack A. Sleep medicine: strategies for change. J Clin Sleep Med 2011;7:577–9.

14. Johnson K, Johnson D. Frequency of sleep apnea in stroke and TIA patients: a meta-analysis. J Clin Sleep Med 2010;6:131–7.

15. Kotzian S, Stanek J, Pinter M, et al. Subjective evaluation of sleep apnea is not sufficient in stroke rehabilitation. Top Stroke Rehabil 2012;19:45–53.

16. Iranzo A, Santamaria J, Berenguer J, et al. Prevalence and clinical importance of sleep apnea in the first night after cerebral infarction. Neurology 2002;58: 911–6.

17. Selic C, Siccoli M, Hermann D, et al. Blood pressure evolution after acute ischemic stroke in patients with and without sleep apnea. Stroke 2005;36: 2614–8.

18. Siccoli M, Valko P, Hermann D, et al. Central periodic breathing during sleep in 74 patients with acute ischemic stroke—neurogenic and cardiogenic factors. J Neurol 2008;255:1687–92.

19. Yan-fang S, Yu-ping W. Sleep-disordered breathing: impact on functional outcome of ischemic stroke patients. Sleep Med 2009;10:717–9.

20. Marshall N, Wong K, Liu P, et al. Sleep apnea as an independent risk factor for all-cause mortality: the Busselton Health Study. Sleep 2008;31:1079–85.

21. Young T, Finn L, Peppard PE, et al. Sleep disordered breathing and mortality: eighteen-year follow-up of the Wisconsin sleep cohort. Sleep 2008;31: 1071–8.

22. Sahlin C, Sandberg O, Gustafson Y, et al. Obstructive sleep apnea is a risk factor for death in patients with stroke: a 10-year follow-up. Arch Intern Med 2008;168:297–301.

23. Yaggi H, Concato J, Kernan W, et al. Obstructive sleep apnea as a risk factor for stroke and death. N Engl J Med 2005;353:2034–41.

24. Leppävuori A, Pohjasvaara T, Vataja R, et al. Insomnia in ischemic stroke patients. Cerebrovasc Dis 2002;142:90–7.

25. Dziewas R, Humpert M, Hopmann B, et al. Increased prevalence of sleep apnea in patients with recurring ischemic stroke compared with first stroke victims. J Neurol 2005;252:1394–8.
26. Martínez-García M, Soler-Cataluña J, Ejarque-Martínez L, et al. Continuous positive airway pressure treatment reduces mortality in patients with ischemic stroke and obstructive sleep apnea: a 5-year follow-up study. Am J Respir Crit Care Med 2009;180:36–41.
27. Martínez-García M, Galiano-Blancart R, Román-Sánchez P, et al. Continuous positive airway pressure treatment in sleep apnea prevents new vascular events after ischemic stroke. Chest 2005;128:2123–9.
28. Wessendorf T, Wang Y, Thilmann A, et al. Treatment of obstructive sleep apnoea with nasal continuous positive airway pressure in stroke. Eur Respir J 2001;18:623–9.
29. Winward C, Sackley C, Metha Z, et al. A population-based study of the prevalence of fatigue after transient ischemic attack and minor stroke. Stroke 2009;40:757–61.
30. Naess H, Lunde L, Brogger J, et al. Fatigue among stroke patients on long-term follow-up. The Bergen Stroke Study. J Neurol Sci 2012;312:138–41.
31. Hermann D, Bassetti C. Sleep-related breathing and sleep-wake disturbances in ischemic stroke. Neurology 2009;73:1313–22.
32. Culebras A, Moore J. Magnetic resonance findings in REM sleep behavior disorder. Neurology 1989;39:1519–23.
33. Lee SJ, Kim JS, Song IU, et al. Poststroke restless legs syndrome and lesion location: anatomical considerations. Mov Disord 2009;24:77–84.
34. Kushida C, Littner M, Morgenthaler T, et al. Practice parameters for the indications for polysomnography and related procedures: an update for 2005. Sleep 2005;28:499–521.
35. Minnerup J, Ritter M, Wersching H, et al. Continuous positive airway pressure ventilation for acute ischemic stroke: a randomized feasibility study. Stroke 2011;43:1137–9.
36. Bravata D, Concato J, Fried T, et al. Continuous positive airway pressure: evaluation of a novel therapy for patients with acute ischemic stroke. Sleep 2011;34:1271–7.
37. Laberge L, Bégin P, Montplaisir J, et al. Sleep complaints in patients with myotonic dystrophy. J Sleep Res 2004;13:95–100.
38. Hilton-Jones D. Myotonic dystrophy—forgotten aspects of an often neglected condition. Curr Opin Neurol 1997;10:399–401.
39. David W, Bundlie S, Mahdavi Z. Polysomnographic studies in amyotrophic lateral sclerosis. J Neurol Sci 1997;152(Suppl 1):S29–35.
40. Amino A, Shiozawa Z, Nagasaka T, et al. Sleep apnoea in well-controlled myasthenia gravis and the effect of thymectomy. J Neurol 1998;245:77–80.
41. Nicolle M, Rask S, Koopman W, et al. Sleep apnea in patients with myasthenia gravis. Neurology 2006;67:140–2.
42. Dahan V, Kimoff R, Petrof B, et al. Sleep-disordered breathing in fatigued postpoliomyelitis clinic patients. Arch Phys Med Rehabil 2006;87:1352–6.
43. Chan C, Mohsenin V, Loke J, et al. Diaphragmatic dysfunction in siblings with hereditary motor and sensory neuropathy (Charcot-Marie-Tooth disease). Chest 1987;91:567–70.
44. Dematteis M, Pépin J, Jeanmart M, et al. Charcot-Marie-Tooth disease and sleep apnoea syndrome: a family study. Lancet 2001;357:267–72.
45. Tantucci C, Bottini P, Fiorani C, et al. Cerebrovascular reactivity and hypercapnic respiratory drive in diabetic autonomic neuropathy. J Appl Physiol 2001;90:889–96.

46. Pinto A, Evangelista T, Carvalho M, et al. Respiratory assistance with a non-invasive ventilator (Bipap) in MND/ALS patients: survival rates in a controlled trial. J Neurol Sci 1995;129(Suppl):19–26.
47. Bourke S, Tomlinson M, Williams T, et al. Effects of non-invasive ventilation on survival and quality of life in patients with amyotrophic lateral sclerosis: a randomised controlled trial. Lancet Neurol 2006;5:140–7.
48. Simonds A. Recent advances in respiratory care for neuromuscular disease. Chest 2006;130:1879–86.
49. Arens R, Muzumdar H. Sleep, sleep disordered breathing, and nocturnal hypoventilation in children with neuromuscular diseases. Paediatr Respir Rev 2010; 11:24–30.
50. Shneerson J, Simonds A. Noninvasive ventilation for chest wall and neuromuscular disorders. Eur Respir J 2002;20:480–7.
51. Smith P, Edwards R, Calverley P. Oxygen treatment of sleep hypoxaemia in Duchenne muscular dystrophy. Thorax 1989;44:997–1001.
52. Martin R, Sufit R, Ringel S, et al. Respiratory improvement by muscle training in adult-onset acid maltase deficiency. Muscle Nerve 1983;6:201–3.
53. Tandberg E, Larsen J, Karlsen K. A community-based study of sleep disorders in patients with Parkinson's disease. Mov Disord 1998;13:895–9.
54. Tan E, Lum S, Fook-Chong S, et al. Evaluation of somnolence in Parkinson's disease: comparison with age-and sex-matched controls. Neurology 2002;58: 465–8.
55. Ghorayeb I, Loundou A, Auquier P, et al. A nationwide survey of excessive daytime sleepiness in Parkinson's disease in France. Mov Disord 2007;22: 1567–72.
56. Scaglione C, Vignatelli L, Plazzi G, et al. REM sleep behaviour disorder in Parkinson's disease: a questionnaire-based study. Neurol Sci 2005;25:316–21.
57. De Cock V, Vidailhet M, Leu S, et al. Restoration of normal motor control in Parkinson's disease during REM sleep. Brain 2007;130:450–6.
58. Ondo W, Vuong K, Jankovic J. Exploring the relationship between Parkinson disease and restless legs syndrome. Arch Neurol 2002;59:421–4.
59. Nomura T, Inoue Y, Miyake M, et al. Prevalence and clinical characteristics of restless legs syndrome in Japanese patients with Parkinson's disease. Mov Disord 2006;21:380–4.
60. Arnulf I, Konofal E, Merino-Andreu M, et al. Parkinson's disease and sleepiness: an integral part of PD. Neurology 2002;58:1019–24.
61. Boeve B, Silber M, Saper C, et al. Pathophysiology of REM sleep behaviour disorder and relevance to neurodegenerative disease. Brain 2007;130: 2770–88.
62. Frauscher B, Iranzo A, Högl B, et al. Quantification of electromyographic activity during REM sleep in multiple muscles in REM sleep behavior disorder. Sleep 2008;31:724–31.
63. Iranzo A, Santamaria J. Severe obstructive sleep apnea/hypopnea mimicking REM sleep behavior disorder. Sleep 2005;28:203–6.
64. Aurora R, Zak R, Maganti R, et al. Best practice guide for the treatment of REM sleep behavior disorder (RBD). J Clin Sleep Med 2010;6:85–95.
65. Ondo W, Vuong K, Khan H, et al. Daytime sleepiness and other sleep disorders in Parkinson's disease. Neurology 2001;57:1392–6.
66. Hobson D, Lang A, Martin W, et al. Excessive daytime sleepiness and sudden-onset sleep in Parkinson disease: a survey by the Canadian Movement Disorders Group. JAMA 2002;287:455–63.

67. Razmy A, Lang A, Shapiro C. Predictors of impaired daytime sleep and wakefulness in patients with Parkinson disease treated with older (ergot) vs newer (nonergot) dopamine agonists. Arch Neurol 2004;61:97–102.
68. Rye D, Bliwise D, Dihenia B, et al. Daytime sleepiness in Parkinson's disease. J Sleep Res 2000;9:63–9.
69. Frucht S, Rogers J, Greene P, et al. Falling asleep at the wheel: motor vehicle mishaps in persons taking pramipexole and ropinirole. Neurology 1999;52: 1908–10.
70. Körner Y, Meindorfner C, Möller J, et al. Predictors of sudden onset of sleep in Parkinson's disease. Mov Disord 2004;19:1298–305.
71. Merino-Andreu M, Arnulf I, Konofal E, et al. Unawareness of naps in Parkinson's disease and in disorders with excessive daytime sleepiness. Neurology 2003; 60:1553–4.
72. Ondo W, Fayle R, Atassi F. Modafinil for daytime somnolence in Parkinson's disease: double blind, placebo controlled parallel trial. J Neurol Neurosurg Psychiatry 2005;76:1636–9.
73. Vetrugno R, Provini F, Cortelli P, et al. Sleep disorders in multiple system atrophy: a correlative video-polysomnographic study. Sleep Med 2004;5:21–30.
74. Iranzo A, Santamaria J, Tolosa E. Continuous positive air pressure eliminates nocturnal stridor in multiple system atrophy. Barcelona Multiple System Atrophy Study Group. Lancet 2000;356:1329–30.
75. Tachibana N, Howard R, Hirsch N, et al. Sleep problems in multiple sclerosis. Eur Neurol 1994;34:320–3.
76. Bamer A, Johnson K, Amtmann D, et al. Prevalence of sleep problems in individuals with multiple sclerosis. Mult Scler 2008;14:1127–30.
77. Krupp L. Fatigue is intrinsic to multiple sclerosis (MS) and is the most commonly reported symptom of the disease. Mult Scler 2006;12:367–8.
78. Bakshi R. Fatigue associated with multiple sclerosis: diagnosis, impact and management. Mult Scler 2003;9:219–27.
79. Clark C, Fleming J, Li D, et al. Sleep disturbance, depression, and lesion site in patients with multiple sclerosis. Arch Neurol 1992;49:641–3.
80. Caminero A, Bartolomé M. Sleep disturbances in multiple sclerosis. J Neurol Sci 2011;309:86–91.
81. Li Y, Munger K, Batool-Anwar S, et al. Association of multiple sclerosis with restless legs syndrome and other sleep disorders in women. Neurology 2012;78: 1500–6.
82. Italian REMS Study Group, Manconi M, Ferini-Strambi L, Filippi M, et al. Multicenter case-control study on restless legs syndrome in multiple sclerosis: the REMS study. Sleep 2008;31:944–52.
83. Littleton E, Hobart J, Palace J. Modafinil for multiple sclerosis fatigue: does it work? Clin Neurol Neurosurg 2010;112:29–31.
84. Stankoff B, Waubant E, Confavreux C, et al. Modafinil for fatigue in MS: a randomized placebo-controlled double-blind study. Neurology 2005;64: 1139–43.
85. Pucci E, Branãs P, D'Amico R, et al. Amantadine for fatigue in multiple sclerosis. Cochrane Database Syst Rev 2007;(1):CD002818.
86. Redline S. Sleep-related breathing disorders in the elderly. Sleep Med Clin 2006;1:247–62.
87. Young T, Shahar E, Nieto F, et al. Predictors of sleep-disordered breathing in community-dwelling adults: the Sleep Heart Health Study. Arch Intern Med 2002;162:893–900.

88. Zhan G, Serrano F, Fenik P, et al. NADPH oxidase mediates hypersomnolence and brain oxidative injury in a murine model of sleep apnea. Am J Respir Crit Care Med 2005;172:921–9.

89. Macey P, Kumar R, Woo M, et al. Brain structural changes in obstructive sleep apnea. Sleep 2008;31:967–77.

90. Yaffe K, Laffan A, Harrison S, et al. Sleep-disordered breathing, hypoxia, and risk of mild cognitive impairment and dementia in older women. JAMA 2011; 306:613–9.

91. Ancoli-Israel S, Palmer B, Cooke J, et al. Cognitive effects of treating obstructive sleep apnea in Alzheimer's disease: a randomized controlled study. J Am Geriatr Soc 2008;56:2076–81.

92. Cooke J, Ancoli-Israel S, Liu L, et al. Continuous positive airway pressure deepens sleep in patients with Alzheimer's disease and obstructive sleep apnea. Sleep Med 2009;10:1101–6.

93. Cooke J, Ayalon L, Palmer BW, et al. Sustained use of CPAP slows deterioration of cognition, sleep, and mood in patients with Alzheimer's disease and obstructive sleep apnea: a preliminary study. J Clin Sleep Med 2009;5:305–9.

94. Montagna P. Fatal familial insomnia: a model disease in sleep physiopathology. Sleep Med Rev 2005;9:339–53.

95. Boeve BF. Update on the diagnosis and management of sleep disturbances in dementia. Sleep Med Clin 2008;3:347–60.

96. Benca R, Obermeyer W, Thisted R, et al. Sleep and psychiatric disorders: a meta-analysis. Arch Gen Psychiatry 1992;49:651–8.

97. Trivedi M, Rush A, Armitage R, et al. Effects of fluoxetine on the polysomnogram in outpatients with major depression. Neuropsychopharmacology 1999;20: 447–59.

98. Peppard P, Szklo-Coxe M, Hla K, et al. Longitudinal association of sleep-related breathing disorder and depression. Arch Intern Med 2006;166:1709–15.

99. Wells R, Freedland K, Carney R, et al. Adherence, reports of benefits, and depression among patients treated with continuous positive airway pressure. Psychosom Med 2007;69:449–54.

100. Kobayashi I, Boarts J, Delahanty D. Polysomnographically measured sleep abnormalities in PTSD: a meta-analytic review. Psychophysiology 2007;44: 660–9.

101. Krakow B, Melendrez D, Johnston L, et al. Sleep-disordered breathing, psychiatric distress, and quality of life impairment in sexual assault survivors. J Nerv Ment Dis 2002;190:442–52.

102. Engdahl B, Eberly R, Hurwitz T, et al. Sleep in a community sample of elderly war veterans with and without posttraumatic stress disorder. Biol Psychiatry 2000; 47:520–5.

103. Ohayon M, Shapiro C. Sleep disturbances and psychiatric disorders associated with posttraumatic stress disorder in the general population. Compr Psychiatry 2000;41:469–78.

104. Mellman T, Kulick-Bell R, Ashlock L, et al. Sleep events among veterans with combat-related posttraumatic stress disorder. Am J Psychiatry 1995;152: 110–5.

105. Krakow B, Germain A, Tandberg D, et al. Sleep breathing and sleep movement disorders masquerading as insomnia in sexual-assault survivors. Compr Psychiatry 2000;41:49–56.

106. Brown T, Boudewyns P. Periodic limb movements of sleep in combat veterans with posttraumatic stress disorder. J Trauma Stress 1996;9:129–36.

107. Raskind M, Peskind E, Kanter E, et al. Reduction of nightmares and other PTSD symptoms in combat veterans by prazosin: a placebo-controlled study. Am J Psychiatry 2003;160:371–3.
108. Taylor FB, Martin P, Thompson C, et al. Prazosin effects on objective sleep measures and clinical symptoms in civilian trauma posttraumatic stress disorder: a placebo-controlled study. Biol Psychiatry 2008;63:629–32.
109. Dierks M, Jordan J, Sheehan A. Prazosin treatment of nightmares related to posttraumatic stress disorder. Ann Pharmacother 2007;41:1013–7.
110. Byers M, Allison K, Wendel C, et al. Prazosin versus quetiapine for nighttime posttraumatic stress disorder symptoms in veterans: an assessment of long-term comparative effectiveness and safety. J Clin Psychopharmacol 2010;30: 225–9.
111. Morin C, Vallières A, Guay B, et al. Cognitive behavioral therapy, singly and combined with medication, for persistent insomnia: a randomized controlled trial. JAMA 2009;301:2005–15.
112. Kripke D, Langer R, Kline L. Hypnotics' association with mortality or cancer: a matched cohort study. BMJ Open 2012;2(1):e000850.
113. Wilson S, Argyropoulos S. Antidepressants and sleep: a qualitative review of the literature. Drugs 2005;65:927–47.
114. Guilleminault C, Davis K, Huynh N. Prospective randomized study of patients with insomnia and mild sleep disordered breathing. Sleep 2008;31:1527–33.
115. Luyster F, Buysse D, Strollo P. Comorbid insomnia and obstructive sleep apnea: challenges for clinical practice and research. J Clin Sleep Med 2010;6:196–204.
116. Krakow B, Ulibarri V, Romero E. Persistent insomnia in chronic hypnotic users presenting to a sleep medical center: a retrospective chart review of 137 consecutive patients. J Nerv Ment Dis 2010;198:734–41.
117. Schutte-Rodin S, Broch L, Buysse D, et al. Clinical guideline for the evaluation and management of chronic insomnia in adults. J Clin Sleep Med 2008;4: 487–504.
118. Headache Classification Subcommittee of the International Headache Society. The international classification of headache disorders. 2nd edition. Cephalalgia; 2004;24(suppl 1):9–160.
119. Goksan B, Gunduz A, Karadeniz D, et al. Morning headache in sleep apnoea: clinical and polysomnographic evaluation and response to nasal continuous positive airway pressure. Cephalalgia 2009;29:635–41.
120. Provini F, Vetrugno R, Lugaresi E, et al. Sleep-related breathing disorders and headache. Neurol Sci 2006;27(Suppl 2):S149–52.
121. Terzaghi M, Ghiotto N, Sances G, et al. Episodic cluster headache: NREM prevalence of nocturnal attacks. Time to look beyond macrostructural analysis? Headache 2010;50:1050–4.
122. Foldvary-Schaefer N, Grigg-Damberger M. Sleep and epilepsy. Semin Neurol 2009;29:419–28.
123. Ochi A, Hung R, Weiss S, et al. Lateralized interictal epileptiform discharges during rapid eye movement sleep correlate with epileptogenic hemisphere in children with intractable epilepsy secondary to tuberous sclerosis complex. Epilepsia 2011;52:1986–94.
124. Vendrame M, Auerbach S, Loddenkemper T, et al. Effect of continuous positive airway pressure treatment on seizure control in patients with obstructive sleep apnea and epilepsy. Epilepsia 2011;52:e168–71.
125. Malow B, Foldvary-Schaefer N, Vaughn B, et al. Treating obstructive sleep apnea in adults with epilepsy: a randomized pilot trial. Neurology 2008;71:572–7.

126. Devinsky O, Ehrenberg B, Barthlen G, et al. Epilepsy and sleep apnea syndrome. Neurology 1994;44:2060–4.
127. Vaughn B, D'Cruz O, Beach R. Improvement of epileptic seizure control with treatment of obstructive sleep apnoea. Seizure 1996;5:73–8.
128. Joncas S, Zadra A, Paquet J, et al. The value of sleep deprivation as a diagnostic tool in adult sleepwalkers. Neurology 2002;58:936–40.

Sleep Disorders

Hypersomnias of Central Origin

Shelby F. Harris, PsyD*, Renee S. Monderer, MD,
Michael Thorpy, MD

KEYWORDS

- Narcolepsy • Cataplexy • Sleep paralysis • Idiopathic hypersomnia
- Kleine-Levin syndrome • Menstrual-related hypersomnia • Recurrent hypersomnias
- Excessive daytime sleepiness

KEY POINTS

- Many patients report symptoms of hypersomnia, yet clear diagnostic and treatment methods are often poorly understood and addressed by treatment providers. Excessive daytime sleepiness (EDS) has many implications, including increased risk of injury at work or home, car accidents, decreased alertness, and lower productivity overall. EDS may also lead to heightened psychological stress with family, friends, and coworkers. Hypersomnia is commonly divided into two categories depending on the origin of the symptomatology; primary or secondary. Narcolepsy is often misdiagnosed at the outset, with many patients waiting nearly 15 years for a proper diagnosis and treatment plan. This review paper will focus on primary hypersomnia of central origin, with a brief discussion of diagnostic criteria, pathophysiology, differential diagnoses, and pharmacological and behavioral treatment. For many patients, a combination of both pharmacological and behavioral methods are necessary, requiring the practitioner to have a thorough understanding of the intricacies of the case presentation and overall goals for the patient. We also present a case study to highlight our key diagnostic and treatment points.

INTRODUCTION

Many patients report symptoms of hypersomnia, yet clear diagnostic and treatment methods are often poorly understood and addressed by treatment providers (**Fig. 1**). Excessive daytime sleepiness (EDS) has many implications, including increased risk of injury at work or home, car accidents, decreased alertness, and lower productivity overall. EDS may also lead to heightened psychological stress with family, friends, and coworkers. Hypersomnia is commonly divided into 2 categories, primary or secondary, depending on the origin of the symptomatology. This review focuses on primary hypersomnia of central origin, with a brief discussion of diagnostic criteria, pathophysiology, differential diagnoses, and pharmacologic and behavioral treatment. A case study is also presented to highlight key diagnostic and treatment points.

Disclosure: Michael Thorpy, MD is a consultant for Teva Pharmaceuticals and Jazz Pharmaceuticals.
Sleep-Wake Disorders Center, Montefiore Medical Center, 111 East 210th Street, Bronx, NY 10467, USA
* Corresponding author.
E-mail address: slharris@montefiore.org

Neurol Clin 30 (2012) 1027–1044
http://dx.doi.org/10.1016/j.ncl.2012.08.002
0733-8619/12/$ – see front matter © 2012 Elsevier Inc. All rights reserved.

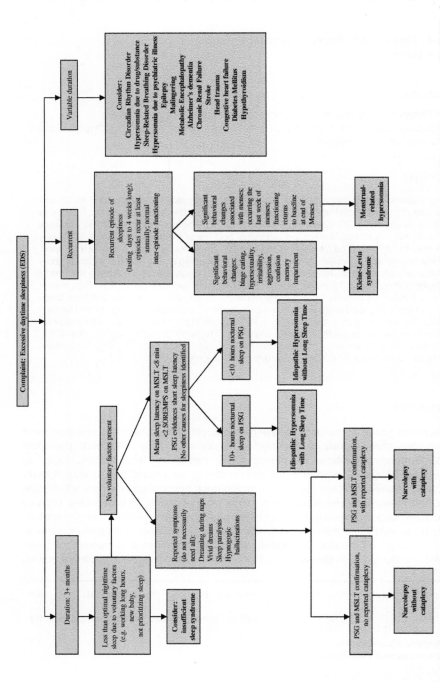

Fig. 1. Diagnostic algorithm for complaint of excessive daytime sleepiness. MSLT, multiple sleep latency test; PSG, polysomnogram; SOREMPS, sleep-onset rapid-eye-movement periods.

NARCOLEPSY

Narcolepsy is a disorder of EDS that is usually associated with cataplexy and other rapid eye movement (REM) phenomena such as sleep paralysis and hypnagogic hallucinations. Sleep regulation and wakefulness are disturbed with rapid transitions between wakefulness and REM sleep, resulting in fragmented sleep and EDS. Narcolepsy occurs with and without cataplexy. Cataplexy is defined as a sudden loss of muscle tone associated with strong emotions.

Epidemiology

The estimated prevalence of narcolepsy is 0.02% to 0.18%. It is slightly more common in Japan, with an estimate of 0.16% to 0.18%, and less common in Israel, with a prevalence as low as 0.002%.[1–5] Men and women are equally affected. Onset can occur at any age, but it most commonly starts in the second decade of life with a second peak seen around 35 years of age.[6] There is often a prolonged latency of about 10 years from the time of symptom onset to diagnosis; however, this latency has become shorter as disease awareness has grown.

Narcolepsy is generally considered a sporadic disease, with only 1% to 4% of cases running in families in an autosomal dominant fashion.[7] Studies of sporadic cases demonstrate the risk to first-degree relatives is 1% to 2%.[8] Studies on monozygotic twins showed a concordance rate of only 25% to 31%, demonstrating that environmental factors contribute significantly.[9]

Clinical Features

Excessive daytime sleepiness

EDS is present in all patients with narcolepsy. This syndrome is usually the first and most disabling feature. It is characterized by a constant background of baseline sleepiness along with lapses into sleep throughout the day. Short naps tend to be refreshing, which is characteristic of narcolepsy; however, within a few hours sleepiness returns. Sleep attacks, defined as sudden onset of sleep or irresistible sleep episodes, can occur throughout the day. Activities that are passive increase the likelihood that sleep will occur. Intense physical or mental activities usually decrease sleepiness; however, in severe cases sleep attacks can occur during activities such as talking, standing up, eating, or driving, which can increase the risk of automobile, home, or industrial accidents.

Sleepiness can present in the form of automatic behaviors, during which the patient performs activities but is unable to recall the event. For example, a patient can drive to a location without remembering the process of getting there. These lapses may account for frequent complaints of memory difficulties in narcolepsy.

Cataplexy

Cataplexy, the sudden loss of bilateral muscle tone elicited by emotions, is pathognomonic for narcolepsy. Emotions that elicit cataplexy usually are positive, such as laughter, excitement, or joy, and less likely negative, such as anger or frustration. Cataplexy can involve nearly all striated muscles or more commonly is localized to certain muscle groups. Notable muscles that are spared include intrinsic eye and ear muscles, and respiratory muscles. During an attack, muscle control can be lost in the knees, face, or neck. Patients often describe knee buckling that can lead to falls, head dropping, facial twitching, jaw dropping, or weakness of the arms. Attacks typically take several seconds to reach full effect, and most patients are able to sit down to prevent a fall. Neurologic examination during a cataplectic attack is notable for loss of reflexes and hypotonia. Occasionally the attacks are accompanied with rhythmic jerking of the facial and neck muscles, and may be mistaken for an epileptic seizure.

The frequency and duration of cataplectic attacks vary dramatically. Episodes can occur once a year to multiple times per day. Most attacks last less than 10 seconds, although, when attacks occur repeatedly, such as when an emotional trigger persists, one may interpret the attacks as a single event. Partial attacks are usually shorter than those that involve all striated muscles. To circumvent attacks, patients may avoid emotional situations, such as social events or other emotionally charged occurrences, ultimately decreasing their quality of life.

Rarely when strong emotional triggers are present, patients can experience multiple episodes in succession that last minutes to hours. Termed *status cataplecticus*, these episodes can be completely disabling and are mostly seen when medication is withdrawn.

Cataplexy usually begins soon after symptoms of daytime sleepiness begin, but it can present months to years later. Patients may be diagnosed with narcolepsy without cataplexy and then later realize that cataplexy is present. Cataplexy tends to improve with advancing age.[10,11]

Sleep paralysis

Sleep paralysis is a transient state of involuntary immobility occurring in transitions between REM sleep and waking. Patients are unable to make gross body movements or speak, but the eyes are open and awareness of surroundings is preserved. Episodes may last a few minutes and remit spontaneously or when interrupted by noise or other external stimuli. Sleep paralysis can be extremely frightening, especially when first experienced. Patients may experience a sensation of difficulty breathing during these episodes and think they are going to die. Often sleep paralysis is accompanied by hypnogogic hallucinations.

About 20% to 50% of narcolepsy patients experience sleep paralysis, but it can occur in the general population and so is not specific to narcolepsy.[12] Episodes generally occur at sleep onset or in the first 2 hours of sleep, but they can occur 6 to 7 hours later or on awakening during later REM transition periods. Events must occur frequently for treatment to be considered.

Hypnogogic hallucinations

Hypnogogic hallucinations are vivid visual, auditory, tactile, or even kinetic perceptions which, like sleep paralysis, occur during the transitions between waking and REM sleep. Typically these hallucinations are unpleasant and accompanied by fear. Examples include a sensation of impending threat, feelings of suffocation, sensations of floating, spinning, or falling, brief sounds, or sudden visual images. Polysomnographic studies show that these hallucinations often occur during REM sleep.

Hypnogogic hallucinations recur in 40% to 80% of patients with narcolepsy with cataplexy. These events are not specific for narcolepsy, as they can occur in the general population in the setting of sleep fragmentation. Hypnogogic hallucinations are easy to distinguish from hallucinations occurring in psychiatric disorders because narcolepsy patients recognize the events as not being real. The timing of events during transitions from waking and sleep also distinguishes them, as hallucinations in psychiatric disorders occur at any time of day.

Fragmented nighttime sleep

Because narcolepsy is a disorder of EDS, this symptom of disturbed nighttime sleep is often overlooked. Narcolepsy patients typically fall asleep quickly, but have difficulty maintaining nighttime sleep. Frequent arousals are often reported with difficulty of falling back to sleep. The total amount of sleep in a 24-hour period is the same as for normal individuals; however, it is distributed throughout the day and night, causing daytime sleep attacks and a fragmented nighttime sleep.[12]

Associated symptoms

Difficulties with memory and concentration are reported in 40% to 50% of narcolepsy patients,[13,14] most likely secondary to a persistent level of sleepiness, sleep attacks, and automatic behaviors.

REM sleep behavior disorder occurs more frequently in narcolepsy with cataplexy (12%–36%) than is typically seen in the general population in the same age group.[15] Patients may report dream-enactment behavior or polysomnography may show REM sleep without atonia. The high prevalence is thought to be secondary to (1) sleep state instability seen in narcolepsy, (2) antidepressants used for cataplexy, or (3) both. Another sleep-associated feature seen is periodic limb movements, but this is likely an isolated polysomnographic finding with little clinical impact. Other REM and non-REM parasomnias, such as sleep talking and sleepwalking, are also more prevalent in this population.

Another related finding in patients with narcolepsy with cataplexy is high body mass index (BMI) or obesity. Initially this was thought to be secondary to inactivity and sleepiness. Another hypothesis focuses on the deficiency of hypocretin/orexin in narcolepsy patients with cataplexy leading to secondary metabolic changes, thus increasing weight.[16]

A high BMI may also predispose patients to develop obstructive sleep apnea. About 25% of narcolepsy patients have this condition.[17] Obstructive sleep apnea is an important comorbidity, as it can significantly worsen daytime sleepiness and is treatable.

The prevalence of depression is reported to be higher in narcolepsy patients (5%–30%) than in the general population.[18] However, this may be a difficult diagnosis to make in narcolepsy because of overlapping symptoms such as lack of energy and daytime sleepiness. This difficulty in diagnosing depression in the presence of narcolepsy accounts for the large variation in the reported prevalence.

Diagnosis

The diagnosis of narcolepsy with cataplexy can be made based on a clear history of EDS and cataplexy along with, whenever possible, either a supportive sleep study or hypocretin-1 levels in the cerebrospinal fluid (CSF) of less than or equal to 110 pg/mL. The sleep study should include nocturnal polysomnography followed by a multiple sleep latency test (MSLT). According to the *International Classification of Sleep Disorders*, second edition (ICSD-2),[19] this sleepiness cannot be better explained by another sleep disorder, medical, psychiatric, or neurologic disorder, or medication or substance use (**Box 1**). The sleep studies assess the severity of sleepiness and rule out other sleep disorders. The diagnosis of narcolepsy without cataplexy can be more difficult to make, and requires a polysomnogram followed by an MSLT.

In narcolepsy (with and without cataplexy), nocturnal polysomnography demonstrates a shortened REM latency in about 50% of patients. The sleep efficiency is often reduced with frequent awakenings and an increased amount of stage N1 sleep, owing to the disturbed nighttime sleep that is often seen in narcolepsy. According to the ICSD-2 criteria, the MSLT should show a mean sleep latency of 8 minutes or less along with 2 or more sleep-onset REM periods (SOREMPs) in the setting of sufficient nocturnal sleep.

A very specific and sensitive way to make the diagnosis is by measuring the CSF hypocretin-1 level, which has been shown to be less than 110 pg/mL in 90% of patients with narcolepsy accompanied by cataplexy.[20] Because a spinal tap is an invasive test, it is typically only used when the MSLT is difficult to interpret, such as

---

Box 1
Differential diagnosis of EDS

Primary Causes

Sleep apnea

Behaviorally induced insufficient sleep time

Narcolepsy with/without cataplexy

Idiopathic hypersomnia

Recurrent hypersomnia (Kleine-Levin syndrome)

Circadian rhythm disorder, shift work disorder

Long sleeper

Secondary Causes

Metabolic encephalopathy

Drug intoxication/withdrawal

Depression

Epilepsy

Hypothyroidism

Diabetes mellitus

Congestive heart failure

Brain tumor

Head trauma

Stroke

Alzheimer dementia

Chronic renal failure

Malingering

---

when patients are on psychoactive drugs or have concurrent sleep disorders. However, CSF hypocretin levels are not readily available and levels are usually only used for research purposes. Low CSF hypocretin-1 levels are seen in just 10% of patients with narcolepsy without cataplexy.[19]

Human leukocyte antigen (HLA) testing can be done in addition to clinical and polysomnographic testing, but is not specific for narcolepsy. Approximately 85% of patients with narcolepsy with cataplexy will be positive for the HLA-DQB1*0602 (and DR2 or DRB1*1501 in Caucasian and Asians), and approximately 40% of patients with narcolepsy without cataplexy will be positive. About 26% of the general population is positive for HLA-DQB1*0602.

Pathophysiology

Hypocretin

The hypocretin system is an excitatory system that is important for sleep-wake regulation. Hypocretin, also known as orexin, is a peptide that was discovered in 1998 by 2 independent research groups, which explains why the peptide is identified by 2 different names.[21,22] In a small number of neurons located in the dorsolateral hypothalamus, the precursor prehypocretin is cleaved to generate the 2 active peptides. The hypocretin-producing neurons project throughout the neuroaxis, including the olfactory bulb, cerebral cortex, thalamus, and hypothalamus, and to cholinergic and monoaminergic sites in the brainstem.[23]

Loss of hypocretin-producing neurons is associated with human narcolepsy with cataplexy.[24,25] Approximately 50,000 to 100,000 hypocretin-containing neurons are lost. Although no definitive studies have been performed, many researchers believe symptoms of narcolepsy begin when the majority of hypocretin cells have degenerated and that the symptoms increase in severity as more cells disappear.[26]

Sleep-wake regulation

The ascending arousal system (AAS) is composed of the cholinergic branch and the monoaminergic branch. The cholinergic branch includes the pedunculopontine tegmental and laterodorsal tegmental nuclei, which project to the thalamic reticular nucleus. During wakefulness and REM sleep, these neurons activate the thalamus to relay sensory signals to the cerebral cortex. The monoaminergic branch includes the locus coeruleus, dorsal and median raphe nuclei, tuberomammillary nuclei, and ventral periaqueductal gray matter, and also projects the cerebral cortex to prepare the cortex to receive input. While awake, both the cholinergic and monoaminergic branches are active and augmented by the hypocretin neurons in the lateral hypothalamus.

These systems are inhibited by the ventrolateral preoptic nucleus (VLPO) during sleep. The phase of the biological clock and duration of wakefulness determine the activity of the VLPO. In non-REM sleep the VLPO inhibits both the cholinergic and monoaminergic branches of the AAS, whereas in REM sleep only the monoaminergic nuclei are inhibited but the cholinergic nuclei are active.

The monoaminergic nuclei also inhibit the VLPO during wakefulness, resulting in a system of reciprocal inhibition. This system has been termed the sleep switch, and functions as a flip-flop switch.[27,28] Both sides of the switch strongly inhibit each other, resulting in a feedback loop with only 2 possible states, sleep and wake. This system prevents intermediate states with quick transitions. Hypocretin is the stabilizer of this switch. In wakefulness, hypocretin reinforces the arousal system to avert unwanted switches into sleep.

The symptoms of narcolepsy can be explained by this "loss of state boundary control,"[29] which is lost in the state of hypocretin deficiency. Wakefulness cannot be maintained for long periods without patients falling asleep. Similarly, cataplexy and sleep paralysis are considered REM phenomena occurring during wakefulness, manifested as expressions of atonia of REM sleep. Hypnogogic hallucinations are the intrusion of dream imagery into wakefulness. In this manner, all of the symptoms of narcolepsy can be explained as a loss of boundary between waking and sleeping.

Autoimmune hypothesis

The strong link between narcolepsy and HLA typing suggests that narcolepsy may be an autoimmune disease. The hypocretin-producing cells have been proposed as a potential target, but no autoantibodies directed at hypocretin-producing cells or hypocretin receptors have been detected.[30] Studies have shown higher levels of anti-streptolysin O and anti-DNAse antibodies in narcolepsy patients in comparison with controls[31,32]; however, there is minimal evidence for an inflammatory process or immune abnormalities in narcolepsy.[33] Case reports have shown that administering intravenous immunoglobulins within a year of onset may reduce the severity of the disease.[34] Another study identifies tribbles homologue 2 (trib2) colocalized with hypocretin-producing cells as a possible autoantigen. Antibodies against trib2 have been detected in higher concentration and higher percentages in narcolepsy patients than in controls.[35] Further research is needed to confirm if narcolepsy is indeed an auto-immune disease.

Pharmacologic Treatments

At present there is no cure or disease-modifying medications for narcolepsy. The goals of treatment are to improve quality of life, EDS, and cataplexy, as well as other REM phenomena. A variety of medications (**Table 1**) can be used to treat these symptoms. Most drugs improve either daytime sleepiness or cataplexy, so often a combination is needed. The only medication that is helpful for both major symptoms is sodium oxybate. It is important to set reasonable expectations for treatment because baseline sleepiness often persists, albeit usually improved, despite treatment.

Treatment of excessive daytime sleepiness

In the past, amphetamines were the main treatment used for EDS. Dextroamphetamine, methamphetamine, and combinations of amphetamine salts (Adderall) are effective in significantly improving daytime alertness; however, side effects often limit their use. Prominent side effects include irritability, headaches, mood changes, decreased appetite, increased blood pressure, and irregular heart beat. Amphetamines (especially methamphetamine) also have a high potential for abuse because of the tolerance and dependence that can develop. Methylphenidate causes fewer side effects overall, but the potential for abuse is still present.

Nowadays modafinil and armodafinil are more commonly used to treat daytime sleepiness. Each is an effective wake-promoting agent with good safety and tolerability measures and low abuse potential. Armodafinil is the R-enantiomer of modafinil, has a longer half-life, and only needs to be given once a day as opposed to modafinil, which is often given twice daily. The most common side effects reported with both modafinil and armodafinil are headaches and nausea. These symptoms are usually mild and resolve after 2 to 4 weeks of use. Of note, women of childbearing age on oral contraceptives should use alternative contraception when taking modafinil or armodafinil, as the metabolism of ethinylestradiol may be increased.

The exact mechanism of action of these medications is unclear. There is evidence that modafinil and armodafinil act through modulation of various neurotransmitters including dopamine, norepinephrine, histamine, glutamate, hypocretin, and serotonin. The wake-promoting effects of these medications may be linked to the stimulation of dopamine release and inhibition of dopamine reuptake.[36,37]

Treatment of cataplexy

Most studies have focused on treatment of cataplexy; however, improvement of cataplexy is usually associated with amelioration of other REM phenomena such as sleep paralysis and hypnogogic hallucinations. Tricyclic antidepressants were initially the most frequently used treatment for cataplexy prior to the development of sodium oxybate. Medications such as protriptyline and clomipramine can be effective in significantly reducing the frequency of cataplectic events; however, side effects can be limiting. Adverse effects such as dry mouth, anorexia, sweating, urinary retention, constipation, impotence, and decreased blood pressure have been reported. Selective serotonin reuptake inhibitors and monoamine oxidase inhibitors can be used for cataplexy as well, but are generally less effective options.

Sodium oxybate is effective in reducing cataplexy, and more recently has been shown to improve daytime alertness in narcolepsy.[38] This medication may also reduce other REM phenomena such as sleep paralysis and hypnogogic hallucinations.[39] The active ingredient, γ-hydroxybutyrate, has strong soporific effects and therefore is

Table 1
Medications used for narcolepsy

Drug Name	Adult Dose	Pediatric Dose[a]	Clinical Use	Side Effects
Dextroamphetamine (Dexedrine)	15–60 mg daily	5–40 mg daily	Daytime sleepiness	Irritability, sweating, headaches, tremors
Methylphenidate (Ritalin)	20–60 mg daily in divided doses	5–60 mg daily in divided doses	Daytime sleepiness	Irritability, sweating, headaches, tremors
Modafinil (Provigil)	200–400 mg daily in divided dose	100–200 mg daily	Daytime sleepiness	Headache, nausea
Armodafinil (Nuvigil)	150–250 mg daily once a day	150 mg daily	Daytime sleepiness	Headache, nausea
Sodium oxybate (Xyrem)	4.5–9 g at night in 2 divided doses	3–9 g at night in 2 divided doses	Cataplexy and daytime sleepiness	Nausea, vomiting, dizziness
Clomipramine (Anafrinil)	25–100 mg daily	25–100 mg daily	Cataplexy	Dry mouth, urinary retention, sweating
Protriptyline (Vivactil)	15–60 mg daily in 3 divided doses	15 mg daily in 3 divided doses	Cataplexy	Dry mouth, urinary retention, sweating
Paroxetine (Paxil)	10–60 mg daily	10–60 mg daily	Cataplexy	Sedation, insomnia, irritability
Phenelzine (Nardil)	15–60 mg daily in divided doses		Cataplexy	Impotence, weight gain, hypertension

[a] There is no medication approved by the Food and Drug Administration to treat narcolepsy or cataplexy in children.

given at night. The mechanism of action of sodium oxybate in narcolepsy is unclear. It appears to have strong effects on dopamine transmission by increasing firing rate and brain content of dopamine.[40] Other neurotransmitters that are affected include opioids, glutamate, γ-aminobutyric acid, and acetylcholine.

Sodium oxybate is generally well tolerated. Because of its sedative properties and short half-life, it is usually given in 2 doses at sleep onset and 2 to 4 hours later. Common side effects include nausea, vomiting, dizziness, and nocturnal enuresis. Because of its strong sedative properties, it should not be taken in conjunction with alcohol or other sedatives to avoid the risk of central nervous system or respiratory depression. Patients and physicians alike are often hesitant to use this medication because of concerns for misuse and abuse; however, data to date show that sodium oxybate is safe and has low risk for dependence or tolerance.[41]

Treatment of fragmented nighttime sleep
Narcolepsy patients wake up frequently at night. Sodium oxybate increases slow-wave sleep and allows patients to sleep more continuously through the night. Alternatively, benzodiazepines or newer nonbenzodiazepines such as zolpidem have been used to consolidate nighttime sleep, but little research has been done in this area.[42]

Future treatments
New treatments to improve the daytime symptoms of narcolepsy are currently being investigated, including histamine-modulating agents and hypocretin agonists. In addition, therapies to potentially modify the disease process are focusing on immunomodulating agents such as intravenous immunoglobulins given close to disease onset. Cell transplantation and gene therapy are potential therapies that may be available in the future.

Nonpharmacologic Treatments

Although little empiric research exists on the use of behavioral management with patients diagnosed with narcolepsy, anecdotally these strategies can make a significant impact on their daily functioning. Scheduling naps, optimizing work periods during times of maximal alertness, strategic caffeine use, following basic sleep hygiene and stimulus control, and knowing limitations can all benefit the patient.[43,44] Education and counseling are paramount in the treatment of narcolepsy, both for the patient and his or her family, friends, and colleagues. The patient should be advised against driving, bathing, swimming, and using any heavy machinery or household appliances during times of sleepiness.

Napping, obtaining sufficient nighttime sleep, and avoiding sugars may help to reduce EDS.[45,46] Many patients report that managing stressful situations are helpful in reducing cataplectic events. Although not formally evaluated, techniques such as planning, worry reduction, counseling, progressive muscle relaxation, and breathing exercises may help reduce and prevent stress and thereby decrease cataplexy. These skills can prove to be more productive than avoiding emotional situations altogether.

Psychotherapeutic strategies for the management of depression, anxiety, and any other psychological issues are recommended. Future research is necessary to fully examine the effectiveness of these strategies.

IDIOPATHIC HYPERSOMNIA
Symptoms

First characterized by Bedrich Roth at the end of the 1950s,[47] idiopathic hypersomnia is generally less common than narcolepsy, is a disorder that is poorly understood, and often has a diagnosis of exclusion when other causes of EDS are ruled out.[19]

Few prevalence studies of idiopathic hypersomnia exist because of the difficulty in making a diagnosis of idiopathic hypersomnia. Symptoms usually start in teenagers or young adults. Some have reported idiopathic hypersomnia to have a female predominance, although it is generally seen equally in both males and females.[48] Although definitive prevalence rates are still unknown owing to limited research on idiopathic hypersomnia overall, narcolepsy appears to be more common than idiopathic hypersomnia, with some suggesting a 10:1[48] ratio and others reporting a 2:1 ratio.[49] This wide variation in narcolepsy-to-idiopathic hypersomnia ratio is likely due to different diagnostic standards between studies.

The primary symptom of idiopathic hypersomnia is EDS, despite a full night of sleep and normal sleep architecture. The current definition of idiopathic hypersomnia is broken up into idiopathic hypersomnia with and without long sleep time.[19] Patients with long sleep time sleep for at least 10 hours at night. These patients rarely awaken during nocturnal sleep, have significant difficulty getting up in the morning, and find naps to be unrefreshing. Patients with idiopathic hypersomnia typically report feelings of "sleep drunkenness," that is, trouble achieving full alertness on awakening in the morning after a full night of sleep. Idiopathic hypersomnia without long sleep time describes patients who sleep less than 10 hours at night with EDS, but are far less likely to report sleep drunkenness. **Box 2** lists the ICSD-2 diagnostic criteria of idiopathic hypersomnia with long sleep time. The differential diagnosis of idiopathic hypersomnia is similar to that of narcolepsy.

Pathophysiology

Little is known about the pathophysiology behind idiopathic hypersomnia, with some researchers suggesting that idiopathic hypersomnia may be related to an abnormal

---

Box 2
ICSD-2 criteria for idiopathic hypersomnia with long sleep time

A. The patient has a complaint of EDS occurring almost daily for at least 3 months.

B. The patient has prolonged nocturnal sleep time (more than 10 hours) documented by interview, actigraphy, or sleep logs. Waking up in the morning or at the end of naps is almost always laborious.

C. Nocturnal polysomnography has excluded other causes of daytime sleepiness.

D. The polysomnogram demonstrates a short sleep latency and a major sleep period that is prolonged to more than 10 hours in duration.

E. If an MSLT is performed following overnight polysomnography, a mean sleep latency of less than 8 minutes is found and fewer than 2 SOREMPs are recorded. Mean sleep latency in idiopathic hypersomnia with long sleep time has been shown to be 6.2 ± 3.0 minutes.

Note: A mean sleep latency on the MSLT of less than 8 minutes can be found in up to 30% of the general population. Both the mean sleep latency on the MSLT and the clinician's interpretation of the patient's symptoms, most notably a clinically significant complaint of sleepiness, should be taking into account in reaching the diagnosis of idiopathic hypersomnia with long sleep time.

F. The hypersomnia is not better explained by another sleep disorder, medical or neurologic disorder, mental disorder, medication use, or substance use disorder.

Note: Of particular importance, head trauma should not be considered to be the cause of the sleepiness.

Adapted from American Academy of Sleep Medicine. International classifications of sleep disorders, diagnostic, and coding manual. 2nd edition. Westchester (IL): American Academy of Sleep Medicine; 2005.

homeostatic sleep drive that decreases overall slow-wave sleep in patients. Others have suggested a circadian disorder in the secretion of melatonin.[50,51] CSF hypocretin levels are normal, and researchers have been unable to associate it with the HLA complex.[52]

Treatment

Treatment of idiopathic hypersomnia generally parallels that of EDS in narcolepsy patients (stimulants and wake-promoting agents such as modafinil and armodafinil), although favorable medication response is not as easy to achieve. The effect of sodium oxybate has not been formally studied in idiopathic hypersomnia. Sleep hygiene, proper diet, and strategic use of caffeine can be useful. Planned naps and increasing time in bed have not been found to be helpful.[49]

RECURRENT HYPERSOMNIA

Recurrent hypersomnia is characterized by episodic periods lasting days or weeks during which the patient reports EDS or extremely extended sleep periods (as long as 15–20 hours), waking only to eat and void. Patients report feeling excessively sleepy and have difficulty with alertness even despite long sleep periods. These episodes appear to spontaneously resolve, with the patient returning to normal behavior, cognition, and alertness. The 2 most common forms of recurrent hypersomnia are Kleine-Levin syndrome (KLS) and menstrual-related hypersomnia. **Box 3** lists the ICSD-2 criteria for recurrent hypersomnia.

Kleine-Levin Syndrome

Symptoms and diagnosis

The best-known recurrent hypersomnia, KLS is a rare disorder with an estimated prevalence of 1 to 2 cases per million people. KLS patients are mostly male adolescents with a mean age of onset at 15 years, with some rare cases beginning as early as age 9 years.[53] Rare familial cases have been reported, with Ashkenazi Jews in the United States and Israel evidencing a large number of cases. Although KLS appears to be genetically transmitted and associated with HLA-DRB1*201, no clear link has been demonstrated.

Hypersomnia is the main symptom of KLS, with total sleep time increasing to well over 12 hours per day. Cognitive impairment is also seen, with symptoms of apathy, confusion, slowness, and amnesia being most prominent. Patients typically report

---

Box 3
ICSD-2 diagnostic criteria for recurrent hypersomnia (including Kleine-Levin syndrome and menstrual-related hypersomnia)

A. The patient experiences recurrent episodes of EDS of 2 days to 4 weeks in duration.

B. Episodes recur at least once a year.

C. The patient has normal alertness, cognitive functioning, and behavior between attacks.

D. The hypersomnia is not better explained by another sleep disorder, medical or neurologic disorder, mental disorder, medication use, or substance use disorder.

Adapted from American Academy of Sleep Medicine. International classifications of sleep disorders, diagnostic, and coding manual. 2nd edition. Westchester (IL): American Academy of Sleep Medicine; 2005.

derealization, a feeling of being in a dream-like, altered state outside of oneself. Other symptoms, though not universally reported, include hypersexuality, depressed mood, and hyperphagia. Males tend to report more hypersexuality, with women having more depressed mood. Interepisode functioning typically returns to baseline, with no notable differences from premorbid abilities and a return to typical sleep needs, cognitive functioning, and appetite.[54]

Pathophysiology
In at least 72% of patients, the first episode is triggered by a high fever or infection. Patients experience an average of 7 to 19 episodes of 10 to 13 days each, relapsing an average of every 3.5 months. Disease course is typically 8 to 14 years, with spontaneous remission in adulthood. The course is longer in men with hypersexuality and a later age of onset.[53]

Electroencephalographic (EEG) slowing during episodes has been noted in a majority of cases,[55] with polysomnography evidencing an increase in slow-wave sleep at first with a decrease in REM sleep in the latter half of an episode, frequent awakenings, and increased stage 1 sleep.[56] Neuroimaging with computed tomography (CT) and magnetic resonance imaging (MRI) have typically been normal, but single-photon emission CT has shown some hypoperfusion in the thalamic, hypothalamic, and frontotemporal regions.[57] One case report noted a significant decrease in hypocretin during episodes, with an interepisode return to baseline values.[58] However, this has yet to be replicated.

Differential diagnosis
Medically based differential diagnoses include checking for alcohol, drug use, tumor, multiple sclerosis, stroke, temporal status epilepticus, Lyme disease, and encephalitis. Psychiatric-related differential diagnoses can be difficult to make, with many patients first presenting for psychiatric treatment before investigation for KLS. Typical psychiatric differential diagnoses include depression, psychotic disorders, and bipolar disorder.

Treatment
No standard treatment has been identified for KLS, although starting on amantadine at the beginning of an episode may help shorten or stop an episode. Lithium, lamotrigine, and valproic acid have also been found to be moderately useful.[59,60]

During episodes, stimulants have not been particularly useful against severe hypersomnia. In some cases, use of stimulants may worsen behavioral and cognitive symptoms. If psychotic symptoms become very pronounced, a brief trial of risperidone may be beneficial. Family supervision is key during episodes. Patients should stay at home when experiencing hypersomnia, with family members ensuring the patient eats a proper amount of food and liquids and also does not experience any suicidal ideation. Alcohol and nicotine should be avoided at all times, with the patient keeping a steady sleep-wake schedule between episodes.

Menstrual-Related Hypersomnia

Prevalence
The prevalence of menstrual-related hypersomnia (MH) is relatively unknown, as few case studies have been published. Two of 235 consecutive patients referred over a 5-year period at the Stanford Sleep Clinic were diagnosed with MH.[61] MH presents mostly during adolescence, although one case of a 42-year-old woman with the disorder was reported.[62] The relationship between hypersomnia symptoms and the hormonal fluctuations of the menstrual cycle distinguishes MH from KLS.

Symptoms

In MH, excessive sleepiness occurs during the premenstrual portion of a woman's cycle, 2 weeks before onset of her period. At onset of menstruation, symptoms quickly resolve. Patients typically report severe hypersomnia for up to 8 days, with reduced intake of food and liquid. Hypersomnia may be preceded by behavioral changes, including irritability or aggression.

Pathophysiology

Limited research exists on the pathophysiology of MH, with some researchers indicating a role for progesterone[63] and others implicating prolactin.[62] Lower percentages of slow-wave sleep with an increased overall total sleep time have been seen. Slow theta activity has been seen on EEG during episodes, with an increase in theta activity evidenced during waking times.[63]

Treatment

Oral contraceptive pills that contain a progestin and estradiol have successfully treated MH.[64] As is the case for KLS, behavioral strategies such as keeping a steady interepisode sleep-wake schedule, avoiding alcohol and nicotine, and having family supervision are indicated.

Case report

A 15-year-old male teenager presented with a complaint of "I sleep all the time," which started 4 years earlier. His sleep was typical for his age up to age 11 years, but things began to change after an upper respiratory infection. He became very sleepy and was sleeping 18 hours per day, for approximately 1 week at a time. He felt disoriented at the time, with no control over his sleep, and did not feel refreshed after sleep episodes. There was no hyperphagia, hypersexuality, or bizarre behavior during the episodes except for prolonged sleeping. The episodes resolved spontaneously, and normal sleep and behavior resumed between episodes. Over the prior 4 years he averaged 2 episodes per year, but more recently had become more sleepy in general.

He slept from 10:30 PM to 6:30 AM on weekdays, and then 11:30 PM to 2 PM on weekends. During school days he also took a late afternoon nap, that lasted for 2 to 3 hours, but sometimes he would continue to sleep through the night until the next morning. His Epworth Sleepiness Score (ESS) was 16/24. The sleepiness had a significant impact on his social and school life. He missed school, and social and sporting activities because of the sleepiness, and he had fallen asleep during class, causing his grades to decline.

He was prescribed Adderall, but this caused significant side effects (shaky, paranoid delusions) and was stopped. His mother (a physician) found that low-dose naltrexone (taken for unclear reasons) seemed to help him stay awake in the morning. Because of his bad response to Adderall, he preferred not to take any medication to improve his alertness in the daytime.

Routine blood chemistry (including thyroid studies) was normal. Urine drug screen was normal. Epstein-Barr (EB) antibodies were positive, indicating a prior infection with EB virus. Other infection antibodies were negative. He had a normal brain MRI. One year earlier he had an overnight polysomnogram and an MSLT. The polysomnogram showed 493 minutes of sleep with a 95% sleep efficiency. The apnea/hypopnea index (number of apneas and hypopneas per hour of sleep) was 0.7, and the MSLT showed a mean sleep latency of 7.8 minutes with no SOREMPs.

He had a normal birth and developmental history, with the only surgery being a tonsillectomy. There was no family history of note. There were no symptoms consistent with sleep apnea, seizures, cataplexy, sleep paralysis, hypnagogic hallucinations, parasomnias, or sleep-related movement disorders.

On examination he weighed 150 lb (68 kg), was 5 ft 9 in (175 cm), with a BMI of 22.1 kg/m^2. The general medical and neurologic examination was normal.

The initial impression was KLS, possibly induced by the EB virus; however, the subsequent development of continuous excessive sleepiness with prolonged sleep episodes was more consistent with a diagnosis of idiopathic hypersomnia with long sleep time (ICD #327.11).

In view of the clear initial features of KLS, the patient was started on amantadine, 100 mg twice daily, and lithium, 300 mg, with gradual weekly titration up to a maximum of 900 mg per 24 hours. Lithium blood levels were drawn every 2 weeks until reaching therapeutic range. Good sleep hygiene with a regular sleep-wake pattern was also advised.

Over the ensuing months the patient attained a lithium dose of 1200 mg/d with a blood level within the normal range. He took both the lithium and amantadine with slight improvement in symptoms, but continued to have EDS and was only able to attend school 3 days per week. After 6 months without clear major improvement in symptoms, the medications were stopped and armodafinil was started, initially at low dose because of his bad reaction to Adderall, and increased slowly to 250 mg/d. He was able to tolerate the medication well with some additional improvement in his daytime alertness. Over the subsequent months his ESS continued to be approximately 12.

PROGNOSIS AND FUTURE DIRECTIONS

Although much has been learned about narcolepsy in the past 10 to 20 years, a significant amount of work still needs to be done. The role of hypocretin in the development of narcolepsy is being elucidated, but more research needs to be done on pathophysiology and susceptibility overall to help target patients potentially at risk. Pharmacotherapy for narcolepsy has come a long way, but medication has been aimed primarily at symptom management. Though helpful for many, these medications are typically not a panacea. Very little research exists on the other forms of hypersomnia (KLS, idiopathic hypersomnia, and MH). Future work should focus on a better understanding of pathophysiology and medication management, as few large-scale studies exist, with most published work comprising case studies.

SUMMARY

Excessive sleepiness is a commonly reported symptom that can greatly affect one's overall quality of life. Although often misunderstood or initially thought of as a symptom of another disorder, having a solid understanding of the diagnoses and therapies for the hypersomnias of central origin can yield beneficial results and avoid the many years of misdiagnosis commonly seen in this population. Pharmacologic methods are often considered as the first-line management of the hypersomnias, with behavioral methods playing a role in both adjunctive and primary treatment as well. Hypersomnias often interfere with occupational and home lives, and working with the patient to help alleviate the symptoms of EDS can make a positive difference in the patient's quality of life.

REFERENCES

1. Silber M, Krahn L, Olson E, et al. The epidemiology of narcolepsy in Olmsted County, Minnesota: a population-based study. Sleep 2002;25:197–202.
2. Longstreth W, Koepsell T, Ton T, et al. The epidemiology of narcolepsy. Sleep 2007;30:13–26.
3. Honda Y. Census of narcolepsy, cataplexy and sleep life among teen-agers in Fujisawa city. J Sleep Res 1979;8:191.

4. Tashiro T, Kanbayashi T, Hishikawa Y. An epidemiological study of narcolepsy in Japanese. In: The Fourth International Symposium of Narcolepsy. Tokyo, 1994. p. 13.

5. Lavie P, Peled R. Narcolepsy is a rare disease in Israel. Sleep 1987;10:608–9.

6. Dauvilliers Y, Montplaisir J, Molinari N, et al. Age at onset of narcolepsy in two large populations of patients in France and Quebec. Neurology 2001;57: 2029–33.

7. Peyerson C, Faraco J, Rogers W, et al. A mutation in a case of early onset narcolepsy and a generalized absence of hypocretin peptides in human narcoleptic brains. Nat Med 2000;6:991–7.

8. Lin L, Hungs M, Mignot E. Narcolepsy and the HLA region. J Neuroimmunol 2001; 117:9–20.

9. Mignot E. Genetic and familial aspects of narcolepsy. Neurology 1998;50:S16–22.

10. Billiard M, Besset A, Cadilhac J. The clinical and polygraphic development of narcolepsy. In: Guilleminault C, Lugaresi E, editors. Sleep/wake disorders: natural history, epidemiology and longterm evolution. New York: Raven Press; 1983. p. 171–85.

11. Rosenthal L, Merlotti L, Young D, et al. Subjective and polysomnographic characteristics of patients diagnosed with narcolepsy. Gen Hosp Psychiatry 1990;12: 191–7.

12. Hishikawa Y, Wakamatsu H, Furuya E, et al. Sleep satiation in narcoleptic patients. Electroencephalogr Clin Neurophysiol 1976;41:1–18.

13. Broughton R, Ghanem Q, Hishikawa Y, et al. Life effects of narcolepsy: relationships to geographic origin and to other patient and illness variables. Can J Neurol Sci 1983;10:100–4.

14. Rogers AE, Rosenberg RS. Tests of memory in narcoleptics. Sleep 1990;13: 42–52.

15. Nightingale S, Orgill J, Ebrahim I, et al. The association between narcolepsy and REM behavior disorder (RBD). Sleep Med 2005;6:253–8.

16. Hara J, Beuchmann C, Nambu T, et al. Genetic ablation of orexin neurons in mice results in narcolepsy, hypophagia, and obesity. Neuron 2001;30:345–54.

17. Sansa G, Iranzo A, Santamaria J. Obstructive sleep apnea in narcolepsy. Sleep Med 2010;11:93–5.

18. Broughton R, Ghanem Q, Hishikawa Y, et al. Life effects of narcolepsy in 180 patients from North America, Asia and Europe compared to matched controls. Can J Neurol Sci 1981;8:299–304.

19. American Academy of Sleep Medicine. International classifications of sleep disorders, diagnostic, and coding manual. 2nd edition. Westchester (IL): American Academy of Sleep Medicine; 2005.

20. Mignot E, Lammers G, Ripley B, et al. The role of cerebrospinal fluid hypocretin measurement in the diagnosis of narcolepsy and other hypersomnias. Arch Neurol 2002;59:1553–62.

21. De Lecea L, Kilduff T, Peyron C, et al. The hypocretins: hypothalamus-specific peptides with neuroexcitatory activity. Proc Natl Acad Sci U S A 1998;95:322–7.

22. Sakurai T, Amemiya A, Ishii M, et al. Orexins and orexin receptors: a family of hypothalamic neuropeptides and G protein-coupled receptors that regulate feeding behavior. Cell 1998;92:573–85.

23. Peyron C, Tighe D, van den Pol A, et al. Neurons containing hypocretin (orexin) project to multiple neuronal systems. J Neurosci 1998;18:9996–10015.

24. Nishino S, Ripley B, Overeem S, et al. Hypocretin (orexin) deficiency in human narcolepsy. Lancet 2000;355:39–40.

25. Thannickal T, Siegal J, Nienhuis R, et al. Pattern of hypocretin (orexin) soma and axon loss, and gliosis, in human narcolepsy. Brain Pathol 2003;13:340–51.

26. Thannickal TC, Nienhuis R, Siegal JM. Localized loss of hypocretin (orexin) cells in narcolepsy without cataplexy. Sleep 2009;32:993–8.

27. Saper C, Chou T, Scammell T. The sleep switch: hypothalamic control of sleep and wakefulness. Trends Neurosci 2001;24:726–31.

28. Saper C, Scammell T, Lu J. Hypothalamic regulation of sleep and circadian rhythms. Nature 2005;437:1257–63.

29. Broughton R, Valley V, Aguirre M, et al. Excessive daytime sleepiness and the pathophysiology of narcolepsy-cataplexy: a laboratory perspective. Sleep 1986;9:205–15.

30. Black J, Silber M, Krahn L, et al. Analysis of hypocretin (orexin) antibodies in patients with narcolepsy. Sleep 2005;28:427–31.

31. Billiard M, Laaberki M, Reygrobellet C, et al. Elevated antibodies to streptococcal antigens in narcoleptic subjects. J Sleep Res 1989;18:201.

32. Montplaisir J, Poirier G, Lapierre O, et al. Streptococcal antibodies in narcolepsy and idiopathic hypersomnia. J Sleep Res 1989;18:271.

33. Mignot E, Guilleminault C, Grumet F, et al. Is narcolepsy an autoimmune disease? In: Smirne S, Francesi M, Ferini-Strambi L, et al, editors. Proceedings of the Third Milano International Symposium, September 18-19. Sleep, hormones, and the immune system. Milan (Italy): Masson; 1992. p. 29–38.

34. Dauvilliers Y, Carlander B, Rivier F, et al. Successful management of cataplexy with intravenous immunoglobulins at narcolepsy onset. Ann Neurol 2004;56:905–8.

35. Cvetkovic V, Bayer L, Dorsaz S, et al. Tribbles homolog 2 as an autoantigen in human narcolepsy. J Clin Invest 2010;120:713–9.

36. Nishino S, Mao J, Sampathkumaran R, et al. Increased dopaminergic transmission mediates the wake-promoting effects of CNS stimulants. Sleep Res Online 1998;1:49–61.

37. Wisor J, Nishino S, Sora I, et al. Dopaminergic role in stimulant-induced wakefulness. J Neurosci 2001;21:1787–94.

38. Black J, Houghton WC. Sodium oxybate improves excessive daytime sleepiness in narcolepsy. Sleep 2006;23:939–46.

39. Mamelak M, Scharf MD, Woods M. Treatment of narcolepsy with gamma-hydroxybutyrate. A review of clinical and sleep laboratory findings. Sleep 1986;9:285–9.

40. Castelli M, Ferrro L, Mocci I, et al. Selective gamma-hydroxybutyric acid receptor ligands increase extracellular glutamate in the hippocampus, but fail to activate G protein and to produce the sedative/hypnotic effects of gamma-hydroxybutyric acid. J Neurochem 2003;87:722–32.

41. Lammers GJ, Bassetti C, Billard M, et al. Sodium oxybate is an effective and safe treatment for narcolepsy. Sleep Med 2010;11:105–6.

42. Thorpy MJ, Snyder M, Aloe FS, et al. Short-term triazolam use improves nocturnal sleep of narcoleptics. Sleep 1992;15:212–6.

43. Mullington J, Broughton R. Scheduled naps in the management of daytime sleepiness in narcolepsy-cataplexy. Sleep 1993;15:444–56.

44. Helmus T, Rosenthal L, Bishop C, et al. The alerting effects of short and long naps in narcoleptic, sleep-deprived and alert individuals. Sleep 1997;20:251–7.

45. Chabas D, Fouton C, Gonzalez J. Eating disorder and metabolism in narcoleptic patients. Sleep 2007;30:1267–73.

46. Bruck D. Food consumption patterns in narcolepsy. Sleep 2003;26(Suppl): A272–3.

47. Roth B, Nevsimalova S, Rechtschaffen A. Hypersomnia with "sleep drunkenness". Arch Gen Psychiatry 1972;26(5):456–62.

48. Aldrich MS. The clinical spectrum of narcolepsy and idiopathic hypersomnia. Neurology 1996;46(2):393–401.

49. Bassetti C, Aldrich MS. Idiopathic hypersomnia. A series of 42 patients. Brain 1997;120(Pt 8):1423–35.

50. Nevsimalova S, Blazejova K, Illnerova H, et al. A contribution to pathophysiology of idiopathic hypersomnia. Suppl Clin Neurophysiol 2000;53:366–70.

51. Sforza E, Gaudreau H, Petit D, et al. Homeostatic sleep regulation in patients with idiopathic hypersomnia. Clin Neurophysiol 2000;111(20):277–82.

52. Heier MS, Evsiukova T, Vilming S, et al. CSF hypocretin-1 levels and clinical profiles in narcolepsy and idiopathic CNS hypersomnia in Norway. Sleep 2007; 30(8):969–73.

53. Arnulf I, Lin L, Gadoth N, et al. Kleine-Levin syndrome: a systematic study of 108 patients. Ann Neurol 2008;63(4):482–93.

54. Arnulf I, Zeitzer JM, File J, et al. Kleine-Levin syndrome: a systematic review of 186 cases in the literature. Brain 2005;128(Pt 12):2763–76.

55. Papacostas SS, Hadjivasilis V. The Kleine Levin syndrome. Report of a case and review of the literature. Eur Psychiatry 2000;15:231–5.

56. Kesler A, Gadoth N, Vainstein G, et al. Kleine Levin syndrome (KLS) in young females. Sleep 2000;23:563–7.

57. Huang YS, Guilleminault C, Kao PF, et al. SPECT findings in the Kleine-Levin syndrome. Sleep 2005;28(8):649–51.

58. Podesta C, Ferraras M, Mozzi M, et al. Kleine-Levin syndrome in a 14-year-old girl; CSF hypocretin-1 measurements. Sleep Med 2006;7(8):649–51.

59. Adlakha A, Chokroverty S. An adult onset patient with Kleine-Levin syndrome responding to valproate. Sleep Med 2009;10:391.

60. Loganathan S, Manjunath S, Jhirwal P, et al. Lithium prophylaxis in Kleine-Levin syndrome. J Neuropsychiatry Clin Neurosci 2009;21:107–28.

61. Guilleminault C, Dement WC. 235 cases of excessive daytime sleepiness. Diagnosis and tentative classification. J Neurol Sci 1977;31:13–27.

62. Bamford CR. Menstrual-associated sleep disorder: an unusual hypersomniac variant associated with both menstruation and amenorrhea with a possible link to prolactin and metoclopramide. Sleep 1993;16:484–6.

63. Billiard M, Guilleminault C, Dement WC. A menstruation-line periodic hypersomnia. Kleine-Levin syndrome or new clinical entity? Neurology 1975;25:436–43.

64. Sachs C, Persson HE, Hagenfeldt K. Menstruation-related periodic hypersomnia: a case study with successful treatment. Neurology 1982;32:1376–9.

Insomnia

Maryann C. Deak, MD*, John W. Winkelman, MD, PhD

KEYWORDS

- Pharmacologic therapy • Cognitive behavioral therapy • For insomnia
- Sleep disturbance

KEY POINTS

- Insomnia is a commonly encountered clinical problem.
- Insomnia can occur independently or in conjunction with a comorbid sleep, medical, neurologic, or psychiatric disorder.
- Insomnia is associated with significant potential consequences at the individual and societal level.
- Insomnia can be treated with cognitive behavioral therapy, pharmacologic treatments, or a combination approach, with each treatment option having advantages and disadvantages.

INTRODUCTION

Insomnia is a disorder commonly encountered in clinical practice in primary care and specialty clinics. Insomnia can be present with or without another sleep, medical, or psychiatric disorder; may have multiple potential contributing factors; and has a variable course. Treatment options include cognitive behavioral therapy (CBT), pharmacologic therapy, or a combination therapy.

Insomnia Definitions

The optimal definition of insomnia has yet to be determined and continues to be the subject of debate. Early definitions focused on difficulty initiating or maintaining sleep and categorization as "transient" or "persistent" based on a duration of more or less than 3 weeks.[1] Currently, insomnia definitions vary based on the classification system. Insomnia is currently defined by three classification systems: (1) the International Classification of Sleep Disorders (ICSD),[2] (2) the World Health Organization's International Classification of Diseases,[3] and (3) the American Psychiatric Association's *Diagnostic and Statistical Manual* (DSM).[4] However, all definitions include the presence of

Division of Sleep Medicine, Harvard Medical School, Sleep Health Centers, Brigham and Women's Hospital, 1505 Commonwealth Avenue, 5th Floor, Brighton, MA 02135, USA
* Corresponding author.
E-mail address: Maryann_Deak@sleephealth.com

Neurol Clin 30 (2012) 1045–1066
http://dx.doi.org/10.1016/j.ncl.2012.08.012
0733-8619/12/$ – see front matter © 2012 Elsevier Inc. All rights reserved.

Clinical approach

Patient presents with an insomnia complaint:

- Identify frequency of symptoms and time course of symptoms, including potential precipitating and perpetuating factors
- Identify potential daytime consequences
- Screen for symptoms of other sleep disorders
- Screen for comorbid medical and psychiatric disorders
- Review sleep habits and identify potential areas for improvement in sleep hygiene
- Identify potential contributing medications or substances

Treatment algorithm:

- Optimize treatment of comorbid disorders
- Evaluate treatment options based on cost, patient preference, comorbid disorders, available treatment options:
  - Cognitive behavioral therapy
    - Individual therapy versus group
    - In-person versus computerized or self-help versions
  - Pharmacologic therapy
    - Consider type of symptoms (eg, sleep onset vs sleep maintenance)
    - Potential side effects in light of patient age and comorbid disorders
  - Combination behavioral and pharmacologic approach

---

disturbed sleep that results in impairment of daytime functioning, with variable requirements for frequency and duration of symptoms. Stated or implied in these definitions is that there has been adequate time and opportunity for sleep.

Disturbed sleep can manifest in several ways. The ICSD-2 defines sleep disturbance as difficulty initiating sleep, difficulty maintaining sleep, early morning awakenings, or sleep that is chronically poor quality or nonrestorative.[2] There are 11 subtypes of insomnia recognized by the ICSD-2. The required duration of symptoms in the ICSD varies by specific subcategory of insomnia. For example, acute insomnia symptoms last less than 3 months by definition, and psychophysiologic insomnia symptoms must last more than 1 month to meet the diagnostic criteria. The DSM-IV manual defines sleep disturbance similarly to ICSD-2, and uses a duration criteria of 1 month.[4] The International Classification of Diseases-10 adds a frequency requirement of the sleep disturbance to occur at least 3 nights a week.[3] Insomnia is generally subcategorized into either primary or comorbid insomnia, with the latter applying to insomnia symptoms in an individual with an underlying medical or psychiatric condition or use of a drug or substance.

The validity and interrater reliability of ICSD-2 and DSM-IV insomnia diagnoses, particularly of the primary insomnias, have recently been called into question.[5] Significant overlap between primary and comorbid insomnia subtypes may be a limitation of these diagnostic classification schemes. Thus, the definition if insomnia will likely continue to evolve. The definition of insomnia is currently under revision for the DSM-V, which has yet to be released. One of the changes proposed includes replacing separate primary and secondary insomnia categories with the general category of insomnia disorder, with specification of comorbid condition.[6] Other proposed revisions include adding sleep dissatisfaction to the definition and adding minimum frequency and duration criteria.

EPIDEMIOLOGY AND RISK FACTORS
Epidemiology

Transient insomnia symptoms are common in the general population. Considering the presence of disturbed sleep alone likely provides an inaccurate picture of the prevalence of clinically relevant insomnia. As a result, prevalence estimates of insomnia should be based on specific diagnostic criteria, taking into account daytime impairment, frequency, and chronicity of symptoms. It is clear that prevalence estimates are considerably higher when considering sleep-related insomnia symptoms alone (approximately 30%) versus more specific criteria that account for frequency of symptoms (16%–21%) or daytime consequences (10%).[7] Even when specific diagnostic criteria are applied, prevalence estimates vary by classification system. One study, which examined International Classification of Diseases-10, ICSD-2, and DSM-IV criteria, found prevalence estimates between 4% and 22% depending on the diagnostic criteria applied.[8]

Populations at Risk

Insomnia is more common in specific patient populations (**Box 1**). Older adults are more likely to experience insomnia symptoms. Between 26% and 70% of older adults report regular occurrence of at least one insomnia symptom, most commonly difficulty maintaining sleep.[9–11] In addition to the presence of medical and psychiatric comorbidities, level of physical activity and social life seem to affect the risk of insomnia in older adults.[11,12] Insomnia is more common in women compared with men, with women being almost 50% more likely to develop insomnia symptoms compared with men (relative risk, 1.41).[13] The difference in insomnia prevalence between men and women increases with age, reaching greatest significance in the postmenopausal period.[13] Insomnia is more common in individuals of lower socioeconomic status and with fewer years of education.[14,15] Ethnicity also seems to impact the prevalence and severity of insomnia symptoms.[16] Although ethnicity-based prevalence estimates are somewhat conflicted, prevalence and severity of insomnia symptoms is greater in young or middle-aged African Americans compared with whites. However, insomnia is more prevalent in older whites compared with African Americans.[17]

Association with Comorbid Disorders

Insomnia is frequently coincident with psychiatric disorders, such as depression and anxiety, and with medical comorbidities. People with insomnia are 10 times more likely to have comorbid depression and 7 times more likely to have comorbid anxiety than

Box 1
Populations at risk for developing insomnia
Older adults
Women
Socioeconomically disadvantaged
Limited education
Psychiatric, neurologic, or medical disorders

those without insomnia.[18] Similarly, insomnia is frequently coincident with medical conditions.[19] Pain disorders, memory problems, and heart disease are all associated with a significantly higher risk of insomnia symptoms when controlling for age and gender.[20]

Insomnia and Neurologic Disorders

Insomnia is common in patients with neurologic disorders, although it may be underestimated (**Table 1**).[21] Neurologic disorders may directly cause insomnia symptoms, although comorbid pain, mood disorders, other sleep disorders, or medications may be important contributors in patients with neurologic disease.

Patients with dementias, such as Lewy body dementia or Alzheimer dementia,[22] frequently experience sleep disturbance, which is a common cause for institutionalization in this population.[23] In Alzheimer dementia, sleep disruption is closely tied to circadian rhythm disruption. Sleep disturbance is common in patients with Parkinson disease, which may be related to nocturnal motor symptoms of Parkinson disease, medications, or comorbid sleep disorders, such as rapid eye movement behavior disorder.[24] Insomnia symptoms are present in more than 50% of patients in the first months after stroke, and may impair recovery poststroke.[25] Causes of insomnia in patients with stroke are often multifactorial with comorbid medical or psychiatric disorders, sleep disorders, such as sleep-disordered breathing, and environmental factors playing a role. Patients with epilepsy often complain of poor sleep, although few studies have examined insomnia in patients with epilepsy.[26] Nocturnal seizures, medication side effects, and high prevalence of comorbid psychiatric disorders are possible contributors.[26] Insomnia is also common in other neurologic disorders, such as traumatic brain injury and multiple sclerosis.[21]

CONSEQUENCES AND CORRELATES OF INSOMNIA

Because insomnia is often a persistent condition,[27] potential consequences of insomnia are significant (**Box 2**). Evidence continues to accumulate regarding the potential impact of insomnia on daytime functioning, health outcomes, and economic factors. Insomnia is associated with lower self-reported quality of life on validated questionnaires.[28] Patient's with insomnia report decreased alertness and fatigue or sleepiness during the day.[29] Objective testing demonstrates reduced performance on cognitive testing[30] and decreased reaction time on psychomotor testing,[31] although other studies have shown that patients with insomnia perform within normative ranges on neuropsychologic testing.[32]

Table 1	
Prevalence of insomnia in neurologic disorders	
Neurologic Disorder	**Prevalence of Insomnia**
Parkinson disease	37%–60%
Alzheimer dementia	25%–35%
Stroke	38%–57%
Epilepsy	25%–52%
Multiple sclerosis	31%–37%
Traumatic brain injury	29%–50%

Data from references.[21,24,26,86]

Box 2
Potential consequences of insomnia

Decreased quality of life

Daytime fatigue or sleepiness

Diminished performance on cognitive testing

Increased absenteeism from work

Higher likelihood of requiring disability benefits or medical leave

Higher risk of developing depression

Higher risk of hypertension and cardiovascular disease

Insomnia is associated with an increased risk of incident psychiatric and health problems. Patients with insomnia lasting at least 2 weeks are between 17% and 50% more likely to develop a major depressive episode.[33] Similar results were noted in a recent meta-analysis, which found that patients with insomnia had a twofold higher risk of developing depression.[34] Moreover, patients with persistent insomnia in the context of depression are 2 to 3.5 times more likely to remain depressed long term.[35] Particularly concerning is the association between short sleep duration and suicidal behavior in adolescents, which is independent of the presence of depressive symptoms. Insomnia is also associated with a higher risk of cardiovascular disease. In a large, prospective, population-based study, patients with a history of acute myocardial infarction who experienced insomnia symptoms, including difficulty initiating sleep, maintaining sleep, or nonrestorative sleep, were significantly more likely to experience a recurrence of myocardial infarction during 11 years of follow-up. The results were adjusted for several demographic and health-related factors, such as blood pressure, diabetes mellitus, smoking, and alcohol consumption.[36] Insomnia may be associated with an increased risk for hypertension,[37] although this relationship is not yet clear.[38]

Finally, insomnia is associated with economic and societal burden. There is a significant association between insomnia and the likelihood of requiring disability benefits or medical leave.[39,40] In addition to costs related to absenteeism from work, insomnia is also associated with poor work performance.[41] When inpatient, outpatient, pharmacy, and emergency room costs are considered, the increased cost during a 6-month period associated with insomnia is estimated at more than $1000 per patient.[42]

CLINICAL ASSESSMENT AND DIAGNOSIS

Insomnia can present in a variety of ways including difficulty initiating sleep, difficulty maintaining sleep, early morning awakenings, or nonrestorative sleep. A thorough and complete history remains the cornerstone of assessment of insomnia (**Box 3**). The clinician should elicit detailed information regarding onset of symptoms, type of sleep disturbance, frequency and severity of symptoms, daytime consequences, factors that worsen or improve symptoms, and treatments previously tried.[43] Possible precipitating factors, such as psychosocial stressors, medical and psychiatric disorders, and medication or substance use, also warrant careful consideration.[44] Presence of maladaptive sleep habits, excessive anxiety surrounding insomnia, and dysfunctional beliefs or attitudes about sleep should be assessed as potential perpetuating factors for insomnia. Medical history and physical examination are also essential to identify

---

Box 3
Important elements of clinical history in the evaluation of insomnia

Symptom onset and duration of symptoms

Type of sleep disturbance (eg, sleep onset, sleep maintenance, early morning awakenings)

Potential precipitating factors (stressors, medical or psychiatric disease, and so forth)

Exacerbating and remitting factors

Daytime consequences

Treatments previously tried

Sleep habits, including sleep hygiene

Sleep-related cognitions (ie, attitudes and beliefs about sleep and insomnia)

Screening for comorbid medical, psychiatric disease

Screening for other sleep disorders

Medications

Substance use

---

possible contributors to symptoms of insomnia.[45] Evaluation of insomnia should include screening for comorbid sleep; medical or psychiatric disorders; review of patient medications; and review of possible substance use including illicit drugs, alcohol, tobacco, and caffeine.[46]

Assessment tools, such as sleep diaries, questionnaires, actigraphy, and polysomnography, can be used to obtain more detailed subjective or objective information regarding sleep. Sleep diaries have long been considered the gold standard for subjective assessment of sleep. Recently, an expert panel established a standardized sleep diary to be used in the research or clinical arena (**Fig. 1**).[47] The essential elements of this sleep diary include assessment of bedtime, time to fall asleep, sleep-onset latency, number and duration of awakenings, time of final awakening, final rise time, and subjective assessment of sleep quality. Questionnaires, such as the Pittsburgh Sleep Quality Index and the Insomnia Severity Index, are used most commonly in research assessment of insomnia, but may serve as a useful guide for clinical assessment of insomnia.[46] Actigraphy is a useful tool for obtaining objective information regarding sleep disturbance and circadian rhythm patterns in patients with insomnia, in addition to evaluating response to treatment.[48] Total sleep time, sleep-onset latency, and the number of wake episodes lasting more than 5 minutes, used in combination, are the most useful parameters in evaluating patients with insomnia with actigraphy.[49] Polysomnography and multiple sleep latency tests are not routinely indicated for evaluation of insomnia in clinical practice unless there is concern for a comorbid sleep disorder, such as obstructive sleep apnea or narcolepsy, based on clinical assessment.[45] However, polysomnography is recommended as a component of standard assessment of insomnia in clinical research (**Fig. 2**).[46]

DIFFERENTIAL DIAGNOSIS

Insomnia can be categorized as either primary insomnia or secondary to another disorder or a use of a substance. Primary insomnia has been categorized into six subtypes by the ICSD-2.[2] Psychophysiologic insomnia must be present for at least 1 month, and is associated with conditioned sleep disturbance, increased arousal in

Today's date	4/5/11							
1. What time did you get into bed?	10:15 p.m							
2. What time did you try to go to sleep?	11:30 p.m							
3. How long did it take you to fall asleep?	55 min.							
4. How many times did you wake up, not counting your final awakening?	3 times							
5. In total, how long did these awakenings last?	1 hour 10 min.							
6. What time was your final awakening?	6:35 a.m.							
7. What time did you get out of bed for the day?	7:20 a.m							
8. How would you rate the quality of your sleep?	☐ Very poor ☒ Poor ☐ Fair ☐ Good ☐ Very good	☐ Very poor ☐ Poor ☐ Fair ☐ Good ☐ Very good	☐ Very poor ☐ Poor ☐ Fair ☐ Good ☐ Very good	☐ Very poor ☐ Poor ☐ Fair ☐ Good ☐ Very good	☐ Very poor ☐ Poor ☐ Fair ☐ Good ☐ Very good	☐ Very poor ☐ Poor ☐ Fair ☐ Good ☐ Very good	☐ Very poor ☐ Poor ☐ Fair ☐ Good ☐ Very good	☐ Very poor ☐ Poor ☐ Fair ☐ Good ☐ Very good
9. Comments (if applicable)	I have a cold							

Fig. 1. Consensus sleep diary. (*From* Carney CE, Buysse DJ, Ancoli-Israel S, et al. The consensus sleep diary: standardizing prospective sleep self-monitoring. Sleep 2012;35(2):287–302; with permission.)

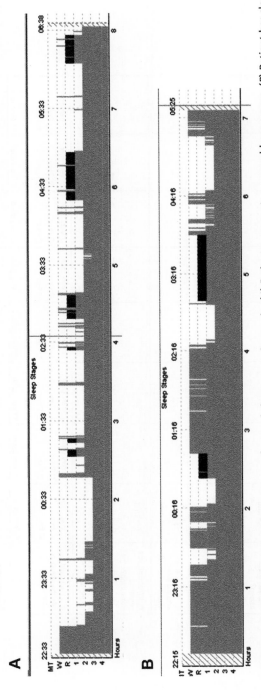

Fig. 2. Polysomnographically derived hypnogram of normal sleep versus insomnia. (*A*) Patient represents a normal hypnogram. (*B*) Patient has sleep-onset and sleep-maintenance insomnia.

bed, or excessive worry about sleep. Adjustment insomnia is characterized by acute, transient insomnia symptoms lasting less than 3 months with an identifiable cause. Paradoxic insomnia lasts at least 1 month and occurs when subjective reports of sleep quantity diverge from objective data, such as polysomnography or actigraphy. Severity of daytime impairment is also less than what would be expected based on subjective reports. Idiopathic insomnia is distinguished by chronic symptoms that begin in childhood without clear cause. Inadequate sleep hygiene occurs when sleep disturbance lasts for a month and is caused by poor sleep habits, such as a highly variable sleep-wake schedule, engaging in stimulating activities before bed, or frequent use of the bed for activities other than sleep. Diagnosis of behavioral insomnia of childhood is based on the child's caregiver's report and is related to the presence of sleep-onset associations or lack of limit setting.

The usefulness of the current diagnostic paradigms for insomnia, particularly primary insomnia, is unclear.[5] In a recent study, the ICSD-2 and DSM-IV diagnoses with the greatest reliability and validity were the secondary insomnia diagnoses, such as insomnia caused by a mental disorder or a medical disorder. Differentiating between primary and secondary insomnia may be a more useful distinction than between subtypes of primary insomnia. There are many potential causes of secondary insomnia symptoms. Insomnia symptoms are common in medical disorders including cardiac, pulmonary, and renal systems.[19] Neurologic disorders, such as Parkinson disease, multiple sclerosis, or stroke are commonly associated with sleep disturbance.[21] Chronic pain is a frequent contributor to insomnia symptoms.[50] Psychiatric conditions, such as depression, bipolar disorder, or anxiety, are frequently associated with disturbed sleep.[18] Substance use, such as alcohol, tobacco, caffeine, and illegal drugs, is a possible contributing factor. A wide range of medications, such as steroids, antidepressants, or thyroid hormone, can contribute to sleep disruption.[51] Insomnia symptoms are a prominent component of other primary sleep disorders, such as obstructive or central sleep apnea, restless legs syndrome, or circadian rhythm disorders. All patients with insomnia should be screened for possible contributing disorders.

PATHOPHYSIOLOGY
Models of Insomnia

Insomnia has long been considered a disorder of hyperarousal at physiologic, cognitive, and emotional levels such that patients with insomnia have a level of alertness and stimulation that interferes with sleep. This notion has been supported by evidence of sympathetic activation in individuals with insomnia, such as increases in basal metabolic rate, levels of circulating catecholamines and cortisol, and beta/gamma activity on electroencephalogram.[52] Several related models have been put forth to provide an explanation for the symptoms and these findings. These models provide the basis for behavioral treatment of insomnia and provide other potential targets for treatment.

The 3P model (**Fig. 3**)[53,54] asserts that individuals are vulnerable to developing insomnia symptoms because of predisposing factors that may be biologic or psychosocial in nature. Sleep disturbance is acutely caused by precipitating factors, such as stressful life events. Finally, insomnia symptoms are perpetuated by compensatory behaviors implemented by the patient, such as spending excessive amounts of time in bed, use of excessive daytime caffeine, and napping. These perpetuating factors are targeted by behavioral therapy techniques for insomnia. The stimulus control model posits that individuals with insomnia are conditioned to associate stimuli that

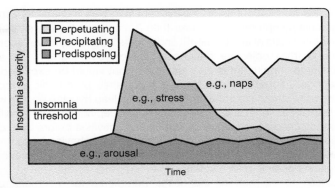

Fig. 3. The 3P Model: predisposing, precipitating, and perpetuating factors contributing to insomnia over time. (*From* Kruger MD, Roth T, Dement WC. Principles and practices of sleep medicine. 5th edition. Philadelphia: Elsevier; 2010. Fig. 77–1; with permission.)

are normally associated with sleep, such as bedtime or bed, with nonsleep activities.[54] The neurocognitive model asserts that insomnia symptoms are caused by conditioned cortical arousal, which results in continued information and memory processing at sleep onset and during sleep.[55] This is evidenced by the presence of beta or gamma activity on electroencephalogram recordings at or around sleep onset in patients with insomnia.

Another theory is composed of the psychobiologic inhibition model of insomnia and the attention-intention-effort pathway.[56] According to this model, sleep is highly regulated by homeostatic and circadian factors, and thus occurs automatically in good sleepers. In the setting of insomnia, sleep is no longer involuntary because of excessive focus on sleep (attention), an overt aim to sleep (intention), and work of trying to sleep (effort). The attention-intention-effort pathway interferes with natural, previously instinctive sleep processes.

The cage exchange model examines the neurobiologic basis for insomnia with a rat model.[57] Rats that are exposed to a psychologic stressor experience symptoms similar to acute insomnia in humans. Neuronal firing patterns in the setting of acute insomnia were examined using the transcription factor Fos. Neuronal activation was increased in the cerebral cortex, limbic system, and parts of the arousal and autonomic systems, simultaneously with activation of sleep-promoting areas. As a result, two systems that typically work in opposition are concurrently activated. The theory posits that deactivation of the limbic-arousal system is a potential target for treatment of acute, stress-induced insomnia.

Finally from the *Drosophila* model of insomnia investigators postulate that individuals are predisposed to developing insomnia based on inherited traits. This notion is supported by modified genes detected in a line of laboratory-selected flies that display behavior and traits similar to human insomnia.[58]

Neuroimaging

In addition to examination of electroencephalographic features, neuronal activation, and genetic patterns, recent work has used neuroimaging as a tool to examine the neurobiologic basis for insomnia. Patients with insomnia were found to have increased global cerebral metabolism during wake and sleep using positron emission tomography, suggesting that insomnia symptoms may be related to continued activity of arousal systems at transitions from wake to sleep.[59] Another study used proton magnetic resonance spectroscopy to examine brain γ-aminobutyric acid (GABA) levels.[60] Patients with primary insomnia had 30% lower average brain GABA levels, which were significantly correlated with increased wake after sleep onset on polysomnography. A follow-up study demonstrated that such GABA deficits were specifically present in the occipital and anterior cingulate cortex.[61] Future work is needed to further explore the neurobiologic basis for insomnia.

TREATMENT

Treatment options for insomnia include CBT, pharmacologic therapy, or a combination approach. Choice of treatment for insomnia is based on careful consideration of the patient's symptoms, comorbid disorders, cost and availability of treatment options, potential risks and benefits of treatment options, and patient preference.

Cognitive Behavioral Therapy

Description

CBT for insomnia (CBTi) addresses psychologic, behavioral, and cognitive factors that perpetuate insomnia symptoms. CBTi generally involves approximately six one-on-one sessions with a specially trained behavioral therapist. Of the techniques applied in CBTi, stimulus control and relaxation training are supported by the highest level of evidence, both being considered standards in the American Academy of Sleep Medicine guidelines.[62] Stimulus control is a collection of techniques designed to re-establish an association between bed and sleep, such as avoiding non–sleep-related activities, such as watching television in bed, getting out of bed when unable to get to sleep and getting into bed only when drowsy, and maintaining a regular sleep schedule.[63] Relaxation training uses such methods as progressive muscle relaxation and meditation to relieve tension and avoid alerting thoughts that prevent sleep. Sleep restriction is recommended as a guideline, and involves limiting time in bed to the amount of time that the patient reports actually being asleep, which initially produces sleep deprivation, and subsequently helps to consolidate sleep.[62,63] In CBTi, behavioral techniques described previously are generally combined with cognitive therapy, which involves addressing exaggerated, nonproductive beliefs about sleep and insomnia, and education about sleep hygiene.[64] The techniques applied in CBTi and the number of sessions required varies based on the needs of an individual patient. In addition, some techniques, such as sleep restriction, may not be appropriate in patients with certain comorbidities, such as epilepsy or bipolar disorder.

Efficacy

CBTi is supported by a high level of evidence, and has been recommended by the US National Institutes of Health and the American Academy of Sleep Medicine.[62,65] Published meta-analyses[66,67] and systematic reviews[63] demonstrate that CBTi improves sleep-onset latency, sleep quality, number of awakenings, and total sleep time (**Fig. 4**). CBTi results in a reduction in sleep-onset latency by approximately 30 minutes and an increase in total sleep time by approximately 30 minutes.[63]

Although medication and CBTi seem to be effective for short-term treatment of insomnia,[67] patients who undergo CBTi may be more likely to achieve sustained benefit over time after discontinuation of therapy.[63,66,68] One study that compared behavioral and pharmacologic therapies found that improvements were maintained over 24 months of follow-up after completion of treatment with the behavioral approach, but not after discontinuation of medication.[69]

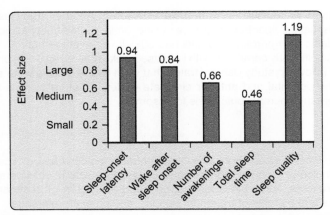

Fig. 4. Efficacy of behavioral therapy for treatment of insomnia. Mean effect size (reported as a standardized z score) across sleep parameters. These effect sizes are pooled across three meta-analyses. (*From* Kruger MD, Roth T, Dement WC. Principles and practices of sleep medicine. 5th edition. Philadelphia: Elsevier; 2010. Fig. 79–1; and *Data from* Morin CM, Culbert JP, Schwartz SM. Nonpharmacological interventions for insomnia: a meta-analysis of treatment efficacy. Am J Psychiatry 1994;151:1172–80; Murtagh DR, Greenwood KM. Identifying effective psychological treatments for insomnia: a meta-analysis. J Consult Clin Psychol 1995;63:79–89; and Smith MT, Perlis ML, Park A, et al. Comparative meta-analysis of pharmacotherapy and behavior therapy for persistent insomnia. Am J Psychiatry 2002;159:5–11.)

CBTi can be used in combination with medication. One study showed that CBTi alone and CBTi in combination with medication resulted in approximately a 60% response rate to treatment, with about 40% of patients achieving long-term remission.[70] Interestingly, the best long-term outcome was achieved when combination therapy was used initially, followed by CBTi alone. CBTi also has been successfully used to assist in the tapering of medication, resulting in discontinuation or reduction in the use of medication in chronic hypnotic users.[71]

Limitations
The primary limitation of CBTi is access. The number of practitioners trained in CBTi is limited, particularly in certain geographic regions. CBTi requires time and a motivated patient. Additionally, CBTi may not be covered by health insurance. Clinicians have devised several alternative strategies to overcome some of the limitations of CBTi. CBTi has been successfully conducted in a group therapy setting or by telephone consultations.[72] Administration of CBTi by trained nurses is another viable option that may be implemented in the primary care setting.[73] Structured Internet-based programs may provide increased flexibility and accessibility to patients.[74] These alternative strategies are best used in conjunction with regular follow-up visits with a treating clinician.

Special populations
CBTi can be used to treat insomnia in patients with comorbid disorders. Patients with major depressive disorder can benefit from CBTi. When used in conjunction with antidepressants, CBTi results in improved remission rates for depression and insomnia.[75] CBTi also benefits sleep in patients with medical comorbidities that are commonly associated with insomnia symptoms, such as cancer.[76] CBTi has been successful in treating insomnia in patients with neurologic disorders, such as traumatic brain injury, multiple sclerosis, and headache.[21]

Pharmacologic Therapy

The use of sleep aids is common in the general population. Based on the 2005 "Sleep in America Poll" conducted by the National Sleep Foundation, 7% of the population use hypnotics prescribed by their doctors. Self-medication is also very common among individuals with disturbed sleep. The same poll found that 9% of individuals use over-the-counter aids for sleep, and 11% use alcohol to help them sleep. Thus, it is important to ask about the use of sleep aids in any evaluation of patients with insomnia symptoms.

There are several medications that have been approved by the US Food and Drug Administration (FDA) for the treatment of insomnia (**Table 2**). Other prescription medications used "off label" for the treatment of insomnia and over-the-counter sleep aids have limited evidence to support their use for the treatment of insomnia. There are potential side effects with the use of pharmacotherapy, and the risks and benefits of hypnotic agents should be carefully weighed for an individual patient. Pharmacologic therapy should be supplemented with behavioral therapy, if possible.[77]

Benzodiazepine receptor agonists

Benzodiazepine receptor agonists (BzRA) are generally considered first-line pharmacologic agents for the treatment of primary insomnia.[77] These medications bind to the GABA-A receptor and are grouped as benzodiazepines or nonbenzodiazepines based on the drug's structure. Benzodiazepines bind nonselectively to any of four alpha

Table 2
FDA-approved medications and indications for treatment of insomnia

Medication	FDA-Approved Indication	Dose Range (mg)	Elimination Half-Life (h)
Benzodiazepine receptor agonists: nonbenzodiazepines			
Zolpidem	Short-term treatment of sleep-onset insomnia	2.5–10	1.4–4.5
Zolpidem CR	Sleep-onset or sleep-maintenance insomnia	6.25–12.5	2.8
Ezcopiclone	Sleep-onset or sleep-maintenance insomnia	1–3	6
Zaleplon	Short-term treatment of sleep-onset insomnia	5–20	1
Benzodiazepine receptor agonists: benzodiazepines			
Estazolam	Short-term treatment of insomnia	0.5–2	10–24
Flurazepam	Short-term treatment of insomnia	15–30	47–100
Temazepam	Short-term treatment of insomnia	7.5–30	4–18
Triazolam	Short-term treatment of insomnia	0.125–0.50	1.5–5.5
Quazepam	Short-term treatment of insomnia	7.5–15	39–73
Antidepressant			
Doxepin	Sleep-maintenance insomnia	3–6	15.3–31
Melatonin receptor agonist			
Ramelteon	Sleep-onset insomnia	8	1–2.6

GABA-A receptor subunits,[78] which results in several potential actions, such as sedation, anxiolysis, amnesia, and muscle relaxation. Nonbenzodiazepine BzRAs are more selective for the α_1 subunit, which mediates sedation and amnesia. Benzodiazepines are generally considered to have greater potential for side effects compared with non-benzodiazepines,[79] although of more importance to the side-effect profile are the administered dose and the half-life of the agent.

Nonbenzodiazepine BzRAs include zolpidem, eszopiclone, and zaleplon. The choice of medication is largely based on the patient's symptoms and the half-life of the medication. Short-acting agents, zolpidem (half-life of 2.5 hours) and zaleplon (half-life of 1 hour), are generally used for sleep-onset insomnia,[80] although zolpidem in the extended-release form is effective in sleep maintenance insomnia. Zaleplon has not been found to produce residual daytime effects if used during middle of the night awakenings when administered 4 hours before awakening.[81] However, zolpidem at approved doses produces daytime effects if administered during middle of the night awakenings and should only be administered at bedtime when the patient has sufficient time to sleep. Eszopiclone, with a half-life of 5 to 6 hours, can be used for sleep-onset and sleep-maintenance insomnia.[80] Nightly use of ezcopiclone and non-nightly use of zolpidem extended release have been tested in long-term studies of 6 months' duration with evidence of continued efficacy without rebound insomnia.[82] Potential side effects of nonbenzodiazepine BzRAs include sedation, dizziness, impairment of motor control, cognitive impairment, headache, amnesia, gastrointestinal symptoms, and unpleasant taste (eszopiclone).[64] Parasomnia behaviors, such as sleep walking or sleep driving, are possible with these medications and potentially dangerous. Abnormal sleep-related behaviors are more likely when hypnotic medications are taken in combination with alcohol or other sedating agents; at times other than the patient's habitual bedtime; or in the setting of untreated sleep disorders, such as restless leg syndrome.[83]

Benzodiazepines approved by the FDA for use in insomnia include estazolam, flurazepam, temazepam, triazolam, and quazepam. Agents with a shorter half-life, such as triazolam (half-life of 2.5 hours), are generally used in the treatment of sleep-onset insomnia. Intermediate half-life agents, such as temazepam, are often used in those with sleep-onset and maintenance insomnia. Longer-acting medications, such as flurazepam (half-life of 47–100 hours) can improve sleep maintenance, but may have greater potential for residual daytime effects. Potential side effects of benzodiazepines include drowsiness, dizziness or lightheadedness, impaired motor control, and cognitive impairment.[84]

Other FDA-approved medications

Ramelteon is a melatonin receptor agonist that is indicated to treat sleep-onset insomnia. Potential side effects include headache, dizziness, drowsiness, fatigue, and nausea.[85] Ramelteon has been tested long term over a 6-month period, and consistently improves sleep-onset latency (but not sleep maintenance) by polysomnography without evidence of daytime residual effects, rebound insomnia, or withdrawal symptoms on discontinuation of treatment.[86] Abuse potential has not been demonstrated with ramelteon and, unlike BzRAs, it is not a scheduled drug. Low-dose ramelteon may be efficacious in treating circadian rhythm disorders.[87]

Doxepin is a sedating antidepressant, which has been approved by the FDA at low doses ($\leq$6 mg) for the treatment of sleep-maintenance insomnia. At these doses, which are significantly lower than those used to treat depression, doxepin acts as a histamine-1 receptor antagonist and has limited anticholinergic effects.[79] Doxepin improves wake after sleep onset, total sleep time, and sleep efficiency.[88] Low-dose doxepin is generally well tolerated in patients with insomnia without evidence of residual daytime effects or anticholinergic effects.[88] Doxepin is not a scheduled substance, and it does not have known potential for abuse.

Non–FDA-approved medications

Several classes of medication, such as sedating antidepressants other than doxepin, antiepileptics, and atypical antipsychotics, are commonly prescribed for treatment of insomnia, although they are not approved by the FDA and evidence to support their use is limited. However, these medications may have use in certain patient populations, particularly in patients with comorbid disorders.

Antidepressants, such as trazodone and mirtazapine, are frequently used for the treatment of insomnia, although at doses significantly lower than antidepressant doses. Mirtazapine may be useful in patients with insomnia and comorbid depression or anxiety.[89] Antidepressants do not have abuse or addiction potential, which provides a potential advantage in patients with a substance abuse history.[64] Potential side effects include drowsiness, dizziness, weight gain, increased suicidal ideation in young adults, cardiac arrhythmias, orthostatic hypotension, and priapism (trazodone).

Antiepileptics, such as gabapentin, pregabalin, and tiagabine, have been used to treat insomnia. These medications may be useful in treating insomnia in certain patient populations, such as patients with generalized anxiety disorder,[90] a history of substance abuse,[91] epilepsy,[92] or chronic pain.[93] Tiagabine increases slow wave sleep, although it does not seem to impact sleep-onset latency or measures of sleep maintenance.[94,95] Possible side effects of these medications include drowsiness, dizziness, cognitive impairment, and mood symptoms.

Atypical antipsychotics, such as olanzapine and quetiapine, are also commonly used in the treatment of insomnia in patients with or without psychiatric conditions.[96,97] These medications seem to increase total sleep time and sleep efficiency.[97] Potential side effects include abnormal lipid regulation, new-onset diabetes mellitus, weight gain, extrapyramidal symptoms, and increased mortality in the elderly.

Pharmacotherapy in comorbid insomnia

Some hypnotic agents have been tested in patients with comorbid psychiatric disorders. Coadministered with an antidepressant, eszopiclone seems to improve insomnia symptoms and mood in patients with depression or anxiety.[98,99] Zolpidem extended release, in combination with an antidepressant, improves sleep quality and next-day symptoms related to sleep in patients with generalized anxiety disorder, but provides no additional improvement in anxiety symptoms compared with placebo.[100]

Treatment of Insomnia in Patients with Neurologic Disorders

Because of the complexity of patients with neurologic disorders, possible causes of insomnia relating to the underlying neurologic disease, comorbid disorders, or medications should be identified and addressed, when possible.[21] There are no pharmacologic therapies that have been approved by the FDA for treatment of insomnia in patients with neurologic disorders. Pharmacologic therapies and CBTi have been used in neurologic patient populations, although evidence is limited.[21] Other behavioral interventions, such as bright light therapy, may be helpful in certain patient populations, such as those with Alzheimer dementia.[101]

Treatment of Insomnia in Older Adults

CBT and pharmacologic therapy have been successfully used to treat insomnia in older adults.[69] Older adults (≥55 years) experience significant improvements in sleep quality, sleep latency, and wake after sleep onset with behavioral intervention.[102] As in younger adults, sleep improvements are better sustained with behavioral therapy compared with pharmacologic therapy after the medication is discontinued.[69]

Several hypnotics, including such BzRAs as eszopiclone, doxepin, and ramelteon, have been specifically tested in older adult populations and were found to be well-tolerated.[103–105] However, there is greater potential for side effects with the use of pharmacologic therapy in older adults, and doses of hypnotic agents may need to be lowered in this patient population. There are data indicating potential increased risk for falls and fractures in older adults taking BzRAs.[106,107] However, this relationship continues to be unclear, because data suggest that insomnia itself increases the risk for falls[108]; although one study controlling for the presence of insomnia found compared with those without insomnia a higher risk of falls in untreated insomnia and ineffectively treated insomnia, and lower risk of falls in effective hypnotic treated insomnia.[109]

FUTURE DIRECTIONS

Further research is needed regarding treatment approaches for insomnia with the goal of developing a catered therapeutic approach that takes into account a patient's clinical presentation, comorbid conditions, and the cost and availability of treatment. Increased data are needed regarding efficacy of alternatives to individual CBTi for situations when CBTi is unavailable or unaffordable. Future research on insomnia will also continue to delineate the relationship between insomnia and comorbid conditions, and the potential bidirectional impact of treatment for either.

SUMMARY

Insomnia is a common disorder with individual and societal consequences. Advances have been made in the understanding of insomnia and its treatment options. However, CBTi and FDA-approved pharmacologic therapies have limitations, the former primarily involving access and the latter involving potential side effects. Further research is needed to optimize management strategies.

Case report

A 42-year-old woman with a history of anxiety and migraine headaches comes to clinic for evaluation of trouble initiating and maintaining sleep. She reports that symptoms began 5 years ago after the birth of her daughter. Although her daughter has been sleeping through the night for the past several years, the patient reports that she continues to have difficulty with sleep. She gets into bed at 8:30 PM (after her daughter goes to sleep). She watches television in bed for an hour. After she turns the lights out at 9:30 PM, she takes approximately 1 hour to fall asleep. She awakens approximately twice a night for an unclear reason, and she is awake for 45 minutes to an hour. She reports that she feels as though her mind "is racing" as she is attempting to return to sleep. She tends to ruminate regarding family and financial concerns. She wakes up at 7 AM with her daughter. After a night of particularly poor sleep, she may take an extended nap in the afternoon for 1 to 2 hours. She feels fatigued during the day, but she denies becoming drowsy or nodding off. The patient finds herself becoming very frustrated with her troubles with sleep, and she worries about her ability to sleep as bedtime approaches. She denies any history of snoring, gasping, or choking episodes, symptoms of restless legs syndrome, leg kicking, or parasomnia behavior. She does not meet criteria for major depression or an anxiety disorder, although she reports "frustration" with her sleep, and irritability, fatigue, and poor concentration after particularly poor nights of sleep. Physical examination including blood pressure, body mass index, and oropharyngeal examination are normal.

Case Discussion

The patient has symptoms consistent with chronic insomnia. Predisposing factors are anxiety, history of migraine headaches, and her tendency to ruminate. Insomnia symptoms seem to have been precipitated by a stressful life event. Perpetuating factors include excessive worry and preoccupation with sleep, spending excessive amounts of time in bed, and performing non–sleep-related activities in bed. The patient is an ideal candidate for CBT. Specific behavioral approaches would include stimulus control techniques including getting into bed only when sleepy, reserving bed for sleep, limiting time in bed to 7 hours, avoidance of daytime napping, and getting out of bed when unable to sleep. Relaxation techniques, such as progressive muscle relaxation, would also likely be helpful for this patient.

REFERENCES

1. Sleep Disorders Centers Ao. Diagnostic classification of sleep and arousal disorders. Sleep 1979;2:5–122.
2. AASM. The international classification of sleep disorders, diagnostic and coding manual. 2nd edition. Westchester (IL): American Academy of Sleep Medicine; 2005.
3. WHO. International classification of diseases (ICD-10). Geneva (Switzerland): World Health Organization; 1991.
4. APA. Diagnostic and statistical manual of mental disorders (DSM-IV-TR). 4th edition. Washington, DC: American Psychiatric Association; 2000.
5. Edinger JD, Wyatt JK, Stepanski EJ, et al. Testing the reliability and validity of DSM-IV-TR and ICSD-2 insomnia diagnoses. Results of a multitrait-multimethod analysis. Arch Gen Psychiatry 2011;68(10):992–1002.
6. Available at: http://www.dsm5.org/ProposedRevisions/Pages/proposedrevision.aspx?rid=65#. Accessed June 1, 2012.
7. Ohayon MM. Epidemiology of insomnia: what we know and what we still need to learn. Sleep Med Rev 2002;6(2):97–111.
8. Roth T, Coulouvrat C, Hajak G, et al. Prevalence and perceived health associated with insomnia based on DSM-IV-TR; international statistical classification of diseases and related health problems, tenth revision; and research diagnostic criteria/international classification of sleep disorders, second edition criteria: results from the America Insomnia Survey. Biol Psychiatry 2011;69(6):592–600.
9. Jaussent I, Dauvilliers Y, Ancelin ML, et al. Insomnia symptoms in older adults: associated factors and gender differences. Am J Geriatr Psychiatry 2011;19(1):88–97.
10. Schubert CR, Cruickshanks KJ, Dalton DS, et al. Prevalence of sleep problems and quality of life in an older population. Sleep 2002;25(8):889–93.
11. Ohayon MM, Zulley J, Guilleminault C, et al. How age and daytime activities are related to insomnia in the general population: consequences for older people. J Am Geriatr Soc 2001;49(4):360–6.
12. Morgan K. Daytime activity and risk factors for late-life insomnia. J Sleep Res 2003;12(3):231–8.
13. Zhang B, Wing YK. Sex differences in insomnia: a meta-analysis. Sleep 2006;29(1):85–93.
14. Gellis LA, Lichstein KL, Scarinci IC, et al. Socioeconomic status and insomnia. J Abnorm Psychol 2005;114(1):111–8.
15. Sekine M, Chandola T, Martikainen P, et al. Explaining social inequalities in health by sleep: the Japanese civil servants study. J Public Health (Oxf) 2006;28(1):63–70.

16. Durrence HH, Lichstein KL. The sleep of African Americans: a comparative review. Behav Sleep Med 2006;4(1):29–44.
17. Jean-Louis G, Magai C, Consedine NS, et al. Insomnia symptoms and repressive coping in a sample of older black and white women. BMC Womens Health 2007;7:1.
18. Taylor DJ, Lichstein KL, Durrence HH, et al. Epidemiology of insomnia, depression, and anxiety. Sleep 2005;28(11):1457–64.
19. Taylor DJ, Mallory LJ, Lichstein KL, et al. Comorbidity of chronic insomnia with medical problems. Sleep 2007;30(2):213–8.
20. Morgan K, Kucharczyk E, Gregory P. Insomnia: evidence-based approaches to assessment and management. Clin Med 2011;11(3):278–81.
21. Mayer G, Jennum P, Riemann D, et al. Insomnia in central neurologic diseases: occurrence and management. Sleep Med Rev 2011;15(6):369–78.
22. Bliwise DL, Mercaldo ND, Avidan AY, et al. Sleep disturbance in dementia with Lewy bodies and Alzheimer's disease: a multicenter analysis. Dement Geriatr Cogn Disord 2011;31(3):239–46.
23. Anderson K. Sleep disturbance and neurological disease. Clin Med 2011;11(3): 271–4.
24. Diederich NJ, McIntyre DJ. Sleep disorders in Parkinson's disease: many causes, few therapeutic options. J Neurol Sci 2012;314(1–2):12–9.
25. Hermann DM, Bassetti CL. Sleep-related breathing and sleep-wake disturbances in ischemic stroke. Neurology 2009;73(16):1313–22.
26. Manni R, Terzaghi M. Comorbidity between epilepsy and sleep disorders. Epilepsy Res 2010;90(3):171–7.
27. Morin CM, Belanger L, LeBlanc M, et al. The natural history of insomnia: a population-based 3-year longitudinal study. Arch Intern Med 2009;169(5): 447–53.
28. Leger D, Scheuermaier K, Philip P, et al. SF-36: evaluation of quality of life in severe and mild insomniacs compared with good sleepers. Psychosom Med 2001;63(1):49–55.
29. Buysse DJ, Thompson W, Scott J, et al. Daytime symptoms in primary insomnia: a prospective analysis using ecological momentary assessment. Sleep Med 2007;8(3):198–208.
30. Haimov I, Hanuka E, Horowitz Y. Chronic insomnia and cognitive functioning among older adults. Behav Sleep Med 2008;6(1):32–54.
31. Edinger JD, Means MK, Carney CE, et al. Psychomotor performance deficits and their relation to prior nights' sleep among individuals with primary insomnia. Sleep 2008;31(5):599–607.
32. Semler CN, Harvey AG. Daytime functioning in primary insomnia: does attentional focus contribute to real or perceived impairment? Behav Sleep Med 2006;4(2):85–103.
33. Buysse DJ, Angst J, Gamma A, et al. Prevalence, course, and comorbidity of insomnia and depression in young adults. Sleep 2008;31(4):473–80.
34. Baglioni C, Battagliese G, Feige B, et al. Insomnia as a predictor of depression: a meta-analytic evaluation of longitudinal epidemiological studies. J Affect Disord 2011;135(1–3):10–9.
35. Pigeon WR, Hegel M, Unutzer J, et al. Is insomnia a perpetuating factor for late-life depression in the IMPACT cohort? Sleep 2008;31(4):481–8.
36. Laugsand LE, Vatten LJ, Platou C, et al. Insomnia and the risk of acute myocardial infarction: a population study. Circulation 2011;124(19):2073–81.

37. Vgontzas AN, Liao D, Bixler EO, et al. Insomnia with objective short sleep duration is associated with a high risk for hypertension. Sleep 2009;32(4):491–7.

38. Phillips B, Buzkova P, Enright P. Insomnia did not predict incident hypertension in older adults in the cardiovascular health study. Sleep 2009;32(1):65–72.

39. Overland S, Glozier N, Sivertsen B, et al. A comparison of insomnia and depression as predictors of disability pension: the HUNT study. Sleep 2008;31(6): 875–80.

40. Sivertsen B, Overland S, Bjorvatn B, et al. Does insomnia predict sick leave? The Hordaland health study. J Psychosom Res 2009;66(1):67–74.

41. Kessler RC, Berglund PA, Coulouvrat C, et al. Insomnia and the performance of US workers: results from the America insomnia survey. Sleep 2011;34(9): 1161–71.

42. Ozminkowski RJ, Wang S, Walsh JK. The direct and indirect costs of untreated insomnia in adults in the United States. Sleep 2007;30(3):263–73.

43. Harvey AG, Spielman AJ. Insomnia: diagnosis, assessment, and outcomes. In: Kryger M, Roth T, Dement W, editors. Principles and practice of sleep medicine. 5th edition. Philadelphia: Elsevier; 2011. p. 838–49.

44. Bastien CH, Vallieres A, Morin CM. Precipitating factors of insomnia. Behav Sleep Med 2004;2(1):50–62.

45. Chesson A Jr, Hartse K, Anderson WM, et al. Practice parameters for the evaluation of chronic insomnia. An American Academy of Sleep Medicine report. Standards of practice committee of the American Academy of Sleep Medicine. Sleep 2000;23(2):237–41.

46. Buysse DJ, Ancoli-Israel S, Edinger JD, et al. Recommendations for a standard research assessment of insomnia. Sleep 2006;29(9):1155–73.

47. Carney CE, Buysse DJ, Ancoli-Israel S, et al. The consensus sleep diary: standardizing prospective sleep self-monitoring. Sleep 2012;35(2):287–302.

48. Morgenthaler T, Alessi C, Friedman L, et al. Practice parameters for the use of actigraphy in the assessment of sleep and sleep disorders: an update for 2007. Sleep 2007;30(4):519–29.

49. Natale V, Plazzi G, Martoni M. Actigraphy in the assessment of insomnia: a quantitative approach. Sleep 2009;32(6):767–71.

50. Tang NK, Goodchild CE, Hester J, et al. Pain-related insomnia versus primary insomnia: a comparison study of sleep pattern, psychological characteristics, and cognitive-behavioral processes. Clin J Pain 2012;28(5):428–36.

51. McCrae CS, Lichstein KL. Secondary insomnia: diagnostic challenges and intervention opportunities. Sleep Med Rev 2001;5(1):47–61.

52. Roth T, Roehrs T, Pies R. Insomnia: pathophysiology and implications for treatment. Sleep Med Rev 2007;11(1):71–9.

53. Spielman AJ, Caruso LS, Glovinsky PB. A behavioral perspective on insomnia treatment. Psychiatr Clin North Am 1987;10(4):541–53.

54. Perlis M, Shaw P, Cano P, et al. Models of insomnia. In: Kryger M, Roth T, Dement W, editors. Principles and practice of sleep medicine. 5th edition. Philadelphia: Elsevier; 2011. p. 850–63.

55. Perlis ML, Giles DE, Mendelson WB, et al. Psychophysiological insomnia: the behavioural model and a neurocognitive perspective. J Sleep Res 1997;6(3): 179–88.

56. Espie CA, Broomfield NM, MacMahon KM, et al. The attention-intention-effort pathway in the development of psychophysiologic insomnia: a theoretical review. Sleep Med Rev 2006;10(4):215–45.

57. Cano G, Mochizuki T, Saper CB. Neural circuitry of stress-induced insomnia in rats. J Neurosci 2008;28(40):10167–84.

58. Seugnet L, Suzuki Y, Thimgan M, et al. Identifying sleep regulatory genes using a *Drosophila* model of insomnia. J Neurosci 2009;29(22):7148–57.

59. Nofzinger EA, Buysse DJ, Germain A, et al. Functional neuroimaging evidence for hyperarousal in insomnia. Am J Psychiatry 2004;161(11):2126–8.

60. Winkelman JW, Buxton OM, Jensen JE, et al. Reduced brain GABA in primary insomnia: preliminary data from 4T proton magnetic resonance spectroscopy (1H-MRS). Sleep 2008;31(11):1499–506.

61. Plante DT, Jensen JE, Schoerning L, et al. Reduced gamma-aminobutyric acid in occipital and anterior cingulate cortices in primary insomnia: a link to major depressive disorder? Neuropsychopharmacology 2012;37(6):1548–57.

62. Morgenthaler T, Kramer M, Alessi C, et al. Practice parameters for the psychological and behavioral treatment of insomnia: an update. An American Academy of Sleep Medicine report. Sleep 2006;29(11):1415–9.

63. Morin CM, Bootzin RR, Buysse DJ, et al. Psychological and behavioral treatment of insomnia: update of the recent evidence (1998-2004). Sleep 2006;29(11):1398–414.

64. Morin CM, Benca R. Chronic insomnia. Lancet 2012;379(9821):1129–41.

65. National Institutes of Health. National Institutes of Health state of the science conference statement on manifestations and management of chronic insomnia in adults, June 13-15, 2005. Sleep 2005;28(9):1049–57.

66. Morin CM, Culbert JP, Schwartz SM. Nonpharmacological interventions for insomnia: a meta-analysis of treatment efficacy. Am J Psychiatry 1994;151(8):1172–80.

67. Smith MT, Perlis ML, Park A, et al. Comparative meta-analysis of pharmacotherapy and behavior therapy for persistent insomnia. Am J Psychiatry 2002;159(1):5–11.

68. Murtagh DR, Greenwood KM. Identifying effective psychological treatments for insomnia: a meta-analysis. J Consult Clin Psychol 1995;63(1):79–89.

69. Morin CM, Colecchi C, Stone J, et al. Behavioral and pharmacological therapies for late-life insomnia: a randomized controlled trial. JAMA 1999;281(11):991–9.

70. Morin CM, Vallieres A, Guay B, et al. Cognitive behavioral therapy, singly and combined with medication, for persistent insomnia: a randomized controlled trial. JAMA 2009;301(19):2005–15.

71. Morin CM, Bastien C, Guay B, et al. Randomized clinical trial of supervised tapering and cognitive behavior therapy to facilitate benzodiazepine discontinuation in older adults with chronic insomnia. Am J Psychiatry 2004;161(2):332–42.

72. Bastien CH, Morin CM, Ouellet MC, et al. Cognitive-behavioral therapy for insomnia: comparison of individual therapy, group therapy, and telephone consultations. J Consult Clin Psychol 2004;72(4):653–9.

73. Espie CA, MacMahon KM, Kelly HL, et al. Randomized clinical effectiveness trial of nurse-administered small-group cognitive behavior therapy for persistent insomnia in general practice. Sleep 2007;30(5):574–84.

74. Ritterband LM, Thorndike FP, Gonder-Frederick LA, et al. Efficacy of an Internet-based behavioral intervention for adults with insomnia. Arch Gen Psychiatry 2009;66(7):692–8.

75. Manber R, Edinger JD, Gress JL, et al. Cognitive behavioral therapy for insomnia enhances depression outcome in patients with comorbid major depressive disorder and insomnia. Sleep 2008;31(4):489–95.

76. Espie CA, Fleming L, Cassidy J, et al. Randomized controlled clinical effectiveness trial of cognitive behavior therapy compared with treatment as usual for persistent insomnia in patients with cancer. J Clin Oncol 2008;26(28): 4651–8.

77. Schutte-Rodin S, Broch L, Buysse D, et al. Clinical guideline for the evaluation and management of chronic insomnia in adults. J Clin Sleep Med 2008;4(5): 487–504.

78. Nutt D. GABAA receptors: subtypes, regional distribution, and function. J Clin Sleep Med 2006;2(2):S7–11.

79. Hall-Porter JM, Curry DT, Walsh JK. Pharmacologic treatment of primary insomnia. Sleep Med Clin 2010;5(4):609–25.

80. Benca RM. Diagnosis and treatment of chronic insomnia: a review. Psychiatr Serv 2005;56(3):332–43.

81. Zammit GK, Corser B, Doghramji K, et al. Sleep and residual sedation after administration of zaleplon, zolpidem, and placebo during experimental middle-of-the-night awakening. J Clin Sleep Med 2006;2(4):417–23.

82. Krystal AD, Erman M, Zammit GK, et al. Long-term efficacy and safety of zolpidem extended-release 12.5 mg, administered 3 to 7 nights per week for 24 weeks, in patients with chronic primary insomnia: a 6-month, randomized, double-blind, placebo-controlled, parallel-group, multicenter study. Sleep 2008;31(1):79–90.

83. Poceta JS. Zolpidem ingestion, automatisms, and sleep driving: a clinical and legal case series. J Clin Sleep Med 2011;7(6):632–8.

84. Holbrook AM, Crowther R, Lotter A, et al. Meta-analysis of benzodiazepine use in the treatment of insomnia. CMAJ 2000;162(2):225–33.

85. Borja NL, Daniel KL. Ramelteon for the treatment of insomnia. Clin Ther 2006; 28(10):1540–55.

86. Mayer G, Wang-Weigand S, Roth-Schechter B, et al. Efficacy and safety of 6-month nightly ramelteon administration in adults with chronic primary insomnia. Sleep 2009;32(3):351–60.

87. Richardson GS, Zee PC, Wang-Weigand S, et al. Circadian phase-shifting effects of repeated ramelteon administration in healthy adults. J Clin Sleep Med 2008;4(5):456–61.

88. Roth T, Rogowski R, Hull S, et al. Efficacy and safety of doxepin 1 mg, 3 mg, and 6 mg in adults with primary insomnia. Sleep 2007;30(11):1555–61.

89. Wiegand MH. Antidepressants for the treatment of insomnia: a suitable approach? Drugs 2008;68(17):2411–7.

90. Montgomery SA, Herman BK, Schweizer E, et al. The efficacy of pregabalin and benzodiazepines in generalized anxiety disorder presenting with high levels of insomnia. Int Clin Psychopharmacol 2009;24(4):214–22.

91. Karam-Hage M, Brower KJ. Gabapentin treatment for insomnia associated with alcohol dependence. Am J Psychiatry 2000;157(1):151.

92. de Haas S, Otte A, de Weerd A, et al. Exploratory polysomnographic evaluation of pregabalin on sleep disturbance in patients with epilepsy. J Clin Sleep Med 2007;3(5):473–8.

93. Saldana MT, Perez C, Navarro A, et al. Pain alleviation and patient-reported health outcomes following switching to pregabalin in individuals with gabapentin-refractory neuropathic pain in routine medical practice. Clin Drug Investig 2012;32(6):401–12.

94. Walsh JK, Zammit G, Schweizer PK, et al. Tiagabine enhances slow wave sleep and sleep maintenance in primary insomnia. Sleep Med 2006;7(2):155–61.

95. Roth T, Wright KP Jr, Walsh J. Effect of tiagabine on sleep in elderly subjects with primary insomnia: a randomized, double-blind, placebo-controlled study. Sleep 2006;29(3):335–41.

96. Wine JN, Sanda C, Caballero J. Effects of quetiapine on sleep in nonpsychiatric and psychiatric conditions. Ann Pharmacother 2009;43(4):707–13.

97. Cohrs S. Sleep disturbances in patients with schizophrenia: impact and effect of antipsychotics. CNS Drugs 2008;22(11):939–62.

98. Fava M, McCall WV, Krystal A, et al. Eszopiclone co-administered with fluoxetine in patients with insomnia coexisting with major depressive disorder. Biol Psychiatry 2006;59(11):1052–60.

99. Pollack M, Kinrys G, Krystal A, et al. Eszopiclone coadministered with escitalopram in patients with insomnia and comorbid generalized anxiety disorder. Arch Gen Psychiatry 2008;65(5):551–62.

100. Fava M, Asnis GM, Shrivastava R, et al. Zolpidem extended-release improves sleep and next-day symptoms in comorbid insomnia and generalized anxiety disorder. J Clin Psychopharmacol 2009;29(3):222–30.

101. Salami O, Lyketsos C, Rao V. Treatment of sleep disturbance in Alzheimer's dementia. Int J Geriatr Psychiatry 2011;26(8):771–82.

102. Irwin MR, Cole JC, Nicassio PM. Comparative meta-analysis of behavioral interventions for insomnia and their efficacy in middle-aged adults and in older adults 55+ years of age. Health Psychol 2006;25(1):3–14.

103. Ancoli-Israel S, Krystal AD, McCall WV, et al. A 12-week, randomized, double-blind, placebo-controlled study evaluating the effect of eszopiclone 2 mg on sleep/wake function in older adults with primary and comorbid insomnia. Sleep 2010;33(2):225–34.

104. Scharf M, Rogowski R, Hull S, et al. Efficacy and safety of doxepin 1 mg, 3 mg, and 6 mg in elderly patients with primary insomnia: a randomized, double-blind, placebo-controlled crossover study. J Clin Psychiatry 2008;69(10):1557–64.

105. Richardson GS, Zammit G, Wang-Weigand S, et al. Safety and subjective sleep effects of ramelteon administration in adults and older adults with chronic primary insomnia: a 1-year, open-label study. J Clin Psychiatry 2009;70(4):467–76.

106. Finkle WD, Der JS, Greenland S, et al. Risk of fractures requiring hospitalization after an initial prescription for zolpidem, alprazolam, lorazepam, or diazepam in older adults. J Am Geriatr Soc 2011;59(10):1883–90.

107. Wang PS, Bohn RL, Glynn RJ, et al. Zolpidem use and hip fractures in older people. J Am Geriatr Soc 2001;49(12):1685–90.

108. Brassington GS, King AC, Bliwise DL. Sleep problems as a risk factor for falls in a sample of community-dwelling adults aged 64-99 years. J Am Geriatr Soc 2000;48(10):1234–40.

109. Avidan AY, Fries BE, James ML, et al. Insomnia and hypnotic use, recorded in the minimum data set, as predictors of falls and hip fractures in Michigan nursing homes. J Am Geriatr Soc 2005;53(6):955–62.

Parasomnias and Their Mimics

Raman K. Malhotra, MD[a], Alon Y. Avidan, MD, MPH[b],*

KEYWORDS

- Parasomnias • Confusional arousals • Sleepwalking • Night terrors • Nightmares
- REM sleep behavior disorder • Sleep paralysis

KEY POINTS

- Parasomnias are abnormal and undesirable motor or verbal events that manifest during sleep or wake-to-sleep transition.
- Features of the clinical history and examination, along with findings from the overnight polysomnogram, are essential to differentiate between different parasomnias and their mimics.
- Disorders of arousal (ie, sleepwalking, sleep terrors, and confusional arousals) arise from nonrapid eye movement sleep (usually stage N3), typically occur during the first third of the night, and usually involve no memory or poor recall of the event by the patient.
- Rapid eye movement (REM) sleep parasomnias, including REM sleep behavior disorder, nightmares, and isolated sleep paralysis, occur out of stage REM sleep and usually involve some recollection of the event or dream content related to the motor activity by the patient.
- Management of parasomnias includes identifying and treating other underlying sleep disorders (such as sleep apnea, periodic leg movements of sleep), educating the patient regarding safety precautions in their home, and possibly pharmacologic treatment specific to the parasomnia or sleep-related motor activity.

INTRODUCTION

Parasomnias are undesirable motor or verbal phenomena that arise from sleep or sleep-wake transition.[1–4] Parasomnias may include abnormal movements, behaviors, sensory phenomena, emotions, and autonomic activity.[2] They are classified into arousal disorders (usually associated with nonrapid eye movement [NREM] slow-wave sleep), parasomnias usually associated with rapid eye movement (REM) sleep, and other parasomnias.

[a] SLUCare Sleep Disorders Center, Department of Neurology and Psychiatry, Saint Louis University School of Medicine, 1438 South Grand Boulevard, St. Louis, MO 63104, USA; [b] Department of Neurology, UCLA Sleep Disorders Center, 710 Westwood Boulevard, Room 1-169/ RNRC, Los Angeles, CA 90095-1769, USA
* Corresponding author.
E-mail address: avidan@mednet.ucla.edu

Neurol Clin 30 (2012) 1067–1094
http://dx.doi.org/10.1016/j.ncl.2012.08.016
0733-8619/12/$ – see front matter © 2012 Elsevier Inc. All rights reserved.

neurologic.theclinics.com

The *International Classification of Sleep Disorders, Second Edition* lists 15 categories of parasomnias[5] divided into disorders of arousal from NREM sleep (confusional arousals, sleepwalking, sleep terrors), parasomnias associated with REM sleep (REM sleep behavior disorder [RBD], recurrent isolated sleep paralysis, and nightmare disorder) and other parasomnias (sleep enuresis, sleep-related eating disorder [SRED], and several others that are not addressed here). **Table 1** presents the key features of the parasomnias discussed in this article with regards to sleep stage propensity, semiology, and suggested treatment.

PATHOPHYSIOLOGY

The current understanding of the cause of parasomnias is that sleep and wakefulness are not mutually exclusive states of being. As one falls asleep and progresses through the various sleep stages, sleep stage shift is not a complete on or off switch phenomenon, but involves reorganization and transition of several neuronal centers for an equivocal stage to declare itself.[1,4] It is during this period of reorganization (a unique state of sleep dissociation) that one encounters an admixture of different states of being. They may overlap or intrude into one another, resulting in complex behaviors, as shown in **Fig. 1**.[1,4,6,7] Disorders of arousal are a consequence of intrusion of wakefulness into NREM sleep. REM parasomnias such as RBD are a corollary of an admixture of wakefulness and REM sleep.[1,7,8] **Fig. 1** shows the interesting corollary in that both patients with narcolepsy and RBD experience abnormalities in REM sleep control: abnormal expression of increased muscle tone during REM sleep, when it is expected to be inhibited in RBD. As is shown in **Fig. 1**, hypnagogic hallucinations are abnormal REM-related visual disturbances that occur during transition from wakefulness into sleep.

Table 1
Key similarities and differentiating features between NREM and REM parasomnias as well as nocturnal seizures

	Confusional Arousals	Sleep Terrors	Sleepwalking	Nightmares	RBD	Nocturnal Seizures
Time	Early	Early	Early-Mid	Late	Late	Any
Sleep stage	SWA	SWA	SWA	REM	REM	Any
EEG discharges	–	–	–	–	–	+
Scream	–	++++	–	++	+	+
CNS activation	+	++++	+	+	+	+
Motor activity	–	+	+++	+	++++	++++
Awakens	–	–	–	+	+	+
Duration (min)	0.5–10	1–10	2–30	3–20	1–10	5–15
Postevent confusion	+	+	+	–	–	+
Age	Child	Child	Child	Child-adult	Older adult	Young adult
Genetics	+	+	+	–	–	±
Organic CNS lesion	–	–	–	–	++	++++

Abbreviation: SWA, slow wave activity or N3 sleep.
Data from Avidan, AY and Kaplish N. The parasomnias: epidemiology, clinical features, and diagnostic approach. Clin Chest Med 2010;31(2):359.

Nocturnal Spells: overlapping states

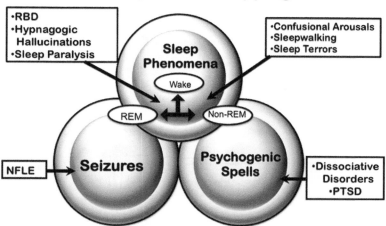

Fig. 1. Overlapping states of being as described by Mahowald and Schenck. Parasomnias are explainable by the notion that sleep and wakefulness are not mutually exclusive states but may dissociate and oscillate rapidly. The abnormal admixture of the 3 states of being (NREM sleep, REM sleep, and wakefulness) may overlap, giving rise to parasomnias. REM parasomnias occur because of the abnormal intrusion of wakefulness into REM sleep, and, likewise, NREM parasomnias such as sleepwalking occur because of abnormal intrusions of wakefulness into NREM sleep. Other nocturnal spells that may be confused with parasomnias include nocturnal frontal lobe epilepsy (NFLE) and psychogenic spells such as posttraumatic stress disorder (PTSD) and dissociated disorders. (*Adapted from* Mahowald MW, Schenck CH. Non-rapid eye movement sleep parasomnias. Neurol Clin 2005;23(4):1078; and Avidan, AY and Kaplish N. The parasomnias: epidemiology, clinical features, and diagnostic approach. Clin Chest Med 2010;31(2):354.)

An alternative hypothesis is that central pattern generators (CPGs), as discussed in **Fig. 2**, lead to deafferentation of the locomotor centers from the generators of the different sleep states.[9] Locomotor centers are present at both spinal and supra spinal levels and this dissociation can explain motor activity or ambulation especially in patients with disorders of arousals.[10]

CPGs, which are located in the brain stem and spinal cord (shown in the yellow regions in **Fig. 2**), are believed to be responsible for involuntary motor behaviors classified into:

a. Oroalimentary automatisms, bruxism, and biting;
b. Ambulatory behaviors, ranging from the classic bimanual-bipedal activity of somnambulism to periodic leg movements; and
c. Various sleep-related events associated with fear, such as sleep terrors, nightmares, and violent behaviors.[10]

CLASSIFICATION OF PARASOMNIAS

The *International Classification of Sleep Disorders* classifies 15 different parasomnias based on the sleep stage during which the parasomnia is most likely to manifest (**Fig. 3**).[11] NREM sleep parasomnias, also known as disorders of arousal (**Box 1**), typically arise from stage N3 sleep, although they can also occur out of stage N1 or N2.

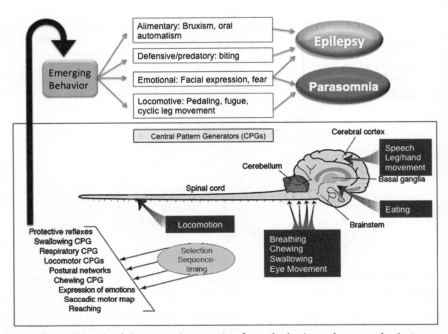

Fig. 2. Along all levels of the neuraxis stemming from the brain to the upper brainstem and spinal cord, several neuronal networks exist that when activated produce different types of behavior (*upper panel*). The network is collectively referred to as CPGs, depicted as the yellow regions in the bottom panel of the diagram. The spectrum of resulting behaviors may be simple and stereotyped, such as rhythmical lip smacking and swallowing, or more polymorphic and complex, such as those generating locomotion and search behaviors. The CPGs may lead to monomorphic spells, which are stereotyped (automatisms), in which the possible cause could be related to nocturnal seizures, or highly complex (locomotive) polymorphic behavior, in which the cause may be a parasomnia. (*Adapted from* Grillner S. The motor infrastructure: from ion channels to neuronal networks. Nat Rev Neurosci 2003;4:573–86; with permission; *data from* Tassinari, CA, Cantalupo G, Högl B, et al. Neuro-ethological approach to frontolimbic epileptic seizures and parasomnias: the same central pattern generators for the same behaviors. Rev Neurol (Paris) 2009;165(10):765.)

They tend to occur during the first third of the night, when stage N3 predominates. They also occur more frequently in childhood because of the higher percentage of stage N3 at these ages, and decrease in frequency with age. Patients do not typically remember the event or have dream recall corresponding to the motor activity, which distinguishes them from REM sleep parasomnias. Motor activity can be simple, benign movements, such as sitting in bed or sleep talking, or can be complex and dangerous, such as walking, driving, fighting, or eating. NREM sleep parasomnias consist of confusional arousals, sleepwalking, and sleep terrors. **Box 2** lists several known factors known to predispose patients to experience these events.

CONFUSIONAL AROUSALS

Confusional arousals consist of mental confusion or confusional behavior during or after arousals from sleep. They occur most often out of stage N3 sleep and during the first third of the night, but can occur out of other stages of NREM sleep and at any time of the night.

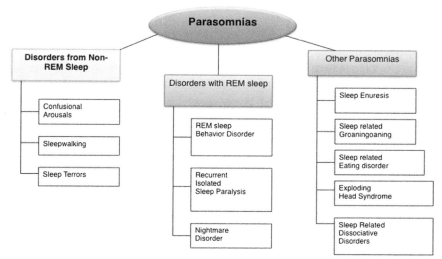

Fig. 3. The *International Classifications of Sleep Disorders, Second Edition* for parasomnias. Disorders from NREM sleep are also known as disorders of arousal. Parasomnias categorized as other parasomnias do not show a strong predilection for NREM or REM sleep. (*Modified after* Avidan, AY and N Kaplish. The parasomnias: epidemiology, clinical features, and diagnostic approach. Clin Chest Med 2010;31(2):355; with permission.)

Epidemiology and Risk Factors

There is no sex difference with confusional arousals, and like other NREM sleep parasomnias, they are more common in children and young adults. Prevalence rate in children 3 to 13 years of age is 17.3%. In children older than 15 years and in adults, prevalence is as high as 6.9%.[12]

Pathophysiology

Exact pathophysiology and localization in the brain have not been confirmed. Areas of the brain in control of arousal, such as the posterior hypothalamus, midbrain reticular area, and the periventricular gray matter, have all been implicated. Confusional arousals may represent a more intense version of symptoms that are experienced when awakening from deep sleep: decreased cognition, reaction time, and attention.[13]

Box 1
Key features common to disorders of arousal

- Typically occur from stage N3 sleep
- Predilection for the first third of the night
- More common in children
- Decrease in frequency with age
- Amnestic or poor recall of the event
- Events have varying behavior, not stereotypic

Box 2
Precipitating factors for disorders of arousal

- Sleep deprivation
- Forced arousal from sleep (noise, full bladder, pain)
- Circadian rhythm disturbances
- Fever or infection
- Medications (central nervous system [CNS] depressants, psychotropics)
- Sleep-disordered breathing
- Periodic leg movements/restless legs syndrome
- Stress
- Menstrual cycle

Data from International classification of sleep disorders. 2nd edition. Westchester (IL): American Academy of Sleep Medicine; 2005.

Key Clinical Features and Diagnosis

Patients experience mental confusion and disorientation to time and space lasting minutes to hours. They have a blunted response to questions and are less interactive with their environment. They have poor memory of the event, with only rare dream recall. They may speak unintelligibly or may perform more complex motor tasks, possibly clumsy, incorrectly, or inappropriately. They can be difficult to fully awaken and may become violent if this is attempted. This parasomnia can be termed sleep drunkenness or morning sleep inertia.[14] Patients may appear awake with their eyes open during the event.[15]

One form of confusional arousal is sexsomnia or sleep sex, where on awakening, the motor activity is sexual in nature. This activity can involve masturbation, molestation, or sexual assault. There is no recollection of the event by the patient. In addition to potentially leading to psychological and physical consequences to their bed partner, sexsomnia may result in shame, guilt, or medicolegal problems for the patient.[16]

Diagnosis is typically made clinically and can be confirmed with overnight, attended polysomnography (PSG). Home videorecording can also be helpful. Overnight PSG can be helpful by either capturing an episode (**Fig. 4**) or by evaluating for causes of sleep fragmentation or arousals that could trigger confusional arousals, such as sleep apnea (**Fig. 5**) or periodic leg movements. It is also useful to evaluate for other possible causes for the motor behavior, such as seizures or RBD. Even if a typical event is not captured during the overnight study, many of these patients have frequent spontaneous arousals from stage N3 sleep or slow-wave sleep fragmentation, suggesting sleep stage instability or a propensity for NREM sleep parasomnias such as confusional arousals (**Fig. 6**). The cyclic alternating pattern (CAP) also may play a role in causing disorders of arousal. CAP is a measure of NREM instability with a high level of arousal oscillation. Patients who have disorders of arousal are found to have increases in CAP rate, number of CAP cycles, and arousals with electroencephalographic (EEG) synchronization.

Treatment

Efforts to wake up the patient or direct the patient are not typically successful during an event. It is recommended to let the episode run its course and ensure that the

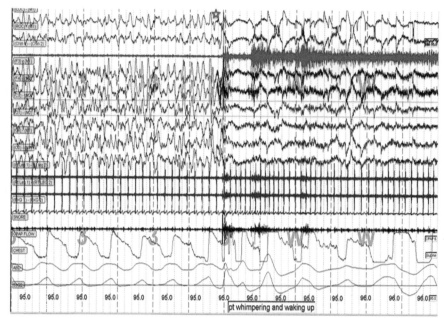

Fig. 4. PSG clip of confusional arousal 60-second epoch of a 35-year-old patient who was undergoing a CPAP titration study to treat obstructive sleep apnea. He had reported episodes of sleep talking and confusion during sleep. There is an awakening from stage N3 sleep followed by the patient starting to whimper and behave confused, consistent with a confusional arousal. EEG shows δ slowing with an arousal, which marks the beginning of the event (*star*). Channels are as follows: electro-oculogram (*left*, LOC-M1; *right*, ROC-M1), chin electromyogram (Chin1-chin2), electroencephalogram (*left*, frontal, F3; central, C3; occipital, O1, left mastoid, M1; and *right*, frontal, F4; central, C4; occipital, O2; right mastoid, M2), left leg EMG (Lt Leg 1-Lt Leg 2), right leg EMG (Rt leg1-Rt leg2), 2 EKG channels (EKG-1, EKG-2), snore channel, CPAP flow, respiratory effort (chest, abdomen [ABD]) and oxygen saturation (Sao₂).

patient is not putting themselves or others in a dangerous situation. To try to prevent episodes from occurring, treating any underlying sleep disorder is important. Ensuring adequate duration of sleep and following good sleep habits are also helpful. Avoiding CNS depressants, alcohol, or other triggers may be necessary. If pharmacologic therapy is warranted, tricyclic antidepressants (TCAs) (clomipramine 25–100 mg at bedtime) or benzodiazepines (clonazepam 0.5–2 mg at bedtime) can be initiated.[17]

Prognosis

In most cases, children outgrow confusional arousals. Many develop sleepwalking. If an underlying cause, such as sleep apnea, is treated or other triggers identified, confusional arousals decrease or disappear.

SLEEPWALKING

Sleepwalking is an arousal disorder culminating in walking around in an altered state with impaired judgment. Sleepwalking occurs most often out of stage N3 sleep and during the first third of the night, but can occur out of other stages of NREM sleep and at any time of the night.

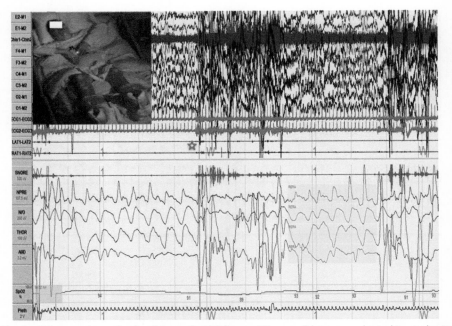

Fig. 5. 120-second epoch of a diagnostic PSG from a 54-year-old man conducted to evaluate for arousals with confusion and singing behavior. The figure shows one of the patient's representative events showing an arousal from slow-wave sleep, as demarcated by the star, with the patient's arms abducted (flapping his arms and described by the technicians to be "quacking like a duck"). Channels are as follows: electro-oculogram (*left*, E1-M2; *right*, E2-M1), chin electromyogram (Chin1-chin2), electroencephalogram (*left*: frontal, F3; central, C3; occipital, O1; left mastoid, M1; and *right*: frontal, F4, central, C4, occipital, O2, right mastoid, M2) 2 ECG channels, 2 limb EMG (LAT, RAT), snore channel, nasal-oral airflow (N/O), nasal pressure signal (NPRE), respiratory effort (thoracic [THOR], abdominal [ABD]) and oxygen saturation (Sao2). *Modified after* Avidan, AY and N Kaplish. The parasomnias: epidemiology, clinical features, and diagnostic approach. Clin Chest Med 2010;31(2):356.

Epidemiology and Risk Factors

No gender difference exists. Prevalence in childhood is as high as 17%, with a peak age of 12 years. Sleepwalking typically decreases in frequency until adulthood, and 3% of adults sleepwalk.[14] Some of the adult sleepwalkers begin to have the condition after childhood (adult-onset sleepwalking). It does seem to run in families, suggesting a genetic component. About 80% of somnambulistic patients have at least 1 family member affected by this parasomnia, and the prevalence of somnambulism is higher in children of parents with a history of sleepwalking.[14,18] A positive association with the HLA-DQB1*05 subtype was found in sleepwalking patients.[19]

Pathophysiology

The pathophysiology of sleepwalking is unknown. The brain is unable to fully awaken from slow-wave sleep. There seems to be incomplete cortical activation in response to an arousing stimulus. One study used transcranial magnetic stimulation to examine brain function in adult sleepwalkers. The study found alterations in sleepwalkers consistent with impaired efficiency of inhibitory circuits during wakefulness, possibly signifying immaturity of neural circuits, synapses, or receptors.[20] Sleepwalkers have

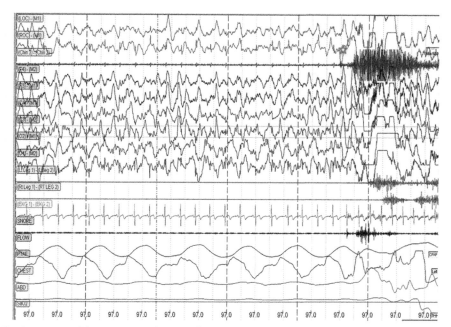

Fig. 6. 17-year-old woman complaining of spells during sleep of ambulating and talking without recollection. A 30-second epoch from her sleep study showing 1 example of the many sponta-neous arousals (*star*) during stage N3 sleep (slow-wave sleep fragmentation), which can be seen frequently in patients with disorders of arousal. Channels are as follows: electro-oculogram (*left*, LOC-M1; *right*, ROC-M1), chin electromyogram (Chin3-chin2), electroencephalo-gram (*left*: frontal, F3; central, C3; occipital, O1; left mastoid, M1; and *right*: frontal, F4; central, C4; occipital, O2; right mastoid, M2), left leg EMG (Lt Leg 1-Lt Leg 2), right leg EMG (Rt Leg1- Rt Leg2), ECG channel (EKG-1, EKG-2), snore channel, thermistor (FLOW), nasal pressure signal (PTAF), respi-ratory effort (chest, abdomen [ABD]) and oxygen saturation (Sao_2).

difficulties maintaining consolidated slow-wave sleep.[21] NREM sleep stage instability, or other sleep disorders such as sleep apnea, periodic leg movements, or restless legs syndrome, commonly cause awakenings, contributing to the development of sleepwalking.

Key Clinical Features and Diagnosis

Episodes usually occur from stage N3 sleep, but may occur out of any NREM sleep stage. They begin abruptly, with the patient having a blank expression with their eyes open. They may appear to be awake, but have decreased awareness of their surroundings and little reactivity. While ambulating, movements are clumsy and slow. Sleep talking or even conversations may be heard. It can be difficult to awaken the patient, and they may react violently to such attempts. At other times, they may listen to instructions and return to bed. They are usually amnestic of the event on awakening in the morning, although they may remember portions of the event.[15] Dreaming is sometimes reported in sleepwalkers, making it difficult to distinguish from RBD. Complex motor activities that have been reported in this state can vary, including driving, cooking, eating, and playing musical instruments.

Diagnosis is usually made clinically, and an overnight sleep study is indicated only in specific cases (**Box 3**).[22] Video, arm leads, and additional EEG leads can be added

> **Box 3**
> **Indications for PSG in evaluation of parasomnias**
>
> - Suspicion of seizures (not confirmed with routine EEG)
> - Behaviors are violent or potentially dangerous
> - Atypical presentation because of age of onset, duration, or semiology
> - Forensic or medicolegal cases
> - Not responsive to conventional therapy
> - Suspicion of another sleep disorder such as sleep apnea

during the study to improve chances of correctly identifying the parasomnia.[22] Although full 18-channel EEG montage had best sensitivity at detecting seizures, a limited 7-channel or 8-channel montage with added temporal leads was superior to a traditional 4-EEG-channel sleep study (central and occipital leads), which had been routinely used in the past.[23] When an overnight study is performed, it is unusual for a sleepwalking episode to be captured in the laboratory. However, the sleep study can be helpful in identifying underlying sleep disorders that may contribute to sleep fragmentation, such as sleep apnea or periodic leg movements. It may also reveal sleep stage instability, with frequent stage shifts or frequent spontaneous arousals from stage N3 sleep (see **Fig. 6**). If an event is captured on sleep study, it can show diffuse rhythmical δ, diffuse δ with intermixed faster frequencies (θ and α), or may be difficult to interpret because of motor artifact.[24]

Treatment

Patients should be instructed to avoid the known triggers (reduce arousals) and any underlying sleep disorders (ie, sleep apnea, periodic leg movement disorder) should be treated. Safety measures and precautions should be put in place (**Box 4**). Often, reassurance is all that is required because sleepwalking may decrease in frequency and resolve in many patients as they get older. Medical treatment may be required if there is fear of injury to the patient or someone else, or if behaviors are disruptive to the family. Treatments include diazepam (2–5 mg) or clonazepam (0.5–2 mg) at bedtime.[24] Trazodone and selective serotonin reuptake inhibitors (SSRIs) are also reported to help in some cases.[25,26]

Prognosis

Sleepwalking decreases with age, which may be because of decreased amounts of slow-wave sleep as we get older, or may be because of full maturation of the brain and its sleep-controlling centers.

> **Box 4**
> **Safety precautions for sleepwalkers**
>
> - Sleep on the first floor
> - Safety gates on stairways
> - Door alarms
> - Secure car keys and weapons
> - Remove oven knobs
> - Clear area of sharp furniture or objects

SLEEP TERRORS

Sleep terrors, also called night terrors, are sudden arousals from NREM sleep associated with intense autonomic and motor symptoms, such as crying or screaming. These events can be dramatic and disturbing to the family, yet the patient may be unfazed by the events.

Epidemiology and Risk Factors

There is no gender difference, but they are more common in children, occurring in up to 6.5%. Prevalence in adults is approximately 2%.[14] Obstructive sleep apnea and other sleep disorders can lead to awakenings from sleep and sleep terrors. Genetic factors play a role, as they do in other disorders of arousal.

Pathophysiology

Pathophysiology is unknown, but is believed to involve mechanisms that control sleep state stability, as in other disorders of arousal.

Clinical Features and Diagnosis

As depicted in **Fig. 7**, on awakening from sleep, patients with sleep terrors have intense autonomic discharge: tachycardia, tachypnea, flushing, diaphoresis, mydriasis, and increased muscle tone. In addition, there is typically screaming or crying initially on awakening and sitting up in bed. The patient does not respond normally and has amnesia for the episode. There can be brief dream fragments or vivid images, which they may remember. During an episode, the person is inconsolable and can be difficult to arouse.[27]

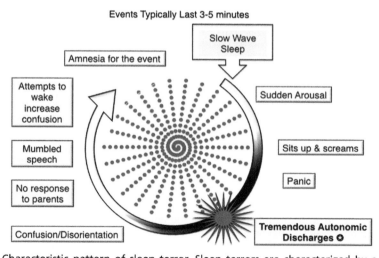

Fig. 7. Characteristic pattern of sleep terror. Sleep terrors are characterized by a sudden arousal associated with a scream, agitation, panic, and heightened autonomic activity (*star*). Inconsolability is almost universal. The child is incoherent and has altered perception of the environment, appearing confused. This behavior may be dangerous and could result in injury. (*Modified after* Avidan, AY and N Kaplish. The parasomnias: epidemiology, clinical features, and diagnostic approach. Clin Chest Med 2010;31(2):361; with permission.)

Diagnosis is made clinically. However, a sleep study may be necessary to evaluate for causes of sleep fragmentation that may lead to sleep terrors, such as sleep apnea or periodic leg movements.[28] A sleep study also helps evaluate for other parasomnias that are on the differential diagnosis such as RBD and seizures. Slow-wave sleep instability with spontaneous arousals is also noted in patients suffering from sleep terrors, as they are in other disorders of arousal. As shown in **Fig. 8**, during a sleep terror, EEG shows δ slowing, and there is an increase in muscle tone, with an increase in respiratory and heart rate.[24]

Differentiation of sleep terrors from an easily confused, but semiologically and sleep stage different parasomnia (REM nightmare) is shown in **Table 2**.

Treatment

Safety precautions, similar to the ones advised in sleepwalking, are important to avoid injuries to the patient or others. Attempts to wake the patient should be avoided because of the possibility of upsetting or confusing them further. The patient should avoid any known triggers for sleep terrors, and underlying sleep disorders should

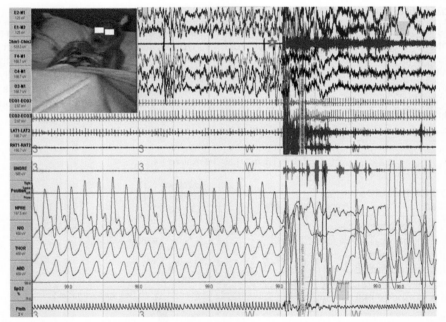

Fig. 8. Two-minute minute epoch of a diagnostic PSG from a 9-year-old boy performed to evaluate arousals associated with screaming and inconsolable crying. The figure shows one of the patient's representative spells showing an arousal with screaming arising out of slow-wave sleep with the patient's arms flexed and held close to the chest (as if afraid and protecting himself). Channels are as follows: electro-oculogram (*left*, E1-M2; *right*, E2-M1), chin electromyogram (Chin1-chin2), electroencephalogram (*right*: frontal, F4; central, C4; occipital, O2; right mastoid, M2) 2 ECG channels, 2 limb EMG (LAT, RAT), snore channel, nasal-oral airflow (N/O), nasal pressure signal (NPRE), respiratory effort (thoracic [THOR], abdominal [ABD]) and oxygen saturation (Sao$_2$). *Modified after* Avidan, AY and N Kaplish. The parasomnias: epidemiology, clinical features, and diagnostic approach. Clin Chest Med 2010;31(2): 358; *Polysomnogram slide courtesy of* Timothy Hoban, MD, Professor of Pediatrics and Neurology, University of Michigan, Ann Arbor, Michigan.

Table 2
Differences between sleep terrors and nightmares

Characteristic	Sleep Terror	Nightmare
Timing during the night	First third (deep slow-wave sleep)	Last third (REM sleep)
Movements	Common	Rare
Severity	Severe	Mild
Vocalizations	Common	Rare
Autonomic discharge	Severe and intense	Mild
Amnesia	Absent	Present
State on waking	Confused/disoriented	Function well
Injuries	Common	Rare
Violence	Common	Rare
Displacement from bed	Common	Very rare

be treated. In most cases, these instructions along with reassurance are all that is necessary because the patient will likely outgrow the sleep terrors. If risk of injury or disruption is sufficient to require treatment, medications that have been shown to be effective include benzodiazepines and imipramine. There have also been reports of trazadone and paroxetine being helpful.[29]

Scheduled awakenings may also be useful if patients that have them at highly predictable times of the night. Parents or family members are instructed to wake the patient 30 minutes before the time that they have their sleep terrors. The patient should be awoken only briefly until their eyes are open or they vocalize, and then put back to sleep.[29] Psychotherapy has also been helpful in patients who suffer from psychopathology.

Prognosis

Sleep terrors typically decrease in frequency as the child grows older, either because of the decreased total sleep time in stage N3 sleep, or because of maturation of the brain.

OTHER PARASOMNIAS
SRED

SRED consists of recurrent episodes of involuntary eating occurring during the main sleep period. This disorder typically involves eating peculiar forms or combinations of food, or possibly dangerous or toxic substances. Like disorders of arousal, most patients do not have full recall of the event. Eating can occur multiple times in 1 night, typically with high caloric foods. Foods may be prepared and cooked, although usually in a sloppy or inappropriate manner.[5]

SRED is commonly associated with sleepwalking, and many have had sleepwalking during childhood. The pathophysiology seems to be similar to the disorders of arousal. Other sleep disorders may also trigger SRED, including obstructive sleep apnea, restless legs syndrome, periodic leg movement disorder, and circadian rhythm disorders. Use of hypnotics along with cessation of smoking or alcohol have also been reported as triggers.[30] There is a female predominance, with the mean age of onset at 22 to 29 years of age. SRED can be distinguished from night eating syndrome (NES), which is characterized by full recall of the eating and absence of bizarre or toxic ingestion. Many have also suggested that SRED and NES may exist along a common spectrum and have many overlapping features.[31]

Treatment includes appropriate management of any underlying sleep disorder. If the patient suffers from other disorders of arousal, recommended treatments for these conditions can help reduce SRED (benzodiazepines and TCAs). Dopamine agonists, SSRIs, and topiramate have all been reported to help improve symptoms, although they lack the support of large trials.[32,33]

Catathrenia

Catathrenia, also called sleep-related groaning, is characterized by expiratory groaning during sleep. Events usually occur nightly and during REM sleep, predominantly in the second half of the night. The sound occurs solely during expiration and sounds like groaning, although the patient does not show emotion or respiratory distress and does not recollect the event. The complaint is usually reported by a bed partner or the affected person may notice hoarseness on awakening. No otolaryngologic or vocal cord abnormalities are found in these cases. There have been some reports of successful use of continuous positive airway pressure (CPAP) in patients with sleep apnea and this condition.[34,35] This is a rare condition with a prevalence of less than 1%, mostly made up of males. There have also been reports of catathrenia secondary to use of sodium oxybate in patients with narcolepsy.[36]

On PSG, as shown in the example in **Fig. 9**, recording sound is required for identifying this condition. The episode generally lasts 2 to 49 seconds, appearing in clusters

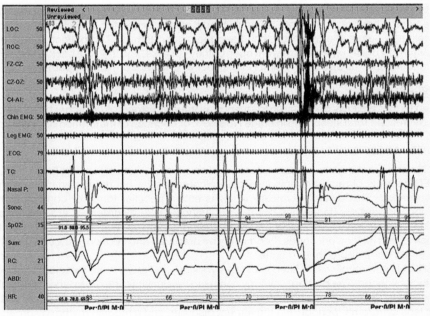

Fig. 9. A 120-second PSG epoch showing 4 episodes of catathrenia. Each episode starts with a deep inhalation followed by a prolonged exhalation with a monotonous sound production as shown by activity in the snore channel. LOC, ROC: ocular channels; FZ-CZ, CZ-OZ, C4-A1: EEG channels; Chin and leg EMG, chin and leg electromyogram channels; ECG, electrocardiogram; Nasal P, nasal flow as measured by nasal pressure transducer signal; Sono, snoring; Spo₂, oxygen saturation; SUM, summation of chest and abdominal respiratory inductance plethysmography (RIP) bands; RC and ABD, chest and abdomen RIP bands; HR, heart rate. (*Modified from* Ramar K and Gay P. Catathrenia: getting the 'cat' out of the bag. Sleep breath 2008;12:292; with permission.)

many times throughout the night during REM sleep. A sudden change in respiratory rhythm is seen in the respiratory channels, usually inspiration followed by a flat line during expiration, ending in arousal on EEG. It is important to distinguish this condition from a central apnea, which it closely resembles, except for the lack of inspiratory signal. No abnormal EEG activity should accompany the vocalizations.[15]

Dissociative Disorder

Dissociative disorders can occur from sleep during transitions between sleep and wake, or within several minutes from awakening from sleep after well-established EEG wakefulness. According to the *Diagnostic and Statistical Manual of Mental Disorders, Fourth Edition*, dissociative disorders are a disruption in the usually integrated functions of consciousness, memory, identity, or perception of the environment. Most patients with sleep-related dissociative disorders also have daytime events and have past history of abuse or psychiatric disease. The condition is more common in females. This condition has also been called pseudoparasomnia.[37]

During an event, patients may scream, run, or engage in violent behaviors lasting minutes to hours, typically longer than disorders of arousal. They may reenact previous sexual or physical abuse situations. The individual is usually amnestic of the event.

PSG shows EEG wakefulness present before, during, and after the episodes if captured during testing. If an event occurs after an arousal from sleep, there must be at least 15 seconds of wakefulness before the activity begins to be consistent with this condition, because many disorders of arousal occur immediately from sleep and have α frequency on EEG during the episode. Treatment typically consists of psychotherapy along with management of other underlying psychiatric disorders such as depression and anxiety.

Exploding Head Syndrome

Exploding head syndrome, also sometimes included in the group of sensory sleep starts, is characterized by a sudden loud noise or sense of explosion in the head either at wake-sleep transition or on waking during the night. The noise can be a loud bang, explosion, or a crash of cymbals, but sometimes less drastic. Patients are typically frightened by their symptoms and concerned about an impending serious health problem. Myoclonic jerks and flashes of light may accompany the sound. They occur more commonly in women, with the median age of onset of 58 years of age. Epidemiology and pathophysiology are unknown, although they are believed to represent a variant of sleep starts.[38] The condition is rarely treated because of its benign nature, but clomipramine, nifedipine, and topiramate have been used.[39,40]

Other Motor Activity During Sleep

Sleep-related movement disorders can sometimes mimic parasomnias. They are different from parasomnias because they are simple, usually stereotyped movements that disturb sleep. One type of sleep-related movement disorder is sleep-related rhythmical movement disorder. In this condition, patients show repetitive, stereotyped, and rhythmical motor behaviors either during sleep or near a nap or bedtime. The behaviors include body rocking, head banging, or head rolling. As shown in **Fig. 10**, the frequency is usually 0.5 to 2 per second, generally lasting less than 15 minutes. The patient may stop the activity if spoken to or distracted. These behaviors mainly occur in infants and children, or adults with developmental delay or other neurologic or psychiatric diseases.[15] No treatment is typically necessary, with the exception of safety precautions in the bedroom if the motor activity could cause

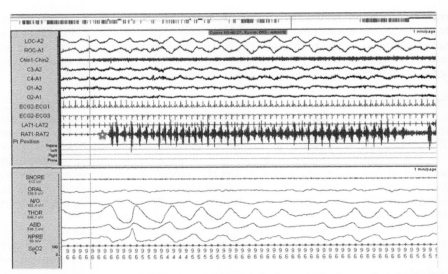

Fig. 10. A 60-second PSG epoch showing unilateral rhythmical movement disorder (*star*) in a patient with untreated obstructive sleep apnea. Channels are as follows: electrooculogram (*left*, E1-M2; *right*, E2-M1), chin electromyogram (Chin1-chin2), electroencephalogram (*right*: frontal, F4; central, C4; occipital, O2; right mastoid, M2) 2 ECG channels, 2 limb EMG (LAT, RAT), snore channel, nasal-oral airflow (N/O), nasal pressure signal (NPRE), respiratory effort (thoracic [THOR], abdominal [ABD]) and oxygen saturation (Sao_2).

harm to the patient. If treatment is necessary, behavioral therapy, hypnosis, and rarely pharmacologic therapy with benzodiazepines have been reported to effective.

Sleep starts, or hypnic jerks, can also mimic parasomnias. These are sudden, brief, simultaneous contractions of the body occurring at sleep onset. They are sometimes associated with a subjective feeling of falling, sensory flash, or sleep-related hallucinations. Sleep starts are common in all ages and sexes. Excessive stimulant use, psychological stress, and sleep deprivation can all increase the frequency of sleep starts.[15] Patients can be reassured regarding the benign nature of sleep starts and do not need medication therapy.

REM PARASOMNIAS
Nightmares

Epidemiology and risk factors
About 10% to 50% of children are affected by nightmares, and up to 75% of the population can remember at least 1 or a few nightmares in the course of their childhood. Prevalence of frequent nightmares, as defined by at least once per week, was 5.1% based on a large community-based cohort of middle-aged Hong Kong Chinese individuals.[41] The frequency of nightmare experiences increases in patients diagnosed with posttraumatic stress disorder, those undergoing medical procedures, and in those with psychological stress caused by major catastrophic events.

Key clinical features and diagnosis
Nightmares manifest as a prolonged and vivid dream pattern that progressively becomes more complex and frightening to the sufferer, terminating in an arousal and vivid recall. Episodes may increase during times of stress, particularly after traumatic events. Certain medications such as β-adrenergic blockers, *L*-dopa, acetyl

cholinesterase inhibitors, and abrupt discontinuation of REM-suppressant medications may induce nightmares. The PSG shows a sudden arousal pattern from REM sleep associated with an increased REM sleep density and variability in heart and respiratory rates.

Treatment
Reassurance is often the only management necessary. However, if offending agents are present, these medications may need to be changed, but for severe and refractory cases, the use of an REM-suppressing agent such as TCAs or SSRIs may be needed.[42-45] Image rehearsal therapy and systematic desensitization and progressive deep muscle relaxation training have been categorized as level A by a recent American Academy of Sleep Medicine best practice guideline.[45]

Recurrent Isolated Sleep Paralysis

Sleep paralysis is the inability to move on awakening and corresponds to lack of voluntary motor function at sleep onset or on awakening.

Epidemiology and risk factors
The episodes may occur at least once in a lifetime in as many as 40% to 50% of normal individuals.

Key clinical features and diagnosis
Sufferers recall a frightening arousal, during which they experience paralysis of skeletal muscles, with the possible exception of respiratory and extraocular movements, although cognition remains intact. Episodes generally last a few minutes and improve spontaneously or on external stimulation. Predisposing features include acute and chronic sleep deprivation and underlying circadian rhythm disturbances, such as jet lag and shift work disorder.

Pathophysiology
The underlying pathophysiology may be related to abnormalities in the mechanism controlling REM sleep muscle atonia.

Treatment
Treatment of sleep paralysis is mainly in the form of reassurance when episodes are infrequent. An example of conservative management is avoidance of an irregular sleep-wake schedule. However, when sleep paralysis is severe, the use of anxiolytic medications and antidepressants such as fluoxetine (as well as other REM-suppressing agents) may be helpful.[46]

RBD

Epidemiology and risk factors
The prevalence of RBD is estimated to be 0.5% of the population.[47] The disorder has a unique gender predilection, affecting male gender by a factor of 9, and has a higher prevalence in patients older than 50 years. Subjective data indicate that as many as 25% of patients with parkinsonism have abnormal dream enactment behaviors suggestive of RBD, whereas formal PSG reports RBD in as many as 47% of patients with Parkinson disease who experience sleep disturbances.[48,49]

Key clinical features and diagnosis
The disorder is uniquely characterized by abnormal elevation of chin or limb muscle tone during REM sleep (**Fig. 11**) and by corresponding complex motor activity associated with elaborate dream enactment, which corresponds with the dream sequence.

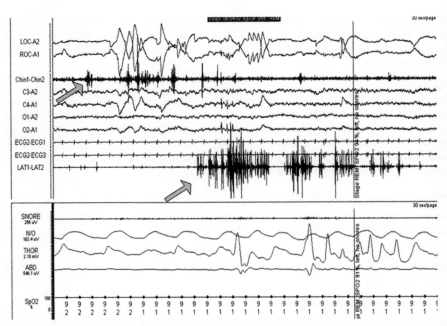

Fig. 11. A 30-second epoch from the diagnostic PSG of an 80-year-old man who was referred to the sleep disorders clinic for evaluation of recurrent violent nighttime awakenings. A typical spell that this patient was experiencing is shown. He was noted to yell, jump from bed, and have complex body movements. The open arrow shows the point during REM sleep at which the patient had abnormal dream enactment behavior associated with REM-associated muscle atonia in the left anterior tibialis muscle. Channels are as follows: electro-oculogram (*left*, LOC-A2; *right*, ROC-A1), chin electromyogram (Chin1-chin2), electroencephalogram (left central, C3-A2; right central, C4-A1; left occipital, O1-A2; right occipital, O2-A1), 2 ECG channels, limb EMG (LAT), snore channel, nasal-oral airflow (N/O), respiratory effort (thoracic [THOR], abdominal [ABD]) and oxygen saturation. (*Modified from* Avidan AY. Sleep disorders in the older patient. Prim Care 2005;32(2):563–86.)

Patients show a spectrum of abnormal dreams, mainly unpleasant and negative themes in which they need to protect themselves. The range of experiences consists of simple verbalizations to singing, yelling, shouting, and screaming to more complex motor phenomena such as walking, running, punching, kicking, jumping, and often agitated and violent behaviors synchronizing with the dream imagery. Often, it is injury to self or bed partner that brings the patient to the attention of the clinician. These complex and polymorphic motor phenomena, which are distinguished from the more stereotyped monomorphic nocturnal seizures, are associated with emotionally charged utterances.[50–53] When awoken from an episode, some patients may have vivid recall and report dream mentation, which correlated with the observed behavior.

The case study in **Box 5** shows a patient with dream enactment behavior and excessive abnormal limb movements that parallel the aggressive dream content. The PSG epoch in **Fig. 11** shows the classic electrographic correlation of the behaviors enacted during dreaming highlighted by the arrows showing excessive chin (Chin1-chin2) and excessive anterior tibialis leg (LAT1-LAT2) electromyographic tone. Antecedal reports of sleep talking, yelling, or limb jerking may be present. With time, the dream content has the potential to become more violent, complex, action-filled, and unpleasant,

---

Box 5
Case study

An 80-year-old man presented with violent dreams reported by his wife of 55 years. He had been noted to move a lot in bed for the past 3 years, but had begun to show aggressive and swift movements against a presumed intruder in the last few months. His wife brought a taperecorded message, which revealed screaming at a supposed intruder saying "You must leave, get out, move away!" A sample of the patient's PSG after presenting to the sleep disorders clinic is shown in **Fig. 11**.

Patients who experience RBD most often experience their spells as soon as they enter REM sleep, which is as early as 90 minutes after sleep onset, but more commonly during the latter half of the night. The spells vary in frequency, from infrequent (ie, once a month) to as frequent as nightly episodes, which leads to significant sleep disruption and more likely results in a referral to the specialist.

---

coinciding with the onset of RBD. If RBD leads to frequent arousals, sleep becomes fragmented, leading to other symptoms such as hypersomnolence. Potential for injury, including facial ecchymosis, skin lacerations, and skull fractures to patient or bed partner, is a major safety concern and warrants immediate and effective pharmacologic intervention.

RBD may be classified into an acute and a chronic form:

1. The acute form of RBD may be seen in the context of medication-related or substance-related, toxic, or metabolic derangements. The most common drug-related and substance-related form includes rapid withdrawal from alcohol, abrupt discontinuation of sedative-hypnotic agents (inducing REM rebound), and examples related to SSRIs, TCAs, monoamine oxidase inhibitors (MAOIs), biperiden, and cholinergic medications.[54–64] Some reports also implicate excessive caffeine consumption (chocolate) as a cause.[65,66] Acute neurologic disorders such as brainstem lesions caused by pontine stroke, multiple sclerosis, subarachnoid hemorrhage, and brainstem neoplasm have all been implicated in the acute form of RBD.[67–70]

2. The chronic form of RBD is typically associated with advanced age as a predisposing factor. This form is idiopathic, generally more frequent, has an onset later in adulthood, progresses over time, and tends to stabilize.

Of the chronic form, about 60% of the cases are idiopathic; the remaining 40% of the cases are associated with underlying neurodegenerative disorders. A spectrum of dementias are implicated in RBD and include the synucleinopathies such as olivopontocerebellar atrophy and diffuse Lewy body disease, with a characteristic α-synuclein inclusion in the nerve cell bodies.

RBD typically begins after age 60 years and may precede clinical manifestation of the underlying neuropathologic lesion process by more than a 10 years.[71–75] Patients with narcolepsy experience a higher incidence of RBD, and presence of RBD in children may indicate the potential onset of evolving narcolepsy.[76] In addition, in patients with narcolepsy, psychiatric medications such as TCAs, SSRIs and MAOIs, which can be used to treat cataplexy, can sometimes trigger or exacerbate RBD in this cohort.[77] As alluded to earlier, RBD is more predominant in men than in women (by a factor of 9), and the reason for this gender predilection is unclear.[70,78,79] Recent data suggest that RBD may be the first sign of childhood narcolepsy in patients with a positive HLA-DQB1 *0602 positive, female gender, in whom cerebrospinal fluid hypocretin level (Hcrt-1) was extremely low.[76,80]

Pathophysiology

RBD is a complex sleep phenomenon with a possible mechanism related to either a reduction of REM atonia or an abnormal augmentation of locomotor intermittent excitatory influences during REM sleep, or both.[51,81]

Fig. 11 shows the underlying pathophysiologic mechanism for RBD, which is proposed to be related to abnormal brainstem control of medullary inhibitory regions. An identical syndrome was reported in cats by the French investigator Jouvet,[82] who experimentally induced bilateral lesions of pontine regions adjacent to the locus coeruleus, inducing absence of the REM-related atonia associated with REM sleep and abnormal motor behaviors during REM sleep. In this experimental model, the animal slept until its first REM sleep episode, during which it jumped, with eyes still closed, and ran around the cage making attack motions. In 1986, Schenck and colleagues[83] described RBD in a new category of sleep disorders, reporting on a series of older patients, mainly men, who presented with aggressive sleep-related behaviors.

Data deduced from single-photon emission computed tomography (SPECT) neuro-imaging reveal a possible mechanism relating to abnormalities in dopaminergic systems showing decreased striatal dopaminergic innervation as well as reduced striatal dopamine transporters.[84–86] In patients with multiple system atrophy and RBD, positron emission tomography as well as SPECT studies indicate reduced nigrostriatal dopaminergic projections.[87] In patients with idiopathic RBD, impaired cortical activation as determined by EEG spectral analysis supports the relationship between RBD and neurodegenerative disorders.[88] **Fig. 12** shows the underlying pathophysiologic mechanism in RBD.

Diagnostic evaluation

PSG reveals abnormal muscle augmentation during REM sleep in excess of the normal REM sleep-related phasic electromyography (EMG) twitches (see **Fig. 11**). The results of the neurologic history and examination may indicate the need for other neuroimaging, looking for structural lesion of underlying neurodegenerative processes. This strategy is especially important if the episodes are acute, follow a neurologic insult, and occur in an otherwise younger patients.[69,89,90]

Differential diagnosis

The differential diagnosis of RBD includes nocturnal frontal lobe seizures, confusional arousals, sleepwalking, sleep terrors, posttraumatic stress disorder, and nightmares. Patients with RBD are often distinguished based on the complex nonstereotypic nature of their episodes, timing later in the night when REM density is highest, and the characteristic patients who are older men.

Treatment

Patients with RBD should be assessed carefully, with meticulous attention to risk for injury during the nocturnal episodes. Environmental safety (level A evidence) is cornerstone and prudent in every patient with likely RBD, especially in those who experience displacement from bed and aggressive spells. Suggested level of pharmacotherapy for RBD is based on clonazepam and melatonin. The former is prescribed in dosages ranging from 0.25 mg to 1 mg by mouth every night at bedtime, achieving improvement in most (90%) patients, with little evidence of tolerance or abuse.[1,91,92] Although clonazepam does not normalize abnormal limb EMG tone during the night, it acts to prevent the arousals associated with the REM sleep disassociation. Treatment of RBD with melatonin may restore REM sleep atonia and was effective in 87% of patients taking 3 to 12 mg at bedtime.[93–95] Melatonin, a dietary supplement,

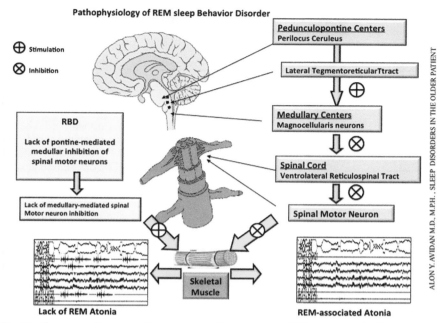

Fig. 12. The normally generalized muscle atonia during REM sleep results from pontine-mediated perilocus coeruleus inhibition of motor activity. This pontine activity exerts an excitatory influence on medullary centers (magnocellularis neurons) via the lateral tegmentoretricular tract. These neuronal groups, in turn, hyperpolarize the spinal motor neuron postsynaptic membranes via the ventrolateral reticulospinal tract. In RBD, the brainstem mechanisms generating the muscle atonia normally seen in REM sleep may be disrupted. The pathophysiology of RBD in humans is based on the cat model. In the cat model, bilateral pontine lesions result in a persistent absence of REM atonia associated with prominent motor activity during REM sleep, similar to that observed in RBD in humans. The pathophysiology of the idiopathic form of RBD in humans is still not well understood but may be related to reduction of striatal presynaptic dopamine transporters. (*Modified from Avidan AY. Sleep disorders in the older patient. Prim Care 2005;32(2):581.*)

is not approved by the US Food and Drug Administration (FDA), has poor regulation in terms of pharmacologic preparation, and side effects have not been widely studied. Other agents that may be helpful for RBD include imipramine (25 mg by mouth every night at bedtime), carbamazepine (100 mg, by mouth 3 times a day) as well as pramipexole or levodopa.[96–98] One recent study described successful amelioration of RBD with sodium oxybate when other treatments are ineffective or poorly tolerated.[99] This finding also suggests that RBD and cataplexy may share a common pathophysiology.[99] Recent data from the Minnesota group[100] suggest the use of an innovative alarm to reduce episodes of RBD in those who may be refractory to traditional pharmacologic agents. **Table 3** summarizes the level of evidence for treating RBD.

Differentiating seizures and parasomnias
Seizures occurring during sleep can closely resemble parasomnias and can pose a diagnostic challenge to the clinician. Nocturnal frontal lobe epilepsy (NFLE) is

Table 3
Evidence-based pharmacotherapy for RBD

Drug[a]	Dose	Level of Recommendation	Special Considerations
Clonazepam	0.25–4.0 mg before bedtime (usual recommended dose is 0.5–2.0 mg)	Suggested[b]	Use with caution in patients with dementia, gait disorders, or concomitant obstructive sleep apnea. Side effects include sedation, impotence, motor incoordination, confusion, and memory dysfunction
Melatonin	3 mg–12 mg before bedtime	Suggested[b]	Effective in patients with α-synucleinopathies, memory problems, and sleep-disordered breathing. Side effects include headaches, sleepiness and delusions/hallucinations
Zopiclone	3.5–7.5 mg before bedtime	May be considered[c]	Side effects include rash and nausea
Yi-Gan San	2.5 gm 3 tid	May be considered[c]	Studied mainly on patients who could not take clonazepam. No side effects were reported when used for the treatment of RBD
Sodium oxybate	Unknown	May be considered[c]	
Donepezil	10–15 mg	May be considered[c]	
Rivastigmine	4.5–6 mg bid	May be considered[c]	Studied mainly on patients with dementia of Lewy body
Temazepam	10 mg	May be considered[c]	
Alprazolam	1–3 mg	May be considered[c]	
Desipramine	50 mg every night at bedtime	May be considered[c]	
Carbamazepine	500–1500 mg every day	May be considered[c]	

[a] Not FDA approved for the treatment of RBD.
[b] Supported by sparse high-grade evidence data, or a substantial amount of low-grade data or clinical consensus.
[c] Supported by low-grade data.
Data from Avidan AY and Zee PC, Handbook of sleep medicine. 2nd edition. Philadelphia: Wolters Kluwer Health/Lippincott Williams & Wilkins; 2011. p. 183.

a good example of this because of its sudden, brief nature of predominantly stereotypic motor activity, which may occur only during sleep and may be missed easily on EEG. **Table 4** shows the distinguishing and common clinical features of NFLE versus NREM and REM sleep parasomnias.[101,102]

Table 4
Differentiating patterns between NFLE and parasomnias: discriminatory components on history

	NFLE	NREM Sleep Parasomnias	REM Parasomnias
Length of event	Typically brief (<1 min)	Longer in duration (5–15 min)	Medium duration (20 s–few minutes)
Motor activity	Stereotyped	Complex, variable	Complex dream enactment (in RBD)
Onset	Within 30 min of sleep	Within 2 h of sleep	Last third of night, during REM sleep
Frequency	Multiple times per a night (clusters of up to 20)	Usually less than 3 times per night	Variable, but rarely more than 1 episode/night
Recall	Can have lucid recall	Amnestic of event	Variable. Dream recall is present if awaken after RBD/nightmare
Other	Presence of aura, dystonic or tonic posturing, abrupt offset	Interaction with environment, wander outside bedroom, slow offset or ending of event	Semiology is that of aggressive behavior toward a supposed intruder, defensive and protective of oneself
Common features of both	Commonly start in childhood, may have vocalizations, motor artifact seen on EEG		RBD: older men

Data from Derry CP, Davey M, Johns M, et al. Distinguishing sleep disorders from seizures: diagnosing bumps in the night. Arch Neurol 2006;63(5):708.

SUMMARY

It is essential for the clinician to understand how to differentiate between each parasomnia or look alikes using features from the history, physical examination, or the overnight sleep study. Historical features such as time of night, age of patient, and recollection of the event are helpful in making the diagnosis. Seizures, rhythmical movement disorder, and dissociative states should always be considered in the differential diagnosis. Sleep study findings may help identify the parasomnia or may uncover underlying sleep disorders that could be triggering the episodes.

Management includes educating the patient and bed partner about safety precautions as well as treating any underlying sleep disorder. Pharmacologic treatment may be necessary in some cases, although the risks of the medications should be considered when making this decision.

REFERENCES

1. Mahowald MW, Ettinger MG. Things that go bump in the night: the parasomnias revisited. J Clin Neurophysiol 1990;7(1):119–43.
2. Broughton R. Behavioral parasomnias. In: Chokroverty S, editor. Sleep disorders medicine. Boston: Butterworth-Heinemann; 1998. p. 635–60.
3. Brooks S, Kushida CA. Behavioral parasomnias. Curr Psychiatry Rep 2002;4(5): 363–8.
4. Mahowald MW, Bornemann MC, Schenck CH. Parasomnias. Semin Neurol 2004;24(3):283–92.

5. American Academy of Sleep Medicine. The international classification of sleep disorders: diagnostic and coding manual. 2nd edition. Westchester (IL): American Academy of Sleep Medicine; 2005. xviii, 297.

6. Avidan AY, Kaplish N. The parasomnias: epidemiology, clinical features, and diagnostic approach. Clin Chest Med 2010;31(2):353–70.

7. Bornemann MA, Mahowald MW, Schenck CH. Parasomnias: clinical features and forensic implications. Chest 2006;130:605–10.

8. Mahowald MW, Schenck CH. Non-rapid eye movement sleep parasomnias. Neurol Clin 2005;23:1077–106.

9. Tassinari CA, et al. Central pattern generators for a common semiology in fronto-limbic seizures and in parasomnias. A neuroethologic approach. Neurol Sci 2005;26(Suppl 3):s225–32.

10. Tassinari CA, Rubboli G, Gardella E, et al. Central pattern generators for a common semiology in fronto-limbic seizures and in parasomnias. A neuroethologic approach. Neurol Sci 2005;26(Suppl 3):s225–32.

11. The international classification of sleep disorders. Westchester (IL): American Academy of Sleep Medicine; 2005.

12. Bjorvatn B, Gronli J, Pallesen S. Prevalence of different parasomnias in the general population. Sleep Med 2010;11(10):1031–4.

13. Broughton RJ. Sleep disorders: disorders of arousal? Enuresis, somnambulism, and nightmares occur in confusional states of arousal, not in "dreaming sleep". Science 1968;159(3819):1070–8.

14. Ohayon MM, Guilleminault C, Priest RG. Night terrors, sleepwalking, and confusional arousals in the general population: their frequency and relationship to other sleep and mental disorders. J Clin Psychiatry 1999;60(4):268–76 [quiz: 277].

15. Anonymous. International classification of sleep disorders. 2nd edition. Westchester (IL): American Academy of Sleep Medicine; 2005.

16. Shapiro CM, Trajanovic NN, Fedoroff JP. Sexsomnia–a new parasomnia? Can J Psychiatry 2003;48(5):311–7.

17. Schenck CH, Mahowald MW. Long-term, nightly benzodiazepine treatment of injurious parasomnias and other disorders of disrupted nocturnal sleep in 170 adults. Am J Med 1996;100(3):333–7.

18. Hublin C, et al. Prevalence and genetics of sleepwalking: a population-based twin study. Neurology 1997;48(1):177–81.

19. Lecendreux M, et al. HLA and genetic susceptibility to sleepwalking. Mol Psychiatry 2003;8(1):114–7.

20. Oliviero A, et al. Functional involvement of cerebral cortex in adult sleepwalking. J Neurol 2007;254(8):1066–72.

21. Guilleminault C, et al. Sleepwalking, a disorder of NREM sleep instability. Sleep Med 2006;7(2):163–70.

22. Kushida CA, et al. Practice parameters for the indications for polysomnography and related procedures: an update for 2005. Sleep 2005;28(4):499–521.

23. Foldvary N, et al. Identifying montages that best detect electrographic seizure activity during polysomnography. Sleep 2000;23(2):221–9.

24. Schenck CH, et al. Analysis of polysomnographic events surrounding 252 slow-wave sleep arousals in thirty-eight adults with injurious sleepwalking and sleep terrors. J Clin Neurophysiol 1998;15(2):159–66.

25. Lillywhite AR, Wilson SJ, Nutt DJ. Successful treatment of night terrors and somnambulism with paroxetine. Br J Psychiatry 1994;164(4):551–4.

26. Balon R. Sleep terror disorder and insomnia treated with trazodone: a case report. Ann Clin Psychiatry 1994;6(3):161–3.

27. Zadra A, Pilon M. NREM parasomnias. Handb Clin Neurol 2011;99:851–68.
28. Guilleminault C, et al. Sleepwalking and sleep terrors in prepubertal children: what triggers them? Pediatrics 2003;111(1):e17–25.
29. Tobin JD Jr. Treatment of somnambulism with anticipatory awakening. J Pediatr 1993;122(3):426–7.
30. Morgenthaler TI, Silber MH. Amnestic sleep-related eating disorder associated with zolpidem. Sleep Med 2002;3(4):323–7.
31. Winkelman JW. Sleep-related eating disorder and night eating syndrome: sleep disorders, eating disorders, or both? Sleep 2006;29(7):876–7.
32. Miyaoka T, et al. Successful treatment of nocturnal eating/drinking syndrome with selective serotonin reuptake inhibitors. Int Clin Psychopharmacol 2003; 18(3):175–7.
33. Howell MJ, Schenck CH. Treatment of nocturnal eating disorders. Curr Treat Options Neurol 2009;11(5):333–9.
34. Guilleminault C, Hagen CC, Khaja AM. Catathrenia: parasomnia or uncommon feature of sleep disordered breathing? Sleep 2008;31(1):132–9.
35. Ott SR, Hamacher J, Seifert E. Bringing light to the sirens of night: laryngoscopy in catathrenia during sleep. Eur Respir J 2011;37(5):1288–9.
36. Poli F, et al. Catathrenia under sodium oxybate in narcolepsy with cataplexy. Sleep Breath 2012;16(2):427–34.
37. Molaie M, Deutsch GK. Psychogenic events presenting as parasomnia. Sleep 1997;20(6):402–5.
38. Evans RW, Pearce JM. Exploding head syndrome. Headache 2001;41(6): 602–3.
39. Jacome DE. Exploding head syndrome and idiopathic stabbing headache relieved by nifedipine. Cephalalgia 2001;21(5):617–8.
40. Palikh GM, Vaughn BV. Topiramate responsive exploding head syndrome. J Clin Sleep Med 2010;6(4):382–3.
41. Li SX, et al. Prevalence and correlates of frequent nightmares: a community-based 2-phase study. Sleep 2010;33(6):774–80.
42. Mahowald MW, Schenck CH. NREM sleep parasomnias. Neurol Clin 1996;14(4): 675–96.
43. Aldrich MS. Sleep medicine. In: Aldrich MS, editor. Sleep medicine, vol. 53. New York: Oxford University Press; 1999.
44. Wise MS. Parasomnias in children. Pediatr Ann 1997;26(7):427–33.
45. Aurora RN, et al. Best practice guide for the treatment of nightmare disorder in adults. J Clin Sleep Med 2010;6(4):389–401.
46. Koran LM, Raghavan S. Fluoxetine for isolated sleep paralysis. Psychosomatics 1993;34(2):184–7.
47. Ohayon MM, Caulet M, Priest RG. Violent behavior during sleep. J Clin Psychiatry 1997;58(8):369–76 [quiz: 377].
48. Comella CL, et al. Sleep-related violence, injury, and REM sleep behavior disorder in Parkinson's disease. Neurology 1998;51:526–9.
49. Eisehsehr I, et al. Sleep in Lennox-Gastaut syndrome: the role of the cyclic alternating pattern (CAP) in the gate control of clinical seizures and generalized polyspikes. Epilepsy Res 2001;46:241–50.
50. Schenck CH, Mahowald MW. REM parasomnias. Neurol Clin 1996;14: 697–720.
51. Mahowald M, Schenck C. REM sleep parasomnias. In: Roth T, Kryger M, Dement W, editors. Principles and practice of sleep medicine. Philadelphia: WB Saunders; 2000. p. 724–37.

52. Schenck CH, Mahowald MW. REM sleep behavior disorder: clinical, developmental, and neuroscience perspectives 16 years after its formal identification in sleep. Sleep 2002;25(2):120–38.

53. Mahowald MW. Parasomnias. Med Clin North Am 2004;88(3):669–78, ix.

54. Tachibana M, Tanaka K, Hishikawa Y, et al. A sleep study of acute psychotic states due to alcohol and meprobamate addiction. Adv in Sleep Research 1975;2:177–205.

55. Passouant P, Cadilhac J, Ribstein M. Les privations de sommeil avec mouvements oculaires par les anti-depresseurs. Rev Neurol (Paris) 1972;127:173–92 [in French].

56. Guilleminault C, et al. Evaluation of short-term and long-term treatment of the narcolepsy syndrome with clomipramine hydrochloride. Acta Neurol Scand 1976;54:71–87.

57. Besset A. Effect of antidepressants on human sleep. Adv Biosci 1978;21:141–8.

58. Shimizu T, Ookawa M, Iijuma S, et al. Effect of clomipramine on nocturnal sleep of normal human subjects. Ann Rev Pharmacopsychiat Res Found 1985;16: 138.

59. Bental E, Lavie P, Sharf B. Severe hypermotility during sleep in treatment of cataplexy with clomipramine. Isr J Med Sci 1979;15:607–9.

60. Akindele MO, Evans JI, Oswald I. Mono-amine oxidase inhibitors, sleep and mood. Electroencephalogr Clin Neurophysiol 1970;29:47–56.

61. Carlander B, et al. REM sleep behavior disorder induced by cholinergic treatment in Alzheimer's disease. J Sleep Res 1996;5(Suppl 1):28.

62. Ross JS, Shua-Haim JR. Aricept-induced nightmares in Alzheimer's disease: 2 case reports. J Am Geriatr Soc 1998;46:119–20.

63. Schenck CH, et al. Prominent eye movements during NREM sleep and REM sleep behavior disorder associated with fluoxetine treatment of depression and obsessive-compulsive disorder. Sleep 1992;15:226–35.

64. Schutte S, Doghramji K. REM behavior disorder seen with venlafaxine (Effexor). Sleep Res 1996;25:364.

65. Stolz SE, Aldrich MS. REM sleep behavior disorder associated with caffeine abuse. Sleep Res 1991;20:341.

66. Vorona RD, Ware JC. Exacerbation of REM sleep behavior disorder by chocolate ingestion: a case report. Sleep Med 2002;3:365–7.

67. Xi Z, Luning W. REM sleep behavior disorder in a patient with pontine stroke. Sleep Med 2009;10(1):143–6.

68. Schenck CH, Mahowald MW. Rapid eye movement sleep parasomnias. Neurol Clin 2005;23(4):1107–26.

69. Plazzi G, Montagna P. Remitting REM sleep behavior disorder as the initial sign of multiple sclerosis. Sleep Med 2002;3(5):437–9.

70. Schenck CH, et al. Rapid eye movement sleep behavior disorder. A treatable parasomnia affecting older adults. JAMA 1987;257(13):1786–9.

71. Pareja JA, et al. A first case of progressive supranuclear palsy and pre-clinical REM sleep behavior disorder presenting as inhibition of speech during wakefulness and somniloquy with phasic muscle twitching during REM sleep. Neurologia 1996;11:304–6.

72. Boeve BF, et al. Association of REM sleep behavior disorder and neurodegenerative disease may reflect an underlying synucleinopathy. Mov Disord 2001; 16:622–30.

73. Boeve BF, et al. Synucleinopathy pathology often underlies REM sleep behavior disorder and dementia or parkinsonism. Neurology 2003;61:40–5.

74. Schenck CH, Bundlie SR, Mahowald MW. Delayed emergence of a parkinsonian disorder in 38% of 29 older men initially diagnosed with idiopathic rapid eye movement sleep behavior disorder. Neurology 1996;46:388–93.

75. Montplaisir J, et al. Sleep and quantitative EEG in patients with progressive supranuclear palsy. Neurology 1997;49:999–1003.

76. Nevsimalova S, et al. REM behavior disorder (RBD) can be one of the first symptoms of childhood narcolepsy. Sleep Med 2007;8(7-8):784–6.

77. Schenck CH, Mahowald MW. Motor dyscontrol in narcolepsy: rapid-eye-movement (REM) sleep without atonia and REM sleep behavior disorder. Ann Neurol 1992;32:3–10.

78. Abad VC, Guilleminault C. Review of rapid eye movement behavior sleep disorders. Curr Neurol Neurosci Rep 2004;4(2):157–63.

79. Ozekmekci S, Apaydin H, Kilic E. Clinical features of 35 patients with Parkinson's disease displaying REM behavior disorder. Clin Neurol Neurosurg 2005;107(4):306–9.

80. Nightingale S, et al. The association between narcolepsy and REM behavior disorder (RBD). Sleep Med 2005;6(3):253–8.

81. Paparrigopoulos TJ. REM sleep behaviour disorder: clinical profiles and pathophysiology. Int Rev Psychiatry 2005;17(4):293–300.

82. Jouvet M, Delorme F. Locus coeruleus et sommeil paradoxal. C R Soc Biol 1965; 159:895–9 [in French].

83. Schenck CH, et al. Chronic behavioral disorders of human REM sleep: a new category of parasomnia. Sleep 1986;9:293–308.

84. Eisensehr I, et al. Reduced striatal dopamine transporters in idiopathic rapid eye movement sleep behavior disorder. Comparison with Parkinson's disease and controls. Brain 2000;123:1155–60.

85. Eisehsehr I, et al. Increased muscle activity during rapid eye movement sleep correlates with decrease of striatal presynaptic dopamine transporters. IPT and IBZM SPECT imaging in subclinical and clinically manifest idiopathic REM sleep behavior disorder, Parkinson's disease, and controls. Sleep 2003;26:507–12.

86. Albin RL, et al. Decreased striatal dopaminergic innervation in REM sleep behavior disorder. Neurology 2000;55:1410–2.

87. Gilman S, et al. REM sleep behavior disorder is related to striatal monoaminergic deficit in MSA. Neurology 2003;61:29–34.

88. Fantini ML, et al. Slowing of electroencephalogram in rapid eye movement sleep behavior disorder. Ann Neurol 2003;53(6):774–80.

89. Bonakis A, et al. REM sleep behaviour disorder (RBD) and its associations in young patients. Sleep Med 2009;10(6):641–5.

90. Stores G. Rapid eye movement sleep behaviour disorder in children and adolescents. Dev Med Child Neurol 2008;50(10):728–32.

91. Schenck CH, Mahowald MW. Polysomnographic, neurologic, psychiatric, and clinical outcome report on 70 consecutive cases with REM sleep behavior disorder (RBD): sustained clonazepam efficacy in 89.5% of 57 treated patients. Cleve Clin J Med 1990;57(Suppl):S9–23.

92. Mahowald MW, Schenck CH. REM sleep behavior disorder. In: Kryger MH, Dement W, Roth T, editors. The principles and practice of sleep medicine. Philadelphia: WB Saunders; 1994. p. 574–88.

93. Takeuchi N, et al. Melatonin therapy for REM sleep behavior disorder. Psychiatry Clin Neurosci 2001;55(3):267–9.

94. Boeve B. Melatonin for treatment of REM sleep behavior disorder: response in 8 patients. Sleep 2001;24(Suppl):A35.

95. Avidan AY, Zee PC. Handbook of sleep medicine. 2nd edition. Philadelphia: Wolters Kluwer Health/Lippincott Williams & Wilkins; 2011. p.

96. Schmidt MH, Koshal VB, Schmidt HS. Use of pramipexole in REM sleep behavior disorder: results from a case series. Sleep Med 2006;7(5):418–23.

97. Fantini ML, et al. The effects of pramipexole in REM sleep behavior disorder. Neurology 2003;61:1418–20.

98. Tan A, Salgado M, Fahn S. Rapid eye movement sleep behavior disorder preceding Parkinson's disease with therapeutic response to levodopa. Mov Disord 1996;11:214–6.

99. Shneerson JM. Successful treatment of REM sleep behavior disorder with sodium oxybate. Clin Neuropharmacol 2009;32(3):158–9.

100. Howell MJ, Arneson PA, Schenck CH. A novel therapy for REM sleep behavior disorder (RBD). J Clin Sleep Med 2011;7(6):639–44 A.

101. Derry CP, et al. NREM arousal parasomnias and their distinction from nocturnal frontal lobe epilepsy: a video EEG analysis. Sleep 2009;32(12):1637–44.

102. Derry CP, et al. Distinguishing sleep disorders from seizures: diagnosing bumps in the night. Arch Neurol 2006;63(5):705–9.

Sleep-Disordered Breathing

Octavian C. Ioachimescu, MD, PhD[a],*, Nancy A. Collop, MD[b]

KEYWORDS

- Sleep-disordered breathing • Obstructive sleep apnea • Snoring
- Central sleep apnea

KEY POINTS

- Obesity is a critical factor in the development of sleep-disordered breathing (SDB).
- Snoring is the most frequent nocturnal symptom suggesting a diagnosis of SDB.
- Other common nighttime symptoms include snorting, gasping, choking, coughing, and witnessed apneas.
- The most frequent diurnal symptom in SDB is excessive daytime sleepiness (EDS).
- Patients suspected of having SDB should undergo a full night of in-laboratory polysomnography (PSG) or in-home oligosomnography (OSG), also called testing with a portable monitor (PM).
- SDB includes a spectrum of disorders; the most common are obstructive sleep apnea (OSA) and central sleep apnea (CSA).

Sleep Disordered Breathing (SDB) spans a spectrum of conditions, including isolated primary snoring (PS), upper airway resistance syndrome (UARS), obstructive sleep apnea (OSA), central sleep apnea (CSA), and obesity hypoventilation syndrome (OHS). OSA implies an intermittent mechanical obstruction of the upper airway during sleep, which leads to reduced airflow to the lungs. CSA is characterized by impaired flow and absent ventilatory effort. UARS describes airflow limitation with frequent arousals from sleep due to flow impairment, whereas PS is generally defined as noisy vibration of the upper airway during sleep without associated alterations in sleep architecture.

Patients suspected of SDB and their bed partners should be subjected to a thorough history, with attention to sleep schedules, daytime symptoms, onset and progression of nocturnal manifestations, exacerbating factors, comorbidities, family history, etc. A targeted physical examination includes assessment of body mass index (BMI), neck circumference, nasal passages, and oropharyngeal area presence of macroglossia, retrognathia, micrognathia, or any palatal abnormalities—all anatomic factors of importance in the pathogenesis of obstructive SDB. PSG and OSG (ie, home sleep

[a] Atlanta Veterans Affairs Medical Center, Emory University School of Medicine, 1670 Clairmont Rd, Decatur, GA, USA; [b] Woodruff Health Sciences Center, Emory University, Atlanta, GA, USA
* Corresponding author.
E-mail address: oioac@yahoo.com

Neurol Clin 30 (2012) 1095–1136
http://dx.doi.org/10.1016/j.ncl.2012.08.003
0733-8619/12/$ – see front matter

testing with a limited number of recording channels) are the modalities of choice to evaluate breathing and potential consequences of impaired airflow during sleep.

Behavioral modifications (avoidance of sleep deprivation, alcohol, sedative medications, and so forth) and positional therapy (ie, avoidance of supine position during sleep) may be of help and potentially sufficient in UARS and PS. A customized, adjustable oral appliance (OA) may be a good therapeutic modality for mild to moderate OSA, whereas in moderate to severe OSA, continuous positive airway pressure (CPAP) or bilevel positive airway pressure (BPAP) may be needed for OSA and occasionally for CSA. Various surgical interventions have been developed, which remain potential considerations in selected cases of OSA, especially of mild to moderate severity. Topical and/or oral agents for nasal congestion and inflammation, radiofrequency ablation of the turbinates, and septoplasty can (1) ameliorate nasal obstruction and (2) help patients with tolerance and adherence to nasal positive airway pressure (PAP) therapy.

NOSOLOGY

The centerpiece of SDB characterization is represented by three types of respiratory events (American Academy of Sleep Medicine [AASM]) 2007 scoring criteria (**Fig. 1**)[1,2]:

- Apnea: complete cessation of flow (ie, flow amplitude ≤10% baseline flow amplitude for more than 90% of the event duration, for ≥10 seconds, as seen in thermistor [preferred], nasal pressure transducer, and/or thoracic or abdominal effort channels).
- Hypopnea (partial apnea): significant reduction in flow, defined as follows: (1) flow amplitude between 10% and 70% of the baseline flow amplitude associated with a 4% oxygen desaturation by pulse oximetry (Centers for Medicare and Medicaid Services [CMS], main AASM, or recommended definition) or (2) flow between 10% and 50% of the baseline flow amplitude associated with a 3% oxygen desaturation by pulse oximetry or an arousal (alternative definition), for more than 90% of the event duration, for ≥10 seconds, as seen in nasal pressure transducer (preferred), thermistor, and/or thoracic or abdominal effort channels.
- Respiratory effort–related arousals (RERAs): defined as a sequence of breaths lasting at least 10 seconds, characterized by increasing respiratory effort or flattening of the nasal pressure waveform leading to an arousal from sleep, as shown by progressively more negative esophageal pressure preceding the arousal and subsequent resumption of normal pressures.[1] RERAs are primarily used to identify patients who may have UARS. Esophageal manometry measuring distal esophageal pressure (Pes) is generally needed to identify UARS. Progressively lower esophageal pressures signify increasing respiratory effort in the setting of dynamic increase in upper airway resistance during sleep.

Apneas and hypopneas are considered obstructive if there is evidence of respiratory effort, central if there is no effort, and mixed if a respiratory event has both obstructive and central features (the first being the central component). These respiratory events are the individual terms of the following diagnostic and severity indices:

- Apnea hypopnea index (AHI) (ie, the combined total number of apneas and hypopneas per hour of sleep)
- Respiratory disturbance index (RDI) (ie, the combined total number of apneas, hypopneas, and RERAs per hour of sleep)

The diagnosis of OSA syndrome (OSAS) in adults is established when the AHI or RDI is 5 or higher plus symptoms, such as EDS, fatigue, nonrefreshing sleep, awaking with

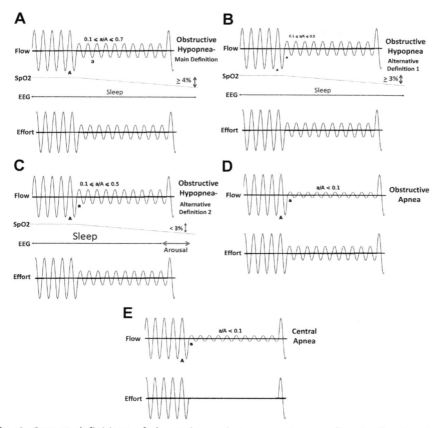

Fig. 1. Current definitions of the main respiratory events, according to the American Academy of Sleep Medicine (AASM) 2007 scoring criteria.

gasping or choking, and bed partner reports of loud snoring or breathing pauses during a patient's sleep.[1] An index (either AHI or RDI) of 5 to 14 is considered mild OSA, an index between 15 and 29 defines moderate OSA, whereas 30 events per hour or more characterize severe OSA. A diagnosis of OSA can also be established without symptoms, but the RDI should be 15 or greater.[1] For children, AHI or RDI cutoff is 1.

KEY CLINICAL FEATURES AND DIAGNOSIS OF SDB
Sleepiness

EDS is a frequent symptom that occurs even in normal individuals and is characterized by a tendency or propensity to fall asleep during periods of desired wakefulness.

In general, EDS may present as

- An abnormal propensity to fall asleep and consequently doze off at inappropriate times or settings, especially in low-stimulus conditions, such as lying on a couch or sitting in a quiet environment, watching television, reading, and so forth.
- Sudden-onset, brief sleep episodes (sleep attacks): these episodes may occur during active situations, such as reading, talking, operating machinery, driving, eating, and so forth.

In patients with SDB, short-duration naps are nonrefreshing and typically patients do not recall dreaming. Impaired memory and concentration may be simply the consequence of a state of drowsiness or periods of microsleep intercalated with wakefulness. **Table 1** lists the main tools used to assess sleepiness in SDB and **Table 2** illustrates a differential diagnosis based on daytime sleepiness as a presenting symptom.

Fatigue

Although it is important to differentiate between EDS and fatigue or lack of energy, asthenia, poor concentration, and tiredness, it is not always easy to ascertain these distinctions. For example, even in obstructive SDB there seem to be certain patient populations who tend to complain more of fatigue versus EDS (premenopausal women, depressed patients, and so forth). Furthermore, CSA can sometimes present predominantly with excessive daytime fatigue as opposed to severe degrees of EDS.

OBSTRUCTIVE SLEEP APNEA

Teaching points
- OSA is a condition characterized by repetitive closure of the upper airway during sleep.

Table 1 Main clinical tools available to evaluate sleepiness in SDB		
Subjective assessment of sleepiness	SSS	SSS measures sleepiness at a specific point in time; varies from 1 ("feeling active and vital; alert wide awake") to 7 ("almost in reverie; sleep onset soon; lost struggle to remain awake").
	KSS	KSS was originally developed to constitute a 1-D scale of sleepiness and was validated against alpha and theta electroencephalogram activity as well as slow eye movement electro-oculogram activity.
	ESS	ESS is the most commonly used scale in clinical practice; it gauges sleepiness as no (0), mild (1), moderate (2), or high (3) chance to fall asleep in 8 specific situations, averaged over a recent period of time (total score: 0–24).
Objective measures of sleepiness	MSLT	The MSLT is currently the standard validated test used to measure objectively one's tendency to fall asleep, based on the assumption (generally true) that the level of sleepiness is well correlated with the sleep latency at that particular point in time.
	MWT	MWT assesses the ability to resist the urge to fall asleep during conducive, soporific conditions and provides an objective measure of the capacity to stay wake. MWT can be used to assess the efficacy or optimize a therapeutic modality (eg, CPAP) or to assess patient's fitness to drive, fly, or work.
	Other tools (mainly used in research)	Pupillometry, driving stimulators, and psychomotor vigilance testing

Table 2
Causes of excessive daytime sleepiness

General Categories	Examples
SDB	OSA, CSA, OHS
Narcolepsy	Narcolepsy with and without cataplexy, due to medical condition, medications, etc.
Idiopathic hypersomnia	With or without long sleep time, due to medical conditions, drugs, etc.
Acute and chronic sleep deprivation	Including behaviorally induced insufficient sleep syndrome
Circadian misalignments	Circadian disorders, shift work, time zone lag, etc.
Psychiatric conditions	Depression, bipolar disorder, etc.
Systemic conditions	Hypothyroidism, chronic fatigue syndrome, fibromyalgia, etc.

- OSAS is defined as 5 respiratory events (apneas, hypopneas, and/or RERAs) per hour of sleep in addition to symptoms attributable to this condition.
- Risk factors for OSA are age, menopause, certain ethnicities, obesity, neck circumference, and nasal and pharyngeal anatomy.
- Typical symptoms in adults include loud snoring, witnessed apneas, gasping, choking, snorting, and frequent awakenings, resulting in poor quality and/or quantity of sleep, intermittent hypoxia, and subsequent EDS or other daytime sequellae. Symptoms in children are more variable.
- PSG is the gold standard test for diagnosis of OSA. A valid alternative diagnostic method is home sleep testing or PM or OSG.
- AHI or RDI is the metric most commonly used to determine the severity of OSA. An index between 5 and 14 represents mild OSA, 15 to 29 is moderate OSA, and 30 or higher is severe OSA.
- PAP is the preferred therapeutic option for moderate to severe OSA and optionally for mild OSA.

Introduction

OSA is a condition characterized by repeated episodes of complete (apnea) or partial (hypopnea and RERA) cessation of airflow due to upper airway closure during sleep.[3] When these respiratory events are associated with EDS, the diagnosis of OSA hypopnea syndrome or OSAS is made.

In 2007, the AASM named an Adult Obstructive Sleep Apnea Task Force, charged to review available evidence and to assembly a set of clinical guidelines for evaluation, management, and follow-up of these patients. The *Clinical Guideline for the Evaluation, Management and Long-Term Care of Obstructive Sleep Apnea in Adults* was published in 2009[4] to better assist physicians who take care of OSA patients. The levels of recommendation were as follows: standard, guideline, or option; whenever available, the strength of recommendations for each component of diagnosis and therapy is listed in light of this 2009 AASM document.

Overall, OSA poses several health risks, from increased perioperative morbidity[5,6] to hypertension,[7] coronary artery disease,[8,9] cardiac dysrrhythmias, sudden death,[10] stroke,[11,12] pulmonary hypertension,[13] and deep vein thrombosis.[14] OSA has been associated in many studies with metabolic syndrome and is thought to contribute or to aggravate some of the metabolic abnormalities.[15] Data from the Sleep Heart Health Study[16] showed abnormal 2-hour glucose tolerance test in 9.3% of patients without OSA versus 15% of those with moderate or severe OSA (odds ratio [OR] 1.44). Marin and colleagues[17] found that untreated, severe OSA is a significant risk factor for the development of nonfatal myocardial infarction and stroke (OR 3.17) compared with healthy participants. The Sleep Heart Health Study[18] found that the OR for developing hypertension was 1.37 in patients with severe OSA versus participants without OSA, even after controlling for BMI, age, alcohol consumption, and smoking status. The Wisconsin Sleep Cohort study,[19] also found a dose-response relationship between the severity of OSA and the presence of hypertension after 4 years of follow-up (OR 2.03 for AHI 5–15 and 2.89 for AHI >15). In other studies, OSA was found an independent risk factor for cerebrovascular disease independent of hypertension, age, or other known cardiovascular risk factors.[12] Many other prospective and cross-sectional studies are also linked SDB to depression and diminished quality of life.[20,21] Alternatively, SDB-caused sleepiness leads to significant morbidity and mortality on the roads and in the workplace. EDS has been shown a risk factor for motor vehicle crushes,[22,23] occupational accidents,[22,24] and impaired cognitive function.[25]

Most of the earlier publications linking SDB and an increase in mortality have been studies on clinic patient samples; this raises a concern for potential referral bias. This concern, however, is at least partially counterbalanced by the evidence from 2 large population-based studies, 1 from the United States and 1 from Australia. The Australian study included residents from a small town of Busselton,[26] who underwent investigation with a home sleep apnea monitoring device (MESAM IV). Mortality was determined after a mean follow-up of 13.4 years and the data were analyzed for a total of 380 participants. Analysis was done after adjustment for age, gender, BMI, mean arterial pressure, total cholesterol, high-density lipoprotein, diabetes, and angina. Patients with history of myocardial infarction and stroke were excluded from the study. The investigators found that mild sleep apnea was not an independent risk factor for higher mortality, but moderate to severe sleep apnea was independently associated with greater risk of all-cause mortality (hazard ratio 6.24) compared with non-OSA participants. Similarly, in the Wisconsin Sleep Cohort (n = 1522) after an 18-year follow-up, Young and colleagues[27] found those with severe SDB had a 3-fold higher hazard ratio for all-cause mortality, after adjustment for age, gender, BMI, and other factors. These 2 studies found either no or negligible association between mild sleep apnea and mortality. Mild OSA, however, may have greater public health significance than moderate to severe OSA, because it is more common, and to determine with certainty this association (ie, to overcome the dilution of a possible smaller effect), further investigation, in larger cohorts, may be needed.

Epidemiology and Risk Factors

Epidemiology

Population-based studies performed in Western countries show that up to 6% of adults (up to 7% of men and up to 5% of women) are likely to have undiagnosed OSAS.[20,28–33] This does not take into account, however, the large proportion of adults with OSA without associated sleepiness. This is an area of controversy and its public health significance remains to be determined; however, many studies have shown adverse health outcomes associated with OSA, regardless of the presence of sleepiness. One of the more recent epidemiologic studies, done in Sao Paulo, Brazil, on more than 1000 participants who were evaluated with questionnaires, full physical examination, and blood work and monitored with actigraphy and PSG, found the prevalence of OSA approximately 15%.[34] Several studies may have underestimated the true prevalence of the disease (eg, studies using pulse oximetry, which used the number of desaturations of >4%/h as a surrogate metric[35]), whereas other publications may have overestimated it (eg, including breath holds during wakefulness or central apneas during sleep[36]). Although prevalence estimates from different countries range between 3% and 28% for mild OSA and 1% and 14% for moderate OSA, the prevalence estimates using similar design and methodology (in Wisconsin and Pennsylvania in the United States, in Spain, and so forth) show that approximately 1 in 5 adults has at least mild OSA and 1 in 15 has at least moderate OSA.[20,28–32,37–40] In adults, there is good evidence that SDB increases in prevalence with age and that it does not correlate well with the presence of daytime sleepiness.[29,30,39,41,42] Little is known today about the natural history, progression, and rate of occurrence of the disease over a given time interval, when studying by age groups. A few population studies have studied OSA progression and focused on changes in AHI over time rather than on incidence. Follow-up data from the Wisconsin Sleep Cohort showed a significant increase in OSA severity (AHI almost doubled) over an 8-year time period. Progression was significantly greater in obese individuals. The 4-year preliminary data from the same study showed that a 10% increase in weight was associated with a 32% increase in AHI and 6-fold risk of developing moderate or severe OSA. A 10% decrease in weight was associated with a 26% decrease in AHI.[20,37] The Cleveland Family Study showed similar trends and numbers.[20,43] Nevertheless, none of the studies provided insight into disease progression in individuals aged 65 and above. For this age category, long-term follow-up (18 years) of SDB in older adults showed little change in AHI with age.[20,43]

Risk factors

Despite a rising awareness about OSA as a prevalent clinical condition, even today, 70% to 80% of those suffering of OSA remain undiagnosed.[44,45] Some of the most important risk factors for OSA are discussed.

Age Irrespective of the methodology, population sample size, geographic location, or diagnostic criteria used, several epidemiologic studies have demonstrated an increased number of respiratory events during sleep in elderly subjects. The EPESE trial[46] showed that more than 50% of elderly individuals (older than 65) had at least 1 chronic sleep complaint, such as trouble falling asleep, waking up, awaking too early, needing to nap, or not feeling rested. Furthermore, the prevalence of SDB ranges from 30% to 70% in this age group versus 2% to 4% in middle-aged adults.[29,30,47,48] With advancing age, sleep is more fragmented and stages N1 and N2 (sleep stages more vulnerable for the development of respiratory instability) are over-represented.

Obesity Obesity and overweight are becoming significantly more common conditions in the modern world, particularly in Western society.[49,50] Obesity, in particular the abdominal (also called truncal or central) type, is a major risk factor for OSA, as shown in several cross-sectional[51–59] and population-based [28,35,38,60–65] studies. Thus, it is not surprising to see a high prevalence of OSA (up to 77%) in bariatric surgery patients.[66–68] In the Wisconsin Sleep Cohort study, investigators found that an increment of 1 SD in BMI was associated with a 4-fold increase in OSA prevalence.[28] The increased risk may be due to anatomic changes of the upper airway (ie, fat and/or muscle deposition around the collapsible portion of the upper airway [collapsible tube theory], reductions in functional residual capacity and vital capacity [tracheal tug theory])[69] or an imbalance between the mechanical load and ventilator drive [neurologic theory]).

Gender Between 2% and 5% of women and 6% to 9% of men have OSA (defined as an AHI of at least 5 and coexistent EDS and/or comorbid cardiovascular disorders [eg, hypertension]).[29,30,70] Although some of the gender differences are age dependent, for men there seems to be a specific predisposition to develop SDB during the age interval of 40 to 55 years.[36,70,71] This may be due to differences in upper airway structure, with more fat in the lateral pharyngeal wall in men versus women, and greater pharyngeal dilator activity in women compared with men. Furthermore, pregnancy is associated with an increase in prevalence of snoring, likely due to the cephalad displacement of the diaphragm and to nasopharyngeal edema[72]; although up to a third of pregnant women snore, overt OSA is not uncommon.[72,73] Hormonal influences likely have an important role in pathogenesis of OSA because (1) disease prevalence is higher in postmenopausal compared with premenopausal women and (2) hormonal therapy (estrogen with or without progesterone) has been associated with lower prevalence of OSA in several epidemiologic studies.

Genetic factors Although familial aggregation observed in several studies may also be related to common lifestyle habits, there are several publications suggesting a genetic predisposition to snoring and OSA, with a global relative risk between 3 and 5, and higher values if both parents are affected.[74–80] Several studies showed that the heritability of the AHI is up to 35%,[78,81,82] suggesting that one-third of the variance is due to genetic factors; approximately 40% of the AHI variance can be explained by obesity, whereas the rest of the variance can be attributed to nongenetic and obesity-independent factors.[83] Among anthropometric factors involved in pathogenesis, craniofacial shape and size of the bones and soft tissues represent another way by which genes may influence predisposition to OSA.[84] Overall, it seems clear that SDB is not due to 1 single genetic mutation or a highly prevalent genotype in the general population.

Overall, genetics may explain several ethnic differences described in epidemiologic studies of OSA.[80] African Americans and Asians seem at higher risk for OSA at a given BMI. A higher prevalence and greater severity of OSA was found in a nonobese Asian population sample versus white individuals.[48] Cephalometric measurements in Asian and white patients with OSA showed that Asians had a narrower cranial base angle, an anthropometric dimension that may signal a propensity to develop SDB.[85] Another study showed that Asians had higher Mallampati grade, smaller thyromental distance, and steeper thyromental plane than white patients, after controlling for BMI and neck circumference.[86]

Smoking In the Wisconsin Sleep Cohort study current smokers had a significantly greater risk of snoring (OR 2.3) and of moderate or severe OSA (OR 4.4) versus never-smokers. Heavy smokers ($\geq$2 packs of cigarettes/d) had the greatest risk of mild SDB (OR 6.7) and of moderate or severe OSA (OR 40.5).[87] Possible mechanisms for the role of smoking in OSA include airway inflammation, smoking related disease, and effects of declining blood nicotine levels on sleep stability. Furthermore, smoking adds to the cardiovascular risk posed by SDB, further complicating the issue of cardiovascular morbidity attributable to OSA.[88]

Alcohol Alcohol has a relaxing action on some of the upper airway dilator muscles, thus increasing upper airway collapsibility, which may lead to OSA in chronic snorers, even in healthy people.[89] It has been shown that ethanol increases the duration and frequency of obstructive respiratory events in patients with OSA.[90,91]

Nasal congestion In the Wisconsin Sleep Cohort,[92] the OR for OSA in individuals with chronic nasal congestion was 1.8. Similar effect size (2-fold increased risk) has been found in the Busselton Health Study.[26] Furthermore, patients with seasonal or allergic rhinitis have been found to have higher AHIs when symptomatic compared with symptom-free periods of time, supporting a role for nasal congestion in OSA.[93]

Other risk factors Several conditions have been identified as additional risk factors for OSA: acromegaly,[94–97] hypothyroidism,[95,98] polycystic ovary syndrome,[99,100] testosterone therapy,[101,102] and so forth (by increasing the amount and density of the soft tissue in and around upper airway and through effects on respiratory centers).

Pathophysiology

Research indicates that both anatomic and neuromuscular factors contribute to the upper airway collapse. Several major theories have been proposed to explain the pathogenesis of OSA.

Anatomic theory

It is plausible that the majority of the patients with OSA have an anatomically small pharyngeal airway. This concept was suggested by tomographic studies,[103] which found reduced cross-sectional area in the nasopharynx, oropharynx, and/or hypopharynx of patients with OSA. Similar studies, done by Schwab and colleagues,[104–106] reported that enlarged tongue and lateral pharyngeal wall size independently increased the risk for OSA. Furthermore, Remmers and colleagues[107] and Isono and colleagues[108] studied patients with general anesthesia and complete muscle paralysis and showed that patients with OSA have higher collapsing pressures and a smaller airway size than normal control subjects (ie, independent of the upper airway dilator muscles). Women tend to have a smaller pharynx and oropharyngeal junctions compared with men but overall tend to have a lower prevalence of OSA, suggesting that anatomic factors may not be sufficient to produce dynamic pharyngeal collapse during sleep. Thus, neuromuscular factors must play a role in protecting the patency of the airway.

Neurologic control theory

There are more than 20 muscles in the human pharynx, generally grouped into phasic (eg, genioglossus) and tonic muscles (eg, tensor palatini). Among oropharyngeal muscles, the genioglossus muscle has been studied the most, mainly due to its potent airway dilator action.

The activity of the pharyngeal dilator muscles is modulated by several factors[109–111]:

1. Output from respiratory centers in the medulla, which leads to inspiratory phasic activation of the genioglossus, preparing the upper airway for negative inspiratory pressure even before the inspiratory flow begins; this suggests coordination at the level of central nervous system (CNS) between upper airway and diaphragm.
2. Falling Pao_2 and transitory elevation of $Paco_2$ are potent stimuli for the central drive to the upper airway and decreasing pharyngeal collapsibility.
3. Negative intrapharyngeal pressure—the most important local stimulus for the activation of the pharyngeal muscles during wakefulness. Topical anesthesia substantially reduces this reflex, whereas CPAP reduces the elecromyographic tonus of the genioglossus muscle to near-normal levels in patients with OSA but has little effect in controls (suggesting that increased upper airway dilator muscle activity even during wake state compensates for a more vulnerable state of the upper airway in OSA patients).
4. State-sensitive activity of the upper airway muscles—transition from wake to sleep is associated with initial fall but with subsequent recovery of genioglossus activity and continued fall in the activity of tensor palatini muscle. During sleep, the

negative pressure reflex is also substantially diminished or lost completely, more so in patients with OSA. This decrease in muscle activity in patients who have anatomically small and collapsible airway leads to dynamic collapse (ie, obstructive respiratory events).

Other factors involved in pathogenesis (other theories)

- It has also been posited that repetitive opening and closing of the upper airway and vibratory trauma lead to muscle and neuronal fiber injury, with subsequent functional sensorimotor dysfunction of these muscles. This could attenuate the response of the muscles to the markedly negative airway pressures generated during periods of airway obstruction.
- Respiratory instability may also contribute to the OSA pathogenesis (eg, loop gain concept from engineering). Loop gain is essentially a metric of the tendency of the control system (respiratory centers) to modulate respiration in response to a stimulus or a signal perturbation. A newer technology using the loop gain concept applied to the respiratory system is the so-called proportional assist ventilation modality.[110,111] Patients with elevated loop gain have a more unstable respiratory system (eg, patients with OSA) than people with loop gain of less than 1, who can stabilize the airway in response to the same signal or perturbation.
- Reduction in lung volumes during sleep (eg, decreased functional residual capacity) as an effect of decubitus position and the effect of intrabdominal content on the diaphragm may lead to loss of tracheal tug on the upper airway, resulting in decreased airway size and higher airway collapse during sleep.

Key Clinical Features and Diagnosis

History

The presence of OSA is often initially suspected on the basis of a patient's daytime experience (sleepiness and fatigue) and on the nighttime bed partner's experience (witnessed snoring and apneas). Characteristic symptoms include (**Box 1**) loud snoring, witnessed apneas, gasping or choking, nocturnal awakenings resulting in poor sleep quality, and EDS, but many times daytime sleepiness is absent. In women, fatigue may be a more common symptom. Moodiness, irritability, lack of concentration, problems with memory, and morning headaches are other common symptoms.[112] Sleepiness, although sometimes difficult to define,[113] is a symptom that is frequently encountered in patients with sleep apnea. Additionally, patients with neurologic disorders may not experience the same symptoms or be able to express similar resultant symptoms as the general population. The spectrum of clinical descriptions usually spans several categories.

Objective

- Behavioral—dozing off, inattention, lack of concentration, frequent yawning, irritability, and hyperactivity in children
- Functional—by assessing activity levels (using accelerometers or actigraphs), performance tests (driving simulators or psychomotor vigilance tests), and polygraphic testing (PSG, portable testing, maintenance of wakefulness test [MWT], multiple sleep latency test [MSLT], pupillometry, cerebral evoked potentials, etc)

Subjective Different scales for sleepiness (eg, Stanford Sleepiness Scale [SSS], Karolinska Sleepiness Scale [KSS], and Epworth Sleepiness Scale [ESS] [see **Table 1**]), fatigue (eg, fatigue severity scale), and so forth. A recent analysis of various parameters' performance in diagnosing SDB[114] has shown that ESS has, unfortunately, an

---

Box 1
Clinical manifestations of OSA

Daytime symptoms

   EDS

   Excessive daytime fatigue

   Morning headaches

   Dry mouth (xerostomia) or sore throat

   Frequent yawning

   Memory and concentration problems

   Increased irritability

Nighttime symptoms

   Loud snoring

   Gasping, chocking, snorting

   Witnessed apneas

   Urinary frequency and polyuria

   Gastroesophageal reflux and/or heartburn

   Frequent arousals

   Sleep maintenance insomnia

   Decreased libido and erectile dysfunction

---

unacceptably high false-negative rate (0.71), which may limit its value in screening for sleep apnea (at least in isolation). Snoring, although strongly associated with OSA, has a positive predictive value of only 63% and a negative predictive value of 56%. Witnessed apneas, similarly to hypersomnolence, have positive and negative predictive values in the range of 40% to 60%. A composite instrument, the Berlin Questionnaire,[115] which is a widely used integrated questionnaire, has false-negative rates up to 38.2%,[114] which also makes it an imprecise tool for screening. Nocturia and enuresis generally suggest benign prostatic hypertrophy in men and overactive bladder or urinary incontinence in women but are also common symptoms in elderly individuals with OSA and generally are ameliorated with effective treatment. Dementia and SDB can coexist; cognitive impairment caused by sleep fragmentation and intermittent hypoxia can be misinterpreted as early sign of dementia in elderly subjects with SDB. Overall, in the elderly, nocturia, sleepiness, and inattention can all increase the risk of accidental falls and subsequent morbidity.

Physical examination

It is important to measure a patient's height and weight and to derive the BMI (ie, weight in kg/height in cm^2). Neck circumference should also be checked because a large cricoid-level neck girth has been associated with OSA. A careful examination of the nose is intended to identify narrow nasal passages, possible deviated septum, hypertrophied nasal turbinate mucosa, and assessment of the internal and external nasal valves with deep inhalation. The overjet is the horizontal distance (in mm) of potential overlap between the central incisors of the maxilla and mandible. The overbite is the vertical distance of overlap (in mm) of the maxillary teeth in relation to the mandibular teeth. Presence of a cross bite, dental malocclusion, retrognathia, or macrognathia should also be looked for carefully. Clinicians should look for a high-arched or narrow hard palate; a low-lying soft palate; long, edematous, low-hanging uvula; tonsillar and adenoid hypertrophy; macroglossia; and temporomandibular joint laxity, all of which may be contributing factors for a small airway cross-sectional area. A fiberoptic upper airway endoscopy in awake, supine patients could facilitate identification of upper airway collapse. A Müller maneuver (sudden inspiratory effort with glottis closed) performed with continuous pressure monitoring can reveal airway collapse at low negative intrathoracic pressures (eg, -6 to -10 cm H_2O). A correlation has been seen between the collapsibility pressures in awake supine patients and the negative pressures during sleep.

The most typical patients with OSA are represented by obese men between 40 and 60 years of age,[28] although this disorder is common at other ages (eg, young children with adenoid and tonsilar hypertrophy) and in both genders (eg, postmenopausal women). Most patients are obese (BMI $\geq$30 kg/m^2). Obesity is also one of the components of the Berlin Questionnaire.[115] Not uncommonly, OSA patients may have a normal physical examination, except for obesity or overweight status, presence of hypertension, and an abnormal oropharyngeal examination. They typically have a crowded or narrow oropharyngeal airway.[4] The OR of having OSA increases by 2.5 for every 1-unit increase in the Mallampati score.[116] Narrow oropharyngeal aperture may be the consequence of retrognathia or micrognathia; macroglossia; enlarged, edematous uvula and soft palate; posterior pharyngeal mucosal edema and cobblestoned appearance; adenotonsillar lymphoid tissue hypertrophy (especially in children); kissing tonsils; high arched palate; and so forth. A neck circumference of more than 17 inches in men (43 cm) and 15 inches in women (38 cm) has been associated with an increased risk of OSA.[4,117,118] Some patients may have pulmonary arterial hypertension, but it is generally mild, except when OSA coexists with a condition leading to daytime hypoxia, such as OHS, parenchymal lung disorders, or a cardiovascular condition (eg, congestive heart failure).

Diagnosis

The use of home-based nocturnal oximetry alone as a screening tool for OSA has a sensitivity of only approximately 31% and can lead to significant underestimation of OSA prevalence[35] and/or severity.[119] Derived from pulse oximetry data, the number of oxygen desaturations per hour (oxygen desaturation index) can be used as a surrogate metric of SDB severity stratification. Clinical impression or symptom-based diagnosis alone lacks the necessary diagnostic accuracy for the disorder; therefore, objective testing by PSG is required in most cases.

Polysomnography PSG is the gold standard test for the diagnosis of OSA.[120] It is also called type I sleep diagnostic testing and is performed in a sleep laboratory, attended by specialized technologists throughout the duration of the study. The complex polygraphic signals collected during this test are generally from 1 of 3 groups: (1) sleep channels (electroencephalogram, electro-oculogram, submental and extremity electromyogram, and so forth), (2) cardiovascular channels (ECG, pulse transit time, and so forth), and (3) respiratory channels (airflow determined by oronasal thermistor or nasal pressure transducer, thoracoabdominal effort by piezoelectric effect or respiratory inductive plethysmography, intercostal muscle or diaphragmatic electromyogram, oximetry, capnography, and so forth).

Oligosomnography Because PSG is laborious, time consuming, and expensive, the sleep medicine field started to explore cheaper, easier, and less complex diagnostic modalities of sleep testing, such as PM. In December 2007, an AASM task force published specific guidelines on the use of PM for the diagnosis of OSA in adults. These guidelines recommended that PMs could be used in the context of a prior comprehensive sleep evaluation done by a sleep specialist in an accredited sleep center, using appropriate equipment, technologies, and quality control programs.[121] The diagnosis of OSA can be made by using comprehensive in-laboratory, attended PSG (type I devices); unattended, comprehensive PSG done in patient homes (type II devices); limited-channel PMs (type III devices); or monitors using at least 3 channels (type IV devices). The authors generically refer to PM devices types III and IV as OSG,[2] pointing to the main difference from the traditional PSG recordings: the number of channels or signals is limited by the technical specifications and the specific device. OSG is generally recommended to be used in an unattended setting as an alternative to PSG for the diagnosis of OSA, in patients with a high pretest probability of moderate to severe OSA (high clinical suspicion) and no comorbid sleep disorders or other major medical or neurologic comorbidities (chronic obstructive pulmonary disease, congestive heart failure, respiratory failure, stroke, and so forth).[121]

MSLT and MWT According to the AASM, MSLT is not routinely indicated in the initial evaluation and diagnosis of OSAS or in assessment of change after treatment with PAP. MSLT may be used if excessive sleepiness persists despite optimal treatment of OSA, to determine objectively how severe it is and to establish a baseline before further therapy is instituted; alternatively, MWT can be used to ascertain the capacity to stay awake during the day in patients on optimal therapy.[120,122,123] According to the AASM, the MWT 40-minute protocol may be used to assess an individual's ability to remain awake when the inability to remain awake constitutes a public or personal safety issue (option). The MWT may be indicated in patients with excessive sleepiness to assess response to treatment (guideline). In general, MSLT and MWT results do not correlate well, because they seem to measure different dimensions of sleepiness.[124]

Treatment

OSA therapy includes medical treatment, behavioral interventions, PAP, dental appliances, and various surgical options. Weight loss can ameliorate or completely reverse OSA in obese patients. Because alcohol and CNS depressants, such as sedatives and opiates, may worsen OSA, such substances should be avoided, if at all possible. Drugs that stimulate respiratory centers, such as progesterone, xanthines, and acetazolamide, do not seem to work in either prevention or treatment of SDB. The same holds true (for now, at least) for several drugs designed to stimulate certain respiratory muscles, and consequently to increase upper airway patency. Hormonal preparations of estrogens, with or without progesterone, may be effective in some perimenopausal or postmenopausal women with OSA, but significant safety concerns remain. Modafinil, a wake-promoting medication, may play a role in treating residual sleepiness in patients compliant with CPAP therapy. Supplemental oxygen has been shown efficacious as a primary treatment of OSA, and it may have a distinct role in patients with sleep apnea who could not tolerate other therapies, although valid concerns related to its potential to lengthen the apneic episodes remain.

Behavioral interventions

Several lifestyle characteristics can place individuals at higher risk for OSA. Modification of these contributory behaviors may have a favorable impact on downstream risks and on subsequent therapy. In any given patient, a comprehensive, multidisciplinary approach is generally preferred and strongly recommended.

Patient education Patient education is of paramount importance in the management of OSA.[4] Patients need to be actively involved in the planning and implementation of the recommended therapeutic interventions. Successful patient education programs include discussions of several components (**Box 2**).

Sleep hygiene and sleep deprivation The Western world seems to be a chronically sleep-deprived society.[125] Beyond the adverse impact of sleep restriction on performance, short sleep duration may also lead to OSA, blunted hypoxic and hypercapnic ventilatory chemoresponsiveness during wakefulness,[126,127] reduced arousal response, and more severe intermittent hypoxia.[126,128] Patients should be encouraged to apply the general principles of good sleep hygiene, although this advice is often unheeded because of social and/or financial pressures.

Weight loss Medical or surgical weight reduction interventions could have a substantial ameliorative impact on OSA.[129–133] A multidisciplinary team approach to weight reduction, encompassing lifestyle and dietary modifications as well as pharmacologic and/or surgical options, may optimize clinical results.[130] Because of the poor long-term success rate of the nonsurgical modalities, bariatric surgery is more frequent in the treatment of these patients, sometimes with excellent results.[134] Most patients referred for bariatric surgery, regardless of whether apnea is suspected, are found to have OSA[68]; it has been suggested that all patients referred for bariatric surgery should have preoperative sleep testing,[66,67] because they tend to have a higher rate of complications after such surgery.[135,136] Smith and colleagues[132] found that dietary instructions targeting weight loss resulted in a 47% decrease in the frequency of apneas for a mean weight loss of 9% over a period of few months. Similarly, Schwartz and coworkers[131] compared the effect of weight loss in a small group of 13 obese patients with 13 age-matched and weight-matched controls who did not undergo any dietary restriction, with no weight loss over a period of 1.5 years; in the intervention group, they found a 60% reduction in the AHI. Finally, there are several surgical weight loss studies that showed greater and consistent decreases in weight and associated reductions in AHI.[109]

Smoking cessation Cigarette smokers tend to have more often difficulty initiating and maintaining sleep, but also difficulty maintaining alertness during the day versus

---

Box 2
The general decalogue of patient education in OSA—points for discussion and clarification, centered on the acronym, BEG (background–expectations–goals)

1. Main findings of the sleep studies (PSG or OSG) (ie, set background)
2. Discussion about disease severity, natural course, and associated comorbidites, especially the ones linked to untreated OSA
3. Pathophysiology of OSA
4. Personalized risk and exacerbating factors; opportunities for risk factor modification
5. Genetic counseling, when indicated
6. Main treatment modalities and available options
7. What results to expect from treatment (ie, set expectations)
8. Outline the patient's role in therapy, address concerns, and set goals
9. Counseling regarding drowsy driving and sleepiness in the workplace
10. Quality of life assessment, questions, and other feedback

never-smokers[137]; furthermore, they have a 4-fold to 5-fold greater OR for moderate or severe SDB.[87] Cigarette smoking may contribute to upper airway dysfunction during sleep through mucosal edema, inflammation, and subsequent increased upper airway resistance. Smoking cessation interventions are an important component of general health measures to complement treatment of SDB.

Alcohol avoidance It is known that alcohol can elicit obstructive apneas in subjects who have PS and increase the apnea frequency and duration in patients with pre-existing OSA.[138,139] Alcohol may also exert an adverse impact on daytime alertness in patients with OSA. The hypnotic effect of this agent is enhanced in the presence of underlying sleepiness. Currently, it is unclear what the impact of alcohol is on the optimal level of PAP needed for patients with OSA.[138,140]

Positional therapy Additional factors, such as positional therapy (ie, avoidance of supine body position during sleep), may be of help. For example, using tennis balls in a back pocket of sleepwear or backpacks has led to modest results.

Pharmacologic treatment of OSA

A recent review of the literature on pharmacologic therapy for OSA found 33 randomized placebo-controlled trials, investigating 27 different drugs, on either OSA severity or on SDB-related symptoms.[141] Although some studies reached statistical significance, they were generally underpowered, over short periods of time, and with overall small effects on ESS, AHI, or oxygen desaturation index.

Among the respiratory stimulants studied, methylxantines, such as aminophylline[142] and theophylline[143]; carbonic anhydrase inhibitors (acetazolamide[144]); and opioid antagonists (naloxone[145] and naltrexone[146]), all seemed to improve OSA severity by a small degree, if any. Medroxyprogesterone, a synthetic analog of progesterone, did not change the AHI in 10 male subjects with OSA over 1-week period trial versus 1 week of placebo.[147] Selective serotonin receptor modulation (eg, 5-HT$_3$ receptor antagonists[148,149]) has been proposed as a potential future therapeutic action on specific respiratory muscles or on their respiratory centers' regulatory areas; such agents are currently in development.

Antihypertensive agents could theoretically improve OSA by interfering with the baroreceptor chemosensitivity and the respiratory centers' activity. The available literature has shown conflicting results: among β-blockers, although propranolol can worsen OSA, metoprolol and atenolol may be beneficial[150,151]; among angiotension-converting enzyme inhibitors, cilazapril and ramipril (similar to spironoloactone) may reduce the AHI of the patients with OSA[150,152–155]; and among calcium channel blockers, isradipine has not been found beneficial.[151]

Older studies found that supplemental oxygen in patients with OSA may significantly increase apnea duration, with associated hypercapnia and respiratory acidosis.[156] Martin and colleagues[156] observed an initial prolongation of apnea duration in a group of eucapnic patients with OSA, in conjunction with a significant reduction in apnea frequency. Gold and colleagues[157] subsequently reported that supplemental oxygen administration was associated with a statistical reduction in apnea frequency, particularly during non–rapid eye movement (NREM) sleep, as well as improved oxyhemoglobin saturation, but apneas were an average 4 to 7 seconds longer. Although the degree and duration of hypoxia that is ultimately harmful remains to be determined,[158] patients with coronary artery disease or cerebrovascular disease and mild OSA, but with severe intermittent oxyhemoglobin desaturations, might benefit from supplemental oxygen.[159,160] Oxygen may also be useful as an adjunct to PAP.[161] Patients with OSA who are sufficiently hypoxemic or borderline-hypoxemic during wakefulness to benefit from supplemental daytime oxygen therapy (with exertion and/or at rest) usually meet the criteria for this therapy during sleep, even if PAP treatment maintains upper airway patency, although PAP itself may improve oxygenation by reducing ventilation-perfusion mismatch.[162]

Some patients with OSAS continue to experience EDS despite optimal therapy (ie, even after normalization of the AHI, oxygen saturation, flow contour, and/or arousal index).[163] For this category of patients, after ensuring optimal treatment, good compliance with the primary therapy, and addressing potential comorbid conditions, adjunctive stimulant therapy may be considered for residual EDS.[4,164,165] Because this therapy is tailored to patient symptoms, which are generally poorly correlated with the disease severity, there is no specific threshold for this indication. Several CNS stimulants are currently available. Although modafinil and R-modafinil (armodafinil) are the only agents that have been studied in OSA patients who have residual EDS after optimal primary therapy, alternatives to this are methylphenidate and various amphetamines, which are generally used in the treatment of narcolepsy and idiopathic hypersomnia. Modafinil is currently considered first-line adjunctive therapy for the treatment of residual EDS after adequate treatment of OSA.[4,164] Its effectiveness has been shown in several randomized trials sponsored by the manufacturer.[166–169] Armodafinil has an apparent longer half-life and seems similarly effective, according to several randomized trials.[170,171] Although reportedly safer than the other stimulants, modafinil should be used with caution in people with a history of arrhythmias or heart disease.[172,173] Side effects are infrequent and include headaches, nausea, vomiting, diarrhea, anorexia, and xerostomia. Addiction related to modafinil has not been unequivocally ruled out. Life-threatening side effects are represented by Stevens-Johnson syndrome or toxic epidermal necrolysis, and, consequently, any rash arising while on this therapy should be a strong reason for seeking medical attention right away and/or for discontinuation of the drug.

Methylphenidate is another CNS stimulant, commonly used to treat attention-deficit hyperactivity disorder, narcolepsy, or traumatic brain injury. Although no clinical trials have been performed in patients with OSAS, methylphenidate is sometimes used off-label as adjunctive therapy to treat residual EDS despite optimal therapy, especially when a stronger stimulative action is needed. Side effects are approximately the same and slightly more common than with modafinil, whereas the addictive potential is clearly higher. Due to its sympathomimetic effect, it should be avoided in patients with known heart disease or cardiac dysrhythmias.

Amphetamines are also potent CNS stimulants, with strong sympathomimetic action. Similarly, the side effects, addictive potential, and unproved clinical efficacy in this clinical setting are similar to the ones of methylphenidate. Amphetamines and their derivatives can lead to irritability, anxiety, tremor, hypertension, and cardiac dysrhythmias. There is a strong risk of addiction and illicit use for amphetamine, dextroamphetamine, and methamphetamine, hence, the controlled substance status and special precautions while monitoring this therapy.

Mechanical therapy

Elevated nasal resistance may facilitate upper airway closure during sleep[174,175] or represent one site of narrowing, because several anatomic areas could be responsible for the impaired airflow in OSA. Although somewhat controversial, approximately 10% of patients with PS or OSA tend to improve after administration of nasal vasoconstrictors. Several devices (recently developed and made available), which mechanically dilate the anterior nasal valve, may reduce the propensity toward OSA. Hoijer and colleagues[176] assessed the effect of an external nasal dilator in 10 snorers, 7 of whom had an apnea index of 5 or higher. Although the average apnea index fell from 18 to 6, and the nadir oxyhemoglobin saturation also improved during sleep, the saturation remained severely reduced in subjects with more advanced disease (ie, higher baseline hypoxic burden). In contrast, Hoffstein and colleagues[177] concluded that dilation of the anterior nasal valve using an external dilator has no impact on SDB, nadir desaturation, or mean oxyhemoglobin saturation, although a reduction in snoring intensity was noted. Using an intranasally applied dilator, Scharf and colleagues[178] reported that a significant number of their participants (total number = 20) had improved sleepiness scores and morning concentration. Using a numeric scale, there were no differences in subjective sleep depth, overall sleep quality, or refreshing quality of sleep. Bed partners reported decreased snoring loudness but no change in snoring regularity. Unfortunately, in this trial there was no objective assessment of sleep and breathing, neither at study onset nor during the treatment period with a nasal dilator. In another study,[179] cyclic alternating pattern sequences in nonapneic snorers were diminished during the use of an intranasally applied dilator, suggesting improved sleep continuity.

Nasopharyngeal airway The concept of nasopharyngeal intubation to maintain upper airway patency during sleep was originally tried in the 1970s[180]; since then, there have been few reports attempting to use it.[181,182] Overall, nasopharyngeal intubation has today limited therapeutic utility in SDB, due to either a lack of tolerance or of efficacy.[182] Nevertheless, in selected patients for whom other therapies have failed, a trial of nasopharyngeal airway may be considered. Another variant of a nasopharyngeal pathway, which could be used in SDB, is represented by the unidirectional nasal valves leading to expiratory PAP, with potential to stent the upper airway susceptible to dynamic collapse. Their efficacy has been reported recently,[183,184] but more validative studies are needed.

Positive airway pressure First described by Sullivan in 1981,[185] CPAP provides the means of pneumatic splinting or stenting the upper airway, by providing intraluminal pressure that is positive in relation to the atmospheric pressure, throughout the respiratory cycle. By 1985, more than 100 patients had used this therapy on a regular basis.[186,187] Since then, evidence supporting the use of CPAP has accumulated exponentially, attesting the improvement in quality of life and patient outcomes. PAP can be delivered in CPAP, BPAP, autotitrating PAP (autoPAP [APAP]), flexible CPAP, adaptive servoventilation (ASV) modes, and so forth. The PAP is applied through either nasal, oral, or oronasal interface (mask).

Nasal CPAP is the treatment of choice for moderate to severe OSA. At the appropriate setting, CPAP is effective, ameliorating daytime sleepiness and fatigue. In a recently published systematic review on the effects of CPAP in OSAS, McDaid and colleagues[188] reviewed the available literature and found a pooled effect on ESS of approximately 2.7 points' reduction (95% CI, −1.9 to −3.4). CPAP is also effective in reducing the frequency of respiratory events (ie, apneas, hypopneas, and RERAs), thus normalizing or ameliorating significantly the AHI.[189,190] As a consequence of this therapeutic modality, upper airway muscle tone decreases with the application of the PAP. Higher levels of PAP may be required in supine position, in rapid eye movement (REM) sleep, after ingestion of alcohol, or after taking different sedative medications. Weight gain may also require an increase in a formerly adequate treatment PAP.

Although CPAP is the preferred option for the treatment of moderate or severe OSA and optional for mild OSA,[4] BPAP or APAP could also be considered in patients intolerant of CPAP or when high pressures are required and the patient experiences difficulty in exhaling against a fixed pressure.[191] An additional indication for BPAP is when there is an element of central hypoventilation, by providing a level of pressure support (PS) (ie, a pressure difference between inspiratory and expiratory pressures).

AutoCPAP or APAP devices were developed with 2 potential uses: (1) to select an effective pressure without the need of an attended in-laboratory PAP titration and (2) to deliver the lowest effective pressure irrespective of the body position, sleep stage, weight changes, medication use, and so forth. AutoCPAP algorithms vary among different devices, but, in general, pressure varies in response to flow (changes in airflow amplitude, airflow limitation, and snoring) or in airway impedance (changes in signal determined by forced oscillation technique). AutoCPAP up-titration may be erroneous in the face of high airflow leaks (mask or mouth leaks), which can simulate respiratory events, and because of the device's inability to differentiate between OSA and CSA (at least by flow-sensing devices). So far, the outcomes of CPAP versus APAP therapy seem similar.[192,193] Recently, autoadjustable bilevel positive airway pressure (autoBPAP) has been introduced, with separate settings for maximum inspiratory PAP, minimum expiratory PAP, and the maximal level of PS (in general between 3 cm H_2O and 8 cm H_2O).

The published criteria for CPAP therapy from the CMS are listed in **Box 3**. CPAP treatment is appropriate for patients with AHI of 15 or greater and for patients with AHI of 5 or greater and concurrent sleepiness or history of hypertension, stroke, ischemic heart disease, cor pulmonale, or mood disorders.

Currently, most patients start CPAP under supervision, usually in a specialized sleep laboratory (ie, CPAP titration study). The purposes of supervision are many-fold: (1) to ensure that patients are educated appropriately about the therapy, (2) to determine the adequacy of CPAP throughout the night, and (3) to evaluate immediate acceptance, tolerance, or problems with the therapy. Economic pressures within the health care systems are challenging this approach, however, and slowly drifting the therapeutic approach in the direction of a less-intensive staffing modality, autoadjustable CPAP, self-titration, or even home initiation of CPAP. Nevertheless, there is no evidence for appropriate safety and efficacy of CPAP titration outside of a medically supervised process.[194] Current evidence supports the use of trained technologists (so-called CPAP coordinators or technologists) to provide patient education, technical aspects of titration, and follow-up. This is especially important in individuals who may have neurologic or cognitive challenges. Recent data from small patient groups have challenged the notion that close medical supervision is needed in neurologically normal individuals, and this may become the target of patient-centered research in the near.[195] The major determinants of CPAP usage are patient understanding of the

---

Box 3
Current CMS criteria for PAP therapy in patients with OSA

AHI ≥15

AHI 5–14 and any of the following:

    EDS

    Hypertension

    Ischemic heart disease (coronary artery disease)

    Stroke (cerebrovascular accidents)

    Insomnia

    Mood disorders

therapy, baseline symptoms, CPAP impact on symptoms, and close professional support, regardless of mask type, CPAP manufacturer, or modality of delivery.

Oral appliances Dental appliances or OAs are customized devices designed to maintain the airway patency during sleep. They fall into 2 general categories: (1) mandibular advancement devices (MADs), which work by protruding the mandible forward, hence are increasing the luminal area of the airway during sleep, and (2) tongue retaining devices, which seem to work by keeping the tongue in place and preventing it occluding the upper airway at the oropharyngeal or laryngopharyngeal level.

When compared with no therapy at all or sham interventions, OAs have been shown effective in diminishing snoring intensity and in decreasing the number of respiratory events, arousals, and oxygen desaturations but not necessarily in normalizing them.[196–198] Although several studies suggest that complete resolution of OSA can be obtained, this seems to apply mostly to patients with mild or moderate OSA (AHI <30) and less so in severe OSA (AHI $\geq$30)[4,198]; other studies have not confirmed the same findings.[196,197] Until further large-scale studies are conducted, the gold standard for primary therapy for OSA patients remains CPAP therapy.[4] The effect of OAs on mortality is currently unknown. Most of the trials conducted have evaluated the effects of MADs and less so the effects and tolerability of tongue retaining devices.

Symptomatically, OAs somewhat improve daytime sleepiness, quality of life, and neurocognitive function. Nevertheless, most of the data come from short-term studies[198,199]; hence, it may be hard to discern how much is placebo effect or ascertainment bias. One randomized crossover trial on 68 patients with OSA (RDI $\geq$10 and at least 2 symptoms or signs of OSA) investigated the efficacy of an MAD versus a control device and showed that, after 4 weeks of therapy, there was a statistically significant/clinically less significant improvement in mean sleep latency (10 vs 9 minutes) and ESS (7 vs 9 global score).[197] When OA was compared with CPAP therapy in one study, it was found that both therapies reduced daytime sleepiness versus baseline (assessed by ESS and Oxford SLEep Resistance (OSLER) test).[200] Both treatments significantly improved subjective and objective sleepiness, cognitive tests, and health-related quality of life. Overall, the reported compliance was higher for MAD, with more than 70% of patients preferring this treatment. Furthermore, 1-night MAD titration had a low negative predictive value for treatment success.[200] OAs also have been reported to improve driving simulator performance, with a magnitude of effect similar to that seen after successful CPAP therapy.[201]

In addition to the efficacy data discussed previously, several studies reported improvements in hemodynamics, neurocognitive function, and quality of life due to OAs.[197,199,202,203] In one Australian study,[197] the effect of an MAD was a reduction in the awake mean systolic and diastolic blood pressures, with the maximal effect noted during the late sleeping period and early morning (approximately 3 mm Hg). In a more recent study by Andren and colleagues,[203] at 3 years of therapy with a dental appliance, systolic and diastolic blood pressures improved by 25 mm Hg and 10 mm Hg, respectively, a magnitude of effect that is much higher than usual interventions and that deserves further scrutiny. Few studies showed that the favorable effects of MADs may persist in the medium term and long term, for at least some patients, although it is currently unclear which patients benefit the most.[198,204–206]

Not surprisingly, most clinical trials comparing MADs to CPAP found the latter superior in normalizing AHI and sleep oxygenation but not necessarily in improving symptoms (eg, EDS), arousal index, or overall sleep architecture.[190,199–201,207] Nevertheless, due to ease of use and comfort, patients generally seem to comply better with the OA therapy.

Recently, in a crossover PSG study from Japan,[208] in which both OAs and CPAP therapy were used, the median baseline AHI was reduced with the OAs from 36 to 12 in 35 patients. In this study, OSA patients with an optimal CPAP of 10.5 cm H_2O or higher were unlikely to respond to OA therapy. This type of predictive model may become in the future clinically useful for identifying the optimal categories of patients who could benefit from OAs for the therapy for OSA.

The most common side effects of OAs are generally seen early during therapy and are represented by dental discomfort (in upper or lower incisors), temporomandibular joint tenderness or pain, either xerostomia or hypersalivation, gingival irritation, and occasionally bruxism.[198] These side effects are generally mild and self-limited. In the long term (ie, >2 years), occlusal changes can occur with OAs.[209,210] In one observational study on 70 patients, with an average follow-up of 7 years, occlusal changes were diagnosed in 86% of patients treated with MADs.[211]

In children, palatal or maxillary expansion can be used as a therapy for those who failed surgical therapy. In one small study, children maintained the benefit for 2 years beyond the orthodontic treatment.[212]

In summary, OAs can be used in mild and moderate OSA, if (1) it is the patient's choice, (2) patient cannot tolerate PAP therapy, or (3) if snoring is the main symptom. In severe OSA, OAs should not be used as first-line therapy, unless major contraindications or intolerance to PAP is encountered.

Surgical therapy

Surgical therapy seems the most logical and likely the most effective modality for patients with OSA due to anatomic causes or obstructing lesions, such as severe adenotonsillar hypertrophy (frequently the case in children).[4] In the absence of an identified anatomic obstruction, there is no consensus for a role of surgery in OSA.[213] Uvulopalatopharyngoplasty (UPPP or U3P) is one of the most common surgical procedures performed in this context and entails resection of the uvula, any redundant retroglossal soft tissue, and palatine tonsillar lymphoid tissue. Radiofrequency ablation and laser-assisted ablation are less-invasive variants of the traditional UPPP. Other surgical procedures used in OSA are septoplasty, rhinoplasty, nasal turbinate reduction, nasal polypectomy, tonsillectomy, adenoidectomy, palatal implants (the so-called Pillar procedure), tongue reduction (partial glossectomy or lingual tonsillectomy), genioglossal advancement/shortening, and maxillomandibular advancement and/or reconstruction.

The main mechanisms by which various surgical procedures work are (1) bypassing the upper airway (eg, tracheostomy); (2) soft tissue removal or trimming (eg, polypectomy, turbinoplasty, UPPP, adenotonsillectomy, midline glossectomy, or basal tongue reduction); and (3) bony and/or soft tissue modifications (eptoplasty, mandibular-maxillary expansion, mandibular advancement, geniglossal advancement or shortening, hyoid myotomy suspention, and so forth).

Relative contraindications to upper airway surgery in OSA are morbid obesity (except for bariatric surgery and tracheostomy), decompensated cardiac or respiratory conditions, alcohol and drug abuse, and psychosis or other unstable mental conditions.[214]

Only a few trials compared surgery to either conservative management modalities or a nonsurgical therapy.[215] Overall, there was no consistent benefit in favor of surgical therapy. Although this could be a true effect, it may also be due to small sample sizes, heterogeneous patient populations, or short-term follow-ups. UPPP is generally effective in approximately half of the patients. It improves the symptoms of OSA, but UPPP achieves a surgical cure rate (ie, postoperative AHI <5) in only a minority of patients[216] and may compromise subsequent CPAP therapy by promoting mouth leaking and reducing the maximal level of pressure tolerated by many patients treated subsequently with CPAP.[217]

Hyoid suspension and genioglossus advancement represent other potential surgical procedures. Riley and colleagues[218,219] have taken a stepwise approach to the surgical treatment of OSA. The approach included a UPPP for retropalatal obstruction alone, genioglossus advancement, and hyoid suspension without UPPP for patients with hypopharyngeal obstruction; and, for obstruction at both sites, all 3 procedures were done. It is unclear if this approach leads to long-term outcome improvement.

Clinical studies comparing OAs versus surgical interventions are also scarce. In one study from Sweden, patients with OSA (AHI 5–25) were randomly assigned to UPPP versus an OA titrated up to 50% of the maximal protrusive distance.[220] One year later, success rate (percentage of subjects with at least 50% reduction in apnea index [AI]) in the MAD group was 81% versus 53% in the UPPP group ($P<.05$). After 4 years of therapy, normalization (AI <5 or AHI <10) was observed in 63% of the MAD group and in 33% of the UPPP group, whereas the compliance rate for MAD was only 62%. Pronounced complaints of nasopharyngeal regurgitation of fluid and difficulty with swallowing after UPPP were reported by 8% and 10%, respectively. Tracheostomy is probably the most definitive surgical procedure for OSA, but it carries its own risks and, understandably, is less preferred by the patients. It remains the modality of choice only after all other less-invasive modalities have been tried and failed.

Central sleep apnea

Key Points Box

- CSA is a condition of SDB characterized by impaired airflow due to reduced or absent ventilatory effort.

- CSA and OSA can often coexist (mixed sleep apnea); there is a significant overlap in clinical presentation, pathophysiology, and treatment of these conditions.

- By convention, mixed sleep apnea is considered primarily a CSA if more than 50% of the respiratory events are central in nature.

- Snoring may be present but is generally less prominent than in OSA.

- There are 2 main categories of CSA: (1) hypercapnic type (central alveolar hypoventilation and CSA secondary to neuromuscular disorders or chronic use of long-acting opioids) and (2) nonhypercapnic type (idiopathic CSA, CSA due to heart failure, sleep-onset periodic breathing, high-altitude CSA, and PAP-emergent or complex CSA).

- CSA can be completely asymptomatic or associated with repetitive nocturnal awakenings, insomnia and EDS or fatigue.

- A definitive diagnosis of CSA requires PSG.

- Therapy is generally tailored to the type and severity of CSA and includes treatment of the underlying disorder, pharmacotherapy for respiratory center stimulation, supplemental oxygen or PAP.

Introduction

CSA is not a single condition but rather several disorders that share clinical and PSG findings. It is important to identify the type and each specific condition's risk factors, clinical course, and therapeutic modalities and to personalize prognosis. CSA is considered a condition of impaired airflow during sleep due to lack of respiratory effort, leading to daytime symptoms, nocturnal hypoxia, and ventilation/CO_2 changes.[221,222] The lack of respiratory effort can be due to reduced central drive ("won't breathe") versus impaired respiratory motor output ("can't breathe") (**Table 3**). CSA can frequently coexist with OSA, because one begets the other.[222–225]

Hypercapnic CSA is characterized by hypoventilation during sleep (ie, higher levels of $Paco_2$), but in many instances it is also characterized by hypercapnia during wake.

Nonhypercapnic CSA is generally associated with increased responsiveness to higher levels of $Paco_2$ and presents with eucapnia or hypocapnia during wakefulness.

Pathophysiology

Respiration has both metabolic and behavioral control feedbacks. Metabolic control involves carotid chemoreceptors responsive to hypoxia, hypercapnia, and acidosis as well as brainstem chemoreceptors responsive to hypercapnia/acidosis. Ventilatory response to these stimuli (chemosensitivity) has some individual variability. Additionally, vagally mediated, stretch receptor–mediated intrapulmonary, chest wall muscle and joint receptors and brain (eg, cortical and limbic system) mechanisms have important roles in controlling respiration. These pathways are active during both wake and sleep, with the exception of the behavioral control, which becomes inactive during sleep. There is greater blunting of ventilatory responses to hypercapnia (vs hypoxia) during sleep. In general, the sleep-wake or wake-sleep transitions are prone to ventilatory instability. During sleep, central events typically happen when rising $Paco_2$ levels trigger a ventilatory overshoot or hyperventilation during the ensuing arousals, which, in turn, make $Paco_2$ fall below what is called *apnea threshold*. Apnea threshold is defined as the arterial partial pressure of CO_2 below which respiratory output ceases and is generally 2 mm Hg to 6 mm Hg lower than the normocapnic $Paco_2$ levels of sleep. Occasional central apneas can be seen at the onset of sleep when levels of $Paco_2$ fluctuate above or below the apnea threshold; these tend to resolve as sleep progresses and deepens and respiratory plant/controller system stabilizes. High-altitude periodic breathing is also more prominent at sleep onset and during NREM

Table 3 CSA types, subtypes, and conditions		
Type	**Subtype**	**Causes**
Hypercapneic	Will not breathe	Medications (CNS depressant agents)
		Brainstem disorders (ischemic or hemorrhagic stroke, tumors, etc)
		OHS
		Congenital central hypoventilation syndrome (PHOX2B mutation)
	Cannot breathe	Myopathies
		Neuromuscular junction disorders (eg, myasthenia gravis) or blockade
		Neuropathies
		Spinal motor neuron pathology (amyotrophic lateral sclerosis and so forth)
		Spinal lesions (infarcts, tumors, trauma, disk compression, etc)
Nonhypercapneic	—	CSR
		High-altitude CSA
		Idiopathic or primary CSA
		Complex or pressure-emergent CSA
		CKD-associated CSA
		Acromegaly-associated CSA

(N) sleep than REM (R) sleep; it can be seen after ascent to high altitude, generally above 4000 m. It is believed that high-altitude CSA is the result of cycles of hypoxia-stimulated hyperventilation, which leads to respiratory alkalosis and hypocapnia, followed by cessation of respiratory output from the brainstem regulators.[226] Risk factors for high-altitude CSA include greater intrinsic hypoxic ventilatory drive, male gender, higher elevation reached, and fast ascent.

Key Clinical Features and Diagnosis of CSA Types

Idiopathic or primary CSA (normocapnic or hypocapnic)

Idiopathic or primary CSA is an uncommon condition, distinct from the other types of CSA syndromes. It is generally found in fewer than 5% of patients undergoing PSG and predominates in men. Pathophysiology of primary CSA is not completely understood, but it is believed that $Paco_2$ plays a major pathophysiologic role. Clinical manifestations primarily include daytime sleepiness, insomnia, frequent nighttime awakenings, and mild snoring. Patients generally have a normal body habitus. Hemodynamic consequences include pulmonary and systemic hypertension, likely related to hypoxia.

PSG generally shows central apnea index of 5 or more per hour of sleep and the respiratory events are mostly observed during N1 and N2 sleep stages. There are several important PSG distinctions between idiopathic CSA and Cheyne-Stokes respiration (CSR). Compared with CSR, cycle duration is typically shorter (20–40 s vs 60–90 s), oxygen desaturations are less severe, arousals occur earlier (at the termination of apnea vs during the peak ventilatory effort), and resumption of breathing is more abrupt and not crescendo, typically with a large-volume breath in idiopathic CSA. Central apnea can also be a result of brainstem dysfunction or compression, such as Arnold-Chiari malformations, and thus a neurologic examination and possibly head imaging should be considered.

Treatment of idiopathic CSA is directed at the likely causes leading to apneas and depends on symptom severity. Primary CSA resolves spontaneously in approximately one-fifth of the patients; consequently, watchful waiting could be considered. Treating upper airway obstruction, such as nasal congestion, might benefit some patients. Supplemental oxygen has also been tried in the treatment of primary CSA[227] to blunt the hypoxia-induced hyperventilation leading to hypocapnia, hence the cyclic pattern. Small amounts of supplemental CO_2 or enlarging the anatomic dead space is also shown beneficial in some studies.[228] The efficacy of CPAP or BPAP to treat idiopathic CSA has also been reported and is attributed to PAP-induced $Paco_2$ stabilization above apnea threshold and normalization of oxygen due to increase in functional residual capacity.[229,230] Pharmacotherapy using zolpidem[231] or acetazolamide[232] has also been used to lower the apnea threshold and abolish the central respiratory events.

Cheyne-Stokes respiration (normocapnic or hypocapnic)

CSR is defined as periodic breathing with recurring episodes of waxing and waning breathing interspersed by central apneas or hypopneas. CSR is generally observed during NREM (N) sleep, and improves or resolves during REM (R) sleep. Both CSA and CSR can be encountered in patients with congestive heart failure (CHF) and brain disease. An early study evaluating the prevalence of SDB in patients with CHF[233] found that 51% of them had an AHI greater than15 per hour; 40% of subjects had CSA and 11% had OSA. Patients with SDB had a higher prevalence of atrial fibrillation and ventricular dysrrhythmias versus controls. A larger, retrospective study[234] of 450 patients with CHF referred to a sleep laboratory for evaluation of SDB found CSA and OSA in 33% and 38% of patients, respectively (defined as AHI >10). Risk factors for

CSA were age, male gender, presence of atrial fibrillation, and hypocapnia, with $Paco_2$ 38 mm Hg.

Optimization of CHF treatment potentially could result in improvement of CSA. A large, randomized, controlled trial assessing the role of CPAP in patients with CSA with a mean AHI of 40 and severe systolic CHF (Canadian Positive Airway Pressure) failed to show any survival benefit.[235] Overall death rate, transplant-free survival, and rates of hospitalization did not differ significantly between the 2 groups. CPAP therapy reduced AHI by approximately half, improved oxygen exchange, and improved ventricular function, as documented by improved left ventricular ejection fraction and neuroendocrine footprint of heart failure (ie, decreased the plasma levels of norepinephrine). One criticism of this trial was that CPAP did not normalize the AHI. In a post hoc analysis of this trial,[236] patients who had central apneas effectively suppressed by CPAP at 3 months (AHI <15) had better transplant-free survival versus the control group.

Newer forms of PAP effective in CSA in patients with CHF have been studied and reported in the past decade.[237,238] In a group of 15 patients with CSR and CHF, treatment with ASV (ie, a type of variable BPAP or closed-loop pressure-preset and volume or flow-cycled mechanical ventilation) reduced daytime sleepiness and improved plasma brain natriuretic peptide and urinary catecholamine levels.[239] In 25 patients with CSR and CHF, ASV was more effective versus CPAP in achieving AHI less than 10. At 6 months, compliance, left ventricular function, and quality of life were all better with ASV.[240]

Opioid-induced CSA (hypercapnic)

Short-acting and long-acting opioids for chronic pain have been used increasingly over the past decades.[241] Unfortunately, CSA can emerge in patients on long-term opioid therapy.[242–245] Other irregular respiratory patterns, including Biot, ataxic, and cluster breathing, have also been described in opioid users. This type of CSA differs from CSR by its lack of crescendo-decrescendo character and generally by shorter cycle times. Prevalence of CSA was found close to 30% among long-term opioid users and seems dose related.[243] Hypercapnic apnea can also occur as a result of brainstem dysfunction, such as brain tumor or compression.

CPAP therapy is effective in controlling OSA in patients on long-term opioid therapy but tends to worsen CSA. ASV for treatment of CSA associated with long-term opioid therapy has been tried[246] and it seems that ASV is effective in controlling SDB of these patients.

Acromegaly and CSA

Acromegaly is caused by overproduction and secretion of growth hormone, often from benign pituitary adenomas. SDB, such as OSA (more often) and CSA, are commonly encountered in these patients.[96,247,248] The pathogenesis of CSA in patients with acromegaly is probably related to upper airway narrowing and reflex inhibition of the respiratory centers as well as increased ventilatory responsiveness to hypercapnia associated with hypersecretion of growth hormone.[96,247]

Somatostatin analogs therapy in acromegaly can induce tumor shrinkage and reduce symptoms in patients not considered surgical candidates. Due to the persistence of skeletal abnormalities in these patients, SDB may persist.[249] In a study assessing the effect of octreotide, a somatostatin analog, on sleep apnea, in 19 patients with active acromegaly, after 6 months of therapy, the severity of both OSA and CSA improved, but SDB was not eliminated in most of the subjects.[250] Surgical therapy for acromegaly can also improve CSA. Trans-sphenoidal adenomectomy improves, at least to some degree and, occasionally in combination with radiotherapy, the CSA.[251–253]

Renal disease and CSA

SDB is frequently encountered in patients with chronic kidney disease (CKD) or end-stage renal disease. Risk factors in this population include volume overload, uremia, pharyngeal airway narrowing, and altered chemoreflex responsiveness during sleep.[254–257] The prevalence of CSA and OSA in patients with end-stage renal disease varies greatly in the available literature, but OSA seems more common in most of the studies.[254,255,258]

Hypocapnia and periodic breathing seen in patients with CKD may be related, at least in part, to the respiratory compensation of chronic metabolic acidosis.[259,260] Nocturnal hemodialysis has been shown to improve CSA as well as OSA in patients with CKD, a finding that is concordant with the pathogenic theories of ventilatory destabilization and upper airway occlusion during sleep in these patients.[259] The influence of hemodialysis (HD) buffer (acetate or bicarbonate) on SDB was assessed in one study[261] using PSG recording, and found that OSA was not different between groups, but those using acetate had significantly more CSA.[261] Furthermore, several case reports showed improvements in sleep apnea after kidney transplantation.[262,263]

Complex or PAP-emergent CSA

Acute application of PAP (generally during PAP titrations) can lead some patients with OSA to develop frequent central apneas or periodic breathing pattern, despite suboptimal treatment of OSA and in the absence of significant mask leaks, a phenomenon called PAP-emergent CSA or complex sleep apnea (CxSA).[264] The long-term clinical consequences of this type of SDB are poorly understood. Several case series have characterized its prevalence, clinical course, and associated risk factors.[264–269] The prevalence of CxSA is estimated at 5% to 6%, based on large retrospective studies.[269,270]

For symptomatic, persistent CxSA, therapy using ASV could be considered.[269] In a prospective randomized crossover trial comparing noninvasive positive pressure ventilation and ASV in subjects with CSA, mixed sleep apnea, or CxSA, mean AHI was 49.4 ± 25.4 (diagnostic study), 41.9 ± 28.1 (on CPAP), 6.8 ± 6.8 (on noninvasive positive pressure ventilation), and 1.6 ± 3.6 (on ASV). ASV was overall more effective in improving the AHI and reducing the RERAs.[268]

A new set of AASM practice parameters for treatment of CSA has been published in 2012,[271] and based on review of the available literature, lists several recommendations for therapy in CSA syndromes (**Table 4**).

Obesity hypoventilation syndrome

OHS is defined by the following criteria: (1) obesity (ie, BMI $\geq$30 kg/m^2); (2) hypercapnia during wakefulness (Paco$_2$ >45 mm Hg) leading to hypoxemia (Pao$_2$ <70 mm Hg), not explained by other conditions; and (3) SDB (in 90% of cases, OSA; in 10% of cases, sleep hypoventilation [ie, Paco$_2$ elevated by more than 10 mm Hg above the levels seen in wakefulness]).[272–274] During sleep, hypercapnia is generally worse than during wake, leading to persistent hypoxia. Furthermore, the hypoxic burden (defined as percent of the total sleep time with Spo$_2$ less than 90%) is generally more significant in OHS versus in pure OSA (42%–70% in OHS vs 9%–47% in OSA). During wakefulness, patients are somnolent and typically wake up with headaches.

Potential pathophysiologic mechanisms in OHS are as follows:

1. Mechanical—increased airway resistance,[275] low lung volumes,[276] reduced chest wall compliance,[277] and respiratory muscle dysfunction,[278] all leading to inability of the ventilator apparatus to compensate for the degree of CO$_2$ production
2. Central—blunted respiratory centers' chemosensitivity[276,279–283]
3. Ventilation-perfusion mismatches due to pulmonary edema[284] or atelectasis[276,285,286]

Table 4	
2012 AASM practice parameters for treatment of CSA syndromes (319)	
Standard recommendations	• CPAP therapy targeting normalization of AHI as the initial treatment of CSA related to CHF
	• Nocturnal supplemental oxygen therapy as treatment of CSA related to CHF
	• ASV therapy targeting normalization of AHI as treatment of CSA related to CHF
Option recommendations	• BPAP therapy in spontaneous timed mode targeting normalization of AHI in the treatment of CSA related to CHF only if there is no response to adequate trials of CPAP, O_2, or ASV
	• Acetazolamide or theophylline in the treatment of CSA related to CHF only after optimization of CHF therapy and if PAP therapy is not tolerated
	• PAP therapy for primary or idiopathic CSA
	• Acetazolamide for primary or idiopathic CSA
	• Zolpidem or triazolam for primary or idiopathic CSA (only if there are no risk factors for respiratory depression)
	• CPAP, supplemental oxygen, bicarbonate buffer in dialysate and nocturnal dialysis in CSA related to end-stage renal disease

4. Hormonal (eg, leptin resistance [leptin, an adipokine that generally stimulates the respiratory centers, seems unable in humans with OHS to increase ventilation as much as the CO_2 production requires it]).[287–289]

Management of OHS primarily involves weight loss,[290–293] BPAP therapy or CPAP,[294–297] average volume-assured PS,[298] and, potentially, supplemental oxygen[299] in a select patient population. Tracheostomy was the first therapy described for treatment of OHS,[300] but it is now reserved for those who are intolerant of other therapies.

Clinical vignette

A 56-year-old man presents with lower extremity weakness and muscle fasciculations of recent onset. A diagnosis of amyotrophic lateral sclerosis is established. He is referred to a sleep specialist for evaluation, because he has moderate snoring and daytime fatigue. His pulmonary function tests, including maximal inspiratory and expiratory pressures, are normal.

Question: What work-up do you recommend and what clinical course do you expect?

Answer: The following considerations are important in this clinical scenario:

• An arterial blood gas analysis is indicated; if CO_2 is normal, hypoventilation is not present.

• A PSG with tidal CO_2 monitoring may show OSA and/or intermittent sleep hypoventilation; although the presence of the latter is of unclear significance, it may herald the need for noninvasive ventilation (BPAP) in the near future.

• Clinical course is highly variable; frequent re-evaluation may identify early signs of neuromuscular weakness affecting the respiratory system.

• Institution of noninvasive ventilation at the time of the earliest signs of ventilatory dysfunction is a life-saving and a life-prolonging measure.

CURRENT CONTROVERSIES AND FUTURE CONSIDERATIONS

Several questions and unknown facts remain for the future:

PS

- What is the optimal method to measure and quantify snoring?
- Does PS evolve in time to more severe forms of SDB, such as UARS, OSA, and OHS?
- Loud snoring has been linked recently to carotid atherosclerosis—does this have an impact on understanding of the cardiovascular pathogenesis in SDB?

OSA

- To what extent is hypoxic burden versus reoxygenation deleterious in OSA?
- What are the ideal biomarkers to be used in diagnosis, risk stratification, and characterization of the susceptibility to significant metabolic, cardiovascular, or neurologic complications in OSA?
- Is there a cardiovascular or neurologic preconditioning to the effects of OSA?
- Who are the patients who benefit from CPAP for OSA?
- Who are the patients who benefit from BPAP for OSA?
- Who are the patients who benefit from oxygen for OSA?
- How can patient adherence to PAP therapy be improved?
- What are the role and efficacy of alternative therapies (surgery, OAs, and so forth) in OSA of various severity degrees?
- It is currently unclear what the optimal algorithm is for SDB diagnosis (PSG vs PM) and therapy (targeting the best outcomes, personalizing risks and benefits, and so forth).

CSA

- What are the risk factors for high-altitude CSA?
- What are the risk factors for CxSA?
- What is the role of PM or OSG in the evaluation of CSA?
- Is there any long-term benefit from PAP therapy for CSA?
- Is there any long-term benefit from pharmacologic therapy for CSA?
- Is there any long-term benefit from oxygen therapy for CSA?
- Can better and safer delivery methods be found and is there any long-term benefit from CO_2 supplementation in CSA?

REFERENCES

1. Iber C, Ancoli-Israel S, Chesson A, et al. The AASM manual for the scoring of sleep and associated events - rules, terminology and technical specifications. 1st edition. Westchester (IL): American Academy of Sleep Medicine; 2007.
2. Kotha K, Ioachimescu OC. Obstructive Sleep Apnea. In: Ioachimescu OC, editor. Contemporary Sleep Medicine (for Physicians, online publication, 1st edition). Sharjah (UAE): Bentham Science Publishers; 2011.
3. Guilleminault C, Tilkian A, Dement WC. The sleep apnea syndromes. Annu Rev Med 1976;27:465–84.
4. Epstein LJ, Kristo D, Strollo PJ Jr, et al. Clinical guideline for the evaluation, management and long-term care of obstructive sleep apnea in adults. J Clin Sleep Med 2009;5(3):263–76.
5. Gupta RM, Parvizi J, Hanssen AD, et al. Postoperative complications in patients with obstructive sleep apnea syndrome undergoing hip or knee replacement: a case-control study. Mayo Clin Proc 2001;76(9):897–905.

6. Kaw R, Golish J, Ghamande S, et al. Incremental risk of obstructive sleep apnea on cardiac surgical outcomes. J Cardiovasc Surg (Torino) 2006;47(6):683–9.

7. Peppard PE, Young T, Palta M, et al. Prospective study of the association between sleep-disordered breathing and hypertension. N Engl J Med 2000; 342(19):1378–84.

8. Schafer H, Koehler U, Ewig S, et al. Obstructive sleep apnea as a risk marker in coronary artery disease. Cardiology 1999;92(2):79–84.

9. Peker Y, Kraiczi H, Hedner J, et al. An independent association between obstructive sleep apnoea and coronary artery disease. Eur Respir J 1999;14(1):179–84.

10. Gami AS, Howard DE, Olson EJ, et al. Day-night pattern of sudden death in obstructive sleep apnea. N Engl J Med 2005;352(12):1206–14.

11. Arzt M, Young T, Finn L, et al. Association of sleep-disordered breathing and the occurrence of stroke. Am J Respir Crit Care Med 2005;172(11):1447–51.

12. Yaggi HK, Concato J, Kernan WN, et al. Obstructive sleep apnea as a risk factor for stroke and death. N Engl J Med 2005;353(19):2034–41.

13. Krieger J, Sforza E, Apprill M, et al. Pulmonary hypertension, hypoxemia, and hypercapnia in obstructive sleep apnea patients. Chest 1989;96(4):729–37.

14. Ambrosetti M, Lucioni A, Ageno W, et al. Is venous thromboembolism more frequent in patients with obstructive sleep apnea syndrome? J Thromb Haemost 2004;2(10):1858–60.

15. Jean-Louis G, Zizi F, Clark LT, et al. Obstructive sleep apnea and cardiovascular disease: role of the metabolic syndrome and its components. J Clin Sleep Med 2008;4(3):261–72.

16. Punjabi NM, Shahar E, Redline S, et al. Sleep-disordered breathing, glucose intolerance, and insulin resistance: the Sleep Heart Health Study. Am J Epidemiol 2004;160(6):521–30.

17. Marin JM, Carrizo SJ, Vicente E, et al. Long-term cardiovascular outcomes in men with obstructive sleep apnoea-hypopnoea with or without treatment with continuous positive airway pressure: an observational study. Lancet 2005; 365(9464):1046–53.

18. Nieto FJ, Young TB, Lind BK, et al. Association of sleep-disordered breathing, sleep apnea, and hypertension in a large community-based study. Sleep Heart Health Study. JAMA 2000;283(14):1829–36.

19. Peppard PE, Young T, Palta M, et al. Longitudinal study of moderate weight change and sleep-disordered breathing. JAMA 2000;284(23):3015–21.

20. Young T, Peppard PE, Gottlieb DJ. Epidemiology of obstructive sleep apnea: a population health perspective. Am J Respir Crit Care Med 2002;165(9): 1217–39.

21. Moyer CA, Sonnad SS, Garetz SL, et al. Quality of life in obstructive sleep apnea: a systematic review of the literature. Sleep Med 2001;2(6):477–91.

22. Engleman HM, Douglas NJ. Sleep, driving and the workplace. Clin Med 2005; 5(2):113–7.

23. Sassani A, Findley LJ, Kryger M, et al. Reducing motor-vehicle collisions, costs, and fatalities by treating obstructive sleep apnea syndrome. Sleep 2004;27(3): 453–8.

24. Lindberg E, Carter N, Gislason T, et al. Role of snoring and daytime sleepiness in occupational accidents. Am J Respir Crit Care Med 2001;164(11):2031–5.

25. Saunamaki T, Jehkonen M. A review of executive functions in obstructive sleep apnea syndrome. Acta Neurol Scand 2007;115(1):1–11.

26. Marshall NS, Wong KK, Liu PY, et al. Sleep apnea as an independent risk factor for all-cause mortality: the Busselton Health Study. Sleep 2008;31(8):1079–85.

27. Young T, Finn L, Peppard PE, et al. Sleep disordered breathing and mortality: eighteen-year follow-up of the Wisconsin sleep cohort. Sleep 2008;31(8): 1071–8.

28. Young T, Palta M, Dempsey J, et al. The occurrence of sleep-disordered breathing among middle-aged adults. N Engl J Med 1993;328(17):1230–5.

29. Bixler EO, Vgontzas AN, Ten HT, et al. Effects of age on sleep apnea in men: I. Prevalence and severity. Am J Respir Crit Care Med 1998;157(1):144–8.

30. Bixler EO, Vgontzas AN, Lin HM, et al. Prevalence of sleep-disordered breathing in women: effects of gender. Am J Respir Crit Care Med 2001;163(3 Pt 1): 608–13.

31. Ip MS, Lam B, Lauder IJ, et al. A community study of sleep-disordered breathing in middle-aged Chinese men in Hong Kong. Chest 2001;119(1):62–9.

32. Ip MS, Lam B, Tang LC, et al. A community study of sleep-disordered breathing in middle-aged Chinese women in Hong Kong: prevalence and gender differences. Chest 2004;125(1):127–34.

33. American Academy of Sleep Medicine Task Force Report. Sleep related breathing disorders in adults:recommendations for syndrome, definition and measurement techniques in clinical research. Sleep 1999;22:667–89.

34. Santos-Silva R, Tufik S, Conway SG, et al. Sao Paulo epidemiologic sleep study: rationale, design, sampling, and procedures. Sleep Med 2009;10(6):679–85.

35. Stradling JR, Crosby JH. Predictors and prevalence of obstructive sleep apnoea and snoring in 1001 middle aged men. Thorax 1991;46(2):85–90.

36. Jennum P, Sjol A. Epidemiology of snoring and obstructive sleep apnoea in a Danish population, age 30-60. J Sleep Res 1992;1(4):240–4.

37. Punjabi NM. The epidemiology of adult obstructive sleep apnea. Proc Am Thorac Soc 2008;5(2):136–43.

38. Bearpark H, Elliott L, Grunstein R, et al. Snoring and sleep apnea. A population study in Australian men. Am J Respir Crit Care Med 1995;151(5):1459–65.

39. Duran J, Esnaola S, Rubio R, et al. Obstructive sleep apnea-hypopnea and related clinical features in a population-based sample of subjects aged 30 to 70 yr. Am J Respir Crit Care Med 2001;163(3 Pt 1):685–9.

40. Udwadia ZF, Doshi AV, Lonkar SG, et al. Prevalence of sleep-disordered breathing and sleep apnea in middle-aged urban Indian men. Am J Respir Crit Care Med 2004;169(2):168–73.

41. Puvanendran K, Goh KL. From snoring to sleep apnea in a Singapore population. Sleep Res Online 1999;2(1):11–4.

42. Gislason T, Almqvist M, Eriksson G, et al. Prevalence of sleep apnea syndrome among Swedish men—an epidemiological study. J Clin Epidemiol 1988;41(6): 571–6.

43. Tishler PV, Larkin EK, Schluchter MD, et al. Incidence of sleep-disordered breathing in an urban adult population: the relative importance of risk factors in the development of sleep-disordered breathing. JAMA 2003;289(17):2230–7.

44. Young T, Evans L, Finn L, et al. Estimation of the clinically diagnosed proportion of sleep apnea syndrome in middle-aged men and women. Sleep 1997;20(9): 705–6.

45. Kapur V, Strohl KP, Redline S, et al. Underdiagnosis of sleep apnea syndrome in U.S. communities. Sleep Breath 2002;6(2):49–54.

46. Foley DJ, Monjan AA, Brown SL, et al. Sleep complaints among elderly persons: an epidemiologic study of three communities. Sleep 1995;18(6):425–32.

47. Ancoli-Israel S, Kripke DF, Klauber MR, et al. Sleep-disordered breathing in community-dwelling elderly. Sleep 1991;14(6):486–95.

48. Young T, Skatrud J, Peppard PE. Risk factors for obstructive sleep apnea in adults. JAMA 2004;291(16):2013–6.
49. Obesity and overweight, 2006. Available at: www.who.int/mediacentre/factsheets/fs311/en/index.html. 2006. Accessed May, 2012.
50. Obesity in US adults: 2007. Available at: http://www.obesity.org/statistics/. 2007. Accessed May, 2012.
51. Katz I, Stradling J, Slutsky AS, et al. Do patients with obstructive sleep apnea have thick necks? Am Rev Respir Dis 1990;141(5 Pt 1):1228–31.
52. Grunstein R, Wilcox I, Yang TS, et al. Snoring and sleep apnoea in men: association with central obesity and hypertension. Int J Obes Relat Metab Disord 1993;17(9):533–40.
53. Davies RJ, Stradling JR. The relationship between neck circumference, radiographic pharyngeal anatomy, and the obstructive sleep apnoea syndrome. Eur Respir J 1990;3(5):509–14.
54. Davies RJ, Ali NJ, Stradling JR. Neck circumference and other clinical features in the diagnosis of the obstructive sleep apnoea syndrome. Thorax 1992;47(2):101–5.
55. Hoffstein V, Mateika S. Differences in abdominal and neck circumferences in patients with and without obstructive sleep apnoea. Eur Respir J 1992;5(4):377–81.
56. Levinson PD, McGarvey ST, Carlisle CC, et al. Adiposity and cardiovascular risk factors in men with obstructive sleep apnea. Chest 1993;103(5):1336–42.
57. Millman RP, Carlisle CC, McGarvey ST, et al. Body fat distribution and sleep apnea severity in women. Chest 1995;107(2):362–6.
58. Shelton KE, Woodson H, Gay S, et al. Pharyngeal fat in obstructive sleep apnea. Am Rev Respir Dis 1993;148(2):462–6.
59. Shinohara E, Kihara S, Yamashita S, et al. Visceral fat accumulation as an important risk factor for obstructive sleep apnoea syndrome in obese subjects. J Intern Med 1997;241(1):11–8.
60. Ferini-Strambi L, Zucconi M, Palazzi S, et al. Snoring and nocturnal oxygen desaturations in an Italian middle-aged male population. Epidemiologic study with an ambulatory device. Chest 1994;105(6):1759–64.
61. Newman AB, Nieto FJ, Guidry U, et al. Relation of sleep-disordered breathing to cardiovascular disease risk factors: the Sleep Heart Health Study. Am J Epidemiol 2001;154(1):50–9.
62. Olson LG, King MT, Hensley MJ, et al. A community study of snoring and sleep-disordered breathing. Prevalence. Am J Respir Crit Care Med 1995;152(2):711–6.
63. Jennum P, Hein HO, Suadicani P, et al. Cardiovascular risk factors in snorers. A cross-sectional study of 3,323 men aged 54 to 74 years: the Copenhagen Male Study. Chest 1992;102(5):1371–6.
64. Jennum P, Sjol A. Snoring, sleep apnoea and cardiovascular risk factors: the MONICA II study. Int J Epidemiol 1993;22(3):439–44.
65. Schmidt-Nowara WW, Coultas DB, Wiggins C, et al. Snoring in a Hispanic-American population. Risk factors and association with hypertension and other morbidity. Arch Intern Med 1990;150(3):597–601.
66. Frey WC, Pilcher J. Obstructive sleep-related breathing disorders in patients evaluated for bariatric surgery. Obes Surg 2003;13(5):676–83.
67. O'Keeffe T, Patterson EJ. Evidence supporting routine polysomnography before bariatric surgery. Obes Surg 2004;14(1):23–6.
68. Bae C, Schauer P, Chand B, et al. Physical examination predictors of obstructive sleep apnea in bariatric surgery candidates. Sleep 2007;30(Suppl):A207.

69. Bliwise DL. Epidemiology of age-dependence in sleep disordered breathing (SDB) in old age: the Bay Area Sleep Cohort (BASC). Sleep Med Clin 2009; 4(1):57–64.

70. Jennum P, Riha RL. Epidemiology of sleep apnoea/hypopnoea syndrome and sleep-disordered breathing. Eur Respir J 2009;33(4):907–14.

71. Flemons WW. Clinical practice. Obstructive sleep apnea. N Engl J Med 2002; 347(7):498–504.

72. Franklin KA, Holmgren PA, Jonsson F, et al. Snoring, pregnancy-induced hypertension, and growth retardation of the fetus. Chest 2000;117(1):137–41.

73. Guilleminault C, Querra-Salva M, Chowdhuri S, et al. Normal pregnancy, daytime sleeping, snoring and blood pressure. Sleep Med 2000;1(4):289–97.

74. Pillar G, Lavie P. Assessment of the role of inheritance in sleep apnea syndrome. Am J Respir Crit Care Med 1995;151(3 Pt 1):688–91.

75. Mathur R, Douglas NJ. Family studies in patients with the sleep apnea-hypopnea syndrome. Ann Intern Med 1995;122(3):174–8.

76. Redline S, Tishler PV, Tosteson TD, et al. The familial aggregation of obstructive sleep apnea. Am J Respir Crit Care Med 1995;151(3 Pt 1):682–7.

77. Ovchinsky A, Rao M, Lotwin I, et al. The familial aggregation of pediatric obstructive sleep apnea syndrome. Arch Otolaryngol Head Neck Surg 2002; 128(7):815–8.

78. Carmelli D, Bliwise DL, Swan GE, et al. Genetic factors in self-reported snoring and excessive daytime sleepiness: a twin study. Am J Respir Crit Care Med 2001;164(6):949–52.

79. Jennum P, Hein HO, Suadicani P, et al. Snoring, family history, and genetic markers in men. The Copenhagen Male Study. Chest 1995;107(5):1289–93.

80. Riha RL, Gislasson T, Diefenbach K. The phenotype and genotype of adult obstructive sleep apnoea/hypopnoea syndrome. Eur Respir J 2009;33(3):646–55.

81. Palmer LJ, Buxbaum SG, Larkin E, et al. A whole-genome scan for obstructive sleep apnea and obesity. Am J Hum Genet 2003;72(2):340–50.

82. Palmer LJ, Buxbaum SG, Larkin EK, et al. Whole genome scan for obstructive sleep apnea and obesity in African-American families. Am J Respir Crit Care Med 2004;169(12):1314–21.

83. Patel SR, Larkin EK, Redline S. Shared genetic basis for obstructive sleep apnea and adiposity measures. Int J Obes (Lond) 2008;32(5):795–800.

84. Schwab RJ, Pasirstein M, Kaplan L, et al. Family aggregation of upper airway soft tissue structures in normal subjects and patients with sleep apnea. Am J Respir Crit Care Med 2006;173(4):453–63.

85. Li KK, Powell NB, Kushida C, et al. A comparison of Asian and white patients with obstructive sleep apnea syndrome. Laryngoscope 1999;109(12):1937–40.

86. Lam B, Ip MS, Tench E, et al. Craniofacial profile in Asian and white subjects with obstructive sleep apnoea. Thorax 2005;60(6):504–10.

87. Wetter DW, Young TB, Bidwell TR, et al. Smoking as a risk factor for sleep-disordered breathing. Arch Intern Med 1994;154(19):2219–24.

88. Lavie L, Lavie P. Smoking interacts with sleep apnea to increase cardiovascular risk. Sleep Med 2008;9(3):247–53.

89. Mitler MM, Dawson A, Henriksen SJ, et al. Bedtime ethanol increases resistance of upper airways and produces sleep apneas in asymptomatic snorers. Alcohol Clin Exp Res 1988;12(6):801–5.

90. Berry RB, Bonnet MH, Light RW. Effect of ethanol on the arousal response to airway occlusion during sleep in normal subjects. Am Rev Respir Dis 1992; 145(2 Pt 1):445–52.

91. Scanlan MF, Roebuck T, Little PJ, et al. Effect of moderate alcohol upon obstructive sleep apnoea. Eur Respir J 2000;16(5):909–13.
92. Young T, Finn L, Kim H. Nasal obstruction as a risk factor for sleep-disordered breathing. The University of Wisconsin Sleep and Respiratory Research Group. J Allergy Clin Immunol 1997;99(2):S757–62.
93. McNicholas WT, Tarlo S, Cole P, et al. Obstructive apneas during sleep in patients with seasonal allergic rhinitis. Am Rev Respir Dis 1982;126(4):625–8.
94. Grunstein RR, Ho KY, Sullivan CE. Sleep apnea in acromegaly. Ann Intern Med 1991;115(7):527–32.
95. Lanfranco F, Motta G, Minetto MA, et al. Neuroendocrine alterations in obese patients with sleep apnea syndrome. Int J Endocrinol 2010;2010:474518.
96. Fatti LM, Scacchi M, Pincelli AI, et al. Prevalence and pathogenesis of sleep apnea and lung disease in acromegaly. Pituitary 2001;4(4):259–62.
97. Mestron A, Webb SM, Astorga R, et al. Epidemiology, clinical characteristics, outcome, morbidity and mortality in acromegaly based on the Spanish Acromegaly Registry (Registro Espanol de Acromegalia, REA). Eur J Endocrinol 2004;151(4):439–46.
98. Winkelman JW, Goldman H, Piscatelli N, et al. Are thyroid function tests necessary in patients with suspected sleep apnea? Sleep 1996;19(10):790–3.
99. Fogel RB, Malhotra A, Pillar G, et al. Increased prevalence of obstructive sleep apnea syndrome in obese women with polycystic ovary syndrome. J Clin Endocrinol Metab 2001;86(3):1175–80.
100. Vgontzas AN, Legro RS, Bixler EO, et al. Polycystic ovary syndrome is associated with obstructive sleep apnea and daytime sleepiness: role of insulin resistance. J Clin Endocrinol Metab 2001;86(2):517–20.
101. Schneider BK, Pickett CK, Zwillich CW, et al. Influence of testosterone on breathing during sleep. J Appl Physiol 1986;61(2):618–23.
102. Liu PY, Yee B, Wishart SM, et al. The short-term effects of high-dose testosterone on sleep, breathing, and function in older men. J Clin Endocrinol Metab 2003; 88(8):3605–13.
103. Haponik EF, Smith PL, Bohlman ME, et al. Computerized tomography in obstructive sleep apnea. Correlation of airway size with physiology during sleep and wakefulness. Am Rev Respir Dis 1983;127(2):221–6.
104. Schwab RJ, Gefter WB, Hoffman EA, et al. Dynamic upper airway imaging during awake respiration in normal subjects and patients with sleep disordered breathing. Am Rev Respir Dis 1993;148(5):1385–400.
105. Schwab RJ, Gefter WB, Pack AI, et al. Dynamic imaging of the upper airway during respiration in normal subjects. J Appl Physiol 1993;74(4):1504–14.
106. Schwab RJ, Gupta KB, Gefter WB, et al. Upper airway and soft tissue anatomy in normal subjects and patients with sleep-disordered breathing. Significance of the lateral pharyngeal walls. Am J Respir Crit Care Med 1995;152(5 Pt 1):1673–89.
107. Remmers JE, Anch AM, deGroot WJ, et al. Oropharyngeal muscle tone in obstructive sleep apnea before and after strychnine. Sleep 1980;3(3–4):447–53.
108. Isono S, Feroah TR, Hajduk EA, et al. Interaction of cross-sectional area, driving pressure, and airflow of passive velopharynx. J Appl Physiol 1997;83(3):851–9.
109. White DP. The pathogenesis of obstructive sleep apnea: advances in the past 100 years. Am J Respir Cell Mol Biol 2006;34(1):1–6.
110. Fogel RB, Malhotra A, White DP. Sleep. 2: pathophysiology of obstructive sleep apnoea/hypopnoea syndrome. Thorax 2004;59(2):159–63.
111. Dempsey JA, Veasey SC, Morgan BJ, et al. Pathophysiology of sleep apnea. Physiol Rev 2010;90(1):47–112.

112. Wenner JB, Cheema R, Ayas NT. Clinical manifestations and consequences of obstructive sleep apnea. J Cardiopulm Rehabil Prev 2009;29(2):76–83.
113. Cluydts R, De VE, Verstraeten E, et al. Daytime sleepiness and its evaluation. Sleep Med Rev 2002;6(2):83–96.
114. Ramachandran SK, Josephs LA. A meta-analysis of clinical screening tests for obstructive sleep apnea. Anesthesiology 2009;110(4):928–39.
115. Netzer NC, Stoohs RA, Netzer CM, et al. Using the Berlin Questionnaire to identify patients at risk for the sleep apnea syndrome. Ann Intern Med 1999;131(7): 485–91.
116. Nuckton TJ, Glidden DV, Browner WS, et al. Physical examination: mallampati score as an independent predictor of obstructive sleep apnea. Sleep 2006; 29(7):903–8.
117. Waite PD. Obstructive sleep apnea: a review of the pathophysiology and surgical management. Oral Surg Oral Med Oral Pathol Oral Radiol Endod 1998;85(4): 352–61.
118. Ioachimescu OC. The diagnosis and severity of obstructive sleep apnea (OSA): a comprehensive analysis of different predictive models. 21st Annual Meeting of the Associated Professional Sleep Societies. Sleep 2007;30(Suppl):A165.
119. Netzer N, Eliasson AH, Netzer C, et al. Overnight pulse oximetry for sleep-disordered breathing in adults: a review. Chest 2001;120(2):625–33.
120. ICSD-2-The international classification of sleep disorders—diagnostic and coding manual. 2nd edition. Westchester (IL): American Academy of Sleep Medicine; 2005.
121. Collop NA, Anderson WM, Boehlecke B, et al. Clinical guidelines for the use of unattended portable monitors in the diagnosis of obstructive sleep apnea in adult patients. Portable monitoring task force of the American Academy of Sleep Medicine. J Clin Sleep Med 2007;3(7):737–47.
122. Littner MR, Kushida C, Wise M, et al. Practice parameters for clinical use of the multiple sleep latency test and the maintenance of wakefulness test. Sleep 2005;28(1):113–21.
123. Arand D, Bonnet M, Hurwitz T, et al. The clinical use of the MSLT and MWT. Sleep 2005;28(1):123–44.
124. Bonnet MH. ACNS clinical controversy: MSLT and MWT have limited clinical utility. J Clin Neurophysiol 2006;23(1):50–8.
125. Bonnet MH, Arand DL. We are chronically sleep deprived. Sleep 1995;18(10): 908–11.
126. Guilleminault C, Rosekind M. The arousal threshold: sleep deprivation, sleep fragmentation, and obstructive sleep apnea syndrome. Bull Eur Physiopathol Respir 1981;17(3):341–9.
127. White DP, Douglas NJ, Pickett CK, et al. Sleep deprivation and the control of ventilation. Am Rev Respir Dis 1983;128(6):984–6.
128. Bowes G, Woolf GM, Sullivan CE, et al. Effect of sleep fragmentation on ventilatory and arousal responses of sleeping dogs to respiratory stimuli. Am Rev Respir Dis 1980;122(6):899–908.
129. Harman EM, Wynne JW, Block AJ. The effect of weight loss on sleep-disordered breathing and oxygen desaturation in morbidly obese men. Chest 1982;82(3): 291–4.
130. Kajaste S, Brander PE, Telakivi T, et al. A cognitive-behavioral weight reduction program in the treatment of obstructive sleep apnea syndrome with or without initial nasal CPAP: a randomized study. Sleep Med 2004;5(2): 125–31.

131. Schwartz AR, Gold AR, Schubert N, et al. Effect of weight loss on upper airway collapsibility in obstructive sleep apnea. Am Rev Respir Dis 1991;144(3 Pt 1): 494–8.

132. Smith PL, Gold AR, Meyers DA, et al. Weight loss in mildly to moderately obese patients with obstructive sleep apnea. Ann Intern Med 1985;103(6 Pt 1):850–5.

133. Suratt PM, McTier RF, Findley LJ, et al. Changes in breathing and the pharynx after weight loss in obstructive sleep apnea. Chest 1987;92(4):631–7.

134. Buchwald H, Avidor Y, Braunwald E, et al. Bariatric surgery: a systematic review and meta-analysis. JAMA 2004;292(14):1724–37.

135. Fernandez AZ Jr, DeMaria EJ, Tichansky DS, et al. Experience with over 3,000 open and laparoscopic bariatric procedures: multivariate analysis of factors related to leak and resultant mortality. Surg Endosc 2004;18(2):193–7.

136. Perugini RA, Mason R, Czerniach DR, et al. Predictors of complication and suboptimal weight loss after laparoscopic Roux-en-Y gastric bypass: a series of 188 patients. Arch Surg 2003;138(5):541–5.

137. Phillips BA, Danner FJ. Cigarette smoking and sleep disturbance. Arch Intern Med 1995;155(7):734–7.

138. Berry RB, Desa MM, Light RW. Effect of ethanol on the efficacy of nasal continuous positive airway pressure as a treatment for obstructive sleep apnea. Chest 1991;99(2):339–43.

139. Gleeson K, Zwillich CW, White DP. The influence of increasing ventilatory effort on arousal from sleep. Am Rev Respir Dis 1990;142(2):295–300.

140. Teschler H, Berthon-Jones M, Wessendorf T, et al. Influence of moderate alcohol consumption on obstructive sleep apnoea with and without AutoSet nasal CPAP therapy. Eur Respir J 1996;9(11):2371–7.

141. Kohler M, Bloch KE, Stradling JR. Pharmacological approaches to the treatment of obstructive sleep apnoea. Expert Opin Investig Drugs 2009;18(5):647–56.

142. Espinoza H, Antic R, Thornton AT, et al. The effects of aminophylline on sleep and sleep-disordered breathing in patients with obstructive sleep apnea syndrome. Am Rev Respir Dis 1987;136(1):80–4.

143. Mulloy E, McNicholas WT. Theophylline in obstructive sleep apnea. A double-blind evaluation. Chest 1992;101(3):753–7.

144. Whyte KF, Gould GA, Airlie MA, et al. Role of protriptyline and acetazolamide in the sleep apnea/hypopnea syndrome. Sleep 1988;11(5):463–72.

145. Atkinson RL, Suratt PM, Wilhoit SC, et al. Naloxone improves sleep apnea in obese humans. Int J Obes 1985;9(4):233–9.

146. Ferber C, Duclaux R, Mouret J. Naltrexone improves blood gas patterns in obstructive sleep apnoea syndrome through its influence on sleep. J Sleep Res 1993;2(3):149–55.

147. Cook WR, Benich JJ, Wooten SA. Indices of severity of obstructive sleep apnea syndrome do not change during medroxyprogesterone acetate therapy. Chest 1989;96(2):262–6.

148. Stradling J, Smith D, Radulovacki M, et al. Effect of ondansetron on moderate obstructive sleep apnoea, a single night, placebo-controlled trial. J Sleep Res 2003;12(2):169–70.

149. Veasey SC, Chachkes J, Fenik P, et al. The effects of ondansetron on sleep-disordered breathing in the English bulldog. Sleep 2001;24(2):155–60.

150. Weichler U, Herres-Mayer B, Mayer J, et al. Influence of antihypertensive drug therapy on sleep pattern and sleep apnea activity. Cardiology 1991;78(2):124–30.

151. Salo TM, Kantola I, Voipio-Pulkki LM, et al. The effect of four different antihypertensive medications on cardiovascular regulation in hypertensive sleep apneic

patients–assessment by spectral analysis of heart rate and blood pressure variability. Eur J Clin Pharmacol 1999;55(3):191–8.

152. Salo TM, Metsala TH, Kantola IM, et al. Ramipril Enhances Autonomic Control in Essential Hypertension: A Study Employing Spectral Analysis of Heart Rate Variation. Am J Ther 1994;1(3):191–7.

153. Bucca CB, Brussino L, Battisti A, et al. Diuretics in obstructive sleep apnea with diastolic heart failure. Chest 2007;132(2):440–6.

154. Pimenta E, Gaddam KK, Oparil S. Mechanisms and treatment of resistant hypertension. J Clin Hypertens (Greenwich) 2008;10(3):239–44.

155. Ziegler MG, Milic M, Sun P. Antihypertensive therapy for patients with obstructive sleep apnea. Curr Opin Nephrol Hypertens 2011;20(1):50–5.

156. Martin RJ, Sanders MH, Gray BA, et al. Acute and long-term ventilatory effects of hyperoxia in the adult sleep apnea syndrome. Am Rev Respir Dis 1982; 125(2):175–80.

157. Gold AR, Schwartz AR, Bleecker ER, et al. The effect of chronic nocturnal oxygen administration upon sleep apnea. Am Rev Respir Dis 1986;134(5):925–9.

158. Sanders MH, Rogers RM. Sleep apnea: when does better become benefit? Chest 1985;88(3):320–1.

159. Hanly P, Sasson Z, Zuberi N, et al. ST-segment depression during sleep in obstructive sleep apnea. Am J Cardiol 1993;71(15):1341–5.

160. Franklin KA, Nilsson JB, Sahlin C, et al. Sleep apnoea and nocturnal angina. Lancet 1995;345(8957):1085–7.

161. Sanders MH, Kern N. Obstructive sleep apnea treated by independently adjusted inspiratory and expiratory positive airway pressures via nasal mask. Physiologic and clinical implications. Chest 1990;98(2):317–24.

162. Piper AJ, Sullivan CE. Effects of short-term NIPPV in the treatment of patients with severe obstructive sleep apnea and hypercapnia. Chest 1994;105(2):434–40.

163. Pepin JL, Viot-Blanc V, Escourrou P, et al. Prevalence of residual excessive sleepiness in CPAP-treated sleep apnoea patients: the French multicentre study. Eur Respir J 2009;33(5):1062–7.

164. Morgenthaler TI, Kapen S, Lee-Chiong T, et al. Practice parameters for the medical therapy of obstructive sleep apnea. Sleep 2006;29(8):1031–5.

165. Veasey SC, Guilleminault C, Strohl KP, et al. Medical therapy for obstructive sleep apnea: a review by the Medical Therapy for Obstructive Sleep Apnea Task Force of the Standards of Practice Committee of the American Academy of Sleep Medicine. Sleep 2006;29(8):1036–44.

166. Black JE, Hirshkowitz M. Modafinil for treatment of residual excessive sleepiness in nasal continuous positive airway pressure-treated obstructive sleep apnea/hypopnea syndrome. Sleep 2005;28(4):464–71.

167. Kingshott RN, Vennelle M, Coleman EL, et al. Randomized, double-blind, placebo-controlled crossover trial of modafinil in the treatment of residual excessive daytime sleepiness in the sleep apnea/hypopnea syndrome. Am J Respir Crit Care Med 2001;163(4):918–23.

168. Pack AI, Black JE, Schwartz JR, et al. Modafinil as adjunct therapy for daytime sleepiness in obstructive sleep apnea. Am J Respir Crit Care Med 2001;164(9): 1675–81.

169. Schwartz JR, Hirshkowitz M, Erman MK, et al. Modafinil as adjunct therapy for daytime sleepiness in obstructive sleep apnea: a 12-week, open-label study. Chest 2003;124(6):2192–9.

170. Roth T, White D, Schmidt-Nowara W, et al. Effects of armodafinil in the treatment of residual excessive sleepiness associated with obstructive sleep apnea/

hypopnea syndrome: a 12-week, multicenter, double-blind, randomized, placebo-controlled study in nCPAP-adherent adults. Clin Ther 2006;28(5): 689–706.

171. Hirshkowitz M, Black JE, Wesnes K, et al. Adjunct armodafinil improves wakefulness and memory in obstructive sleep apnea/hypopnea syndrome. Respir Med 2007;101(3):616–27.

172. Hou RH, Langley RW, Szabadi E, et al. Comparison of diphenhydramine and modafinil on arousal and autonomic functions in healthy volunteers. J Psychopharmacol 2007;21(6):567–78.

173. Wong YN, Simcoe D, Hartman LN, et al. A double-blind, placebo-controlled, ascending-dose evaluation of the pharmacokinetics and tolerability of modafinil tablets in healthy male volunteers. J Clin Pharmacol 1999;39(1):30–40.

174. Lavie P, Fischel N, Zomer J, et al. The effects of partial and complete mechanical occlusion of the nasal passages on sleep structure and breathing in sleep. Acta Otolaryngol 1983;95(1–2):161–6.

175. Suratt PM, Turner BL, Wilhoit SC. Effect of intranasal obstruction on breathing during sleep. Chest 1986;90(3):324–9.

176. Hoijer U, Ejnell H, Hedner J, et al. The effects of nasal dilation on snoring and obstructive sleep apnea. Arch Otolaryngol Head Neck Surg 1992;118(3):281–4.

177. Hoffstein V, Mateika S, Metes A. Effect of nasal dilation on snoring and apneas during different stages of sleep. Sleep 1993;16(4):360–5.

178. Scharf MB, Brannen DE, McDannold M. A subjective evaluation of a nasal dilator on sleep & snoring. Ear Nose Throat J 1994;73(6):395–401.

179. Scharf MB, McDannold MD, Zaretsky NT, et al. Cyclic alternating pattern sequences in non-apneic snorers with and without nasal dilation. Ear Nose Throat J 1996;75(9):617–9.

180. Cornblatt B, Obuchowski M, Roberts S, et al. Cognitive and behavioral precursors of schizophrenia. Dev Psychopathol 1999;11(3):487–508.

181. Afzelius LE, Elmqvist D, Hougaard K, et al. Sleep apnea syndrome—an alternative treatment to tracheostomy. Laryngoscope 1981;91(2):285–91.

182. Nahmias JS, Karetzky MS. Treatment of the obstructive sleep apnea syndrome using a nasopharyngeal tube. Chest 1988;94(6):1142–7.

183. Berry RB, Kryger MH, Massie CA. A novel nasal expiratory positive airway pressure (EPAP) device for the treatment of obstructive sleep apnea: a randomized controlled trial. Sleep 2011;34(4):479–85.

184. Patel AV, Hwang D, Masdeu MJ, et al. Predictors of response to a nasal expiratory resistor device and its potential mechanisms of action for treatment of obstructive sleep apnea. J Clin Sleep Med 2011;7(1):13–22.

185. Sullivan CE, Issa FG, Berthon-Jones M, et al. Reversal of obstructive sleep apnoea by continuous positive airway pressure applied through the nares. Lancet 1981;1(8225):862–5.

186. Grunstein RR. Sleep-related breathing disorders. 5. Nasal continuous airway pressure treatment for obstructive sleep apnoea. Thorax 1995;50(10):1106–13.

187. Grunstein RR, Hedner J, Grote L. Treatment options for sleep apnoea. Drugs 2001;61(2):237–51.

188. McDaid C, Duree KH, Griffin SC, et al. A systematic review of continuous positive airway pressure for obstructive sleep apnoea-hypopnoea syndrome. Sleep Med Rev 2009;13(6):427–36.

189. Patel SR, White DP, Malhotra A, et al. Continuous positive airway pressure therapy for treating sleepiness in a diverse population with obstructive sleep apnea: results of a meta-analysis. Arch Intern Med 2003;163(5):565–71.

190. Giles TL, Lasserson TJ, Smith BH, et al. Continuous positive airways pressure for obstructive sleep apnoea in adults. Cochrane Database Syst Rev 2006;(3): CD001106.

191. Reeves-Hoche MK, Hudgel DW, Meck R, et al. Continuous versus bilevel positive airway pressure for obstructive sleep apnea. Am J Respir Crit Care Med 1995;151(2 Pt 1):443–9.

192. Fietze I, Glos M, Moebus I, et al. Automatic pressure titration with APAP is as effective as manual titration with CPAP in patients with obstructive sleep apnea. Respiration 2007;74(3):279–86.

193. Nussbaumer Y, Bloch KE, Genser T, et al. Equivalence of autoadjusted and constant continuous positive airway pressure in home treatment of sleep apnea. Chest 2006;129(3):638–43.

194. Zozula R, Rosen R. Compliance with continuous positive airway pressure therapy: assessing and improving treatment outcomes. Curr Opin Pulm Med 2001;7(6):391–8.

195. Fitzpatrick MF, Alloway CE, Wakeford TM, et al. Can patients with obstructive sleep apnea titrate their own continuous positive airway pressure? Am J Respir Crit Care Med 2003;167(5):716–22.

196. Mehta A, Qian J, Petocz P, et al. A randomized, controlled study of a mandibular advancement splint for obstructive sleep apnea. Am J Respir Crit Care Med 2001;163(6):1457–61.

197. Gotsopoulos H, Chen C, Qian J, et al. Oral appliance therapy improves symptoms in obstructive sleep apnea: a randomized, controlled trial. Am J Respir Crit Care Med 2002;166(5):743–8.

198. Cistulli PA, Gotsopoulos H, Marklund M, et al. Treatment of snoring and obstructive sleep apnea with mandibular repositioning appliances. Sleep Med Rev 2004;8(6):443–57.

199. Ferguson KA, Cartwright R, Rogers R, et al. Oral appliances for snoring and obstructive sleep apnea: a review. Sleep 2006;29(2):244–62.

200. Gagnadoux F, Fleury B, Vielle B, et al. Titrated mandibular advancement versus positive airway pressure for sleep apnoea. Eur Respir J 2009;34(4): 914–20.

201. Hoekema A, Stegenga B, Bakker M, et al. Simulated driving in obstructive sleep apnoea-hypopnoea; effects of oral appliances and continuous positive airway pressure. Sleep Breath 2007;11(3):129–38.

202. Barnes M, McEvoy RD, Banks S, et al. Efficacy of positive airway pressure and oral appliance in mild to moderate obstructive sleep apnea. Am J Respir Crit Care Med 2004;170(6):656–64.

203. Andren A, Sjoquist M, Tegelberg A. Effects on blood pressure after treatment of obstructive sleep apnoea with a mandibular advancement appliance - a three-year follow-up. J Oral Rehabil 2009;36(10):719–25.

204. Schmidt-Nowara W, Lowe A, Wiegand L, et al. Oral appliances for the treatment of snoring and obstructive sleep apnea: a review. Sleep 1995;18(6):501–10.

205. Marklund M, Sahlin C, Stenlund H, et al. Mandibular advancement device in patients with obstructive sleep apnea: long-term effects on apnea and sleep. Chest 2001;120(1):162–9.

206. Marklund M, Stenlund H, Franklin KA. Mandibular advancement devices in 630 men and women with obstructive sleep apnea and snoring: tolerability and predictors of treatment success. Chest 2004;125(4):1270–8.

207. Lim J, Lasserson TJ, Fleetham J, et al. Oral appliances for obstructive sleep apnoea. Cochrane Database Syst Rev 2006;(1):CD004435.

208. Tsuiki S, Kobayashi M, Namba K, et al. Optimal positive airway pressure predicts oral appliance response to sleep apnoea. Eur Respir J 2010;35(5): 1098–105.
209. Pantin CC, Hillman DR, Tennant M. Dental side effects of an oral device to treat snoring and obstructive sleep apnea. Sleep 1999;22(2):237–40.
210. Rose EC, Staats R, Virchow C Jr, et al. Occlusal and skeletal effects of an oral appliance in the treatment of obstructive sleep apnea. Chest 2002;122(3):871–7.
211. Almeida FR, Lowe AA, Otsuka R, et al. Long-term sequellae of oral appliance therapy in obstructive sleep apnea patients: part 2. Study-model analysis. Am J Orthod Dentofacial Orthop 2006;129(2):205–13.
212. Villa MP, Rizzoli A, Miano S, et al. Efficacy of rapid maxillary expansion in children with obstructive sleep apnea syndrome: 36 months of follow-up. Sleep Breath 2011;15(2):179–84.
213. Loube DI, Gay PC, Strohl KP, et al. Indications for positive airway pressure treatment of adult obstructive sleep apnea patients: a consensus statement. Chest 1999;115(3):863–6.
214. Holty JE, Guilleminault C. Surgical options for the treatment of obstructive sleep apnea. Med Clin North Am 2010;94(3):479–515.
215. Sundaram S, Bridgman SA, Lim J, et al. Surgery for obstructive sleep apnoea. Cochrane Database Syst Rev 2005;(4):CD001004.
216. Khan A, Ramar K, Maddirala S, et al. Uvulopalatopharyngoplasty in the management of obstructive sleep apnea: the Mayo clinic experience. Mayo Clin Proc 2009;84(9):795–800.
217. Mortimore IL, Bradley PA, Murray JA, et al. Uvulopalatopharyngoplasty may compromise nasal CPAP therapy in sleep apnea syndrome. Am J Respir Crit Care Med 1996;154(6 Pt 1):1759–62.
218. Riley R, Powell N, Guilleminault C. Maxillofacial surgery and nasal CPAP: a comparison of treatment for obstructive sleep apnea syndrome. Chest 1990; 98:1421–5.
219. Riley R, Powell N, Guilleminault C. Obstructive sleep apnea syndrome: a review of 306 consecutively treated surgical patients. Otolaryngol Head Neck Surg 1993;108:117–25.
220. Walker-Engstrom ML, Tegelberg A, Wilhelmsson B, et al. 4-Year follow-up of treatment with dental appliance or uvulopalatopharyngoplasty in patients with obstructive sleep apnea: a randomized study. Chest 2002;121(3):739–46.
221. White DP. Central sleep apnea. Med Clin North Am 1985;69(6):1205–19.
222. White DP. Pathogenesis of obstructive and central sleep apnea. Am J Respir Crit Care Med 2005;172(11):1363–70.
223. Badr MS, Toiber F, Skatrud JB, et al. Pharyngeal narrowing/occlusion during central sleep apnea. J Appl Physiol 1995;78(5):1806–15.
224. Sankri-Tarbichi AG, Rowley JA, Badr MS. Expiratory pharyngeal narrowing during central hypocapnic hypopnea. Am J Respir Crit Care Med 2009; 179(4):313–9.
225. Sankri-Tarbichi AG, Richardson NN, Chowdhuri S, et al. Hypocapnia is associated with increased upper airway expiratory resistance during sleep. Respir Physiol Neurobiol 2011;177(2):108–13.
226. White DP, Gleeson K, Pickett CK, et al. Altitude acclimatization: influence on periodic breathing and chemoresponsiveness during sleep. J Appl Physiol 1987;63(1):401–12.
227. Franklin KA, Eriksson P, Sahlin C, et al. Reversal of central sleep apnea with oxygen. Chest 1997;111(1):163–9.

228. Szollosi I, Jones M, Morrell MJ, et al. Effect of CO_2 inhalation on central sleep apnea and arousals from sleep. Respiration 2004;71(5):493–8.

229. Issa FG, Sullivan CE. Reversal of central sleep apnea using nasal CPAP. Chest 1986;90(2):165–71.

230. Hommura F, Nishimura M, Oguri M, et al. Continuous versus bilevel positive airway pressure in a patient with idiopathic central sleep apnea. Am J Respir Crit Care Med 1997;155(4):1482–5.

231. Quadri S, Drake C, Hudgel DW. Improvement of idiopathic central sleep apnea with zolpidem. J Clin Sleep Med 2009;5(2):122–9.

232. DeBacker WA, Verbraecken J, Willemen M, et al. Central apnea index decreases after prolonged treatment with acetazolamide. Am J Respir Crit Care Med 1995; 151(1):87–91.

233. Javaheri S, Parker TJ, Liming JD, et al. Sleep apnea in 81 ambulatory male patients with stable heart failure. Types and their prevalences, consequences, and presentations. Circulation 1998;97(21):2154–9.

234. Sin DD, Fitzgerald F, Parker JD, et al. Risk factors for central and obstructive sleep apnea in 450 men and women with congestive heart failure. Am J Respir Crit Care Med 1999;160(4):1101–6.

235. Bradley TD, Logan AG, Kimoff RJ, et al. Continuous positive airway pressure for central sleep apnea and heart failure. N Engl J Med 2005;353(19):2025–33.

236. Arzt M, Floras JS, Logan AG, et al. Suppression of central sleep apnea by continuous positive airway pressure and transplant-free survival in heart failure: a post hoc analysis of the Canadian Continuous Positive Airway Pressure for Patients with Central Sleep Apnea and Heart Failure Trial (CANPAP). Circulation 2007;115(25):3173–80.

237. Teschler H, Dohring J, Wang YM, et al. Adaptive pressure support servo-ventilation: a novel treatment for Cheyne-Stokes respiration in heart failure. Am J Respir Crit Care Med 2001;164(4):614–9.

238. Allam JS, Olson EJ, Gay PC, et al. Efficacy of adaptive servoventilation in treatment of complex and central sleep apnea syndromes. Chest 2007;132(6):1839–46.

239. Pepperell JC, Maskell NA, Jones DR, et al. A randomized controlled trial of adaptive ventilation for Cheyne-Stokes breathing in heart failure. Am J Respir Crit Care Med 2003;168(9):1109–14.

240. Philippe C, Stoica-Herman M, Drouot X, et al. Compliance with and effectiveness of adaptive servoventilation versus continuous positive airway pressure in the treatment of Cheyne-Stokes respiration in heart failure over a six month period. Heart 2006;92(3):337–42.

241. Novak S, Nemeth WC, Lawson KA. Trends in medical use and abuse of sustained-release opioid analgesics: a revisit. Pain Med 2004;5(1):59–65.

242. Teichtahl H, Prodromidis A, Miller B, et al. Sleep-disordered breathing in stable methadone programme patients: a pilot study. Addiction 2001;96(3):395–403.

243. Wang D, Teichtahl H, Drummer O, et al. Central sleep apnea in stable methadone maintenance treatment patients. Chest 2005;128(3):1348–56.

244. Walker JM, Farney RJ, Rhondeau SM, et al. Chronic opioid use is a risk factor for the development of central sleep apnea and ataxic breathing. J Clin Sleep Med 2007;3(5):455–61.

245. Webster LR, Choi Y, Desai H, et al. Sleep-disordered breathing and chronic opioid therapy. Pain Med 2008;9(4):425–32.

246. Javaheri S, Malik A, Smith J, et al. Adaptive pressure support servoventilation: a novel treatment for sleep apnea associated with use of opioids. J Clin Sleep Med 2008;4(4):305–10.

247. Grunstein RR, Ho KY, Berthon-Jones M, et al. Central sleep apnea is associated with increased ventilatory response to carbon dioxide and hypersecretion of growth hormone in patients with acromegaly. Am J Respir Crit Care Med 1994;150(2):496–502.

248. Weiss V, Sonka K, Pretl M, et al. Prevalence of the sleep apnea syndrome in acromegaly population. J Endocrinol Invest 2000;23(8):515–9.

249. Tolis G, Angelopoulos NG, Katounda E, et al. Medical treatment of acromegaly: comorbidities and their reversibility by somatostatin analogs. Neuroendocrinology 2006;83(3–4):249–57.

250. Grunstein RR, Ho KK, Sullivan CE. Effect of octreotide, a somatostatin analog, on sleep apnea in patients with acromegaly. Ann Intern Med 1994;121(7):478–83.

251. Sze L, Schmid C, Bloch KE, et al. Effect of transsphenoidal surgery on sleep apnoea in acromegaly. Eur J Endocrinol 2007;156(3):321–9.

252. Pekkarinen T, Partinen M, Pelkonen R, et al. Sleep apnoea and daytime sleepiness in acromegaly: relationship to endocrinological factors. Clin Endocrinol (Oxf) 1987;27(6):649–54.

253. Pelttari L, Polo O, Rauhala E, et al. Nocturnal breathing abnormalities in acromegaly after adenomectomy. Clin Endocrinol (Oxf) 1995;43(2):175–82.

254. de Oliveira Rodrigues CJ, Marson O, Tufic S, et al. Relationship among end-stage renal disease, hypertension, and sleep apnea in nondiabetic dialysis patients. Am J Hypertens 2005;18(2 Pt 1):152–7.

255. Tada T, Kusano KF, Ogawa A, et al. The predictors of central and obstructive sleep apnoea in haemodialysis patients. Nephrol Dial Transplant 2007;22(4):1190–7.

256. Beecroft JM, Hoffstein V, Pierratos A, et al. Nocturnal haemodialysis increases pharyngeal size in patients with sleep apnoea and end-stage renal disease. Nephrol Dial Transplant 2008;23(2):673–9.

257. Beecroft JM, Duffin J, Pierratos A, et al. Decreased chemosensitivity and improvement of sleep apnea by nocturnal hemodialysis. Sleep Med 2009;10(1):47–54.

258. Beecroft J, Duffin J, Pierratos A, et al. Enhanced chemo-responsiveness in patients with sleep apnoea and end-stage renal disease. Eur Respir J 2006; 28(1):151–8.

259. Hamilton RW, Epstein PE, Henderson LW, et al. Control of breathing in uremia: ventilatory response to CO_2 after hemodialysis. J Appl Physiol 1976;41(2):216–22.

260. Wilcox I, McNamara SG, Dodd MJ, et al. Ventilatory control in patients with sleep apnoea and left ventricular dysfunction: comparison of obstructive and central sleep apnoea. Eur Respir J 1998;11(1):7–13.

261. Jean G, Piperno D, Francois B, et al. Sleep apnea incidence in maintenance hemodialysis patients: influence of dialysate buffer. Nephron 1995;71(2):138–42.

262. Langevin B, Fouque D, Leger P, et al. Sleep apnea syndrome and end-stage renal disease. Cure after renal transplantation. Chest 1993;103(5):1330–5.

263. Beecroft JM, Zaltzman J, Prasad R, et al. Impact of kidney transplantation on sleep apnoea in patients with end-stage renal disease. Nephrol Dial Transplant 2007;22(10):3028–33.

264. Morgenthaler TI, Kagramanov V, Hanak V, et al. Complex sleep apnea syndrome: is it a unique clinical syndrome? Sleep 2006;29(9):1203–9.

265. Dernaika T, Tawk M, Nazir S, et al. The significance and outcome of continuous positive airway pressure-related central sleep apnea during split-night sleep studies. Chest 2007;132(1):81–7.

266. Lehman S, Antic NA, Thompson C, et al. Central sleep apnea on commencement of continuous positive airway pressure in patients with a primary diagnosis of obstructive sleep apnea-hypopnea. J Clin Sleep Med 2007;3(5):462–6.

267. Kuzniar TJ, Pusalavidyasagar S, Gay PC, et al. Natural course of complex sleep apnea–a retrospective study. Sleep Breath 2008;12(2):135–9.
268. Morgenthaler TI, Gay PC, Gordon N, et al. Adaptive servoventilation versus noninvasive positive pressure ventilation for central, mixed, and complex sleep apnea syndromes. Sleep 2007;30(4):468–75.
269. Javaheri S, Smith J, Chung E. The prevalence and natural history of complex sleep apnea. J Clin Sleep Med 2009;5(3):205–11.
270. Endo Y, Suzuki M, Inoue Y, et al. Prevalence of complex sleep apnea among Japanese patients with sleep apnea syndrome. Tohoku J Exp Med 2008; 215(4):349–54.
271. Aurora RN, Chowdhuri S, Ramar K, et al. The treatment of central sleep apnea syndromes in adults: practice parameters with an evidence-based literature review and meta-analyses. Sleep 2012;35(1):17–40.
272. Littleton SW, Mokhlesi B. The pickwickian syndrome-obesity hypoventilation syndrome. Clin Chest Med 2009;30(3):467–78, viii.
273. Mokhlesi B, Kryger MH, Grunstein RR. Assessment and management of patients with obesity hypoventilation syndrome. Proc Am Thorac Soc 2008; 5(2):218–25.
274. Mokhlesi B, Tulaimat A, Faibussowitsch I, et al. Obesity hypoventilation syndrome: prevalence and predictors in patients with obstructive sleep apnea. Sleep Breath 2007;11(2):117–24.
275. Lin CC, Wu KM, Chou CS, et al. Oral airway resistance during wakefulness in eucapnic and hypercapnic sleep apnea syndrome. Respir Physiol Neurobiol 2004;139(2):215–24.
276. Piper AJ, Grunstein RR. Big breathing: the complex interaction of obesity, hypoventilation, weight loss, and respiratory function. J Appl Physiol 2010;108(1): 199–205.
277. Sharp JT, Henry JP, Sweany SK, et al. The total work of breathing in normal and obese men. J Clin Invest 1964;43:728–39.
278. Koenig SM. Pulmonary complications of obesity. Am J Med Sci 2001;321(4): 249–79.
279. Lopata M, Freilich RA, Onal E, et al. Ventilatory control and the obesity hypoventilation syndrome. Am Rev Respir Dis 1979;119(2 Pt 2):165–8.
280. Lopata M, Onal E. Mass loading, sleep apnea, and the pathogenesis of obesity hypoventilation. Am Rev Respir Dis 1982;126(4):640–5.
281. Han F, Chen E, Wei H, et al. The role of breathing control disorder in the development of carbon dioxide retention in patients with obesity hypoventilation syndrome. Zhonghua Nei Ke Za Zhi 1999;38(7):466–9 [in Chinese].
282. Bradley CA, Fleetham JA, Anthonisen NR. Ventilatory control in patients with hypoxemia due to obstructive lung disease. Am Rev Respir Dis 1979;120(1):21–30.
283. Kaw R, Hernandez AV, Walker E, et al. Determinants of hypercapnia in obese patients with obstructive sleep apnea: a systematic review and metaanalysis of cohort studies. Chest 2009;136(3):787–96.
284. Kaltman AJ, Goldring RM. Role of circulatory congestion in the cardiorespiratory failure of obesity. Am J Med 1976;60(5):645–53.
285. Crummy F, Piper AJ, Naughton MT. Obesity and the lung: 2. Obesity and sleep-disordered breathing. Thorax 2008;63(8):738–46.
286. Piper AJ, Grunstein RR. Obesity hypoventilation syndrome: mechanisms and management. Am J Respir Crit Care Med 2011;183(3):292–8.
287. Phipps PR, Starritt E, Caterson I, et al. Association of serum leptin with hypoventilation in human obesity. Thorax 2002;57(1):75–6.

288. Yee BJ, Cheung J, Phipps P, et al. Treatment of obesity hypoventilation syndrome and serum leptin. Respiration 2006;73(2):209–12.
289. Kalra SP. Central leptin insufficiency syndrome: an interactive etiology for obesity, metabolic and neural diseases and for designing new therapeutic interventions. Peptides 2008;29(1):127–38.
290. Sugerman HJ, Fairman RP, Lindeman AK, et al. Gastroplasty for respiratory insufficiency of obesity. Ann Surg 1981;193(6):677–85.
291. Sugerman HJ, Fairman RP, Sood RK, et al. Long-term effects of gastric surgery for treating respiratory insufficiency of obesity. Am J Clin Nutr 1992;55(Suppl 2): 597S–601S.
292. Sugerman HJ. Bariatric surgery for severe obesity. J Assoc Acad Minor Phys 2001;12(3):129–36.
293. Olson AL, Zwillich C. The obesity hypoventilation syndrome. Am J Med 2005; 118(9):948–56.
294. Perez de Llano LA, Golpe R, Ortiz PM, et al. Short-term and long-term effects of nasal intermittent positive pressure ventilation in patients with obesity-hypoventilation syndrome. Chest 2005;128(2):587–94.
295. Mokhlesi B. Positive airway pressure titration in obesity hypoventilation syndrome: continuous positive airway pressure or bilevel positive airway pressure. Chest 2007;131(6):1624–6.
296. Berry RB, Chediak A, Brown LK, et al. Best clinical practices for the sleep center adjustment of noninvasive positive pressure ventilation (NPPV) in stable chronic alveolar hypoventilation syndromes. J Clin Sleep Med 2010;6(5):491–509.
297. Perez de Llano LA, Golpe R, Piquer MO, et al. Clinical heterogeneity among patients with obesity hypoventilation syndrome: therapeutic implications. Respiration 2008;75(1):34–9.
298. Storre JH, Seuthe B, Fiechter R, et al. Average volume-assured pressure support in obesity hypoventilation: a randomized crossover trial. Chest 2006; 130(3):815–21.
299. Wijesinghe M, Williams M, Perrin K, et al. The effect of supplemental oxygen on hypercapnia in subjects with obesity-associated hypoventilation: a randomized, crossover, clinical study. Chest 2011;139(5):1018–24.
300. Hensley MJ, Read DJ. Intermittent obstruction of the upper airway during sleep causing profound hypoxaemia. A neglected mechanism exacerbating chronic respiratory failure. Aust N Z J Med 1976;6(5):481–6.

Restless Legs Syndrome and Periodic Leg Movements of Sleep

David B. Rye, MD, PhD[a],*, Lynn Marie Trotti, MD, MSc[a,b]

KEYWORDS

- Restless legs • Periodic leg movements • Supraspinal • Flexor withdrawal
- Dopamine • Iron

KEY POINTS

- Restless legs syndrome (RLS) is a common, complex disease.
- RLS is a clinical diagnosis with many supportive features that facilitate its recognition in ambiguous clinical scenarios.
- There are many, proven, effective treatments, including dopaminergic agents and gabapentin and its derivatives.
- Genetic factors, iron deficiency, pregnancy, and many common medical disorders influence RLS expressivity.
- Disinhibition of spinal sensorimotor circuits is central to expression of the sensory symptoms and motor signs (periodic leg movements while awake and asleep) of RLS.

INTRODUCTION

Restless legs syndrome (RLS) is defined by a compelling urge to move the legs that worsens with inactivity, is relieved by movement or counterstimuli, and is most aggravating in the evening and at night. Seminal descriptions of RLS noted additional key features: (1) a prevalence of at least 5%; (2) a subpopulation of patients who perceive RLS sensations as pain; (3) a proclivity to affect pregnant women; (4) heritability; and (5) favorable responses to iron supplementation and sympathectomy. A second advance came with recognition that periodic limb movements in sleep (PLMS) are present in 85% to 95% of patients. A third major advance has come with showing that pharmacologic agents acting at D_2 and D_3 dopamine receptors, opiates, and

Disclosure: In the past 3 years Dr Rye has consulted for or served on advisory committees for UCB Pharma, Impax Laboratories, Jazz Pharmaceuticals, and Merck. Dr Trotti has been an advisor to UCB Pharma.
[a] Program in Sleep, Department of Neurology, Emory University School of Medicine, 101 Woodruff Circle, WMRB – Office 6113, Atlanta, GA 30322, USA; [b] Program in Sleep, Department of Neurology, Emory University School of Medicine, 1841 Clifton Road NE, WWHC – 5th floor, Atlanta, GA 30329, USA
* Corresponding author.
E-mail addresses: drye@emory.edu; lbecke2@emory.edu

derivatives of gabapentin relieve both the sensory (RLS) and motor (PLMS) symptoms. A fourth advance has been showing reductions in brain iron in a subpopulation of RLS cases. The fifth seminal advance has been identification that multiple genetic loci in several genes account for most of the population-attributable risk of RLS and PLMS (**Fig. 1**).

DIFFERENTIAL DIAGNOSIS

RLS is a clinical diagnosis that includes: (1) an intense urge to move the legs that is uncomfortable; (2) a worsening at rest; (3) relief with movement; and (4) a diurnal preference for the evening and night.[1] Self-administered questionnaires inquiring about these consensus criteria show sensitivities and specificities of approximately 0.75. False-positive results arise from common conditions that mimic RLS.[2–4] With careful attention to diagnostic and supportive criteria and the medication history, both past and present, RLS can usually be distinguished from mimics. For instance, in radiculopathy, there may be discomfort in the legs provoked by sitting or lying down, but there is no urge to move or response to dopaminergics.[5] Neuropathy can cause uncomfortable leg sensations with a nocturnal predominance, albeit less pronounced than in RLS, but typically without an associated urge to move or improvement with movement.[5] In addition, while neuropathy is most often symmetric and predominantly

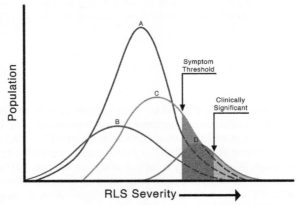

Fig. 1. Expressivity of RLS symptoms is influenced by genetic and environmental/medical factors. (A) Representative of an adult population of northern European descent. The area under the curve to the right of the arrow designated "Symptom threshold" defines the proportion of the population affected by RLS symptoms. The area under the curve to the right of the arrow marked "Clinically significant" represents the proportion in whom symptoms are frequent or intense enough to necessitate treatment. The remaining curves depict populations in whom expressivity varies from this baseline population. (B) Representative of adolescent northern Europeans or adult populations of Asian descent, whose diatheses to RLS are substantially lower because of age-related or genetic factors, respectively. (C) Represents the nearly 50% of northern Europeans who are homozygous for the susceptibility variant in the BTBD9 gene, and thus, a correspondingly greater proportion who surpass the RLS symptom and clinically significant thresholds. (D) Represents the small population of patients with end-stage renal disease requiring dialysis, and in whom RLS is nearly ubiquitous. (*Reprinted from* Trotti LM, Bhadriraju S, Rye DB. An update on the pathophysiology and genetics of restless legs syndrome. Curr Neurol Neurosci Rep 2008;8(4):282; with permission.)

affects the feet, RLS often shows asymmetry and typically spares the feet. The urge to move of RLS is similar to that encountered in neuroleptic-induced akathisia, but akathisia is typically an inner, psychic restlessness that does not preferentially affect the legs, does not have a circadian pattern of symptom expression, and is not associated with unpleasant sensations that accompany the urge to move.[6] Nocturnal leg cramps have a circadian pattern and preferentially affect the legs, but are not associated with an urge to move and do not improve with movement.[6] The syndrome of painful legs and moving toes (PLMT) bears a remarkable resemblance to RLS, as emphasized in original descriptions by Marsden and colleagues,[7,8] and we believe that PLMT and RLS/PLMS are part of the same phenotypic spectrum.

EPIDEMIOLOGY AND RISK FACTORS

Variability in symptom expressivity is the rule rather than the exception. Symptoms begin as mild and infrequent and slowly progress, thereby delaying most diagnoses until the fourth to sixth decades of life. RLS prevalence in populations of European descent ranges from 3% to 15%.[9,10] Clinically significant RLS (ie, symptoms that are deemed frequent or severe enough to require treatment) is less common, occurring in about 1.6% to 2.8% of these populations.[10]

Symptoms of RLS and PLMS show a circadian propensity,[11–13] and are also influenced by age, sex, pregnancy, genetic factors, and common medical conditions. RLS affects 2% of school-aged children,[14] 3% of 30-year-olds, and 20% aged 80 years and older.[15] Women are affected more often than men in a roughly 2:1 ratio and show greater night-to-night variability in PLMS.[16] Nearly 1 in 3 pregnant women experience RLS in their third trimester,[17,18] and the risk of RLS increases linearly with the number of live births (odds ratio [OR] = 3.57 for >3 births).[19] Familial aggregation of RLS is well documented, and the proportion of phenotypic variation attributable to genes (ie, heritability) is 54% to 83%.[20,21] Prevalence in non-Europeans is notably low 0.1% in Singapore,[22] 0.9% in South Korea,[23] 2.0% in Ecuador,[24] 3.2% in Turkey,[25] and 3.3% in Japan[26]), implicating genetic, environmental, or sociocultural factors in expressivity or reporting. The frequency that RLS is encountered in many common medical conditions (ostensibly, secondary RLS) exceeds that expected by chance and includes iron deficiency,[27] frequent blood donation,[28] end-stage renal disease (ESRD),[29] rheumatologic disorders,[30] diabetes,[31] pulmonary hypertension,[32] chronic obstructive pulmonary disease,[33,34] obstructive sleep apnea,[35] liver disease,[36] Crohn's[37] and celiac disease,[38,39] gastric surgery,[40] and irritable bowel syndrome.[41] Neurologic conditions associated with RLS include migraine,[42,43] Parkinson disease (PD),[44–49] spinocerebellar ataxias types 1, 2, and 3,[50–53] and multiple sclerosis.[53]

Genetic linkage studies have identified several regions of interest,[54] but only RLS1 on chromosome 12 is common to French Canadian, Icelandic, and German families and implicates neuronal nitric oxide synthase (NOS1).[55] Genome-wide association studies have identified multiple single-nucleotide polymorphisms (SNPs), pointing to potential involvement of 6 different gene products: *BTBD9*, *Meis1*, *PTPRD*, *MAP2K5*, *LBXCOR1*, and *TOX3*.[2,56–59] The at-risk SNPs in each instance are common, present within noncoding, intronic, or intergenic regions, and the implicated genes are widely expressed in the central nervous system and other organs.[60] Association of a single SNP (rs3923809) in an intron of *BTBD9* increases risk of RLS and PLMS by 70% to 80%. Because this at-risk variant is common (nearly one-half of those of northern European ancestry carry 2 copies), it accounts for at least 50% of the population-attributable risk for RLS/PLMS. Biologic plausibility of these variants derives from: (1) a dose-dependency between the *BTBD9* variant and decrements in iron stores[2]; (2) the *Meis1* variant appearing causal to functional decrements in iron homeostasis[61]; (3) dose-dependency between the *BTBD9 and Meis1* risk variants and number of PLMS[2] (personal observations); and (4) the disparate frequencies of the at-risk alleles in various ethnic groups closely tracking the different RLS prevalences worldwide[60] (http://www.hapmap.org). Genetic manipulations of the homolog of BTBD9 in *Drosophila* suggest causality because the resultant mutants show RLS-like features that are reversible with pramipexole and associated with brain reductions in dopamine and influence iron metabolism in cultured cells[62]

The expressivity of RLS is influenced by a substantial genetic component, and further affected by circadian, medical/neurologic, environmental, and additional genetic factors through mechanisms that remain poorly defined.

PATHOPHYSIOLOGY

There is extensive overlap in the pathophysiologic substrates of RLS and PLMS because they frequently coexist, respond to, and are aggravated by the same medications and share common electrophysiologic characteristics and susceptibility genes. The neural networks implicated in their expression are many and diverse, and include both the peripheral and central nervous systems. The characteristics of both the sensory disturbances and wake-related and sleep-related movements in RLS favor a final common pathway that resides in the spinal cord. As a site of convergence for peripheral sensory afferents and descending tracts that modulate sensorimotor and autonomic excitability, the spinal cord provides a utilitarian substrate that: (1) accounts for much of what has been gleaned from clinical experience and electrophysiologic investigations of RLS/PLMS; and (2) justifies the logic of beginning ones neurologic examination of individuals being evaluated for RLS/PLMS from the periphery and ascending to the cranium.

Spinal Cord

PLMS involve flexion of the hip and knee, dorsiflexion of the ankle, and extension of the great toe, which resemble the spinal defense reflex mechanism designed to withdraw the limb from painful stimuli. This primitive, pathologic reflex belies heightened excitability in neural elements comprising the flexor-reflex arc. In patients with RLS, the threshold to elicit this flexor-reflex is reduced during sleep, and it is exaggerated as manifest in reflex spread to muscles beyond the segmental nerve root stimulated.[63,64] This situation likely reflects failure of presynaptic and postsynaptic inhibitory mechanisms acting within the spinal cord, a pattern also evident when PLMS occur alone (eg, absent sensory symptoms of RLS).[65] There are many supraspinal brain circuits that may contribute to this disinhibition of spinal cord sensorimotor and autonomic networks. Wherever their origin, they are exquisitely responsive to D_2-like dopamine and opiate receptor agonists. Spinal D_3 dopamine receptors dampen the flexor-reflex[66] and sympathetic tone,[67] and intrathecal opiates abolish otherwise medically refractory RLS.[68–70] These findings emphasize the central role of spinal cord networks in the pathophysiology of RLS/PLMS. The spinal cord is also the most reliable site from which a disparate array of diseases can elicit RLS or PLMS lacking RLS sensory symptoms.[49,71–75]

Peripheral Nerves

The sensory component of RLS suggests involvement of the peripheral nervous system, especially the small caliber A-δ-fibers and C-fibers, which carry pain signals and mediate somatosympathetic reflexes. Although associations between diffuse, small-fiber axonopathies and RLS have been described,[76,77] they are most evident in some hereditary neuropathies,[78,79] or are limited to selective, small case series in which the neuropathy was subclinical and evident only by electrophysiologic[80] or microscopic[81] examination, conventional electromyograms and nerve conduction velocities, somatosensory evoked potentials, and sympathetic skin responses are usually normal in idiopathic RLS[82–85] and PLMS in isolation.[86,87] The prevalence of RLS in patients with acquired neuropathies is no greater than that in the population, except in those with genetic predispositions to RLS.[79] That RLS can acutely worsen when a diffuse neuropathy develops, or preferentially lateralize to the leg or foot after damage to a spinal root or peripheral nerve, injury or surgery to a soft or bony tissue, or a thrombosed vein, in our clinical experiences, emphasizes that the peripheral nervous system modulates RLS expressivity. The mechanisms acting in the periphery that precipitate the sensory RLS experience and the neural substrates that convey them remain unknown. They are likely to involve ectopic or ephaptic excitation in damaged peripheral nerves and abnormal impulse generation in their sensory or sympathetic components. Pharmacologics effective for neuropathic pain such as gabapentin and its derivatives might derive their efficacy from actions on peripheral nerves.[88] Sympathetic mechanisms in the periphery are likely also important mediators, given the complete relief from painful RLS (ie, asthenia crurum dolorosa) experienced by 3 of 4 Ekbom's patients[89] after lumbar sympathetic ganglia blockade.

Supraspinal Networks

The influence of supraspinal pathways on expression of RLS/PLMS is supported by many observations. Coactivation of axial and upper limb muscles with PLMS[83] implicates brain regions above the foramen magnum. Neural hyperexcitability reflective of generalized disinhibition is evident in spinal sensorimotor circuits,[63–65] the brainstem,[86,90,91] and motor cortex.[92,93] Premotor circuits in each of these regions converge and modulate the spinal sensorimotor apparatus. Converging lines of evidence emphasize that monoaminergic (ie, noradrenergic, serotonergic, and dopaminergic) pathways descending from the brainstem potently gate ascending sensory impulses (such as those occurring in RLS) via postsynaptic actions on dorsal horn neurons or presynaptic actions on the terminal axons of dorsal root afferents.[67,94–97] A dopaminergic diencephalospinal pathway originating from the posterior hypothalamic A11 cell group is of interest given the efficacy of D_2-like dopamine receptor agonists in alleviating RLS/PLMS.[67] Electrical[94] and pharmacologic[98] manipulations of A11 are antinociceptive and suppress neuropathic hypersensitivity, respectively. Lesioning of the A11 cell group in animals yields a phenotype reminiscent of RLS/PLMS.[99–101] Supraspinally mediated disinhibition of A-δ-fiber, high-threshold mechanoreceptor input (a hallmark sign of a hyperalgesic type of neuropathic pain) manifests in patients with RLS as a static mechanical hyperalgesia.[102] Disinhibition of A-δ-fiber contributions to spinal reflexes also manifests as prolongation of the cutaneous silent period in RLS.[103] Hypersensitivity to pain in RLS might involve alternate, supraspinal, dopamine-sensitive basal ganglia, insular and anterior cingulate cortical, and thalamic circuits.[104,105] Although the basal ganglia, in particular, have often been implicated in RLS/PLMS, there are few concrete data that establish cause and effect. Lesioning of the internal globus pallidus to treat medically refractory PD improved RLS sensory symptoms, and preferentially benefited the contralateral leg, in a single patient.[106] Bilateral subthalamic nucleus stimulation produces inconsistent affects on RLS in patients with coincident PD,[107,108] whereas deep brain stimulation of the thalamic ventralis intermedius nucleus does not benefit patients with RLS with coexistent essential tremor.[109] RLS with PLMS and PLMS in isolation are common with any lesion that interrupts descending supraspinal pathways, most of which gate sensorimotor reflexes, such as in the setting of subcortical strokes[110] and, especially, subcortical and infratentorial demyelinating lesions in multiple sclerosis.[75,111]

RLS and PLMS are best conceptualized as complex traits that are influenced not by a single brain circuit, but rather by any one of a multitude of peripheral and central nervous system pathways that converge on the spinal cord.

Iron and Dopamine

Theories about the origin of RLS/PLMS have long been dominated by discussions of iron deficiency and the efficacy of dopaminomimetics in relieving both RLS sensory symptoms and its motor signs (PLMS).[112] An intimate interplay between systemic and brain iron and central dopaminergic tone is supported by clinical investigations, several neuroimaging modalities, analyses of autopsy tissue and cerebrospinal fluid, and experimental models of dietary iron deficiency.[27,112–114]

That brain iron deficiency is a unifying mechanism causal to idiopathic and many (if not all) secondary cases of RLS/PLMS does not translate smoothly to the bedside. First, clinical experience with iron-deficient states and epidemiologic considerations are unambiguous that systemic iron deficiency is neither sufficient nor necessary to produce RLS/PLMS. A small cross-sectional study, for example, found RLS in only 40% of patients with documented iron deficiency.[115] Although RLS can emerge or worsen in nearly one-third of pregnant women, iron parameters bear little to no relation to symptoms that otherwise resolve quickly on delivery (despite the attendant loss of blood, and presumably iron).[18,116–118] Similarly, although RLS has been noted in frequent blood donors,[28] a systematic study failed to find a relationship of RLS to donation of 3 or less units of blood in 2000 donors.[119,120] Neither was an association between RLS and iron deficiency found in the only large, rigorous, population-based study of RLS that used sensitive serologic measures to detect early iron deficiency.[121] Second, 1 open-label study,[122] and 2 randomized, double-blind, placebo-controlled studies[123,124] of intravenous (IV) iron for RLS failed to show efficacy. Much of the inconsistency between the iron deficiency hypothesis of RLS and these realities likely reflects a selection bias for more severely affected individuals more likely to present to specialized centers. Pathologically low iron stores as revealed by serum ferritin, for example, are more frequently encountered in these settings than they are in the general population: 25% in 113 patients with RLS in 1 retrospective study,[125] and 14.6% and 44.4% with values of 15 ng/mL or less and 40 ng/mL or less, respectively, in 437 of our patients with RLS. An additional counterweight to the hypothesis that iron deficiency is universal to RLS/PLMS is the fact that each RLS susceptibility allele in the *BTBD9* gene predicts 13% lower ferritin per copy, yet this variant accounts for only 50% of the population-attributable risk.[2] Systemic or brain iron deficiency is a recognizable and reversible state that modulates expression of RLS in a proportion of, but not all, individuals with idiopathic RLS. There remain few data to go on to guide selection of patients who are deserving of treatment with iron, and which mode of delivery and formulation of iron should be used.

Given the efficacy of levodopa and dopamine agonists in relieving RLS/PLMS, and the basal ganglia being a principal arbiter of hypokinetic and hyperkinetic movement disorders, the original hypothesis of RLS/PLMS pathophysiology focused around a hypodopaminergic state in nigrostriatal circuits. This hypothesis has endured because: (1) natural nadirs in the synthesis, release, and signaling of dopamine coincide with the peak time for RLS/PLMS symptoms[126]; (2) iron is a cofactor for the rate-limiting enzyme in the synthesis of dopamine (ie, tyrosine hydroxylase [TH])[127,128]; and (3) dietary iron deficiency impairs the recycling and signaling of synaptic dopamine in the basal ganglia.[129–131] Evidence of a hypodopaminergic state in the basal ganglia occurring independently of, or because of, iron deficiency, and that is relevant to the RLS population at large, has not emerged. Because D_2-like ($D_{2,3,4}$) receptors are the principal autoreceptors and inhibitory, they seem best poised to mediate the benefits observed with the low doses of dopaminomimetics used in RLS/PLMS. Interest in the D_3 receptor derives from the efficacy of the newer, D_3-preferring agonists in alleviating RLS/PLMS, the preferential affinity that this receptor subtype shows for endogenous dopamine, and that spinal reflexes[66,67] and sleep behavior[132,133] of mice lacking a functional D_3 receptor[66,67] recapitulate many features of RLS. Dietary models of iron deficiency show an excess in extracellular dopamine in the basal ganglia because of disordered presynaptic mechanisms governing the release of dopamine (eg, reductions in the dopamine-transporter and D_2-like receptors) as opposed to its synthesis.[129–131] Supportive of a hyperdopaminergic versus hypodopaminergic state are metabolic profiles of cerebrospinal fluid,[134] and analyses of RLS autopsy tissue and animals and cell lines depleted of iron.[135] The molecular and anatomic networks by which deficiencies in iron contribute to RLS/PLMS, and whether this occurs primarily, if not exclusively, by way of dopamine signaling abnormalities, and nigrostriatal versus diencephalospinal circuits, remain areas of active investigation.

CLINICAL FEATURES AND DIAGNOSIS
RLS

The 4 RLS diagnostic criteria are sufficient for a diagnosis, but several supportive features can prove useful in confirming a diagnosis in ambiguous cases.[136] These features include PLMS, a favorable response to dopaminergic therapy, and a family history. Empiric trials of dopamine agonists can improve diagnostic accuracy.[137,138] In addition, a history of intolerance to, or symptom exacerbation with, a variety of over-the-counter and prescribed medications often proves a useful diagnostic clue. Exacerbation of both the signs (PLMs)[139,140] and symptoms[141,142] of RLS have been noted with serotonin, and especially, norepinephrine reuptake inhibitors. Symptom worsening with nonspecific antihistamines (eg, diphenhydramine), sympathomimetics (eg, ephedrine and pseudoephedrine), and antidopaminergics (eg, metaclopramide and prochlorperazine) is common but by no means universal. Antagonism with normal dopamine signaling also is likely to underlie symptom worsening with typical and atypical antipsychotics. Dramatic worsening of RLS/PLMs after regional and spinal anesthesia is likely caused by the use of sympathomimetic amines to support blood pressure in these scenarios.[143–147]

Periodic Leg Movements and Other Motor Stereotypies

PLMS are an objective sign of RLS and an important tool to its understanding. Nearly all patients with RLS experience periodic leg movements while awake (PLMW) or asleep (PLMS). These movements (originally coined nocturnal myoclonus) are involuntary, highly stereotyped, and have a relatively constant intermovement interval centered around 22 seconds. They occur at a rate of more than 5/h from anterior tibialis surface electrodes (used in routine polysomnography [PSG]) in 80% of patients with RLS, increasing to 88% on 2 consecutive recording nights.[148] PLMS detected by ambulatory accelerometry manifest at a rate of more than 5/h from a single leg on at least 1 of 5 nights in 91% of patients with RLS.[16] Enhanced sensitivity with additional recording nights emphasizes that the night-to-night variability is significant, and particularly so in younger, less severely affected patients, and women.

A PLMS index (PLMSI; PLMS per hour) greater than 5/h is generally considered significant. PLMS are conventionally taught to be nonspecific, occurring in other conditions such as narcolepsy, rapid eye movement sleep behavior disorder, and in seemingly asymptomatic individuals. Prevalences for PLMS range from 5% to 11% for rates 5/h or greater,[149] to 4.3% for African Americans and 9.3% for European Americans meeting a threshold of 15 PLMS/h on a single PSG.[150] There are no population-based or longitudinal data that tell us what proportion of individuals with PLMS fulfill, or develop, a portion or all of the diagnostic criteria for RLS. Asymptomatic PLMS are often a precursor to RLS,[151–154] are more common in families with RLS,[155] and are more prevalent and abundant in ethnic groups who have the highest frequencies of RLS/PLMS risk alleles (eg, North Americans of European vs African descent).[150,156] The BTBD9 RLS risk variant is a more powerful predictor of PLMS in individuals who experience symptoms atypical of RLS or none at all.[2] Quantification of PLMW (>15/h) occurring during bouts of wakefulness after sleep onset shows good specificity (~90%) for diagnosing RLS.[157] A combination of PLMSI of more than 5/h and the 4 consensus RLS symptoms improves diagnostic certainty substantially (positive predictive value of >95%).[158] Assessment of PLMS, and particularly PLMW, is useful as a supportive diagnostic tool as well as an objective means of assessing treatment response in RLS.

PSG is expensive and incapable of capturing between-night variability in PLMW, and PLMS, so that accelerometric monitoring has seen increased use. Miniaturized accelerometers placed on the big toe, ankle, or foot capture movement as opposed to electromyographic activity, avoid the expense of PSG, and can be conducted in the home environment over multiple nights. The PAM-RL triaxial accelerometer (Respironics, Murrysville, PA) has proved useful for diagnostic purposes and in clinical trials. It provides an accurate naturalistic assessment of PSG-derived PLMSI (Pearson correlation $r = 0.87$, $P<.0001$),[159] discriminates between PLMS and random nocturnal motor activity,[160] and is sensitive to treatment effects.[161,162] Further practical advantages include reliability and durability,[2] and engagement of the patient in their assessment and care.

The potential diagnostic usefulness of voluntary and involuntary movements manifest by patients with RLS during the waking state has not been comprehensively assessed. In our clinical experience, many patients show stereotypies in their feet and legs, which involve volitional, repetitive foot tapping, flexion and extension at the knee, and abduction and adduction at the hip. Less frequently (~3%–5% in our tertiary referral center), these movements are nonvolitional and pathologic, and have the appearance of a dyskinesia,[163] fanning or clawing of the toes as described in PLMT, brief myoclonic jerks in isolated muscles of the feet, or a flexor-withdrawal sequence emulating a PLMW.

TREATMENT

Achieving symptom relief in RLS demands a thorough clinical evaluation to rule out coexisting conditions that enhance its expressivity (**Box 1**). There is an absence of evidence-based medicine as to the positive or negative effects of lifestyle and diet on RLS/PLMS. However, sleep restriction, tobacco, alcohol, and caffeine have all been implicated in worsening of RLS[164] and should be avoided.[165] Medications known or suspected to worsen RLS should be discontinued when feasible. These medications include the nonspecific antihistamines (eg, diphenhydramine and meclizine), dopamine antagonists (eg, metaclopramide), antidepressants, neuroleptics, and lithium.[142,164,166,167] Of the selective serotonin (SSRI), norepinephrine (SNRI), and

---

Box 1
Factors known or likely to enhance expressivity of RLS (see text for details)

Lifestyle

    Irregular sleep-wake schedule

    Sleep restriction

    Soporific environment

    Dietary: caffeine, alcohol, biogenic amines

    Activity: too little, or overly strenuous physical activity

    Habits: nicotine

Pharmacologic

    Antihistamines: over-the-counter cold remedies, nasal decongestants, sleeping aids, and antidepressants with antihistaminergic actions (eg, desyrel and mirtazapine)

    Antidopaminergics: metoclopramide, promethazine, and typical and atypical neuroleptics

    Antidepressants: tricyclics and second-generation serotonin, and, especially, norepinephrine reuptake inhibitors

Metabolic

    Iron deficiency

    Folate deficiency

Structural

    Neuropathies: acquired and familial; axonal and demyelinating radiculopathies

    Myelopathies: heritable, acquired, and compressive/traumatic; varicose veins/venous insufficiency

    Musculoskeletal abnormalities or injuries

---

mixed reuptake inhibitors, mirtazapine has the highest rate of new or worsened RLS (occurring in 28% of treated patients, vs 9% of patients treated with any SSRI or SNRI).[142] If comorbid depression requires treatment, we prefer agents with the least norepinephrine reuptake blockade, and often prescribe bupropion given its relative selectivity for the dopamine transporter. By itself, bupropion might improve RLS.[168,169] Proton pump inhibitors (PPIs) can aggravate RLS by interfering with iron absorption secondary to increased duodenal pH.[170] This phenomenon can emerge within weeks of a PPI being prescribed, suggesting that the curve describing the relationship of systemic iron availability to RLS severity might be steep in some individuals.

Iron deficiency is another common factor that influences RLS expressivity. It should be routinely assessed for at initial evaluation and at yearly follow-up. Because many (~two-thirds of our clinic population) iron-deficient patients with RLS do not show coexisting anemia (ie, they have preanemic iron deficiency), and ferritin being an acute-phase reactant prone to false increases, a complete serum iron panel (iron, total iron-binding capacity, percent transferrin saturation, and ferritin) is preferred. We are particularly vigilant in assessing serum iron parameters in patients with comorbid gastrointestinal diseases (eg, gastric stapling or bypass and celiac disease) in whom iron deficiency is common and seems contributory to RLS.[38–41] We also regularly assess for vitamin B_{12} and folate because their malabsorption can also occur in these conditions, and theoretically interfere with dopamine synthesis because each is required for the biosynthesis of tetrahydrobiopterin (a cofactor for TH).[171] One small open-label study of oral folate to treat RLS in the setting of documented deficiencies of folate reported good results.[172] However, in idiopathic, primary RLS, folate and vitamin B_{12} deficiencies are no more common than observed in the population.[173,174]

The RLS Foundation treatment algorithm recommends iron repletion when ferritin is less than 20 ng/mL and repletion on a case-by-case basis when the ferritin is between 20 and 50 ng/mL.[165] Although an expert guideline, data proving efficacy with supplementation are still mixed. A randomized, controlled trial of oral iron sulfate in patients with RLS did not benefit sleep or RLS,[175] although improvement was noted in the subset of patients whose iron parameters showed the greatest increases. Consistent with this experience, 1 controlled trial of oral iron in patients with RLS with low to normal ferritin did significantly reduce symptom severity.[176] Although a ferritin of 50 ng/mL or less does not seem to diminish the efficacy of dopaminergic therapy for RLS,[177] very low ferritins of 20 ng/mL or less do increase the risk of treatment complications, specifically, augmentation.[178] If reduced iron stores are suspected or confirmed, first educate the patient on factors that interfere with absorption of dietary or supplemental sources of iron. Dietary iron comes in 2 sources: heme iron and nonheme iron. The former is derived from animal sources and in red more than white meat, and is efficiently absorbed because of its solubility. Nonheme iron, derived from vegetables and grains, is less efficiently absorbed in the presence of phytates, oxalates, and phenols, metallic elements (eg, magnesium, manganese, zinc, calcium, and copper), with which it competes for absorption, and in alkalinized environments, in which it has a proclivity to form insoluble complexes. Thus, dietary or supplemental iron should preferably be ingested on an empty stomach devoid of nutritional supplements, antacids, or beverages containing tannic acid (eg, teas, coffees, and many red wines). Ascorbic acid (ie, vitamin C)-containing supplements or foods/juices significantly enhance absorption of nonheme iron. Several formulations of both nonheme and heme iron are available for oral supplementation and include ferrous sulfate, ferrous gluconate, and ferrous fumarate. Dosing that provides 100 to 200 mg of elemental iron per day is preferred over conventional, daily multivitamins and prenatal vitamins that contain 27 to 65 mg of iron. Many preparations cause constipation, diarrhea, nausea, and abdominal pain. These side effects can be minimized by reducing the amount of elemental iron, by taking the iron with food, lowering the dose of iron, or using a preparation with a low amount of elemental iron such as ferrous gluconate.[179] The time to repletion of iron with a goal of ferritin greater than 50 ng/mL and a transferrin saturation greater than 20% is highly variable, but is generally 4 to 6 weeks.

Several IV formulations of iron are also available. Of these formulations, iron dextran has the highest rate of serious anaphylaxis (0.6–0.7%) and other adverse events, present in up to 50% of patients.[180] Iron sucrose and ferric gluconate have lower rates of anaphylaxis (0.002% and 0.04%, respectively) and adverse events (36% and 35%),[180] although outside chronic renal failure, their use is off-label, and the single negative study of iron sucrose in RLS raises questions about its efficacy relative to iron dextran. We reserve use only for those patients whose iron deficiency is unambiguous (eg, ferritin <10 ng/mL, transferrin saturations <15%, or iron <25 μg/dL [females]/ 45 μg/dL [males]) and who are refractory to pharmacologic interventions, and in whom the risks associated with RLS-related sleep restriction to less than 3 to 4 h/night exceed those posed by a course of IV iron. The usefulness of IV iron is well established only in patients with ESRD.[181] In a study of 1 g of iron dextran in 10 patients with RLS, there were 4 nonresponders and there were few, if any, complete responders as assessed for PLMS (44 ± 27% reduction in PLMS).[122] One placebo-controlled study of patients with RLS with normal systemic iron status reported no benefit in an interim analysis and was therefore halted prematurely.[123] In a second study of IV iron sucrose in RLS with mild-to-moderate evidence of systemic iron deficiency, some positive symptom benefit was shown, but not at all time points or in all patients.[124]

When pharmacologic treatment of RLS is needed, the first-line pharmacologic agents are dopaminergic agents. Clinical trials establishing their efficacies excluded individuals with suspected iron deficiency because this was a presumed cause of secondary RLS (eg, ferritin <15–20 ng/mL), and these populations were two-thirds women, and the results might therefore not be generalizable. The medication class in which there is the largest published experience includes the dopamine agonists, which were the first agents approved by the US Food and Drug Administration (FDA) for RLS treatment. Gabapentin and its derivatives are beginning to gain favor as potential first-line agents because they avoid the complications of augmentation and impulse control disorders (ICDs) attributed to dopamine agonists (see section on prognosis). In a direct comparison with the dopamine agonist pramipexole, pregabalin showed equal or superior efficacy on subjective and objective metrics and was well tolerated.[182] Because the dopaminergics, gabapentinoids, and opioids are likely to exert beneficial effects on RLS at unique anatomic sites, in combination they may offer some practical benefits to monotherapy. In practice, it is not uncommon that agents from different therapeutic classes are used in combination, especially in severely affected patients (eg, **Box 2**, **Fig. 2**).

Dopamine agonists alleviate RLS symptoms in 70% to 90% of patients.[183] Placebo effects are notable,[184] consistent with evolving views that they are common in disorders such as RLS, in which supraspinal top-down and dopaminergic mechanisms are implicated.[185] Pramipexole is a nonergot-derived dopamine D_3 receptor and D_2 receptor agonist with proven efficacy for both RLS and PLMS.[186–190] The mean effective daily dose ranges from 0.25 to 1 mg,[191] although little added benefit is evident beyond 0.5 mg. Pramipexole is exclusively excreted by the kidneys, and should therefore be titrated more slowly in the setting of impaired creatinine clearances and ESRD. Ropinirole is another nonergot-derived dopamine agonist that also acts preferentially on D_3 and D_2 receptor subtypes, and is effective for RLS and PLMS.[192–196] The mean effective daily dose of ropinirole is approximately 2 mg.[191] Ropinirole is metabolized through the CYP1A2 isoenzyme of the cytochrome P450 system, and has important drug interactions with inhibitors and inducers (including nicotine) of this system. Because of this situation, warfarin levels can be increased by concomitant use of ropinirole, making pramipexole a potentially safer choice. Because plasma concentrations for both pramipexole and ropinirole peak nearly 2 hours after ingestion, it is critical to dose them several hours before symptom onset. Split dosing around the evening meal and again at bedtime seems to enhance compliance and ensures that efficacy is initiated and maintained throughout rest and sleep periods. A direct comparison of these 2 agents has not been conducted, although 1 industry-sponsored meta-analysis[197] suggests a slight superiority for pramipexole in relieving RLS, and a more favorable side effect profile. Cabergoline is an ergot-derived dopamine agonist that is a particularly effective RLS treatment given its long elimination half-life.[198–201] However, because ergot-derived dopamine agonists carry some risk for valvular heart disease, albeit minor,[202] cabergoline is not considered a first-line RLS therapy.

Transdermal dopamine agonists have also been investigated for the treatment of RLS, given the rationale that continuous drug administration could maintain more stable plasma levels,[203] thereby benefiting patients with daytime symptoms with

---

Box 2
Case example

A 63-year-old woman self-referred in 2006 by way of the RLS Foundation's *Nightwalkers* newsletter for treatment of her RLS. Symptoms first emerged during the third trimester of her third pregnancy at the age of 27 years. They resolved on delivery, and over the years occurred sporadically, until she was 59 years old, when they were frequent and intense enough to warrant treatment. Symptoms predominated in her right leg. Pramipexole brought relief for about 3 years, but tolerance to medication was followed by temporal expansion of symptoms to the early afternoon, and spatial extension to her arms (ie, augmentation). She was prescribed 1 mg of ropinirole 2 hours before bedtime but believed that her symptoms were inadequately managed. She experienced frequent afternoon symptoms, did not typically fall asleep until 1:00 AM, and often awakened 4 to 5 hours later with RLS symptoms (eg, symptom rebound). NyQuil, and especially NyQuil-D caused acute symptom exacerbation. Several family members with RLS included a son, and a maternal uncle and cousin. Her past medical history was significant for a herniated disk and right L5 radiculopathy, which was treated surgically (in 1978), a C5-C6 herniated disk repair (1999), and hysterectomy for uterine cancer (2006). She experienced panic attacks and anxiety, which were managed with citalopram (20 mg), and psychophysiologic insomnia, which she attributed to years of poorly controlled RLS, for which she took zolpidem on an as-needed basis. She was prescribed lansoprazole for gastroesophageal reflux. Her examination was significant for flexor-withdrawal-like, nonvolitional movements in her right big toe and ankle (eg, PLMW), and 3+ tendon reflexes throughout, with no pathologic spread or sensorimotor features suggestive of a myelopathy, radiculopathy, or neuropathy.

Laboratory tests revealed preanemic iron deficiency (iron = 56 μg/dL; ferritin = 22 ng/ ml, and a transferrin saturation of 17%), with normal serum cyanocobalamin and thyroid-stimulating hormone levels.

She was initially managed with an increased and split dosing of 1-mg ropinirole tablets, a first dose at dinnertime and a second dose at midnight, carbidopa-levodopa 25/100 on an as-needed basis (no more than 3 times a week) for symptom breakthrough in the afternoon, and oral iron supplementation. Because of reemergence/worsening of her augmentation during the first year, a dose escalation to 4 mg total of ropinirole was recommended, but was limited to 3.0 mg by nausea and evening somnolence. Repeat iron studies confirmed adequate iron repletion (iron = 109 μg/dL; ferritin = 78 ng/ml, and a transferrin saturation of 39%), which remained stable on 1 slow-release ferrous sulfate tablet providing 45 mg of elemental iron.

In 2008, the patient was started back on pramipexole 0.125 mg at dinnertime and repeated at bedtime, with overall improvement that lasted another year. Simultaneously, she was moved from citalopram to 10 mg of the more potent and selective serotonin reuptake blocker S-(+)-enantiomer escitalopram (eg, to avoid the theoretic aggravating affects of any noradrenaline reuptake blockade). Over the ensuing 3 years, because of augmentation, her dose was slowly titrated upwards to 0.25 mg at noon, 0.25 mg at dinnertime, and 0.25 mg at 10:00 pm. On her most recent visits, 6 years since presenting, her International Restless Legs Study Group (IRLSSG) rating scale score was 21 (on a 40-point scale), despite treatment. Augmentation had been troublesome, with no problems with impulse control. Gabapentin enacarbil (600 mg) at dinnertime was therefore added to her regimen and the pramipexole weaned. Augmentation completely resolved, but she noted continued benefit to sleep maintenance and RLS with 0.25 mg of pramipexole in the later evening (presumably because of synergism reflective of different mechanistic sites of drug action). Her IRLSSG rating scale score had improved to 7, and PLMW were less obvious on examination, and diffuse hyperreflexia remained (presumably signs of supraspinal disinhibition operable in RLS; see text for details).

---

a more favorable side effect profile.[204] Pilot, open-label, and controlled trials support the use of rotigotine.[204–208] Rotigotine is available in many European countries, and has been reintroduced in the United States after reformulation to prevent its crystallization within the patch substrate. Factors that render it unique from oral dopamine

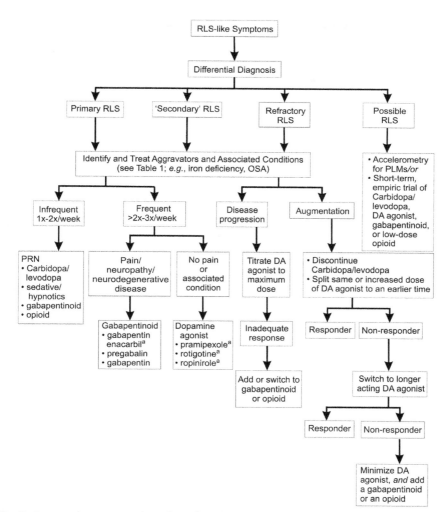

Fig. 2. Proposed treatment algorithm of RLS based on clinical experience and best available evidence (see text for details). DA, dopamine agonist; OSA, obstructive sleep apnea; [a] drugs approved by the FDA for treatment of moderately severe RLS. See **Table 1** for specific agents within a specified pharmacologic class and their recommended dose ranges.

agonists include published long-term safety and efficacy data, a substantial proportion of symptom-free patients (39%) amongst the 43% who remained on therapy at 5 years, and a lower rate of symptom augmentation at the 1-mg to 3-mg doses approved by the European Medicines Agency.[208,209] Adverse effects associated with dopamine agonists include nausea, somnolence, headache, dizziness, rhinitis, and peripheral edema.

Levodopa can also be used for the treatment of RLS, although it is more likely to cause symptom augmentation when compared with the dopamine agonists.[210] For patients with sporadic symptoms who need a rescue medication as opposed to a daily prophylactic medication, levodopa (100–200 mg) is a reasonable choice because of its rapid onset of action. Side effects of levodopa are similar to those of the dopamine agonists and include hypotension, hallucinations, sleepiness, and gastrointestinal discomfort.

Controlled clinical trials have also shown efficacy for gabapentin and its derivatives (eg, pregabalin and gabapentin enacarbil) in the treatment of RLS/PLMS (**Table 1**). Mean effective daily doses of gabapentin are 1855 mg/d, divided into 2 daily doses,[88] with benefit more evident in patients experiencing painful RLS. Open-label[211] and controlled trials with pregabalin also yield clinical and PSG-based improvements in RLS, with 90% efficacy observed at 123.9 mg/d,[212] and a mean effective dose in another study of 322.5 mg/d.[213] The prodrug gabapentin enacarbil offers a pharmacokinetic advantage over gabapentin because of its superior absorption and a longer duration of action, and has recently been approved by the FDA at a single dosage of 600 mg for the treatment of moderate-to-severe RLS, with efficacy demonstrable up to 64 weeks.[214–217] The most commonly reported adverse effects with these gabapentinoids include somnolence, dizziness, and dyscoordination.

A systematic review by an expert task force of the Movement Disorders Society (MDS) identified several other medications as likely efficacious in RLS.[191] These medications included oxycodone, carbamazepine, valproic acid, and clonidine.[191] Given concerns about long-term opioid use, Walters and colleagues[218] reviewed their experience with 36 patients who had attempted opioid monotherapy for RLS. Of these patients, 20 remained on monotherapy for an average of almost 6 years. Of the

Table 1
Pharmacologic treatments for RLS

First-line:	
Dopamine agonists	
Pramipexole	0.25–0.75 mg
Ropinirole	0.25–4.0 mg
Rotigotine	1–3 mg
Second-line:	
Gabapentin enacabril	600 mg
Gabapentin[a]	800–3000 mg
Pregabalin[a]	75–350 mg
Levodopa[a]	100–200 mg
Third-line[a]:	
Oxycodone	5–30 mg
Carbamazepine	200–400 mg
Valproic acid	600 mg
Clonidine	0.1–0.5 mg
Cabergoline	0.5–2.0 mg
Investigational[a]:	
Methadone	10–40 mg
Tramadol	50–200 mg
Clonazepam	0.25–1.0 mg
Zolpidem	2.5–10.0 mg
Amantadine	100–300 mg
Transdermal lisuride	3–6 mg every other day

[a] Use of these medications constitutes off-label use in the United States.

one-third of patients not remaining on monotherapy, 8 had discontinued because of side effects, 7 had an incomplete response, and only 1 patient developed tolerance and addiction. When 7 of the 20 patients who remained on monotherapy were studied with PSG, new sleep apnea had emerged in 2, and a third showed exacerbation of previously diagnosed apnea.[218] Thus, opioids may have long-term effectiveness for some patients with RLS, but side effects and sleep-disordered breathing may be limiting. Clonidine was shown to be effective for RLS, but not PLMS, in a single small, controlled trial.[219] Other medications considered investigational include methadone, tramadol, clonazepam, zolpidem, and amantadine.[191]

Several nonpharmacologic or nonprescription interventions have also been investigated for use in RLS. A small randomized, controlled trial comparing pneumatic with sham compression devices, both used for at least 1 hour a day before typical symptom onset, significantly attenuated RLS severity.[220] In patients with comorbid venous insufficiency, endovascular laser ablation significantly reduces RLS symptoms.[221] Several groups have investigated acupuncture for RLS, but the data are insufficient to support its routine use.[222] Magnesium and folate supplementation do not have sufficient evidence to support their use except as experimental or adjunct therapies.[191] Exercise (aerobic and lower body conditioning) may reduce RLS symptoms,[223] but is still considered investigational.[191]

TREATMENT (SPECIAL CLINICAL SITUATIONS)

Patients with ESRD have a high prevalence of RLS, ranging from 6.6% and 62% of dialysis patients, with similar prevalence in patients receiving peritoneal dialysis and hemodialysis.[224] Dialysis itself does not relieve RLS, but renal transplantation frequently does.[225,226] As with idiopathic RLS, dopaminergic medications are considered first-line therapy for patients with ESRD.[224] Pramipexole and levodopa are both effective.[224,227] Nondopaminergic therapies used in primary RLS also benefit uremic patients, including clonazepam, gabapentin, and clonidine.[224] Because gabapentin is renally excreted, it is critical to limit its dosing to the postdialysis time period and not nightly. RLS in pregnancy presents a particular challenge. Nonpharmacologic therapies are preferable. Iron deficiency should be corrected when identified, and some advocate for magnesium supplementation based on anecdotal cases of IV magnesium for tocolysis coincidentally relieving RLS.[228] Contributions of iron, vitamin B_{12}, or folate deficiencies to pregnancy-related RLS are unclear, yet lower serum folates have been associated with RLS in the third trimester,[116] and folate added to multivitamin and iron supplementation showed superiority in alleviating pregnancy-related RLS.[172] If pharmacologic treatments are required, several of the opioids and anticonvulsants are FDA class B and have a more extensive record of safety in pregnant humans[229] than the more commonly used RLS medications inclusive of dopamine agonists and gabapentin (FDA class C). When use is limited to the third trimester coincident with RLS being most common and potentially troublesome, the lowest efficacious doses of oxycodone, hydroxymorphone, and methadone seem preferable to hydrocodone, propoxyphene, codeine, and tramadol, which are considered FDA class C.

PROGNOSIS

The prognosis of RLS is generally good with recognition and treatment. Although expressivity is variable and remissions are encountered, clinical experience and cross-sectional data suggest that progression with aging (manifest as both increased frequency and intensity of symptoms) is slow and inexorable. However, longitudinal data are notably absent. The most commonly encountered symptoms to be aware of as they relate to prognosis are those associated with medication use. Augmentation is a troubling clinical phenomenon, which follows a period of effective pharmacologic intervention and then tolerance, and manifests as spatial and temporal spread of RLS symptoms that are more bothersome than those appearing at disease onset. Augmentation needs to be distinguished from symptom rebound, which is symptom emergence at a time consistent with the half-life of the drug. Rebound is encountered more frequently with dopaminergic agents with shorter half-lives and typically manifests late in the sleep period or early in the morning. It occurs in at least one-quarter of patients treated with levodopa,[230] yet it is rarely a clinically relevant problem. Management includes switching to an agent with a longer half-life, or a second dose being taken immediately at bedtime. In the instance of augmentation, increased severity manifests as either the occurrence of symptoms by at least 4 hours earlier in the day, or 2 of the following: symptom spread to previously unaffected body parts; quicker symptom onset with inactivity; increase in symptom intensity; shorter duration of treatment effect; or the appearance of PLMW.[231] The most specific feature of augmentation is emergence of RLS earlier in the day, whereas the most sensitive is an increase in symptom intensity.[210] Augmentation can range from a minor problem to a severe clinical complication. It occurs predominantly with dopaminergic medications, but can also occur with tramadol.[232] Estimates of augmentation rates are limited by the short duration of most RLS clinical trials (weeks to months) compared with the months to years usually required for its emergence, and only recently available scales to evaluate it.[191,233] However, data suggest that augmentation rates with levodopa are as high as 60% to 73%,[233,234] whereas those for pramipexole are lower (8%–56%); reliable rates for ropinirole have not been published.[234] It is our clinical experience that augmentation with ropinirole is at least as common as that reported for pramipexole. Risk for augmentation is higher amongst individuals free of neuropathy who have previously experienced augmentation with dopaminergics, a family history of RLS,[235] and those with serum ferritins less than 20 ng/mL.[178] Mild cases of augmentation are managed by dosing earlier in the day[234] or by split dosing. For more severe cases, the patient should be moved to a different medication, typically a gabapentin derivative or an opiate.[234] In our and others'[236] experience, methadone (10–40 mg) in divided doses is an effective alternative in severe, refractory RLS, and particularly in severe cases of augmentation. Changing from 1 dopamine agonist to another is controversial[234] but can be beneficial.[165] To avoid the development of tolerance and augmentation, a strategy of rotation amongst agents from various drug classes (eg, dopaminergics, opiates, gabapentin, and even benzodiazepines) has been advocated.[237]

ICDs and compulsive behaviors associated with the treatment of RLS with dopaminergic agents are limited almost solely to case reports.[238–242] Cross-sectional, questionnaire-based surveys by mail[243,244] or face-to-face interview[245] of a collective 283 patients with RLS treated with dopaminergic medications suggest a rate of 8.5% of any repetitive stereotyped behavior (inclusive of ICD/obsessions/compulsions/motor tics) to 2.8% for any increase in gambling behavior (gambling noted to be pathologic in only a single individual). The degree of impulsivity is generally not deleterious or resolves with discontinuation or reduction in dosage. Careful assessment of 1 large controlled study comparing ICDs in sleep apneic patients and untreated patients with RLS with patients with RLS prescribed dopaminergic medication is particularly informative.[246] First, whereas compulsive shopping and pathologic gambling were more common in RLS versus those with sleep apnea, only compulsive shopping was more common in treated versus untreated patients with RLS. Second, the mean pramipexole dosage at which ICDs emerged (1.2 mg) exceeded the FDA approved dosage of 0.25 to 0.75 mg. Third, treated patients with RLS were more likely (62% vs 37%) to have a preexisting psychiatric diagnosis. Thus, consistent with the experience that vulnerability to ICDs in PD is increased by high novelty-seeking personality traits, depression, male sex, substance abuse, and younger age at disease onset,[247,248] compulsive shopping in RLS may be influenced by preexistent psychiatric disease, and gambling reflective of an underlying diathesis to impulsivity or risk-taking that accompanies the complex RLS trait. A recent study of 50 medication-free patients with RLS and 60 age-matched controls confirmed higher rates of depressive symptoms in RLS, but not of ICDs.[249] Patients should be alerted to this potentially serious complication, although prospective, longitudinal studies with validated measures of impulse control are needed to clarify any cause-effect relationship.

TREATMENT IN SPECIAL SITUATIONS

Patients with ESRD have a high prevalence of RLS, ranging from 6.6% and 62% of dialysis patients, with similar prevalence in patients receiving peritoneal dialysis and hemodialysis.[224] Dialysis itself does not relieve the symptoms of RLS, but renal transplantation frequently does.[225,226] As with idiopathic RLS, dopaminergic medications are considered first-line therapy for patients with ESRD.[224] Pramipexole and levodopa are both effective in this population.[224,227] Nondopaminergic therapies used in primary RLS have also been studied and shown to be beneficial in uremic patients, including clonazepam, gabapentin, and clonidine.[224] Because gabapentin is renally excreted, it is critical to limit its dosing to the postdialysis period and not nightly.

RLS in pregnancy presents a particular challenge because medications typically used in the treatment of RLS are not considered safe in pregnancy. RLS medications that are FDA class C (for which animal data show harm but no human data exist, or for which neither animal nor human data exist) include ropinirole, pramipexole, levodopa, clonidine, and gabapentin. Medications that are pregnancy class D (having evidence of fetal risk in human studies) include carbamazepine and some benzodiazepines. In addition, infants born to mothers taking benzodiazepines or opioids near the end of pregnancy are at risk for withdrawal symptoms.[250,251] Thus, nonpharmacologic therapies should be used when possible. Iron deficiency should be corrected when present in pregnancy and some investigators propose the use of magnesium for the treatment of RLS based on cases of RLS improving when pregnant women are given IV magnesium for tocolysis.[228] Contributions of iron, vitamin B_{12}, or folate deficiencies to pregnancy-related RLS are unclear, yet attention to serum folate status might be most relevant. Lower serum folate levels as opposed to ferritin or vitamin B_{12} have been associated with RLS in the third trimester,[116] and addition of folate to multivitamin and iron supplementation showed superiority in alleviating pregnancy-related RLS.[172] Similarly, although no differences in serologic measures of ferritin, vitamin B_{12} or folate were noted in another study of pregnant women with RLS, RLS was less frequently observed in those taking prenatal vitamins.[117]

REFERENCES

1. Allen R, Hening W, Montplaisir J, et al. Restless legs syndrome: diagnostic criteria, special considerations, and epidemiology: a report from the RLS diagnosis and epidemiology workshop at the National Institutes of Health. Sleep Med 2003;4:101–19.
2. Stefansson H, Rye DB, Hicks A, et al. A genetic risk factor for periodic limb movements in sleep [see comment]. N Engl J Med 2007;357(7):639–47.

3. Hening WA. Subjective and objective criteria in the diagnosis of the restless legs syndrome. Sleep Med 2004;5(3):285–92.

4. Hening WA, Allen RP, Washburn M, et al. The four diagnostic criteria for restless legs syndrome are unable to exclude confounding conditions ("mimics"). Sleep Med 2009;10(9):976–81.

5. Benes H, Walters AS, Allen RP, et al. Definition of restless legs syndrome, how to diagnose it, and how to differentiate it from RLS mimics. Mov Disord 2007; 22(Suppl 18):S401–8.

6. Chaudhuri KR, Rye DB, Muzerengi S. Differential diagnosis of RLS. In: Chaudhuri KR, Ferini-Strambi L, Rye DB, editors. Restless legs syndrome. Oxford (United Kingdom): Oxford University Press; 2008. p. 35–43.

7. Spillane JD, Nathan PW, Kelly RE, et al. Painful legs and moving toes. Brain 1971;94(3):541–56.

8. Dressler D, Thompson PD, Gledhill RF, et al. The syndrome of painful legs and moving toes. Mov Disord 1994;9(1):13–21.

9. Hening W, Walters A, Allen R, et al. Impact, diagnosis and treatment of restless legs syndrome (RLS) in a primary care population: the REST (RLS epidemiology, symptoms, and treatment) primary care study. Sleep Med 2004;5:237–46.

10. Allen RP, Walters AS, Montplaisir J, et al. Restless legs syndrome prevalence and impact: REST general population study. Arch Intern Med 2005;165(11):1286–92.

11. Michaud M, Dumont M, Selmaoui B, et al. Circadian rhythm of restless legs syndrome: relationship with biological markers. Ann Neurol 2004;55:372–80.

12. Duffy J, Lowe A, Winkelman J, et al. Peak circadian occurrence of PLMs during the biological nighttime [abstract]. Sleep 2005;28(Suppl):A275.

13. Baier P, Trenkwalder C. Circadian variation in restless legs syndrome. Sleep Med 2007;8(6):645–50.

14. Picchietti D, Stevens H. Early manifestations of restless legs syndrome in childhood and adolescence. Sleep Med 2007;22:297–300.

15. Phillips B, Young T, Finn L, et al. Epidemiology of restless legs symptoms in adults. Arch Intern Med 2000;160:2137–41.

16. Trotti LM, Bliwise D, Greer SA, et al. Correlates of PLMs variability over multiple nights and impact upon RLS diagnosis. Sleep Med 2009;10(6):668–71.

17. Lamberg L. Sleeping poorly while pregnant may not be "normal". JAMA 2006; 295(12):1357–61.

18. Manconi M, Govoni V, De Vito A, et al. Restless legs syndrome and pregnancy. Neurology 2004;63:1065–9.

19. Berger K, Luedemann J, Trenkwalder C, et al. Sex and the risk of restless legs syndrome in the general population. Arch Intern Med 2004;164:196–202.

20. Desai A, Cherkas L, Spector T, et al. Genetic influences in self-reported symptoms of obstructive sleep apnoea and restless legs syndrome: a twin study. Twin Res 2004;7:589–95.

21. Ondo WG, Vuong KD, Wang Q. Restless legs syndrome in monozygotic twins. Neurology 2000;55(9):1404–6.

22. Tan E, Seah A, See S, et al. Restless legs syndrome in an Asian population: a study in Singapore. Mov Disord 2001;16:577–9.

23. Cho SJ, Hong JP, Hahm BJ, et al. Restless legs syndrome in a community sample of Korean adults: prevalence, impact on quality of life, and association with DSM-IV psychiatric disorders. Sleep 2009;32(8):1069–76.

24. Castillo PR, Kaplan J, Lin SC, et al. Prevalence of restless legs syndrome among native South Americans residing in coastal and mountainous areas. Mayo Clin Proc 2006;81(10):1345–7.

25. Sevim S, Dogu O, Camdeviren H, et al. Unexpectedly low prevalence and unusual characteristics of RLS in Mersin, Turkey. Neurology 2003;61(11): 1562–9.

26. Inoue Y, Ishizuka T, Arai H. Surveillance on epidemiology and treatment of restless legs syndrome in Japan. J New Rem Clim 2000;49:244–54.

27. Earley C, Allen R, Beard J, et al. Insight into the pathophysiology of restless legs syndrome. J Neurosci Res 2000;62(5):623–8.

28. Silber M, Richardson J. Multiple blood donations associated with iron deficiency in patients with restless legs syndrome. Mayo Clin Proc 2003;78:52–4.

29. Winkelman JW, Chertow GM, Lazarus JM. Restless legs syndrome in end-stage renal disease. Am J Kidney Dis 1996;28(3):372–8.

30. Hening WA, Caivano CK. Restless legs syndrome: a common disorder in patients with rheumatologic conditions. Semin Arthritis Rheum 2008;38(1):55–62.

31. Merlino G, Fratticci L, Valente M, et al. Association of restless legs syndrome in type 2 diabetes: a case-control study. Sleep 2007;30(7):866–71.

32. Minai OA, Malik N, Foldvary N, et al. Prevalence and characteristics of restless legs syndrome in patients with pulmonary hypertension. J Heart Lung Transplant 2008;27(3):335–40.

33. Kaplan Y, Inonu H, Yilmaz A, et al. Restless legs syndrome in patients with chronic obstructive pulmonary disease. Can J Neurol Sci 2008;35(3):352–7.

34. Lo Coco D, Mattaliano A, Lo Coco A, et al. Increased frequency of restless legs syndrome in chronic obstructive pulmonary disease patients. Sleep Med 2009; 10(5):572–6.

35. Benediksdottir B, Arnardottir E, Janson C, et al. Prevalence of restless legs syndrome among patients with obstructive sleep apnea before and after CPAP treatment, compared to the general population–the Icelandic Sleep Apnea Cohort (ISAC) study. Sleep 2012;35:A265.

36. Franco RA, Ashwathnarayan R, Deshpandee A, et al. The high prevalence of restless legs syndrome symptoms in liver disease in an academic-based hepatology practice. J Clin Sleep Med 2008;4(1):45–9.

37. Weinstock LB, Bosworth BP, Scherl EJ, et al. Crohn's disease is associated with restless legs syndrome. Inflamm Bowel Dis 2009;16(2):275–9.

38. Manchanda S, Davies CR, Picchietti D. Celiac disease as a possible cause for low serum ferritin in patients with restless legs syndrome. Sleep Med 2009;10(7):763–5.

39. Weinstock LB, Walters AS, Mullin GE, et al. Celiac disease is associated with restless legs syndrome. Dig Dis Sci 2009;55(6):1667–73.

40. Banerji NK, Hurwitz LJ. Restless legs syndrome, with particular reference to its occurrence after gastric surgery. Br Med J 1970;4(5738):774–5.

41. Weinstock LB, Fern SE, Duntley SP. Restless legs syndrome in patients with irritable bowel syndrome: response to small intestinal bacterial overgrowth therapy. Dig Dis Sci 2008;53(5):1252–6.

42. Cologno D, Cicarelli G, Petretta V, et al. High prevalence of dopaminergic premonitory symptoms in migraine patients with restless legs syndrome: a pathogenetic link? Neurol Sci 2008;29(Suppl 1):S166–8.

43. Rhode AM, Hosing VG, Happe S, et al. Comorbidity of migraine and restless legs syndrome–a case-control study. Cephalalgia 2007;27(11):1255–60.

44. Poewe W, Hogl B. Akathisia, restless legs, and periodic limb movements in sleep in Parkinson's disease. Neurology 2004;63(Suppl 3):S12–6.

45. Nomura T, Inoue Y, Miyake M, et al. Prevalence and clinical characteristics of restless legs syndrome in Japanese patients with Parkinson's disease. Mov Disord 2006;21(3):380–4.

46. Gomez-Esteban JC, Zarranz JJ, Tijero B, et al. Restless legs syndrome in Parkinson's disease. Mov Disord 2007;22(13):1912–6.

47. Calzetti S, Negrotti A, Bonavina G, et al. Absence of comorbidity of Parkinson disease and restless legs syndrome: a case-control study in patients attending a movement disorders clinic. Neurol Sci 2009;30:119–22.

48. Lee J, Shin H, Kim K, et al. Factors contributing to the development of restless legs syndrome in patients with Parkinson disease. Mov Disord 2009;24(4): 579–82.

49. Trotti LM, Rye DB. Functional anatomy and treatment of RLS/PLMS emerging after spinal cord lesions. Sleep 2007;30:A306.

50. Abele M, Burk K, Laccone F, et al. Restless legs syndrome in spinocerebellar ataxia types 1, 2, and 3. J Neurol 2001;248(4):311–4.

51. Schöls L, Haan J, Riess O, et al. Sleep disturbance in spinocerebellar ataxias. Is the SCA3 mutation a cause of restless leg syndrome? Neurology 1998;51: 1603–7.

52. Tuin I, Voss U, Kang JS, et al. Stages of sleep pathology in spinocerebellar ataxia type 2 (SCA2). Neurology 2006;67(11):1966–72.

53. Manconi M, Fabbrini M, Bonanni E, et al. High prevalence of restless legs syndrome in multiple sclerosis. Eur J Neurol 2007;14(5):534–9.

54. Winkelmann J, Polo O, Provini F, et al. Genetics of restless legs syndrome (RLS): state-of-the-art and future directions. Mov Disord 2007;22(Suppl 18):S449–58.

55. Winkelmann J, Lichtner P, Schormair B, et al. Variants in the neuronal nitric oxide synthase (nNOS, NOS1) gene are associated with restless legs syndrome. Mov Disord 2008;23(3):350–8.

56. Winkelmann J, Schormair B, Lichtner P, et al. Genome-wide association study of restless legs syndrome identifies common variants in three genomic regions [see comment]. Nat Genet 2007;39(8):1000–6.

57. Vilarino-Guell C, Farrer MJ, Lin SC. A genetic risk factor for periodic limb movements in sleep. N Engl J Med 2008;358(4):425–7.

58. Schormair B, Kemlink D, Roeske D, et al. PTPRD (protein tyrosine phosphatase receptor type delta) is associated with restless legs syndrome. Nat Genet 2008; 40(8):946–8.

59. Winkelmann J, Czamara D, Schormair B, et al. Genome-wide association study identifies novel restless legs syndrome susceptibility loci on 2p14 and 16q12.1. PLoS Genet 2011;7(7):e1002171.

60. Mignot E. A step forward for restless legs syndrome [comment]. Nat Genet 2007;39(8):938–9.

61. Catoire H, Dion PA, Xiong L, et al. Restless legs syndrome-associated MEIS1 risk variant influences iron homeostasis. Ann Neurol 2011;70(1):170–5.

62. Freeman A, Pranski E, Miller RD, et al. Sleep fragmentation and motor restlessness in a Drosophila model of restless legs syndrome. Curr Biol 2012;22(12): 1142–8.

63. Bara-Jimenez W, Aksu M, Graham B, et al. Periodic limb movements in sleep: state-dependent excitability of the spinal flexor reflex. Neurology 2000;54(8): 1609–16.

64. Aksu M, Bara-Jimenez W. State dependent excitability changes of spinal flexor reflex in patients with restless legs syndrome secondary to chronic renal failure. Sleep Med 2002;3(5):427–30.

65. Rijsman RM, Stam CJ, de Weerd AW. Abnormal H-reflexes in periodic limb movement disorder; impact on understanding the pathophysiology of the disorder. Clin Neurophysiol 2005;116(1):204–10.

66. Clemens S, Hochman S. Conversion of the modulatory actions of dopamine on spinal reflexes from depression to facilitation in D3 receptor knock-out mice. J Neurosci 2004;24:11337–45.

67. Clemens S, Rye D, Hochman S. Restless legs syndrome: revisiting the dopamine hypothesis from the spinal cord perspective. Neurology 2006;67(1): 125–30.

68. Jakobsson B, Ruuth K. Successful treatment of restless legs syndrome with an implanted pump for intrathecal drug delivery. Acta Anaesthesiol Scand 2002; 46(1):114–7.

69. Lindvall P, Ruuth K, Jakobsson B, et al. Intrathecal morphine as a treatment for refractory restless legs syndrome. Neurosurgery 2008;63(6):E1209 [author reply: E1209].

70. Ross DA, Narus MS, Nutt JG. Control of medically refractory restless legs syndrome with intrathecal morphine: case report. Neurosurgery 2008;62(1): E263 [discussion: E263].

71. Yokota T, Hirose K, Tanabe H, et al. Sleep-related periodic leg movements (nocturnal myoclonus) due to spinal cord lesion. J Neurol Sci 1991;104:13–8.

72. Dickel M, Renfrow S, Moore P, et al. Rapid eye movement sleep periodic leg movements in patients with spinal cord injury. Sleep 1994;17(8):733–8.

73. Lee M, Choi Y, Lee S. Sleep-related periodic leg movements associated with spinal cord lesions. Mov Disord 1996;11(6):719–22.

74. de Mello M, Lauro F, Silva A, et al. Incidence of periodic leg movements and of the restless legs syndrome during sleep following acute physical activity in spinal cord injury subjects. Spinal Cord 1996;34(5):294–6.

75. Manconi M, Rocca M, Ferini-Strambi L, et al. Restless legs syndrome is a common finding in multiple sclerosis and correlates with cervical cord damage. Mult Scler 2008;14(1):86–93.

76. Rutkove S, Matheson J, Logigian E. Restless legs syndrome in patients with polyneuropathy. Muscle Nerve 1996;19(5):670–2.

77. Ondo W, Jankovic J. Restless legs syndrome: clinicoetiologic correlates. Neurology 1996;47:1435–41.

78. Gemignani F, Marbini A, Di Giovanni G, et al. Charcot-Marie-Tooth disease type 2 with restless legs syndrome [see comment]. Neurology 1999;52(5):1064–6.

79. Hattan E, Chalk C, Postuma R. Is there a higher risk of restless legs syndrome in peripheral neuropathy? Neurology 2009;72(11):955–60.

80. Iannaccone S, Zucconi M, Marchettini P, et al. Evidence of peripheral axonal neuropathy in primary restless legs syndrome. Mov Disord 1995;10(1):2–9.

81. Polydefkis M, Allen R, Hauer P, et al. Subclinical sensory neuropathy in late-onset restless legs syndrome. Neurology 2000;55(8):1115–21.

82. Montplaisir J, Godbout R, Boghen D, et al. Familial restless legs with periodic movements in sleep: electrophysiologic, biochemical, and pharmacologic study. Neurology 1985;35:130–4.

83. Provini F, Vetrugno R, Meletti S, et al. Motor pattern of periodic limb movements during sleep. Neurology 2001;57(2):300–4.

84. Ferreri F, Rossini P. Neurophysiological investigations in restless legs syndrome and other disorders of movement during sleep. Sleep Med 2004;5:397–9.

85. Tyvaert L, Laureau E, Hurtevent J, et al. A-delta and C-fibres function in primary restless legs syndrome. Neurophysiol Clin 2009;39(6):267–74.

86. Wechsler L, Stakes J, Shahani B, et al. Periodic leg movements of sleep (nocturnal myoclonus): an electrophysiological study. Ann Neurol 1986;19: 168–73.

87. Smith R, Gouin P, Minkley P, et al. Periodic limb movement disorder is associated with normal motor conduction latencies when studied by central magnetic stimulation–successful use of a new technique. Sleep 1992;15(4):312–8.

88. Garcia-Borreguero D, Larrosa O, de la Llave Y, et al. Treatment of restless legs syndrome with gabapentin: a double-blind, cross-over study. Neurology 2002; 59:1573–9.

89. Ekbom K. Restless legs. Acta Med Scand Suppl 1945;158:1–123.

90. Wechsler L, Stakes J, Shahani B, et al. Nocturnal myoclonus, restless legs syndrome, and abnormal electrophysiological findings. Ann Neurol 1987;21:515.

91. Briellmann R, Rosler K, Hess C. Blink reflex excitability is abnormal in patients with periodic leg movements in sleep. Mov Disord 1996;11(6):710–4.

92. Scalise A, Cadore IP, Gigli GL. Motor cortex excitability in restless legs syndrome. Sleep Med 2004;5(4):393–6.

93. Nardone R, Ausserer H, Bratti A, et al. Cabergoline reverses cortical hyperexcitability in patients with restless legs syndrome. Acta Neurol Scand 2006;114(4): 244–9.

94. Fleetwood-Walker S, Hope P, Mitchell R. Antinociceptive actions of descending dopaminergic tracts on cat and rat dorsal horn somatosensory neurones. J Physiol (Lond) 1988;399:335–48.

95. Garraway S, Hochman S. Modulatory actions of serotonin, norepinephrine, dopamine, and acetylcholine in spinal cord deep dorsal horn neurons. J Neurophysiol 2001;86:2183–94.

96. Millan MJ, Colpaert FC. alpha2 Receptors mediate the antinociceptive action of 8-OH-DPAT in the hot-plate test in mice. Brain Res 1991;539:342–6.

97. Yoshimura M, Furue H. Mechanisms for the anti-nociceptive actions of the descending noradrenergic and serotonergic systems in the spinal cord. J Pharmacol Sci 2006;101(2):107–17.

98. Wei H, Viisanen H, Pertovaara A. Descending modulation of neuropathic hypersensitivity by dopamine D2 receptors in or adjacent to the hypothalamic A11 cell group. Pharmacol Res 2009;59(5):355–63.

99. Ondo WG, He Y, Rajasekaran S, et al. Clinical correlates of 6-hydroxydopamine injections into A11 dopaminergic neurons in rats: a possible model for restless legs syndrome. Mov Disord 2000;15(1):154–8.

100. Qu S, Le W, Zhang X, et al. Locomotion is increased in a11-lesioned mice with iron deprivation: a possible animal model for restless legs syndrome. J Neuropathol Exp Neurol 2007;66(5):383–8.

101. Zhao H, Zhu W, Pan T, et al. Spinal cord dopamine receptor expression and function in mice with 6-OHDA lesion of the A11 nucleus and dietary iron deprivation. J Neurosci Res 2007;85(5):1065–76.

102. Stiasny-Kolster K, Magerl W, Oertel W, et al. Static mechanical hyperalgesia without dynamic tactile allodynia in patients with restless legs syndrome. Brain 2004;127:773–82.

103. Han JK, Oh K, Kim BJ, et al. Cutaneous silent period in patients with restless leg syndrome. Clin Neurophysiol 2007;118(8):1705–10.

104. Rye D, Freeman A. Pain and its interaction with thalamocortical excitability states. In: Lavigne G, Choinière M, Sessle B, et al, editors. Sleep and pain. Seattle (WA): IASP Press; 2007. p. 77–97.

105. Wood PB. Role of central dopamine in pain and analgesia. Expert Rev Neurother 2008;8(5):781–97.

106. Rye D, DeLong M. Amelioration of sensory limb discomfort of restless legs syndrome by pallidotomy. Ann Neurol 1999;46(5):800–1.

107. Kedia S, Moro E, Tagliati M, et al. Emergence of restless legs syndrome during subthalamic stimulation for Parkinson disease. Neurology 2004; 63(12):2410–2.
108. Driver-Dunckley E, Evidente VG, Adler CH, et al. Restless legs syndrome in Parkinson's disease patients may improve with subthalamic stimulation. Mov Disord 2006;21(8):1287–9.
109. Ondo W. VIM deep brain stimulation does not improve pre-existing restless legs syndrome in patients with essential tremor. Parkinsonism Relat Disord 2006; 12(2):113–4.
110. Lee SJ, Kim JS, Song IU, et al. Poststroke restless legs syndrome and lesion location: anatomical considerations. Mov Disord 2009;24(1):77–84.
111. Ferini-Strambi L, Filippi M, Martinelli V, et al. Nocturnal sleep study in multiple sclerosis: correlations with clinical and brain magnetic resonance imaging findings. J Neurol Sci 1994;125:194–7.
112. Allen R. Dopamine and iron in the pathophysiology of restless legs syndrome (RLS). Sleep Med 2004;5(4):385–91.
113. Allen R, Earley C. The role of iron in restless legs syndrome. Mov Disord 2007; 22(Suppl 18):S440–8.
114. Connor J. Pathophysiology of restless legs syndrome: evidence for iron involvement. Curr Neurol Neurosci Rep 2008;8(2):162–6.
115. Akyol A, Kiylioglu N, Kadikoylu G, et al. Iron deficiency anemia and restless legs syndrome: is there an electrophysiological abnormality? Clin Neurol Neurosurg 2003;106:23–7.
116. Lee K, Zaffke M, Baratte-Beebe K. Restless legs syndrome and sleep disturbance during pregnancy: the role of folate and iron. J Womens Health Gend Based Med 2001;10(4):335–41.
117. Tunc T, Karadag Y, Dogulu F, et al. Predisposing factors of restless legs syndrome in pregnancy. Mov Disord 2007;22(5):627–31.
118. Dzaja A, Wehrle R, Lancel M, et al. Elevated estradiol plasma levels in women with restless legs during pregnancy. Sleep 2009;32(2):169–74.
119. Burchell BJ, Allen RP, Miller JK, et al. RLS and blood donation. Sleep Med 2009; 10(8):844–9.
120. Becker PM. Bleed less than 3: RLS and blood donation. Sleep Med 2009;10(8): 820–1.
121. Berger K, von Eckardstein A, Trenkwalder C, et al. Iron metabolism and the risk of restless legs syndrome in an elderly general population–the MEMO study. J Neurol 2002;249:1195–9.
122. Earley C, Heckler D, Allen R. The treatment of restless legs syndrome with intravenous iron dextran. Sleep Med 2004;5:231–5.
123. Earley CJ, Horska A, Mohamed MA, et al. A randomized, double-blind, placebo-controlled trial of intravenous iron sucrose in restless legs syndrome. Sleep Med 2009;10(2):206–11.
124. Grote L, Leissner L, Hedner J, et al. A randomized, double-blind, placebo controlled, multi-center study of intravenous iron sucrose and placebo in the treatment of restless legs syndrome. Mov Disord 2009;24(10): 1445–52.
125. Aul EA, Davis BJ, Rodnitzky RL. The importance of formal serum iron studies in the assessment of restless legs syndrome. Neurology 1998;51(3):912.
126. Freeman A, Rye D. Dopamine in behavioral state control. In: Sinton C, Perumal P, Monti J, editors. The neurochemistry of sleep and wakefulness. Cambridge (United Kingdom): Cambridge University Press; 2008. p. 179–223.

127. Ramsey A, Hillas P, Fitzpatrick P. Characterization of the active site iron in tyrosine hydroxylase redox states of the iron. J Biol Chem 1996;271:24395–400.
128. Nagatsu I. Tyrosine hydroxylase: human isoforms, structure and regulation in physiology and pathology. Essays Biochem 1995;30:15–35.
129. Nelson C, Erikson K, Pinero DJ, et al. In vivo dopamine metabolism is altered in iron-deficient anemic rats. J Nutr 1997;127(12):2282–8.
130. Bianco LE, Wiesinger J, Earley CJ, et al. Iron deficiency alters dopamine uptake and response to L-DOPA injection in Sprague-Dawley rats. J Neurochem 2008; 106(1):205–15.
131. Bianco L, Unger E, Earley C, et al. Iron deficiency alters the day-night variation in monoamine levels in mice. Chronobiol Int 2009;26(3):447–63.
132. Hue GE, Decker MJ, Solomon IG, et al. Increased wakefulness and hyper-responsivity to novel environments in mice lacking functional dopamine D3 receptors. Soc Neurosci 2003;616:16.
133. Beckford G. The functional organization and behavioral relevance of the A11 hypothalamospinal dopaminergic system. Atlanta (GA): Emory; 2008.
134. Allen RP, Connor JR, Hyland K, et al. Abnormally increased CSF 3-ortho-meth-yldopa (3-OMD) in untreated restless legs syndrome (RLS) patients indicates more severe disease and possibly abnormally increased dopamine synthesis. Sleep Med 2009;10(1):123–8.
135. Connor JR, Wang XS, Allen RP, et al. Altered dopaminergic profile in the putamen and substantia nigra in restless leg syndrome. Brain 2009;132(Pt 9):2403–12.
136. Perez-Diaz H, Iranzo A, Rye DB, et al. Restless abdomen: a phenotypic variant of restless legs syndrome. Neurology 2011;77(13):1283–6.
137. Benes H, von Eye A, Kohnen R. Empirical evaluation of the accuracy of diagnostic criteria for restless legs syndrome. Sleep Med 2009;10(5):524–30.
138. Stiasny-Kolster K, Kohnen R, Moller JC, et al. Validation of the "L-DOPA test" for diagnosis of restless legs syndrome. Mov Disord 2006;21(9):1333–9.
139. Salin-Pascual R, Galicia-Polo L, Drucker-Colin R. Sleep changes after 4 consecutive days of venlafaxine administration in normal volunteers. J Clin Psychiatry 1997;58(8):348–50.
140. Yang C, White DP, Winkelman JW. Antidepressants and periodic leg movements of sleep. Biol Psychiatry 2005;58(6):510–4.
141. Page RL 2nd, Ruscin JM, Bainbridge JL, et al. Restless legs syndrome induced by escitalopram: case report and review of the literature. Pharmacotherapy 2008;28(2):271–80.
142. Rottach KG, Schaner BM, Kirch MH, et al. Restless legs syndrome as side effect of second generation antidepressants. J Psychiatr Res 2008;43(1):70–5.
143. Fox EJ, Villanueva R, Schutta HS. Myoclonus following spinal anesthesia. Neurology 1979;29(3):379–80.
144. Lee MS, Lyoo CH, Kim WC, et al. Periodic bursts of rhythmic dyskinesia associated with spinal anesthesia. Mov Disord 1997;12(5):816–7.
145. Nadkarni AV, Tondare AS. Localized clonic convulsions after spinal anesthesia with lidocaine and epinephrine. Anesth Analg 1982;61(11):945–7.
146. Watanabe S, Sakai K, Ono Y, et al. Alternating periodic leg movement induced by spinal anesthesia in an elderly male. Anesth Analg 1987;66(10):1031–2.
147. Hogl B, Frauscher B, Seppi K, et al. Transient restless legs syndrome after spinal anesthesia: a prospective study. Neurology 2002;59(11):1705–7.
148. Montplaisir J, Boucher S, Poirier G, et al. Clinical, polysomnographic, and genetic characteristics of restless legs syndrome: a study of 133 patients diagnosed with new standard criteria. Mov Disord 1997;12:61–5.

149. Bixler E, Kales A, Vela-Bueno A, et al. Nocturnal myoclonus and nocturnal myoclonic activity in the normal population. Res Commun Chem Pathol Pharmacol 1982;36(1):129–40.
150. Scofield H, Roth T, Drake C. Periodic limb movements during sleep: population prevalence, clinical correlates, and racial differences. Sleep 2008;31(9):1221–7.
151. Allen R, Earley C. Augmentation of the restless legs syndrome with carbidopa/levodopa. Sleep 1996;19:205–13.
152. Picchietti MA, Picchietti DL. Restless legs syndrome and periodic limb movement disorder in children and adolescents. Semin Pediatr Neurol 2008;15(2):91–9.
153. Santamaria J, Iranzo A, Tolosa E. Development of restless legs syndrome after dopaminergic treatment in a patient with periodic leg movements in sleep. Sleep Med 2003;4:153–5.
154. Walters A, Picchietti D, Hening W, et al. Variable expressivity in familial restless legs syndrome. Arch Neurol 1990;47:1219–20.
155. Birinyi PV, Allen RP, Hening W, et al. Undiagnosed individuals with first-degree relatives with restless legs syndrome have increased periodic limb movements. Sleep Med 2006;7(6):480–5.
156. O'Brien LM, Holbrook CR, Faye Jones V, et al. Ethnic difference in periodic limb movements in children [see comment]. Sleep Med 2007;8(3):240–6.
157. Michaud M, Soucy J, Chabli A, et al. SPECT imaging of striatal pre- and post-synaptic dopaminergic status in restless legs syndrome with periodic leg movements in sleep. J Neurol 2002;249:164–70.
158. Rye D, Bliwise D, Iranzo A, et al. A novel 2-step diagnostic approach for RLS disease classification. Sleep 2004;27(Suppl S):306–7.
159. Sforza E, Johannes M, Claudio B. The PAM-RL ambulatory device for detection of periodic leg movements: a validation study [see comment]. Sleep Med 2005;6(5):407–13.
160. Tuisku K, Holi M, Wahlbeck K, et al. Quantitative rest activity in ambulatory monitoring as a physiological marker of restless legs syndrome: a controlled study. Mov Disord 2003;18:442–8.
161. Tuisku K, Holi M, Wahlbeck K, et al. Actometry in measuring the symptom severity of restless legs syndrome. Eur J Neurol 2005;12:385–7.
162. Rye D, Allen R, Carson S, et al. Ropinirole decreases bedtime periodic leg movements in patients with RLS: results of a 12-week US study. Sleep 2005;28(Suppl S):A270.
163. Hening W, Walters A, Kavey N, et al. Dyskinesias while awake and periodic movements in sleep in restless legs syndrome: treatment with opioids. Neurology 1986;36:1363–6.
164. Hening WA. Current guidelines and standards of practice for restless legs syndrome. Am J Med 2007;120(1 Suppl 1):S22–7.
165. Silber M, Ehrenberg B, Allen R, et al. An algorithm for the management of restless legs syndrome. Mayo Clin Proc 2004;79:916–22.
166. Hornyak M, Feige B, Riemann D, et al. Periodic leg movements in sleep and periodic limb movement disorder: prevalence, clinical significance and treatment. Sleep Med Rev 2006;10(3):169–77.
167. Urbano MR, Ware JC. Restless legs syndrome caused by quetiapine successfully treated with ropinirole in 2 patients with bipolar disorder. J Clin Pharmacol 2008;28(6):704–5.
168. Kim S, Shin I, Kim J, et al. Bupropion may improve restless legs syndrome: a report of three cases. Clin Neuropharmacol 2005;28(6):298–301.

169. Lee J, Erdos J, Wilkoosz M, et al. Bupropion as a possible treatment option for restless legs syndrome. Ann Pharmacother 2009;43(2):370–4.
170. Smith HS, Dhingra R, Ryckewaert L, et al. Proton pump inhibitors and pain. Pain Physician 2009;12(6):1013–23.
171. Numata Y, Kato T, Nagatsu T, et al. Effects of stereochemical structures of tetrahydrobiopterin on tyrosine hydroxylase. Biochim Biophys Acta 1977;480(1):104–12.
172. Botez M, Lambert B. Folate deficiency and restless legs syndrome in pregnancy. N Engl J Med 1977;297(12):670.
173. O'Keeffe S, Gavin K, Lavan J. Iron status and restless legs syndrome in the elderly. Age Ageing 1994;23:200–3.
174. Bachmann C, Guth N, Helmshmied K, et al. Homocysteine in restless legs syndrome. Sleep Med 2008;9(4):388–92.
175. Davis BJ, Rajput A, Rajput ML, et al. A randomized, double-blind placebo-controlled trial of iron in restless legs syndrome. Eur Neurol 2000;43(2):70–5.
176. Wang J, O'Reilly B, Venkataraman R, et al. Efficacy of oral iron in patients with restless legs syndrome and a low-normal ferritin: a randomized, double-blind, placebo-controlled study. Sleep Med 2009;10(9):973–5.
177. Morgan JC, Ames M, Sethi KD. Response to ropinirole in restless legs syndrome is independent of baseline serum ferritin. J Neurol Neurosurg Psychiatr 2008;79(8):964–5.
178. Trenkwalder C, Hogl B, Benes H, et al. Augmentation in restless legs syndrome is associated with low ferritin. Sleep Med 2008;9(5):572–4.
179. Umbreit J. Iron deficiency: a concise review. Am J Hematol 2005;78(3):225–31.
180. Silverstein SB, Rodgers GM. Parenteral iron therapy options. Am J Hematol 2004;76(1):74–8.
181. Sloand J, Shelly M, Feigin A, et al. A double-blind, placebo-controlled trial of intravenous iron dextran therapy in patients with ESRD and restless legs syndrome. Am J Kidney Dis 2004;43:663–70.
182. Becker P, Patrick F, Dubrava S, et al. Effect of pregabalin on sleep disturbances in patients with restless legs syndrome (Willis-Ekbom disease). Sleep 2012;35:A257.
183. Happe S, Trenkwalder C. Role of dopamine receptor agonists in the treatment of restless legs syndrome. CNS Drugs 2004;18(1):27–36.
184. Fulda S, Wetter TC. Where dopamine meets opioids: a meta-analysis of the placebo effect in restless legs syndrome treatment studies. Brain 2008;131(Pt 4):902–17.
185. Diederich NJ, Goetz CG. The placebo treatments in neurosciences: new insights from clinical and neuroimaging studies. Neurology 2008;71(9):677–84.
186. Montplaisir J, Nicolas A, Denesle R, et al. Restless legs syndrome improved by pramipexole: a double-blind randomized study. Neurology 1999;52:938–43.
187. Montplaisir J, Denesle R, Petit D. Pramipexole in the treatment of restless legs syndrome: a follow-up study. Eur J Neurol 2000;7(Suppl 1):27–31.
188. Winkelman JW, Sethi KD, Kushida CA, et al. Efficacy and safety of pramipexole in restless legs syndrome. Neurology 2006;67(6):1034–9.
189. Ferini-Strambi L, Aarskog D, Partinen M, et al. Effect of pramipexole on RLS symptoms and sleep: a randomized, double-blind, placebo-controlled trial. Sleep Med 2008;9:874–81.
190. Partinen M, Hirvonen K, Jama L, et al. Efficacy and safety of pramipexole in idiopathic restless legs syndrome: a polysomnographic dose-finding study–the PRELUDE study. Sleep Med 2006;7(5):407–17.

191. Trenkwalder C, Hening WA, Montagna P, et al. Treatment of restless legs syndrome: an evidence-based review and implications for clinical practice. Mov Disord 2008;23(16):2267–302.
192. Adler CH, Hauser RA, Sethi K, et al. Ropinirole for restless legs syndrome: a placebo-controlled crossover trial. Neurology 2004;62(8):1405–7.
193. Walters AS, Ondo WG, Dreykluft T, et al. Ropinirole is effective in the treatment of restless legs syndrome. TREAT RLS 2: a 12-week, double-blind, randomized, parallel-group, placebo-controlled study. Mov Disord 2004;19(12):1414–23.
194. Allen R, Becker PM, Bogan R, et al. Ropinirole decreases periodic leg movements and improves sleep parameters in patients with restless legs syndrome. Sleep 2004;27(5):907–14.
195. Bliwise DL, Freeman A, Ingram CD, et al. Randomized, double-blind, placebo-controlled, short-term trial of ropinirole in restless legs syndrome. Sleep Med 2005;6(2):141–7.
196. Bogan RK, Fry JM, Schmidt MH, et al. Ropinirole in the treatment of patients with restless legs syndrome: a US-based randomized, double-blind, placebo-controlled clinical trial. Mayo Clin Proc 2006;81(1):17–27.
197. Quilici S, Abrams K, Nicolas A, et al. Meta-analysis of the efficacy and tolerability of pramipexole versus ropinirole in the treatment of restless legs syndrome. Sleep Med 2008;9(7):715–26.
198. Stiasny-Kolster K, Benes H, Peglau I, et al. Effective cabergoline treatment in idiopathic restless legs syndrome (RLS): a randomized, double-blind, placebo-controlled, multicenter dose-finding study followed by an open long-term extension. Neurology 2004;63(12):2272–9.
199. Benes H, Heinrich CR, Ueberall MA, et al. Long-term safety and efficacy of cabergoline for the treatment of idiopathic restless legs syndrome: results from an open-label 6-month clinical trial. Sleep 2004;27(4):674–82.
200. Oertel WH, Benes H, Bodenschatz R, et al. Efficacy of cabergoline in restless legs syndrome: a placebo-controlled study with polysomnography (CATOR). Neurology 2006;67(6):1040–6.
201. Trenkwalder C, Benes H, Grote L, et al. Cabergoline compared to levodopa in the treatment of patients with severe restless legs syndrome: results from a multi-center, randomized, active controlled trial. Mov Disord 2007;22(5):696–703.
202. Zanettini R, Antonini A, Gatto G, et al. Valvular heart disease and the use of dopamine agonists for Parkinson's disease. N Engl J Med 2007;356(1):39–46.
203. Benes H. Transdermal lisuride: short-term efficacy and tolerability study in patients with severe restless legs syndrome. Sleep Med 2006;7(1):31–5.
204. Stiasny-Kolster K, Kohnen R, Schollmayer E, et al. Patch application of the dopamine agonist rotigotine to patients with moderate to advanced stages of restless legs syndrome: a double-blind, placebo-controlled pilot study. Mov Disord 2004;19(12):1432–8.
205. Oertel WH, Benes H, Garcia-Borreguero D, et al. Rotigotine transdermal patch in moderate to severe idiopathic restless legs syndrome: a randomized, placebo-controlled polysomnographic study. Sleep Med 2010;11(9):848–56.
206. Oertel WH, Benes H, Garcia-Borreguero D, et al. One year open-label safety and efficacy trial with rotigotine transdermal patch in moderate to severe idiopathic restless legs syndrome. Sleep Med 2008;9:865–73.
207. Hening WA, Allen RP, Ondo WG, et al. Rotigotine improves restless legs syndrome: a 6-month randomized, double-blind, placebo-controlled trial in the United States. Mov Disord 2010;25(11):1675–83.

208. Oertel W, Trenkwalder C, Benes H, et al. Long-term safety and efficacy of roti-gotine transdermal patch for moderate-to-severe idiopathic restless legs syndrome: a 5-year open-label extension study. Lancet Neurol 2011;10(8): 710–20.

209. Benes H, Garcia-Borreguero D, Ferini-Strambi L, et al. Augmentation in the treat-ment of restless legs syndrome with transdermal rotigotine. Sleep Med 2012; 13(6):589–97.

210. Paulus W, Trenkwalder C. Less is more: pathophysiology of dopaminergic-therapy-related augmentation in restless legs syndrome. Lancet Neurol 2006; 5(10):878–86.

211. Sommer M, Bachmann CG, Liebetanz KM, et al. Pregabalin in restless legs syndrome with and without neuropathic pain. Acta Neurol Scand 2007;115(5): 347–50.

212. Allen R, Chen C, Soaita A, et al. A randomized, double-blind, 6-week, dose-ranging study of pregabalin in patients with restless legs syndrome. Sleep Med 2010;11(6):512–9.

213. Garcia-Borreguero D, Larrosa O, Williams AM, et al. Treatment of restless legs syndrome with pregabalin: a double-blind, placebo-controlled study. Neurology 2010;74(23):1897–904.

214. Kushida C, Ellenbogen A, Becker P, et al. A randomized, double-blind, placebo-controlled study to assess the efficacy and tolerability of XP13512 1200 mg in patients with restless legs syndrome. Neurology 2008;70(11):A409.

215. Kushida CA, Walters AS, Becker P, et al. A randomized, double-blind, placebo-controlled, crossover study of XP13512/GSK1838262 in the treatment of patients with primary restless legs syndrome. Sleep 2009;32(2):159–68.

216. Winkelman JW, Bogan RK, Schmidt MH, et al. Randomized polysomnography study of gabapentin enacarbil in subjects with restless legs syndrome. Mov Disord 2011;26(11):2065–72.

217. Lee DO, Ziman RB, Perkins AT, et al. A randomized, double-blind, placebo-controlled study to assess the efficacy and tolerability of gabapentin enacarbil in subjects with restless legs syndrome. J Clin Sleep Med 2011;7(3):282–92.

218. Walters AS, Winkelmann J, Trenkwalder C, et al. Long-term follow-up on restless legs syndrome patients treated with opioids. Mov Disord 2001;16(6):1105–9.

219. Wagner ML, Walters AS, Coleman RG, et al. Randomized, double-blind, placebo-controlled study of clonidine in restless legs syndrome. Sleep 1996; 19(1):52–8.

220. Lettieri CJ, Eliasson AH. Pneumatic compression devices are an effective therapy for restless legs syndrome: a prospective, randomized, double-blinded, sham-controlled trial. Chest 2009;135(1):74–80.

221. Hayes CA, Kingsley JR, Hamby KR, et al. The effect of endovenous laser abla-tion on restless legs syndrome. Phlebology 2008;23(3):112–7.

222. Cui Y, Wang Y, Liu Z. Acupuncture for restless legs syndrome. Cochrane Data-base Syst Rev 2008;(4):CD006457.

223. Aukerman MM, Aukerman D, Bayard M, et al. Exercise and restless legs syndrome: a randomized controlled trial. J Am Board Fam Med 2006;19(5): 487–93.

224. Kavanagh D, Siddiqui S, Geddes CC. Restless legs syndrome in patients on dialysis. Am J Kidney Dis 2004;43(5):763–71.

225. Winkelmann J, Stautner A, Samtleben W, et al. Long-term course of restless legs syndrome in dialysis patients after kidney transplantation. Mov Disord 2002; 17(5):1072–6.

226. Molnar MZ, Novak M, Ambrus C, et al. Restless legs syndrome in patients after renal transplantation. Am J Kidney Dis 2005;45(2):388–96.
227. Miranda M, Kagi M, Fabres L, et al. Pramipexole for the treatment of uremic restless legs in patients undergoing hemodialysis. Neurology 2004;62(5):831–2.
228. Bartell S, Zallek S. Intravenous magnesium sulfate may relieve restless legs syndrome in pregnancy. J Clin Sleep Med 2006;2(2):187–8.
229. Djokanovic N, Garcia-Bournissen F, Koren G. Medications for restless legs syndrome in pregnancy. J Obstet Gynaecol Can 2008;30(6):505–7.
230. Guilleminault C, Cetel M, Philip P. Dopaminergic treatment of restless legs and rebound phenomenon. Neurology 1993;43(2):445.
231. Garcia-Borreguero D, Allen RP, Kohnen R, et al. Diagnostic standards for dopaminergic augmentation of restless legs syndrome: report from a World Association Of Sleep Medicine-International Restless Legs Syndrome Study Group consensus conference at the Max Planck Institute. Sleep Med 2007;8(5):520–30.
232. Earley CJ, Allen RP. Restless legs syndrome augmentation associated with tramadol. Sleep Med 2006;7(7):592–3.
233. Garcia-Borreguero D, Kohnen R, Hogl B, et al. Validation of the Augmentation Severity Rating Scale (ASRS). Sleep Med 2007;8:455–63.
234. Garcia-Borreguero D, Allen RP, Benes H, et al. Augmentation as a treatment complication of restless legs syndrome: concept and management. Mov Disord 2007;22(Suppl 18):S476–84.
235. Ondo W, Romanyshyn J, Vuong K, et al. Long-term treatment of restless legs syndrome with dopamine agonists. Arch Neurol 2004;61:1393–7.
236. Ondo WG. Methadone for refractory restless legs syndrome. Mov Disord 2005;20(3):345–8.
237. Kurlan R, Richard I, Deeley C. Medication tolerance and augmentation in restless legs syndrome: the need for drug class rotation. J Gen Intern Med 2006;21(12):C1–4.
238. Tippmann-Peikert M, Park JG, Boeve BF, et al. Pathologic gambling in patients with restless legs syndrome treated with dopaminergic agonists. Neurology 2007;68(4):301–3.
239. Quickfall J, Suchowersky O. Pathological gambling associated with dopamine agonist use in restless legs syndrome. Parkinsonism Relat Disord 2007;13(8):535–6.
240. Evans AH, Stegeman JR. Punding in patients on dopamine agonists for restless leg syndrome. Mov Disord 2009;24(1):140–1.
241. Salas RE, Allen RP, Earley CJ, et al. A case of compulsive behaviors observed in a restless legs syndrome patient treated with a dopamine agonist. Sleep 2009;32(5):587–8.
242. Kolla BP, Mansukhani MP, Barraza R, et al. Impact of dopamine agonists on compulsive behaviors: a case series of pramipexole-induced pathological gambling. Psychosomatics 2010;51(3):271–3.
243. Driver-Dunckley ED, Noble BN, Hentz JG, et al. Gambling and increased sexual desire with dopaminergic medications in restless legs syndrome. Clin Neuropharmacol 2007;30(5):249–55.
244. Pourcher E, Remillard S, Cohen H. Compulsive habits in restless legs syndrome patients under dopaminergic treatment. J Neurol Sci 2010;290(1–2):52–6.
245. Ondo WG, Lai D. Predictors of impulsivity and reward seeking behavior with dopamine agonists. Parkinsonism Relat Disord 2008;14(1):28–32.

246. Cornelius J, Tippmann-Piekert M, Slocumb N, et al. Impulse control disorders with use of dopaminergic agents in restless legs syndrome: a case-control study. Sleep 2010;33(1):81–7.
247. Voon V, Thomsen T, Miyasaki JM, et al. Factors associated with dopaminergic drug-related pathological gambling in Parkinson disease. Arch Neurol 2007; 64(2):212–6.
248. Potenza MN, Voon V, Weintraub D. Drug Insight: impulse control disorders and dopamine therapies in Parkinson's disease. Nat Clin Pract Neurol 2007;3(12): 664–72.
249. Bayard S, Yu H, Langenier MC, et al. Decision making in restless legs syndrome. Mov Disord 2010;25(15):2634–40.
250. Chesson AL Jr, Wise M, Davila D, et al. Practice parameters for the treatment of restless legs syndrome and periodic limb movement disorder. An American Academy of Sleep Medicine report. Standards of Practice Committee of the American Academy of Sleep Medicine. Sleep 1999;22(7):961–8.
251. Trotti LM, Bhadriraju S, Rye DB. An update on the pathophysiology and genetics of restless legs syndrome. Curr Neurol Neurosci Rep 2008;8(4):281–7.

Circadian Rhythm Sleep Disorders

Lirong Zhu, MD, PhD, Phyllis C. Zee, MD, PhD*

KEYWORDS

- Circadian rhythm • Light • Melatonin • Sleep phase • Shift work • Jet lag

KEY POINTS

- The endogenous human circadian rhythm is genetically determined. This near 24-hour oscillation is generated by a central clock located in the suprachiasmatic nucleus of the hypothalamus, and regulates the timing of most physiologic and behavioral cycles, including sleep and wake.
- Light is the strongest synchronizing agent for the circadian clock. However, nonphotic signals, such as melatonin and both social and physical activity, can also affect timing of circadian rhythms.
- The ability of synchronizing agents to shift the timing of circadian rhythms depends on the time, intensity, and duration of exposure.
- Circadian rhythm sleep disorders (CRSDs) are characterized by a persistent or recurrent pattern of sleep disturbance (difficulty falling asleep or staying asleep and excessive sleepiness) resulting from alterations of the circadian timekeeping system and/or misalignment of the endogenous circadian rhythm and the external environment. CRSDs include delayed sleep phase disorder, advanced sleep phase disorder, irregular sleep-wake rhythm, free-running disorder, shift-work disorder, and jet lag.
- Effective treatment of CRSDs requires a multimodal approach using the principles of sleep hygiene, timed exposure to light and melatonin, and avoidance of bright light at inappropriate times.

OVERVIEW OF HUMAN CIRCADIAN BIOLOGY

Circadian rhythms are ubiquitous in all living organisms, and nearly all physiologic functions, most notably sleep and wake cycles, exhibit circadian rhythmicity. Circadian rhythms are endogenous and persist in the absence of environmental time cues. The suprachiasmatic nucleus (SCN), a paired structure in the anterior hypothalamus,[1] is the site of a master circadian clock. It is composed of a network of approximately 20,000 neurons in humans and displays a self-sustained circadian (near 24-hour) rhythm in neuronal firing.[2–5] The SCN plays a pivotal role in coordinating

Department of Neurology, Circadian Rhythms and Sleep Research Lab, Northwestern University, 710 North Lake Shore Drive, 5th Floor, Chicago, IL 60611, USA
* Corresponding author.
E-mail address: p-zee@northwestern.edu

Neurol Clin 30 (2012) 1167–1191
http://dx.doi.org/10.1016/j.ncl.2012.08.011
0733-8619/12/$ – see front matter © 2012 Elsevier Inc. All rights reserved.
neurologic.theclinics.com

circadian rhythmicity by communicating timing information to oscillators in tissues elsewhere in the brain, and almost all the peripheral tissues and organs.[6–9] As a result, virtually every physiologic and behavioral parameter follows the roughly 24-hour (circadian) rhythms, among which the sleep-wake cycle is the most apparent. Either disruption of the endogenous circadian control mechanism or misalignment between internal circadian rhythms with the 24-hour outside environment would result in circadian rhythm disorders with adverse consequences in sleep and many other aspects of human health, including metabolism dysfunction, cognitive impairment, cardiovascular abnormalities, and gastrointestinal and genitourinary dysfunctions.[10,11]

In humans, the endogenous period of the circadian oscillation is slightly longer than 24 hours.[12] Evidence from animal and human studies demonstrates a genetic basis for the generation of circadian rhythms. A molecular machinery (transcription-translation feedback loops) drives circadian rhythms in both SCN and peripheral cells at transcription, translation, and posttranslational levels.[13,14] The CLOCK-BMAL1 heterodimer is a transcriptional activator that binds to the E-box located upstream of the *Period* (*Per*), *Cryptochrome* (*Cry*), *Retinoid-related Orphan Receptor* (*Ror*), and *Rev-Erb* genes.[15,16] After transcription and translation, these proteins accumulate in the cytoplasm. In the cytoplasm, PER is phosphorylated by several isoforms of casein kinase I (CKI), including CKIδ and CKIε, which regulates the stability of PER and subcellular localization.[17–19] After PER reaches a critical level, it permits dimerization with CRY and nuclear translocation. In the nuclear, CRY suppresses CLOCK-BMAL1–induced transcription of *Per*, *Cry*, *Ror*, and *Rev-Erb* in a negative feedback loop (see Ref.[20] for a review). PER2 activates *Bmal* transcription.[21] ROR and REV-ERB translocate to the nucleus independently and bind to the *Bmal* promoter. ROR activates *Bmal* transcription while REV-ERB inhibits it, which generates a rhythmic level of BMAL1.[16,22] Most clock component messenger RNA and protein have a 24-hour oscillating rhythm except for CLOCK, CKIδ, and CKIε (see Ref.[23] for a review).

The endogenous circadian rhythm is synchronized or entrained to the 24-hour rhythm of the external environments daily by synchronizing agents, including light, physical activity, social behaviors, and melatonin. Among these, light is the most influential entraining agent.[24] The phase-shifting effect of light on the circadian rhythm depends on the intensity, duration, and time of light exposure (**Fig. 1**). A phase-response curve (PRC) is a graph of the amount of the phase shift plotted against the circadian time of administration of the stimulus. Exposure of light in the biological evening or early night will delay the circadian pacemaker, causing the circadian cycle to shift late relative to clock time. By contrast, exposure of light in the biological morning will advance the circadian pacemaker, resulting in the circadian cycle to shift early relative to clock time.[24] The melanopsin-containing retinal ganglion cell is the primary circadian photoreceptor and is most sensitive to blue light.[25,26] The photic information reaches the SCN through a direct pathway, the retinohypothalamic tract,[27] and an indirect pathway, from the optic tract to the intergeniculate leaflet and then to the SCN via the geniculohypothalamic tract.[28]

The SCN signals the pineal gland via the superior cervical ganglion to inhibit the production of melatonin, an important entraining agent produced by the pineal gland.[29] In darkness, this inhibition effect is removed and the release of melatonin feeds back to inhibit the firing rate of SCN neurons, permitting the sleep drive.[30,31] Similar to light, timed administration of melatonin can phase-shift the circadian clock according its PRC that is nearly opposite in phase with the PRC for light exposure (see **Fig. 1**).[32] Exogenous melatonin advances the circadian rhythm when administered in the biological early evening before the nadir of core body temperature, but delays the circadian rhythm when administered in the biological morning after the nadir of core

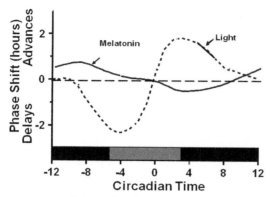

Fig. 1. Phase-response curves to light and melatonin. Circadian time point 0 is the timing of the nadir of the circadian core temperature rhythm. Light exposure before the temperature nadir results in a delay of circadian rhythms, whereas light exposure after the temperature nadir causes phase advances. Note that there is a dead zone in the middle of the day where bright light exposure has no effect on the timing of circadian rhythms. By contrast, melatonin administered in the beginning of the night advances the circadian rhythm, whereas melatonin in the morning delays the circadian rhythm. (*Data from* Lewy AJ, Bauer VK, Ahmed S, et al. The human phase response curve (PRC) to melatonin is about 12 hours out of phase with the PRC to light. Chronobiol Int 1998;15:71–83; and Khalsa SB, Jewett ME, Cajochen C, et al. A phase response curve to single bright light pulses in human subjects. J Physiol 2003;549:945–52; *Reprinted from* Zee PC, Manthena P. The brain's master circadian clock: implications and opportunities for therapy of sleep disorders. Sleep Med Rev 2007;11(1):59–70; with permission.)

body temperature.[33] Physical activity has also been shown to have phase-shifting effects.[34,35]

The sleep-wake cycle is regulated by a complex interaction between the homeostatic process (a drive for sleep that builds up during wakefulness and declines during sleep) and circadian process (a sleep-wake independent 24-hour oscillatory rhythm that modulates sleep propensity). The circadian drive for sleep is the highest at the end of biological night and lowest at the end of biological day. In the entrained situation, when homeostatic drive for sleep dissipates with sleep, the circadian drive for sleep increases in a compensatory manner to facilitate the consolidation of sleep. Conversely, when homeostatic drive for sleep increases with wakefulness during the biological day, the circadian drive for sleep decreases and helps the consolidation of wakefulness.[36] Therefore, proper alignment between the homeostatic and circadian processes is critical for optimal sleep quality and performance.

INTRODUCTION TO CIRCADIAN RHYTHM SLEEP DISORDERS

Circadian rhythm sleep disorders (CRSDs) arise from a chronic or recurrent pattern of sleep and wake disturbance that is due to dysfunction of the circadian clock system, or misalignment between the timing of the endogenous circadian rhythm and externally imposed social and work cycles, resulting in clinically significant functional impairments.[37] CRSDs can be categorized according to their postulated underlying mechanisms: (1) the endogenous circadian clock itself is altered (delayed sleep phase disorder [DSPD], advanced sleep phase disorder [ASPD], irregular sleep-wake rhythm [ISWR], and free-running disorder); (2) the external environment and/or social circumstances are altered relative to the endogenous circadian clock (jet lag and shift-work disorder [SWD]).

The diagnosis of CRSD is based on a detailed history of the patient's sleep and wake pattern, and diagnostic tools, such as a sleep diary and actigraphy. In addition, assessment of the timing of physiologic circadian rhythm markers, such as core temperature and melatonin, are useful diagnostic tools that can be used to confirm the diagnosis. Actigraphy watches are typically worn on the nondominant wrist for 7 to 14 days to record patterns of rest/activity cycles. Melatonin rhythm and body temperature rhythm are reliable biological phase markers of the endogenous circadian rhythm and exhibit distinct phase relationships with the sleep-wake rhythm. Regulated by the SCN, and under dim light conditions, the pineal gland begins to secrete mela-tonin (dim-light melatonin onset [DLMO]) about 2 to 2.5 hours before sleep onset. The nadir of the core body temperature rhythm occurs approximately 2 hours before habitual sleep offset.[38]

Because patients with CRSD commonly present with symptoms of insomnia and/or excessive sleepiness, circadian abnormalities should be considered in the differential diagnosis or as a comorbid condition in all patients with sleep and wake disturbances (**Fig. 2**). **Table 1** summarizes the common clinical features and treatment approaches for CRSD. The management of CRSD requires a multimodal approach because bio-logical, behavioral, and environmental factors all can contribute to the development and severity of presenting symptoms.

DELAYED SLEEP PHASE DISORDER (DELAYED SLEEP PHASE SYNDROME, DELAYED SLEEP PHASE TYPE)

DSPD is a sleep disorder in which there is a stable delay of the major sleep episode relative to the required sleep-wake clock time. This delayed pattern leads to chronic symptoms of insomnia and excessive sleepiness associated with impairment in daytime functioning.

Epidemiology and Risk Factors

DSPD is the most common CRSD, with an estimated prevalence of 0.17% in the general population[39] and 7% to 16% among adolescents.[40,41] It has been estimated that 5% to 10% of chronic insomnia patients in sleep clinics have DSPD.[42] Several studies indicate a genetic predisposition for DSPD. For example, a length polymor-phism in hPER3 is correlated significantly with extreme diurnal preference.[43-45] Asso-ciation of circadian chronotypes of diurnal preference have been reported with polymorphisms in hCLOCK,[46] hPER1,[47] and hPER2,[48] and a missense variation of S408N in hCKIε[49] was found to play a protective role in DSPD and free-running disorder. A polymorphism of Arylalkylamine N-acetyltransferase[50] and the frequency of HLA-DR1 were found to be significantly higher in the patients with DSPD when compared with healthy controls.[51]

Pathophysiology

In addition to genetic vulnerability, physiologic, behavioral and environmental factors likely play important roles in the development of DSPD. Several mechanisms have been proposed. (1) An unusually long endogenous circadian period[52] may alter the relationship between sleep onset or offset with the timing of other endogenous circa-dian rhythms. For example, patients with DSPD have been shown to have a greater interval between sleep offset and nadir of core body temperature.[53,54] (2) Alteration in entrainment mechanisms may occur. DSPD patients have been shown to have

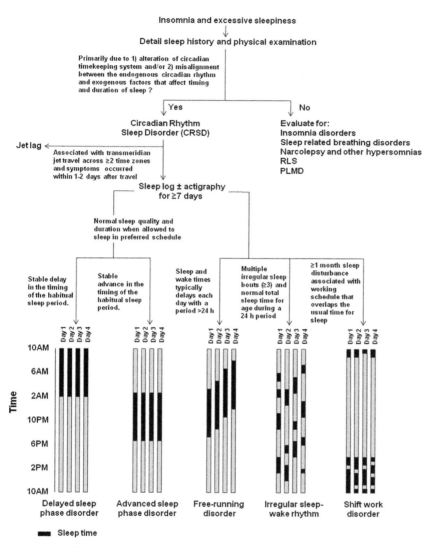

Fig. 2. Clinical approach to the diagnosis of circadian rhythm sleep disorders (CRSD). A history of sleep and wake disturbance resulting from alteration of circadian timing and function is the mainstay of the clinical diagnosis. It is important to consider other sleep disorders and mood disorders in the differential diagnosis of most CRSDs. The pattern of sleep and wake disturbance differs among the various types of CRSDs as illustrated here. PLMD, periodic limb movement disorder; RLS, restless legs syndrome.

a hypersensitivity of melatonin suppression to light at night.[55] There is also evidence that the advance portion of the PRC to light in DSPD patients may be smaller than usual.[56] (3) The homeostatic process may be altered, indicated by the alterations in slow-wave activity[54] and sleep propensity in response to sleep deprivation.[57,58]

Table 1
Overview of clinical features and treatment of circadian rhythm sleep disorders (CRSD)[a]

Disorder	Clinical Features	Treatment
Delayed sleep phase disorder (DSPD)	Stable delay of the major sleep period, resulting in difficulty falling asleep at night and difficulty waking up in the morning	Bright-light therapy 2000–2500 lux for 2 h at or 2–3 h before habitual rise time, 0.5–3 mg melatonin 5–7 h before sleep time
Advanced sleep phase disorder (ASPD)	Stable advance of the major sleep period, resulting in difficulty staying awake in the evening and difficulty maintaining sleep in the morning	Bright-light therapy 2000–2500 lux for 2 h in evening (around 7–9 PM)
Non–24-h sleep-wake disorder (N24HSWD)	Chronic and steady 1–2 h daily delay of sleep and wake schedule resulting in insomnia, difficulty waking up in the morning, and excessive daytime sleepiness	Blind: 0.5 mg melatonin 1 h before preferred bedtime. Sighted: morning bright-light therapy at rise time and/or night melatonin administration
Irregular sleep-wake rhythm (ISWR)	Absence of a clearly discernible sleep-wake circadian rhythm, resulting in insomnia and/or excessive daytime sleepiness	Increase daytime light exposure and social activity. Minimize nighttime light and noise exposure. Evening melatonin administration combined with daytime light exposure

[a] Sleep hygiene is an important component in treating CRSD.

(4) Behavioral factors precipitate and perpetuate DSPD. For example, the delayed sleep and wake times of patients with DSPD is often associated with less light exposure in the phase-advance portion of the PRC curve (morning) and more light exposure in the phase-delay portion of the PRC curve (evening).

Clinical Features and Diagnosis

With work, school, or social constraints, patients with DSPD typically present with symptoms of chronic difficulty falling asleep before between 2 and 6 AM and inability to wake up in the morning. When allowed to choose their natural preferred schedules, their sleep is usually of normal quality and duration for age. When attempting to comply with their school and occupational obligations, sleep duration is curtailed, resulting in chronic partial sleep deprivation and associated excessive daytime sleepiness and impairment of daily functioning.

The diagnosis of DSPD is largely based on obtaining a detailed sleep history of a sleep and wake pattern that is chronically and stably delayed. A sleep diary and/or wrist actigraphy (**Fig. 3**A) for at least 7 consecutive days (longer if possible) is indicated to establish the habitually delayed sleep/wake pattern. In addition, biological markers of circadian timing can be useful and are desirable if available. DLMO (**Fig. 3**B) and nadir of core body temperature have been used in clinical practice and demonstrate, as expected, a delayed phase. Nocturnal polysomnography is not indicated unless there is suspicion of concomitant disorders such as sleep-disordered breathing and other causes of insomnia or daytime sleepiness.[59] DSPD is strongly associated with anxiety and depression, so screening for mood disorders should be considered in all patients.[60,61]

Treatment

The management of DSPD requires a combined approach using behavioral techniques, manipulation of light/dark exposure and, in some patients, pharmacologic agents. The treatment of DSPD includes adherence to good sleep habits, regular sleep and wake times, chronotherapy, timed bright-light therapy, and pharmacotherapy. Chronotherapy is a treatment whereby the sleep and wake times are progressively delayed by about 3 hours every 2 days until a final earlier bedtime schedule is achieved and maintained.[56] Although effective, adherence is generally poor because of the requirement for the strict scheduling of social, school, and work activities as well as very careful control of the time of light exposure. Despite its challenges, chronotherapy is particularly useful in treating children and adolescents.

Timed bright-light therapy is one of the most commonly used treatments for DSPD. Exposure to light in the biological evening or early night phase delays circadian rhythms, whereas exposure to light in the morning results in phase advances.[24] Therefore, bright light of 2000 to 2500 lux for 2 hours in the biological morning combined with avoidance of bright-light exposure in the biological night can effectively achieve earlier sleep and wake times in DSPD patients.[62] Exposure to bright light between 7 and 9 AM is usually effective for most DSPD patients. However, for patients who are more severely delayed (whose endogenous sleep time is after 3 AM and wake time after 9 AM), the time of morning light exposure should be given later in the morning (shortly after awakening) to avoid light exposure before the nadir of core body temperature, which could further delay circadian rhythms. Compliance with light therapy can be challenging, because of the inability of patients to awaken in the morning for light exposure and the need to restructure their social and professional activities around the light regimen. Light therapy in the morning should be accompanied by avoidance of bright light in the evening by using sunglasses or decreasing ambient light intensity.

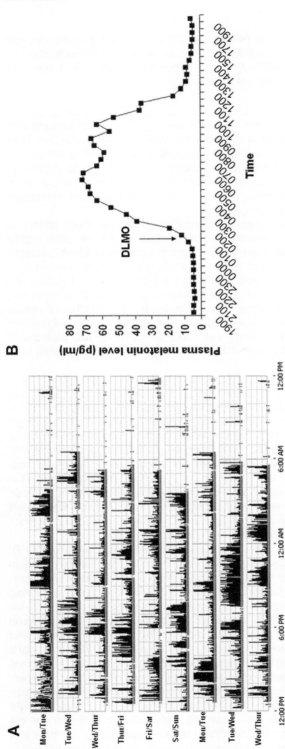

Fig. 3. Actogram of a patient with DSPD. (A) Actogram derived from actigraphy data obtained over 9 days in a patient with severe DSPD. The yellow lines depict light exposure. The high-amplitude dense bars are representative of wakefulness, and no to low activity time is representative of sleep. Note that average sleep onset is 5 to 6 AM and wake time is from noon to 1 PM. Note the stable delay of the sleep-wake rhythm in relation to the conventional sleep time and wake-up time. (B) The 24-hour plasma melatonin level rhythm of this patient. The dim-light melatonin onset (DLMO) was defined as an absolute threshold at 10 pg/mL. The DLMO of this patient is delayed, at 1:23 AM (which is approximately 5 hours later than would be expected in nondelayed persons).

Because of some of the practical limitations of chronotherapy and timed bright-light therapy, the benefit of taking melatonin in the evening has been investigated. The effectiveness of melatonin administration in the evening in the treatment of DSPD has been demonstrated in several studies.[63–67] Appropriately timed melatonin (in the early evening) has been shown to decrease sleep latency, increase sleep duration, and improve function in DSPD patients.[59,65] One small placebo-controlled study in DSPD patients showed that administration of melatonin, 0.3 or 3 mg about 6 hours before their sleep time, resulted in the largest phase advances of sleep and wake times.[64] Although melatonin is indicated as a treatment for DSPD, large randomized placebo-controlled studies are still needed to establish a standard clinical approach for its use.

In addition to light and melatonin, treatment of DSPD should also include proper sleep hygiene, such as adherence to regular sleep-wake times and structured social and physical activity schedules, and address other factors, such as comorbid psychopathology and other sleep disorders.

ADVANCED SLEEP PHASE DISORDER (ADVANCED SLEEP PHASE SYNDROME, ADVANCED SLEEP PHASE TYPE)

ASPD is a sleep disorder in which there is a stable advance of the major sleep period, characterized by habitual and involuntary sleep onset and wake-up times that are several hours earlier than the desired or conventional clock time.

Epidemiology and Risk Factors

ASPD is more common among middle-aged and older adults. The estimated prevalence of ASPD is about 1% in middle-aged adults.[39] A genetic basis has been clearly demonstrated in familial ASPD. Missense mutations located in 2 different genes have been reported to cosegregate with the ASPD phenotype in families with ASPD:S662G located within the CKIε binding region in h*PER2* and T44A in *CKIδ*.[68,69] The S662G mutation was found to result in hypophosphorylation of PER2 by CKIε,[68] which shortens the circadian period.

Pathophysiology

In addition to the genetic factors in familial ASPD, a shortened endogenous circadian period has been postulated to be involved in sporadic cases.[70] Other proposed mechanisms include alterations of entrainment mechanisms, such as increased retinal response to light in the morning,[71] or increased early-morning light exposure, both of which can perpetuate the advanced circadian phase.

Clinical Features and Diagnosis

Patients with ASPD typically present with complaints of sleepiness in the late afternoon or early evening, and difficulty maintaining asleep in the early-morning hours. Most report sleep onset between 6 and 9 PM and wake time of 2 to 5 AM. Even when sleep time is voluntarily delayed owing to social and occupational obligations, patients continue to wake up earlier than desired, resulting in chronic partial sleep deficiency.

The diagnosis of ASPD largely relies on a detailed sleep history of a stable advance in sleep and wake times. When allowed to sleep at their advanced endogenous sleep time, sleep quality and duration are normal for age. A sleep diary and/or wrist actigraphy (**Fig. 4**A) for at least 7 consecutive days is recommended to establish the habitual advanced sleep/wake pattern. Measurement of DLMO is desirable if available, and can help confirm the advanced circadian rhythm (**Fig. 4**B). Nocturnal

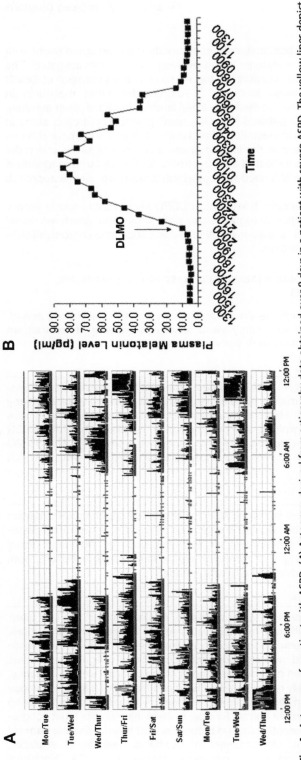

Fig. 4. Actogram of a patient with ASPD. (*A*) Actogram derived from actigraphy data obtained over 9 days in a patient with severe ASPD. The yellow lines depict light exposure. The high-amplitude dense bars are representative of wakefulness, and no to low activity time is representative of sleep. Note that average sleep onset is 8 to 9 PM and wake time is from 4 to 5 AM. Note the stable advance of the sleep-wake rhythm in relation to the conventional sleep time and wake-up time. (*B*) The 24-hour plasma melatonin level rhythm of this patient. The DLMO was defined as an absolute threshold at 10 pg/mL. The DLMO of this patient is advanced, at 7:30 PM (which is approximately 2–3 hours earlier than would be expected in nonadvanced persons).

polysomnography is not indicated, except when the history suggests the presence of other sleep disorders, such as sleep apnea (common in older adults).

Treatment

A combined approach with timed bright-light exposure for 2 hours in the evening, planned sleep and wake scheduling, and adherence to good sleep hygiene is recommended by the American Association of Sleep Medicine (AASM) Practice Parameters.[59] Bright-light exposure in the evening, typically between 7 and 9 PM, has been shown to delay the phase of circadian rhythms and improve sleep efficiency.[72,73] Melatonin can theoretically delay circadian rhythms if taken in the early biological morning, but clinical evidence of its efficacy or safety for the treatment of ASPD is lacking. Although hypnotic agents can be useful for the management of sleep maintenance symptoms associated with ASPD, they are not approved by the Food and Drug Administration (FDA) for the treatment of ASPD.

NON–24-HOUR SLEEP-WAKE DISORDER (FREE-RUNNING DISORDER, NONENTRAINED TYPE, HYPERNYCHTHEMERAL SYNDROME)

Non–24-hour sleep-wake disorder (N24HSWD) is characterized by a chronic or recurring pattern of sleep and wake times that are not stably entrained to the 24-hour environmental cycle. There is typically a predicable drift over weeks (usually to later and later times) of sleep onset and wake times.

Epidemiology, Risk Factors, and Pathophysiology

N24HSWD affects approximately 50% of blind people and is thought to be rare in sighted persons.[74] Sighted patients with N24HSWD are generally evening chronotypes, or may have a history of DSPD. The largest case series of N24HSWD in sighted subjects reported 57 cases identified over a 10-year period.[75] The etiology of N24HSWD in the blind is the absence or near absence of light perception. The mechanism(s) responsible in sighted individuals is less clear. The primary risk factor in sighted persons appears to be a long circadian period that is beyond the range of entrainment to a 24-hour cycle.[76] Other mechanisms include: (1) decreased response of the circadian clock to light, (2) alteration and reduction of environmental or social cues because of social withdrawal induced by psychiatric illness,[77] (3) mutation in the CK1ε gene.[49] Of note, N24HSWD has been reported in sighted individuals following traumatic brain injury,[78,79] but the mechanism is poorly understood.

Clinical Features and Diagnosis

Patients with N24HSWD typically complain of insomnia, difficulty waking up in the morning, excessive daytime sleepiness, and inability to meet their social and occupational obligations. Because the timing of the sleep-wake cycle is progressively changing (usually to later and later times), there is a history of both symptomatic and asymptomatic episodes. At times when the endogenous circadian rhythm is in phase with the conventional sleep and wake time their sleep is usually normal, whereas when the nonentrained circadian pacemaker is out of phase with the conventional sleep and wake schedules, they have symptoms of insomnia and excessive sleepiness.

The diagnosis is established primarily by a detailed sleep history and a sleep diary with or without concurrent actigraphy for at least 14 days (**Fig. 5**). Actigraphy is particularly useful because, depending on the length of the endogenous circadian period, a clear nonentrained pattern may not be evident for several weeks. Most sighted

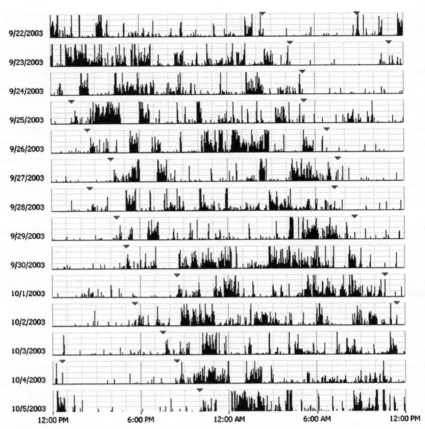

Fig. 5. Actogram of a patient with non–24-hour sleep-wake disorder (N24HSWD), derived from actigraphy data obtained over 14 days in a sighted patient with N24HSWD. The high-amplitude dense bars are representative of wakefulness, and no to low activity time is representative of sleep. Note the daily drift to later times of the sleep-wake pattern with a period that is slightly longer than 24 hours.

persons with N24HSWD have an evening chronotype, and may exhibit episodes of delayed sleep phase. Unlike patients with DSPD, however, patients with N24HSWD cannot maintain a stable delayed sleep-wake pattern. It is important to make the distinction between DSPD and N24HSWD because treatment of DSPD with chronotherapy may precipitate the development of N24HSWD.[80]

Treatment

The goal of treatment of N24HSWD is to improve sleep quality and daytime function by establishing stable entrainment of the sleep-wake pattern to the 24-hour external cycle. In the blind, the primary approach is a combination of good sleep hygiene, structured social, school and work schedules, and low-dose melatonin (0.5 mg) 1 hour before their preferred sleep time.[81–83] Many blind patients, whose circadian period is close to 24 hours, are able to maintain entrainment with even lower nightly doses of 20 to 300 μg.

A practical approach is to start with a higher dose of melatonin (3–5 mg) for the first month 1 to 2 hours before bedtime. Once entrainment is established, a lower dose of 0.5 mg can be used for maintenance therapy. For sighted patients, the addition of bright-light exposure in the morning shortly after awakening is a very useful option. Vitamin B12 has also been proposed as a treatment,[84] but the evidence from case reports is inconclusive, and B12 is not recommended by the AASM Practice Parameters.[59]

IRREGULAR SLEEP-WAKE RHYTHM DISORDER (IRREGULAR SLEEP-WAKE TYPE, IRREGULAR SLEEP-WAKE DISORDER)

Irregular sleep-wake rhythm disorder (ISWRD) is characterized by temporal disorganization of the circadian sleep-wake rhythm, resulting in multiple short sleep and wake bouts occurring throughout the 24-hour cycle.

Epidemiology, Risk Factors, and Pathophysiology

The exact prevalence of the ISWR in the general population is unknown, but is commonly reported in institutionalized residents, particularly in those with dementia, children with mental retardation, and individuals with traumatic brain injury.[85–89] The most accepted etiology is a dysfunction of the central circadian clock system resulting from neurodegeneration or injury. In addition, decreased exposure to synchronizing agents, such as light and structured activities during the day in institutionalized patients, can decrease the strength of an already weakened circadian oscillation and thus exacerbate the temporal disorganization of sleep-wake behaviors.[90] Other external factors such as nighttime noise and adverse effect of medications can further disrupt sleep and increase daytime naps.

Clinical Presentation and Diagnosis

Patients with ISWR or their caregivers typically report chronic symptoms of difficulty maintaining sleep during the night and excessive daytime sleepiness. The diagnosis is made primarily by a careful history of a minimum of 3 irregular sleep-wake bouts occurring in a 24-hour cycle recorded for at least 7 days, preferably longer by sleep diary and/or actigraphy. The sleep and wake episodes occur in short intervals of 1 to 4 hours throughout the 24 hours. Total sleep time per day may be normal for age. Poor sleep hygiene, voluntary irregular sleep-wake schedules, and other medical or mental disorders with similar clinical presentation must be considered in the differential diagnosis.

Treatment

The goal of the treatment of ISWR patients is to consolidate sleep during the night and maintain wakefulness during the daytime. A multimodal approach consisting of structured activities during the day, increasing daytime light exposure, and addressing nighttime noise and nocturia are basic for all patients with ISWRD.[59] Exposure to bright light of 3000 to 5000 lux for 2 hours in the morning for 4 weeks improved daytime alertness, decreased napping, consolidated nighttime sleep, and reduced nocturnal agitation.[91]

Several randomized controlled studies showed that the combination of increasing daytime light exposure and social activity, evening melatonin administration, structured physical activity, and minimizing nighttime light and noise exposure are helpful in improving the robustness of rest/activity rhythms and reducing the nighttime awakenings in institutionalized residents with disrupted sleep/wake patterns.[92–95] However, the evidence for the efficacy of melatonin as a single treatment has been at best inconsistent in older adults and in patients with dementia,[95,96] and is thus not recommended. Treatment with melatonin alone was found to be associated with withdrawn behavior and mood disturbance in one study.[95] However, melatonin may be more effective in children with ISWR and mental retardation. Melatonin, 3 mg administered in the evening, increased nighttime sleep duration, improved sleep efficiency, and reduced daytime naps in these children.[97]

SHIFT-WORK DISORDER

SWD occurs when work hours are scheduled during the habitual sleep time, resulting in chronic complaints of insomnia and excessive daytime sleepiness and consequent impairment of function, temporarily associated with the unconventional work schedules.

Epidemiology, Risk Factors, and Pathophysiology

Most shift workers do not have SWD. The estimated prevalence of SWD is approximately 10% in night and rotating shift workers.[98] Factors that influence the ability to cope with shift work include age, type of work schedule, domestic responsibilities, diurnal preference, commute time, and other sleep disorders (eg, sleep apnea, narcolepsy).[99,100] Sleep disturbance is most commonly associated with night or early-morning shifts.[101,102]

Clinical Presentation and Diagnosis

SWD is characterized by symptoms of insomnia and excessive sleepiness when patients sleep or work at an adverse circadian phase relative to their endogenous circadian sleep and wake propensity rhythm. These impairments persist despite optimizing environmental conditions for sleep. As a result, most patients, particularly night workers, are chronically sleep deprived by 1 to 4 hours per day.[101] Chronic partial sleep deprivation associated with SWD can result in reduced alertness and performance capacity. Excessive sleepiness usually occurs during the shift (mainly night or early morning) when the circadian propensity for sleep is high. These symptoms may persist on days off or for several days after the last work shift. In addition, the unconventional work schedule often interferes with family time and impairs social relationships.

Other symptoms of SWD include chronic fatigue, malaise, mood disorder, gastrointestinal problems, and decreased libido. Risk of alcohol and substance abuse is increased, as is the risk of weight gain, hypertension, cardiovascular disease, and breast and endometrial cancer.[98] In addition to the medical comorbidities, SWD is associated with significant loss of productivity, increased health care utilization, and increased risk for personal and public safety.

The diagnosis of SWD is reliant on obtaining a careful sleep and work history that documents the chronic impairments in sleep and functioning that occur in relation to the shift-work schedule. A sleep diary and/or actigraphy for at least 7 days, but preferably longer, are useful tools to determine the relationship between sleep and work.[59,103] Polysomnography is not specifically indicated, but is recommended to evaluate for other comorbid sleep disorders such as sleep-disordered breathing, primary hypersomnias, and parasomnias.

Treatment

The goal of treatment is to improve sleep quality, alertness and performance at work, and overall quality of life. Although symptomatic management may be necessary during the course of adaptation to shift work, the ideal approach is to ensure good sleep hygiene and to realign circadian rhythms with the work schedule. Short-acting hypnotic medications can be used to treat associated insomnia, but they are not FDA-approved specifically for the treatment of SWD.[104–109] Appropriate alignment of circadian rhythms will improve sleep quality, increase alertness and performance during the shift, and safety (**Fig. 6**). The bulk of the treatment data comes from night-shift workers. In night workers, the aim is to induce a delay shift of circadian rhythms, so that alertness is highest during the night (work) and sleep propensity is highest during the late morning and afternoon.

Bright-light exposure (continuous or intermittent), 2500 to 9500 lux started early during the night shift and terminated approximately 2 hours before the end of the shift (induces a phase delay) and/or wearing dark glasses or blue light–blocking glasses to avoid light exposure in the morning after the night shift (avoiding advance shift)

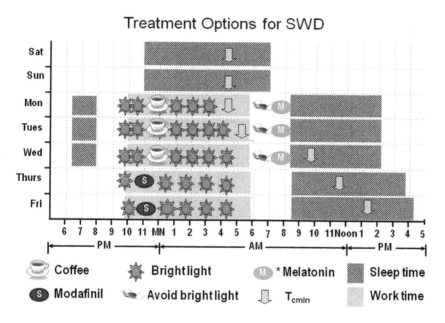

Fig. 6. Treatment options for the management of shift-work disorder (SWD). This example illustrates the timing of light exposure and the use of pharmacologic agents, either alone or in combination, for the management of SWD. The habitual preshift sleep time of this 42-year-old man is 11 PM to 7 AM. The new work shift requires that he work from 10 PM to 6 AM for 4 to 5 days per week. Circadian alignment can be achieved by manipulating light and dark exposure. To delay his circadian rhythm, bright-light exposure (continuous or intermittent) should start early in the shift and stop about 1 to 2 hours before the shift ends, with sunglasses worn to avoid advancing circadian rhythms in the morning. If needed, melatonin taken before bedtime may help improve sleep quality. To address the issue of excessive sleepiness, a scheduled 1- to 2-hour nap before the shift work, if possible a short 30-minute nap in the middle of the shift, and/or caffeine can help decrease sleepiness at work. If sleepiness persists, modafinil, 200 mg and armodafinil, 150 mg have been shown to improve alertness during work and are approved by the FDA for the treatment of excessive sleepiness in patients with SWD.

facilitate circadian rhythm adaptation.[110–113] The combination of bright-light exposure at work and avoidance of bright light in the morning is the most effective approach.[111,113,114] However, there is some concern about the use of dark goggles when driving because of the alerting effect of bright light.[115] Melatonin can potentially induce a delay shift of circadian rhythms when administered in the morning in night workers. Although administration of melatonin before bedtime in night-shift SWD patients has been shown to improve daytime sleep duration,[116] it does not appear to significantly improve alertness.

Excessive sleepiness is perhaps the most debilitating problem for many patients with SWD, and can persist despite therapies aimed at improving sleep quality. A short 1- to 2-hour nap 2 to 3 hours before the shift work or even naps of relatively short duration (20 minutes) at work, when possible, can decrease sleepiness. Wake-promoting agents such as caffeine and modafinil can also be used to improve alertness and performance during the night shift.[117–119] The combination of naps and intermittent low-dose caffeine can further improve alertness during work. Modafinil is approved by the FDA for the treatment of excessive sleepiness associated with SWD. Modafinil, 200 mg taken at the beginning of the shift, has been shown to decrease sleepiness and improve performance on Psychomotor Vigilance Test in patients with SWD. However, it should be noted that residual sleepiness on average remained in the pathologic range.[117] A similar effect was observed in one recent study using armodafinil, 150 mg.[120] **Fig. 6** provides an example to illustrate timely treatment strategy for SWD.

Jet Lag

Jet lag is characterized by symptoms of difficulty falling asleep or staying asleep, daytime sleepiness, and general malaise attributable to a temporary misalignment of the internal circadian system with the external physical environment associated with rapid travel across multiple time zones.

Clinical Presentation and Diagnosis

The diagnosis of jet lag as a disorder is established by a history of symptoms of insomnia and excessive sleepiness that is temporally associated with travel across more than 2 time zones. The severity of the clinical symptoms depends on the direction of travel and the number of time zones crossed. These symptoms typically subside within a few days or up to 1 week. However, for frequent travelers the symptoms and functional impairments can be chronic and severe, prompting them to seek treatment.

In general, it is more difficult to adapt to eastward travel. For eastward travelers, the symptoms at the destination include difficulty falling asleep, excessive daytime sleepiness, and decreased daytime performance, especially in the morning. For westward travelers, falling asleep is less problematic than maintaining sleep, and early-evening sleepiness and decreased performance are especially troublesome. Other common associated symptoms of jet lag include (1) altered appetite and gastrointestinal function, (2) general malaise, (3) fatigue, and (4) mood disturbance. Other sleep disorders causing insomnia and/or excessive daytime sleepiness should be considered.

Treatment

The main treatment goal for jet lag is to accelerate realignment of the endogenous circadian rhythm to the destination's time zone. Circadian adaptation after eastward travel requires advancing the phase of circadian rhythms, whereas westward travel usually requires a phase delay. Phase advancement after eastward traveling is more difficult than phase delay after westward traveling, because the endogenous period of human circadian rhythms is slightly longer than 24 hours.[121]

Circadian synchronizing agents such as timed bright-light exposure and exogenous melatonin are recommended. The timing of light exposure depends primarily on the direction of travel and the number of time zones crossed. For example, for eastward flights, one can begin to advance the timing of circadian rhythms by exposure to bright light on awakening and avoiding light exposure in the evening.[122,123] On the other hand, at the destination one should avoid bright light too early in the morning, but increase exposure to light in the late morning and afternoon for the first 2 to 3 days. If flying westward, at the destination one should stay awake during the daylight hours, increase light exposure in the afternoon and early evening, and avoid napping before bedtime at the destination.

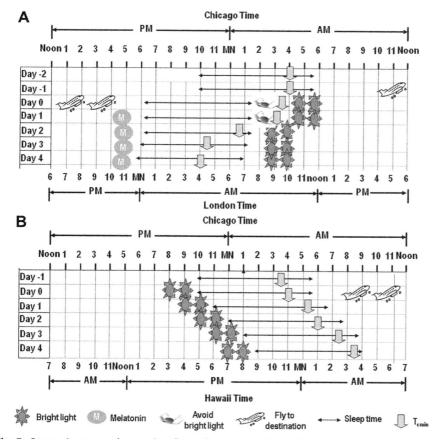

Fig. 7. Strategies to accelerate circadian adaption to jet lag. (*A*) An example of a treatment strategy for jet lag associated with an eastward flight over 6 time zones (from Chicago to London). Adjustment requires an equal number of hours of phase advance. On arrival, the traveler should avoid bright light in the early-morning hours (before 9 AM) for the first 2 days so that light does not decrease before nadir of the core body temperature (which will induce a phase delay), and exposure to bright light after 9 AM to induce phase advances. In addition, melatonin, 1 to 5 mg taken at 18:00 local time on the departure day and at local bedtime (22:00–23:00) on arrival for 4 days has been shown to be effective.[124] (*B*) Treatment strategy for jet lag associated with a westward flight over 5 time zones (from Chicago to Hawaii). The subject should be exposed as much as light as possible in the late afternoon and early evening at the destination, which will result in the required phase delay.

Although there are no FDA-approved pharmacologic therapies for jet lag, results from several studies support the use of melatonin (0.5–5 mg) for alleviating jet lag symptoms with eastward travel.[124,125] One recent placebo-controlled study showed that bedtime administration of ramelteon (1 mg), a melatonin receptor agonist, reduced sleep latency in subjects traveling eastward across 5 time zones.[126] However, this effect was only seen under dim-light conditions, indicating that light is still the most powerful stimulus for phase resetting of circadian rhythms.

Other pharmacologic agents, including caffeine, armodafinil, and short-acting hypnotics, have been studied for the management symptoms of insomnia and excessive sleepiness associated with jet lag. Wake-promoting agents, such as caffeine and armodafinil (150 mg), have been shown to have beneficial effects on alertness and fatigue when flying eastward.[124,127] Short-acting hypnotics, such as zolpidem, 10 mg given for 3 consecutive nights immediately after travel, may be effective for improving sleep quality and duration.[124,128] **Fig. 7** provides examples to illustrate the treatment strategy for jet lag with respect to eastward and westward travel.

Case study

A 17-year-old male high school student presents with complaints of difficulty falling asleep at night and excessive daytime sleepiness of about a year's duration. The constant tiredness during the day has significantly affected his school performance and mood. He is often irritable, and feels depressed and anxious most of the time. About 3 months ago, his primary care physician prescribed zolpidem, 10 mg for insomnia and estacilopram for depression. When he takes zolpidem, he is able to fall asleep on most nights, but still feels very sleepy during the day, especially until noon.

A sleep diary he completed showed that his bedtime is about 10 PM on school days, but sleep onset was on average between 2 to 3 AM. He would lay in bed, working or watching movies on his laptop. Once asleep, he sleeps soundly. He gets on average about 4 hours of sleep on school nights, and it's a huge struggle to get him to wake up, even at 7:30 AM for his 8 AM class (which he misses 3 days a week). He often takes a 1- to 2-hour nap after he comes back home after school. On weekends, he stays up until 3 AM and wakes up without an alarm around 1 PM. The remainder of the sleep history is unremarkable.

The most likely diagnosis is delayed sleep phase disorder. The history and sleep diary show a stable delay of his desired sleep period in relation to the conventional sleep time and wake-up time required for school. If allowed to sleep at his natural delayed schedule on weekends, his sleep duration and quality are relatively normal for his age. In fact, the long sleep duration on weekends may indicate "recovery sleep" because of the sleep deficiency during the week. Other sleep disorders including narcolepsy or sleep apnea are very unlikely based on the history. However, depression and anxiety disorders are common comorbid conditions, and may also require treatment.

Bright-light therapy in the morning, avoidance of bright light in the evening within 3 hours of bedtime, and enforcement of a structured sleep and wake schedule, alone or if needed with early-evening low-dose (0.5–3 mg) melatonin (8 PM, which is approximately 6–7 hours before his sleep time of 2–3 AM) and sleep hygiene are recommended treatments for him. Light therapy in the morning (full spectrum or blue enriched) should begin on a weekend or vacation. The initial time to initiate light exposure should be between 9 and 10 AM (shortly after the nadir of the core temperature rhythm), and the timing can be moved earlier by 30 minutes every 2 to 3 days or an hour per week, until his desired wake time is achieved. To avoid bright light in the evening, he was instructed to use amber-colored blue light–blocking glasses. If these methods are insufficient or compliance is poor with light exposure, the addition of good sleep hygiene, including moderating caffeine intake, exercise, and eliminating his afternoon nap, can help him maintain the regularity of his sleep and wake cycles, and also decrease sleep latency by increasing the homeostatic drive for sleep at night.

SUMMARY

CRSD is a group of sleep disorders sharing a common underlying etiology of circadian dysfunction primarily caused by alterations in the central pacemaker and/or its entrainment mechanisms, or by external changes in the physical or social/work environment that lead to circadian misalignment. The most evident manifestation of the circadian disturbance is the prominent changes in sleep and wake function. However, recent evidence clearly shows that circadian dysfunction not only impairs sleep and wake performance but also negatively affects the function of multiple organ systems, and increases the risk for cardiovascular, metabolic, cognitive, and mood disorders. Given the importance of circadian function in health and disease development, it is important to consider CRSDs in the differential diagnosis of most sleep disorders. The challenge now is to develop more precise and clinically practical diagnostic tools for the various CRSDs, and to conduct large, multicenter, controlled studies of treatment approaches to establish strong evidence-based clinical guidelines.

REFERENCES

1. Stephan FK, Zucker I. Circadian rhythms in drinking behavior and locomotor activity of rats are eliminated by hypothalamic lesions. Proc Natl Acad Sci U S A 1972;69:1583–6.
2. Green DJ, Gillette R. Circadian rhythm of firing rate recorded from single cells in the rat suprachiasmatic brain slice. Brain Res 1982;245:198–200.
3. Groos G, Hendriks J. Circadian rhythms in electrical discharge of rat suprachiasmatic neurones recorded in vitro. Neurosci Lett 1982;34:283–8.
4. Hofman MA, Fliers E, Goudsmit E, et al. Morphometric analysis of the suprachiasmatic and paraventricular nuclei in the human brain: sex differences and age-dependent changes. J Anat 1988;160:127–43.
5. Swaab DF, Fliers E, Partiman TS. The suprachiasmatic nucleus of the human brain in relation to sex, age and senile dementia. Brain Res 1985;342:37–44.
6. McNamara P, Seo SB, Rudic RD, et al. Regulation of CLOCK and MOP4 by nuclear hormone receptors in the vasculature: a humoral mechanism to reset a peripheral clock. Cell 2001;105:877–89.
7. Storch KF, Lipan O, Leykin I, et al. Extensive and divergent circadian gene expression in liver and heart. Nature 2002;417:78–83.
8. Yamazaki S, Numano R, Abe M, et al. Resetting central and peripheral circadian oscillators in transgenic rats. Science 2000;288:682–5.
9. Fukuhara C, Tosini G. Peripheral circadian oscillators and their rhythmic regulation. Front Biosci 2003;8:d642–51.
10. Young ME, Bray MS. Potential role for peripheral circadian clock dyssynchrony in the pathogenesis of cardiovascular dysfunction. Sleep Med 2007; 8:656–67.
11. Klerman EB. Clinical aspects of human circadian rhythms. J Biol Rhythms 2005; 20:375–86.
12. Czeisler CA, Duffy JF, Shanahan TL, et al. Stability, precision, and near-24-hour period of the human circadian pacemaker. Science 1999;284:2177–81.
13. Yagita K, Tamanini F, van Der Horst GT, et al. Molecular mechanisms of the biological clock in cultured fibroblasts. Science 2001;292:278–81.
14. Dunlap JC. Molecular bases for circadian clocks. Cell 1999;96:271–90.
15. Gekakis N, Staknis D, Nguyen HB, et al. Role of the CLOCK protein in the mammalian circadian mechanism. Science 1998;280:1564–9.

16. Preitner N, Damiola F, Lopez-Molina L, et al. The orphan nuclear receptor REV-ERBalpha controls circadian transcription within the positive limb of the mammalian circadian oscillator. Cell 2002;110:251–60.

17. Eide EJ, Virshup DM. Casein kinase I: another cog in the circadian clockworks. Chronobiol Int 2001;18:389–98.

18. Akashi M, Tsuchiya Y, Yoshino T, et al. Control of intracellular dynamics of mammalian period proteins by casein kinase I epsilon (CKIepsilon) and CKIdelta in cultured cells. Mol Cell Biol 2002;22:1693–703.

19. Vanselow K, Vanselow JT, Westermark PO, et al. Differential effects of PER2 phosphorylation: molecular basis for the human familial advanced sleep phase syndrome (FASPS). Genes Dev 2006;20:2660–72.

20. Ko CH, Takahashi JS. Molecular components of the mammalian circadian clock. Hum Mol Genet 2006;15(Spec No 2):R271–7.

21. Shearman LP, Sriram S, Weaver DR, et al. Interacting molecular loops in the mammalian circadian clock. Science 2000;288:1013–9.

22. Guillaumond F, Dardente H, Giguere V, et al. Differential control of Bmal1 circadian transcription by REV-ERB and ROR nuclear receptors. J Biol Rhythms 2005;20:391–403.

23. Toh KL. Basic science review on circadian rhythm biology and circadian sleep disorders, vol. 37. Singapore: Annals of the Academy of Medicine; 2008. p. 662–8.

24. Czeisler CA, Allan JS, Strogatz SH, et al. Bright light resets the human circadian pacemaker independent of the timing of the sleep-wake cycle. Science 1986; 233:667–71.

25. Freedman MS, Lucas RJ, Soni B, et al. Regulation of mammalian circadian behavior by non-rod, non-cone, ocular photoreceptors. Science 1999;284:502–4.

26. Ruby NF, Brennan TJ, Xie X, et al. Role of melanopsin in circadian responses to light. Science 2002;298:2211–3.

27. Moore RY, Speh JC, Card JP. The retinohypothalamic tract originates from a distinct subset of retinal ganglion cells. J Comp Neurol 1995;352:351–66.

28. Pickard GE. Bifurcating axons of retinal ganglion cells terminate in the hypothalamic suprachiasmatic nucleus and the intergeniculate leaflet of the thalamus. Neurosci Lett 1985;55:211–7.

29. Reppert SM, Perlow MJ, Ungerleider LG, et al. Effects of damage to the suprachiasmatic area of the anterior hypothalamus on the daily melatonin and cortisol rhythms in the rhesus monkey. J Neurosci 1981;1:1414–25.

30. Jin X, von Gall C, Pieschl RL, et al. Targeted disruption of the mouse Mel(1b) melatonin receptor. Mol Cell Biol 2003;23:1054–60.

31. Liu C, Weaver DR, Jin X, et al. Molecular dissection of two distinct actions of melatonin on the suprachiasmatic circadian clock. Neuron 1997;19:91–102.

32. Lewy AJ, Bauer VK, Ahmed S, et al. The human phase response curve (PRC) to melatonin is about 12 hours out of phase with the PRC to light. Chronobiol Int 1998;15:71–83.

33. Lewy AJ, Ahmed S, Jackson JM, et al. Melatonin shifts human circadian rhythms according to a phase-response curve. Chronobiol Int 1992;9:380–92.

34. Buxton OM, Frank SA, L'Hermite-Baleriaux M, et al. Roles of intensity and duration of nocturnal exercise in causing phase delays of human circadian rhythms. Am J Physiol 1997;273:E536–42.

35. Van Reeth O, Sturis J, Byrne MM, et al. Nocturnal exercise phase delays circadian rhythms of melatonin and thyrotropin secretion in normal men. Am J Physiol 1994;266:E964–74.

36. Dijk DJ, Czeisler CA. Paradoxical timing of the circadian rhythm of sleep propensity serves to consolidate sleep and wakefulness in humans. Neurosci Lett 1994;166:63–8.

37. The international classification of sleep disorders: diagnostic and coding manual, ICSD-2. 2nd edition. Westchester (IL): American Academy of Sleep Medicine; 2005.

38. Benloucif S, Guico MJ, Reid KJ, et al. Stability of melatonin and temperature as circadian phase markers and their relation to sleep times in humans. J Biol Rhythms 2005;20:178–88.

39. Schrader H, Bovim G, Sand T. The prevalence of delayed and advanced sleep phase syndromes. J Sleep Res 1993;2:51–5.

40. Pelayo RP, Thorpy MJ, Glovinski P. Prevalence of delayed sleep phase syndrome among adolescents. Sleep Res 1988;17:392.

41. Regestein QR, Monk TH. Delayed sleep phase syndrome: a review of its clinical aspects. Am J Psychiatry 1995;152:602–8.

42. Weitzman ED, Czeisler CA, Coleman RM, et al. Delayed sleep phase syndrome. A chronobiological disorder with sleep-onset insomnia. Arch Gen Psychiatry 1981;38:737–46.

43. Archer SN, Carpen JD, Gibson M, et al. Polymorphism in the PER3 promoter associates with diurnal preference and delayed sleep phase disorder. Sleep 2010;33:695–701.

44. Pereira DS, Tufik S, Louzada FM, et al. Association of the length polymorphism in the human Per3 gene with the delayed sleep-phase syndrome: does latitude have an influence upon it? Sleep 2005;28:29–32.

45. Archer SN, Robilliard DL, Skene DJ, et al. A length polymorphism in the circadian clock gene Per3 is linked to delayed sleep phase syndrome and extreme diurnal preference. Sleep 2003;26:413–5.

46. Katzenberg D, Young T, Finn L, et al. A CLOCK polymorphism associated with human diurnal preference. Sleep 1998;21:569–76.

47. Carpen JD, von Schantz M, Smits M, et al. A silent polymorphism in the PER1 gene associates with extreme diurnal preference in humans. J Hum Genet 2006;51:1122–5.

48. Carpen JD, Archer SN, Skene DJ, et al. A single-nucleotide polymorphism in the 5'-untranslated region of the hPER2 gene is associated with diurnal preference. J Sleep Res 2005;14:293–7.

49. Takano A, Uchiyama M, Kajimura N, et al. A missense variation in human casein kinase I epsilon gene that induces functional alteration and shows an inverse association with circadian rhythm sleep disorders. Neuropsychopharmacology 2004;29:1901–9.

50. Hohjoh H, Takasu M, Shishikura K, et al. Significant association of the arylalkyl-amine N-acetyltransferase (AA-NAT) gene with delayed sleep phase syndrome. Neurogenetics 2003;4:151–3.

51. Hohjoh H, Takahashi Y, Hatta Y, et al. Possible association of human leucocyte antigen DR1 with delayed sleep phase syndrome. Psychiatry Clin Neurosci 1999;53:527–9.

52. Ozaki N, Iwata T, Itoh A, et al. Body temperature monitoring in subjects with delayed sleep phase syndrome. Neuropsychobiology 1988;20:174–7.

53. Uchiyama M, Okawa M, Shibui K, et al. Altered phase relation between sleep timing and core body temperature rhythm in delayed sleep phase syndrome and non-24-hour sleep-wake syndrome in humans. Neurosci Lett 2000;294:101–4.

54. Watanabe T, Kajimura N, Kato M, et al. Sleep and circadian rhythm disturbances in patients with delayed sleep phase syndrome. Sleep 2003;26:657–61.

55. Aoki H, Ozeki Y, Yamada N. Hypersensitivity of melatonin suppression in response to light in patients with delayed sleep phase syndrome. Chronobiol Int 2001;18:263–71.

56. Czeisler CA, Richardson GS, Coleman RM, et al. Chronotherapy: resetting the circadian clocks of patients with delayed sleep phase insomnia. Sleep 1981; 4:1–21.

57. Uchiyama M, Okawa M, Shibui K, et al. Poor recovery sleep after sleep deprivation in delayed sleep phase syndrome. Psychiatry Clin Neurosci 1999;53:195–7.

58. Uchiyama M, Okawa M, Shibui K, et al. Poor compensatory function for sleep loss as a pathogenic factor in patients with delayed sleep phase syndrome. Sleep 2000;23:553–8.

59. Morgenthaler TI, Lee-Chiong T, Alessi C, et al. Practice parameters for the clinical evaluation and treatment of circadian rhythm sleep disorders. An American Academy of Sleep Medicine report. Sleep 2007;30:1445–59.

60. Schrader H, Bovim G, Sand T. Depression in the delayed sleep phase syndrome. Am J Psychiatry 1996;153:1238.

61. Shirayama M, Shirayama Y, Iida H, et al. The psychological aspects of patients with delayed sleep phase syndrome (DSPS). Sleep Med 2003;4:427–33.

62. Rosenthal NE, Joseph-Vanderpool JR, Levendosky AA, et al. Phase-shifting effects of bright morning light as treatment for delayed sleep phase syndrome. Sleep 1990;13:354–61.

63. Dahlitz M, Alvarez B, Vignau J, et al. Delayed sleep phase syndrome response to melatonin. Lancet 1991;337:1121–4.

64. Mundey K, Benloucif S, Harsanyi K, et al. Phase-dependent treatment of delayed sleep phase syndrome with melatonin. Sleep 2005;28:1271–8.

65. Nagtegaal JE, Kerkhof GA, Smits MG, et al. Delayed sleep phase syndrome: a placebo-controlled cross-over study on the effects of melatonin administered five hours before the individual dim light melatonin onset. J Sleep Res 1998;7: 135–43.

66. Oldani A, Ferini-Strambi L, Zucconi M, et al. Melatonin and delayed sleep phase syndrome: ambulatory polygraphic evaluation. Neuroreport 1994;6:132–4.

67. Nagtegaal JE, Laurant MW, Kerkhof GA, et al. Effects of melatonin on the quality of life in patients with delayed sleep phase syndrome. J Psychosom Res 2000; 48:45–50.

68. Toh KL, Jones CR, He Y, et al. An hPer2 phosphorylation site mutation in familial advanced sleep phase syndrome. Science 2001;291:1040–3.

69. Xu Y, Padiath QS, Shapiro RE, et al. Functional consequences of a CKIdelta mutation causing familial advanced sleep phase syndrome. Nature 2005;434:640–4.

70. Jones CR, Campbell SS, Zone SE, et al. Familial advanced sleep-phase syndrome: a short-period circadian rhythm variant in humans. Nat Med 1999; 5:1062–5.

71. Rufiange M, Dumont M, Lachapelle P. Correlating retinal function with melatonin secretion in subjects with an early or late circadian phase. Invest Ophthalmol Vis Sci 2002;43:2491–9.

72. Lack L, Wright H. The effect of evening bright light in delaying the circadian rhythms and lengthening the sleep of early morning awakening insomniacs. Sleep 1993;16:436–43.

73. Campbell SS, Dawson D, Anderson MW. Alleviation of sleep maintenance insomnia with timed exposure to bright light. J Am Geriatr Soc 1993;41:829–36.

74. Sack RL, Lewy AJ, Blood ML, et al. Circadian rhythm abnormalities in totally blind people: incidence and clinical significance. J Clin Endocrinol Metab 1992;75:127–34.

75. Hayakawa T, Uchiyama M, Kamei Y, et al. Clinical analyses of sighted patients with non-24-hour sleep-wake syndrome: a study of 57 consecutively diagnosed cases. Sleep 2005;28:945–52.

76. Uchiyama M, Shibui K, Hayakawa T, et al. Larger phase angle between sleep propensity and melatonin rhythms in sighted humans with non-24-hour sleep-wake syndrome. Sleep 2002;25:83–8.

77. Reid KJ, Zee PC. Circadian rhythm disorders. Semin Neurol 2009;29:393–405.

78. Boivin DB, James FO, Santo JB, et al. Non-24-hour sleep-wake syndrome following a car accident. Neurology 2003;60:1841–3.

79. Ayalon L, Borodkin K, Dishon L, et al. Circadian rhythm sleep disorders following mild traumatic brain injury. Neurology 2007;68:1136–40.

80. Oren DA, Wehr TA. Hypernychthemeral syndrome after chronotherapy for delayed sleep phase syndrome. N Engl J Med 1992;327:1762.

81. Sack RL, Brandes RW, Kendall AR, et al. Entrainment of free-running circadian rhythms by melatonin in blind people. N Engl J Med 2000;343:1070–7.

82. Lewy AJ, Bauer VK, Hasler BP, et al. Capturing the circadian rhythms of free-running blind people with 0.5 mg melatonin. Brain Res 2001;918:96–100.

83. Hack LM, Lockley SW, Arendt J, et al. The effects of low-dose 0.5-mg melatonin on the free-running circadian rhythms of blind subjects. J Biol Rhythms 2003;18: 420–9.

84. Kamgar-Parsi B, Wehr TA, Gillin JC. Successful treatment of human non-24-hour sleep-wake syndrome. Sleep 1983;6:257–64.

85. Hoogendijk WJ, van Someren EJ, Mirmiran M, et al. Circadian rhythm-related behavioral disturbances and structural hypothalamic changes in Alzheimer's disease. Int Psychogeriatr 1996;8(Suppl 3):245–52 [discussion: 269–72].

86. Witting W, Kwa IH, Eikelenboom P, et al. Alterations in the circadian rest-activity rhythm in aging and Alzheimer's disease. Biol Psychiatry 1990;27:563–72.

87. Pollak CP, Stokes PE. Circadian rest-activity rhythms in demented and nondemented older community residents and their caregivers. J Am Geriatr Soc 1997;45:446–52.

88. Palm L, Blennow G, Wetterberg L. Correction of non-24-hour sleep/wake cycle by melatonin in a blind retarded boy. Ann Neurol 1991;29:336–9.

89. Wagner DR. Disorders of the circadian sleep-wake cycle. Neurol Clin 1996;14: 651–70.

90. Zee PC, Vitiello MV. Circadian rhythm sleep disorder: irregular sleep wake rhythm type. Sleep Med Clin 2009;4:213–8.

91. Mishima K, Okawa M, Hishikawa Y, et al. Morning bright light therapy for sleep and behavior disorders in elderly patients with dementia. Acta Psychiatr Scand 1994;89:1–7.

92. Dowling GA, Burr RL, Van Someren EJ, et al. Melatonin and bright-light treatment for rest-activity disruption in institutionalized patients with Alzheimer's disease. J Am Geriatr Soc 2008;56:239–46.

93. McCurry SM, Gibbons LE, Logsdon RG, et al. Nighttime insomnia treatment and education for Alzheimer's disease: a randomized, controlled trial. J Am Geriatr Soc 2005;53:793–802.

94. Martin JL, Marler MR, Harker JO, et al. A multicomponent nonpharmacological intervention improves activity rhythms among nursing home residents with disrupted sleep/wake patterns. J Gerontol A Biol Sci Med Sci 2007;62:67–72.

95. Riemersma-van der Lek RF, Swaab DF, Twisk J, et al. Effect of bright light and melatonin on cognitive and noncognitive function in elderly residents of group care facilities: a randomized controlled trial. JAMA 2008;299:2642–55.

96. Gehrman PR, Connor DJ, Martin JL, et al. Melatonin fails to improve sleep or agitation in double-blind randomized placebo-controlled trial of institutionalized patients with Alzheimer disease. Am J Geriatr Psychiatry 2009;17:166–9.

97. Pillar G, Shahar E, Peled N, et al. Melatonin improves sleep-wake patterns in psychomotor retarded children. Pediatr Neurol 2000;23:225–8.

98. Drake CL, Roehrs T, Richardson G, et al. Shift work sleep disorder: prevalence and consequences beyond that of symptomatic day workers. Sleep 2004;27: 1453–62.

99. Harma MI, Hakola T, Akerstedt T, et al. Age and adjustment to night work. Occup Environ Med 1994;51:568–73.

100. Folkard S, Monk TH, Lobban MC. Short and long-term adjustment of circadian rhythms in 'permanent' night nurses. Ergonomics 1978;21:785–99.

101. Knauth P, Landau K, Droge C, et al. Duration of sleep depending on the type of shift work. Int Arch Occup Environ Health 1980;46:167–77.

102. Akerstedt T. Work hours, sleepiness and the underlying mechanisms. J Sleep Res 1995;4:15–22.

103. Morgenthaler T, Alessi C, Friedman L, et al. Practice parameters for the use of actigraphy in the assessment of sleep and sleep disorders: an update for 2007. Sleep 2007;30:519–29.

104. Hart CL, Ward AS, Haney M, et al. Zolpidem-related effects on performance and mood during simulated night-shift work. Exp Clin Psychopharmacol 2003;11: 259–68.

105. Moon CA, Hindmarch I, Holland RL. The effect of zopiclone 7.5 mg on the sleep, mood and performance of shift workers. Int Clin Psychopharmacol 1990; 5(Suppl 2):79–83.

106. Hart CL, Haney M, Nasser J, et al. Combined effects of methamphetamine and zolpidem on performance and mood during simulated night shift work. Pharmacol Biochem Behav 2005;81:559–68.

107. Van Camp RO. Zolpidem in fatigue management for surge operations of remotely piloted aircraft. Aviat Space Environ Med 2009;80:553–5.

108. Monchesky TC, Billings BJ, Phillips R, et al. Zopiclone in insomniac shiftworkers. Evaluation of its hypnotic properties and its effects on mood and work performance. Int Arch Occup Environ Health 1989;61:255–9.

109. Walsh JK, Schweitzer PK, Anch AM, et al. Sleepiness/alertness on a simulated night shift following sleep at home with triazolam. Sleep 1991;14:140–6.

110. Dawson D, Campbell SS. Timed exposure to bright light improves sleep and alertness during simulated night shifts. Sleep 1991;14:511–6.

111. Crowley SJ, Lee C, Tseng CY, et al. Combinations of bright light, scheduled dark, sunglasses, and melatonin to facilitate circadian entrainment to night shift work. J Biol Rhythms 2003;18:513–23.

112. Boivin DB, James FO. Circadian adaptation to night-shift work by judicious light and darkness exposure. J Biol Rhythms 2002;17:556–67.

113. Eastman CI, Stewart KT, Mahoney MP, et al. Dark goggles and bright light improve circadian rhythm adaptation to night-shift work. Sleep 1994;17:535–43.

114. Campbell SS, Dijk DJ, Boulos Z, et al. Light treatment for sleep disorders: consensus report. III. Alerting and activating effects. J Biol Rhythms 1995;10: 129–32.

115. Cajochen C. Alerting effects of light. Sleep Med Rev 2007;11:453–64.

116. Bjorvatn B, Stangenes K, Oyane N, et al. Randomized placebo-controlled field study of the effects of bright light and melatonin in adaptation to night work. Scand J Work Environ Health 2007;33:204–14.
117. Czeisler CA, Walsh JK, Roth T, et al. Modafinil for excessive sleepiness associated with shift-work sleep disorder. N Engl J Med 2005;353:476–86.
118. Muehlbach MJ, Walsh JK. The effects of caffeine on simulated night-shift work and subsequent daytime sleep. Sleep 1995;18:22–9.
119. Babkoff H, French J, Whitmore J, et al. Single-dose bright light and/or caffeine effect on nocturnal performance. Aviat Space Environ Med 2002;73:341–50.
120. Czeisler CA, Walsh JK, Wesnes KA, et al. Armodafinil for treatment of excessive sleepiness associated with shift work disorder: a randomized controlled study. Mayo Clin Proc 2009;84:958–72.
121. Boulos Z, Campbell SS, Lewy AJ, et al. Light treatment for sleep disorders: consensus report. VII. Jet lag. J Biol Rhythms 1995;10:167–76.
122. Burgess HJ, Crowley SJ, Gazda CJ, et al. Preflight adjustment to eastward travel: 3 days of advancing sleep with and without morning bright light. J Biol Rhythms 2003;18:318–28.
123. Eastman CI, Gazda CJ, Burgess HJ, et al. Advancing circadian rhythms before eastward flight: a strategy to prevent or reduce jet lag. Sleep 2005;28:33–44.
124. Beaumont M, Batejat D, Pierard C, et al. Caffeine or melatonin effects on sleep and sleepiness after rapid eastward transmeridian travel. J Appl Physiol 2004; 96:50–8.
125. Srinivasan V, Spence DW, Pandi-Perumal SR, et al. Jet lag: therapeutic use of melatonin and possible application of melatonin analogs. Travel Med Infect Dis 2008;6:17–28.
126. Zee PC, Wang-Weigand S, Wright KP Jr, et al. Effects of ramelteon on insomnia symptoms induced by rapid, eastward travel. Sleep Med 2010;11:525–33.
127. Rosenberg RP, Bogan RK, Tiller JM, et al. A phase 3, double-blind, randomized, placebo-controlled study of armodafinil for excessive sleepiness associated with jet lag disorder. Mayo Clin Proc 2010;85:630–8.
128. Jamieson AO, Zammit GK, Rosenberg RS, et al. Zolpidem reduces the sleep disturbance of jet lag. Sleep medicine 2001;2:423–30.

Pediatric Sleep-Wake Disorders

Suresh Kotagal, MD[a,b,c],*, Amit Chopra, MD[a]

KEYWORDS

- Developmental aspects • Clinical assessment • Obstructive sleep apnea
- Hypoventilation syndromes • Narcolepsy • Restless legs syndrome • Parasomnias
- Behavioral insomnia of childhood

KEY POINTS

- Sleep-wake function evolves continuously from infancy to adolescence.
- Sleep paralysis and hypnagogic hallucinations may not be readily apparent in childhood narcolepsy.
- Precocious puberty and obesity and hypocretin deficiency are associated with narcolepsy-cataplexy of childhood.
- Obstructive sleep apnea hypopnea that occurs in syndromes with mental retardation or neuromuscular disorders such as Down syndrome may necessitate treatment with a positive airway pressure breathing device after surgical measures like adenotonsillectomy.
- Delayed sleep phase syndrome is a common circadian rhythm sleep disorder of adolescents.
- Restless legs syndrome is often underrecognized. It may be associated with attention-deficit disorder and systemic iron deficiency.
- Frequently recurring nonrapid eye movement parasomnias like confusional arousals and sleep walking may necessitate investigation for triggers such as obstructive sleep apnea, periodic limb movements, and anxiety.
- Sleep initiation and maintenance difficulties are common in attention-deficit disorder, depression and anxiety. A bidirectional relationship exists between sleep and these psychiatric disorders.

INTRODUCTION

Childhood sleep-wake problems are common; in a questionnaire survey of 332 children of 11 to 15 years of age, Ipsiroglu and associates[1] observed that 28% of the children had snoring, insomnia, or a parasomnia. In another prospective study of 359 mother-child pairs who were followed from birth till 36 months of age and administered sleep questionnaires at 6, 12, 24, and 36 months, the prevalence of sleep disorders at each assessment point was 10%.[2] Childhood sleep disorders can have

[a] The Center for Sleep Medicine, Mayo Clinic, Rochester, MN, USA; [b] Department of Neurology, Mayo Clinic, Rochester, MN, USA; [c] Department of Pediatrics, Mayo Clinic, Rochester, MN, USA
* Corresponding author. Division of Child Neurology, Mayo Clinic, 200 First Street Southwest, Rochester, MN 55905.
E-mail address: kotagal.suresh@mayo.edu

Neurol Clin 30 (2012) 1193–1212
http://dx.doi.org/10.1016/j.ncl.2012.08.005
0733-8619/12/$ – see front matter © 2012 Elsevier Inc. All rights reserved.

neurologic.theclinics.com

a significant impact on the quality of life. Many disorders are also easily treatable, which underscores the importance of why they should be recognized and treated promptly. This article addresses developmental aspects of childhood sleep, their clinical assessment, and some important categories of sleep-wake disorders.

DEVELOPMENTAL ASPECTS OF SLEEP

In the preterm infant of 28 to 30 weeks' postconceptional age, wakefulness can be differentiated from sleep on the electroencephalogram (EEG), which shows periods of discontinuity or quiescence alternating with periods of cortical activity (ie, trace discontinue).[3] Concurrent with progressive maturation of cortical synaptic function, the EEG evolves from a discontinuous to a continuous pattern by 32 to 34 weeks' postconceptional age. Also, the bursts of EEG activity becomes progressively synchronous between the 2 hemispheres. Another characteristic feature of the EEG of the preterm infant is the presence of spindle δ brushes, which are fast, 10-Hz to 20-Hz waveforms that are superimposed on slower, 0.3-Hz to 1.5-Hz activity. Spindle δ brushes resolve by 40 to 42 weeks' postconceptional age. Between 32 and 40 weeks, quiet sleep starts progressive organization into alternating periods of high and low voltage (trace alternans). At around 32 weeks' postconceptional age, about 80% of sleep is of the active or rapid eye movement (REM) type, whereas about 20% is of the non-REM (NREM) type, also termed quiet sleep. By 40 weeks' postconceptional age, active sleep decreases to about 50% of the total, with a corresponding increase in the proportion of quiet sleep. Active sleep is associated with irregular breathing, phasic electromyographic activity, reduced muscle tone, and low-voltage electroencephalographic activity. Cerebral blood flow and metabolism are higher in active sleep compared with quiet sleep. By 46 to 50 weeks' postconceptional age, sleep spindles and K-complexes start to appear, with differentiation into stages N2 and N3 of NREM sleep. N3 is also termed slow-wave sleep. It is characterized by the generalized slow-wave activity in the 0.5 to 2 Hz range. The bulk of N3 occurs during the first third of the night. Growth hormone release is closely tied to N3 sleep, with suppression of the latter stage being associated with impaired release of growth hormone.[4] The release of cortisol is suppressed during N3 sleep, but surges in the early morning hours, close to the habitual awakening time.[4] The proportion of REM sleep continues to gradually decrease, with the result that by 3 years of age, it represents only 20% to 25% of total sleep.

Before the age of 3 months, the passage from wakefulness is initially into REM sleep. However, after this age and through the rest of childhood, the physiologic transition is from wakefulness into NREM sleep, with REM sleep appearing 90 to 140 minutes later. The conventional sleep-onset time in preadolescents is usually around 8:00 PM to 8:30 PM. Around adolescence, there is a physiologic delay in sleep-onset time, which shifts to around 10:30 PM to 11:00 PM.[5] Teenage girls generally have their final morning awakening about half an hour earlier than boys. When juxtaposed with early high-school start times of around 7:30 AM, it is easy to understand why most teenagers are chronically sleep deprived.

ASSESSMENT OF CHILDHOOD SLEEP-WAKE COMPLAINTS
Sleep History

The sleep history is provided by the patient, parent, or guardian. It is crucial to the planning of appropriate diagnostic procedures and arriving at a specific diagnosis. Questions relevant to infants and preschool-age children are shown in **Box 1**. In

---

Box 1
The pediatric sleep-wake history

- The sleeping environment (eg, crib, bassinet, parent's bed)
- The sleeping position (eg, prone or supine, semiupright, arching of the neck)
- Habitual need for sleep aids (eg, pacifier, rocking, patting)
- The times of going to bed, sleep onset, and the final morning awakening (on school nights and during weekends and holidays)
- Sensation of restlessness in the legs before sleep onset, intrusive thoughts or worries that might interfere with sleep onset
- Habitual snoring, mouth breathing, observed apnea, restless sleep, sweating, gastroesophageal reflux, and abnormal behavior at night suggestive of seizures or parasomnias
- Daytime irritability, inattentiveness, hyperactivity, or sleepiness
- Number of daytime naps and their duration, association with dreaming
- Medications that may affect sleep-wake function (eg, sedatives, stimulants)
- Interventions that the parents have used to improve the child's sleep

---

adolescents, one should also inquire about activities that might interfere with going to bed at a reasonable hour, such as after-school employment, and resorting to vigorous exercise, heavy meals, caffeine, cell phones, computers, television, nicotine, and illicit substances in the late evening/bedtime. Patients with restless legs syndrome (RLS) may experience an urge to move their limbs, a feeling of "bugs or spiders crawling on their legs" in the evening hours, exacerbation of this discomfort when the limbs are kept immobile, and have relief with movement. Daytime sleepiness assessment should include questions about taking involuntary naps in the classroom, automatic behavior, and the impact of sleepiness on driving, cataplexy, hypnagogic hallucinations, medications used to promote alertness, academic function and behavioral and mood problems, and the number of school days missed because of sleepiness.

The Pediatric Daytime Sleepiness Scale (PDSS) is a simple, validated questionnaire that can be administered to children in the 11-year to 14-year age group.[6] It has 8 items, with each rated on a 0 to 4 scale. The scale provides a numerical score for sleepiness: the 50th percentile score on the PDSS is 16, the 75th percentile is 20, and the 90th percentile is 23. Participants who reported low school achievement, high absenteeism, low school enjoyment, low total sleep time, and frequent illnesses all had higher levels of sleepiness as measured by this scale.[6] Another survey tool that is commonly used in clinical practice is the Children's Sleep Habits Questionnaire.[7] This is a 45-item, validated questionnaire that is completed by parents of 4-year-olds to 11-year-olds. The questions pertain to sleep-wake function in the preceding 2 weeks, such as the "child sleeps too little" or "the child suddenly falls asleep in the middle of active behavior." The items represent several domains that present as sleep complaints, such as bedtime resistance, sleep-onset delay, sleep duration, sleep anxiety, night awakenings, parasomnias, breathing disturbance, and daytime sleepiness. Responses are rated as occurring rarely (0–1 time/wk; 1 point), sometimes (2–4 nights/wk; 2 points), or usually (5–7 nights/wk; 3 points). Scores of 41 or greater correlate with presence of a sleep disorder. The internal consistency estimate for this questionnaire in a community (nonclinic sample) of 4-year-olds to 10-year-olds is 0.36 to 0.70. The test-retest reliability over a 2-week period is 0.62 to 0.79.[7]

Sleep-Related Examination

Height, weight, and body mass index (calculated as weight in kilograms divided by the square of height in meters) are recorded because obstructive sleep apnea (OSA) may be associated with failure to thrive during infancy, and with obesity in adolesence.[8] The blood pressure should be measured because long-standing and severe OSA may be associated with hypertension. Patients with OSA may show craniofacial abnormalities such as micrognathia, dental malocclusion, macroglossia, myopathic face and midface hypoplasia, deviated nasal septum, swollen inferior turbinates, tonsillar hypertrophy, and mouth breathing.[9,10] Consultation with a pediatric otolaryngologist is required to exclude adenoidal hypertrophy. Inattentiveness, irritability, and mood swings may occur because of prefrontal cortex disinhibition as a consequence of daytime sleepiness. OSA related to brainstem abnormalities like the Chiari type I or II malformations can be associated with hoarseness of voice, decreased gag reflex, posttussive headache, and changes in the amplitude of the jaw jerk relative to that of other tendon reflexes. Neuromuscular disorders like myotonic dystrophy can be associated with chronic obstructive hypoventilation from a combination of palatal muscle weakness, high arched palate, and diminished chest wall–abdominal excursion.[11,12] The parent-child interaction should be observed not only for clues toward parental anxiety and reluctance to set limits on inappropriate behaviors that perpetuate insomnia in toddlers but also for subtle clues to a child maltreatment syndrome. Home videos, if available, may be invaluable in the assessment of RLS, parasomnias, and nocturnal seizures.

Sleep Laboratory Investigations

Space constraints limit addressing this issue in any detail. The reader is encouraged to review additional articles for technical guidelines pertaining to sleep laboratory investigations such as actigraphy, nocturnal polysomnography, and the multiple sleep latency test (MSLT).[13–16]

COMMON CHILDHOOD SLEEP DISORDERS
Sleep-Disordered Breathing

The spectrum of sleep-disordered breathing in childhood ranges from snoring without sleep disruption (primary snoring) to the upper airway resistance syndrome (UARS) (snoring that disrupts sleep continuity but without apnea or oxygen desaturation) to classic OSA and obstructive hypoventilation (apnea, oxygen desaturation, plus hypercarbia). As per the 2007 sleep scoring manual of the American Academy of Sleep Medicine,[17] the duration of obstructive apnea events in adults needs to be 10 seconds or longer, whereas in children the events need to be 5 seconds or more. A 3% oxygen desaturation threshold is used when scoring childhood obstructive apnea events rather than the 4% desaturation requirement for adults. Also, in contrast to adults, children tend to show fewer frank OSA events and more of partial airway occlusion with consequent respiratory event–related arousals.

Primary snoring

Between 10% and 12% of children snore on a habitual basis.[18] Snoring without associated apnea and oxygen desaturation is called primary snoring. There are neuropsychological consequences of primary snoring as well; a study of 87 children aged 5 to 7 years[19] found that compared with age-matched nonsnoring children, those with primary snoring performed worse on neuropsychologic measures of attention and had more social problems and anxious or depressive symptoms.

OSA

OSA is characterized by partial or complete upper airway occlusion, with associated impaired air exchange despite persistence of thoracic and abdominal respiratory effort. It generally occurs in association with transient oxygen desaturation of 3%.[20] In some instances, there is an additional component of hypoventilation caused by shallow abdominal and chest wall motion, which leads to hypercarbia. Community-based studies have determined the prevalence of childhood OSA to be 1.1% to 2.9%.[21,22] The most common causes for OSA are adenotonsillar hypertrophy, craniofacial anomalies like micrognathia or maxillary hypoplasia, neuromuscular disorders such as myotonic dystrophy or congenital nonprogressive myopathies, and obesity.[23] Repetitive occlusion of the upper airway during sleep with resultant oxygen desaturation provokes cortical arousals, and suppression of REM and N3 sleep. Nocturnal symptoms of childhood OSA include habitual snoring, restless sleep with snort arousals, bed wetting, excessive sweating, mouth breathing, choking sounds, and parasomnias such as confusional arousals and sleep walking. Parents may report snoring that is interrupted by silent pauses, which then terminate with snorting sounds. A metabolic syndrome may develop as a consequence of OSA. This syndrome is generally characterized by insulin resistance, hyperglycemia, hypertension, dyslipidemia, abdominal obesity, and proinflammatory and prothrombotic states.[8] The daytime symptoms of OSA include inattentiveness, impaired academic performance, hyperactivity, and sleepiness.[24,25] UARS is a variant of upper airway obstruction in which no frank apneas or oxygen desaturation occur, but the airway narrowing and increased respiratory effort lead to recurrent arousals, fragmented sleep, and daytime sleepiness.[25] Some patients show subtle posterior displacement of the tongue, narrow nostrils, or a high arched palate, but others might not show any craniofacial anomalies. The nocturnal polysomnogram may appear superficially normal, with the exception of snoring and increased EEG arousals of 3 or more seconds (normally fewer than 10 to 12 per hour of sleep). Simultaneously obtained intraluminal pressures from an esophageal balloon show an increase in the intrathoracic negative pressure during UARS episodes. Infants with OSA often present with stridor and laryngomalacia and may have a higher incidence of congenital anomalies of the upper airway, such as choanal atresia.

Nocturnal polysomnography is not required to confirm the diagnosis in patients who already show the classic symptoms of OSA with marked tonsillar hypertrophy; overnight oximetry in the home environment that documents recurrent oxygen desaturation is sufficient for establishing the diagnosis in these patients.[26] However, nocturnal polysomnography is indicated when the diagnosis is uncertain or less obvious. It is also indicated when OSA is suspected in patients with multiple neurologic handicaps such as in Down syndrome or cerebral palsy, and when the patient needs to be considered for nonsurgical treatment, such as a continuous positive airway pressure (PAP) device.

Mild OSA (apnea-hypopnea index [AHI] less than 3) can be treated with topical nasal corticosteroids at bedtime. In a randomized, double-blind crossover trial of intranasal budesonide 32 μg in each nostril at bedtime for mild OSA, there was significant improvement in polysomnographic measures and adenoid size after 6 weeks in 48 children who received the topical steroid compared with 32 children on the placebo arm.[27]

For moderate (AHI >3) or severe OSA (AHI >10), the first step in management of OSA is usually adenotonsillectomy, to which most patients respond in a modestly favorable manner. Patients younger than 3 years old and those with severe OSA should be monitored closely in the intensive care unit for postoperative respiratory compromise from upper airway edema. There should be a clinical, and if necessary, a polysomnographic reevaluation 2 to 3 months after adenotonsillectomy. Supraglottoplasty is a common surgical procedure during infancy.[28] In children weighing more than 14 kg, if there is residual OSA, a PAP breathing device should be considered. These devices are approved for use by the US Food and Drug Administration in children weighing more than 14 kg. A variety of masks and pressure delivery devices, such as continuous PAP (CPAP), bilevel PAP device, bilevel PAP device with expiratory relief, are now available. Adherence rate to PAP therapy after 3 months is estimated to be around 60%.[29] Bilevel PAP with expiratory relief is not superior to CPAP from the standpoint of adherence at 3 months.[29] Weight-reduction measures are indicated in obese patients. Orthodontic consultation and the use of oral appliances during sleep are indicated in those with retrognathia and tongue prolapse.[30] Rapid maxillary distraction is a nonsurgical technique that is used in OSA with associated high arched palate and consequent narrowing of the nasal passages.[31]

Central hypoventilation syndromes

Defective automatic control of breathing during sleep as a result of brainstem dysfunction is characteristic of this category of disorders, which present in infancy or childhood. Head injury, bulbar poliomyelitis, syringobulbia, Chiari types I and II malformation,[32] and inborn errors of metabolism (eg, Leigh syndrome) are some underlying conditions. Polysomnography may reveal central sleep apnea, oxygen desaturation, shallow respiratory effort, and increased levels of end tidal CO_2. Except for surgical decompression in Chiari malformation and syringobulbia-associated hypoventilation, the management is similar to that of primary congenital central alveolar hypoventilation.

Congenital central alveolar hypoventilation syndrome is a disorder in which there is no obvious brainstem structural explanation for the defective central control of breathing during sleep.[33,34] Onset of symptoms is during infancy or early childhood. The respiratory rate and depth are initially normal during wakefulness, but shallow breathing (hypoventilation), hypercarbia, and oxygen desaturation appear when asleep. Respiratory rate and depth are more impaired in NREM sleep compared with REM sleep. Ventilatory challenge with inhalation of a mixture of 5% CO_2 and 95% O_2 fails to evoke the physiologic, 3-fold to 5-fold increase in minute volume. Common sites of neuronal loss and reactive gliosis include the arcuate nucleus in the medulla, the ventrolateral nucleus of the tractus solitarius, nucleus ambiguus, nucleus retroambigualis, the chemosensitive ventral medullary surface, and the nucleus parabrachialis in the dorsolateral pons. Between 15% and 20% of patients with congenital central alveolar hypoventilation have coexisting Hirschsprung disease or neural crest tumors such as neuroblastoma or ganglioneuroma.[35,36]

Mutations in the PHOX2B gene have been identified in more than 90% of patients with central hypoventilation syndrome.[37] They generally consist of expansions of the polyalanine tail in this gene, although expansions of nonpolyalanine repeats have also been implicated.[38] Tumors of the neural crest show increased prevalence in those with nonpolyalanine expansions. Mutations in the PHOX2B gene are transmitted in an autosomal-dominant manner. Mosaicism occurs in 5% to 10% of the parents, which emphasizes the importance of molecular testing in parents of affected children.[38]

There is no satisfactory treatment of congenital central alveolar hypoventilation, although acetazolamide and theophylline enhance chemoreceptivity of the brainstem respiratory neurons to a modest degree. Home ventilation via tracheostomy and diaphragmatic pacing are other therapeutic modalities. Patients may die during infancy or childhood. It is recommended that patients with congenital central hypoventilation syndrome undergo an annual hospital admission for a comprehensive, multidisciplinary evaluation that includes 72-hour Holter monitoring, echocardiogram, evaluation of autonomic dysregulation affecting other organ systems, and imaging for neural crest tumors when appropriate.[38]

Central sleep apnea

This syndrome is composed of respiratory events in which there is absence of inspiratory effort during the event. The duration of the central apnea events needs to be 20 seconds or longer; alternatively, they may last at least 2 missed breaths (or the duration of 2 missed breaths as determined by the baseline breathing pattern) and are associated with arousals, awakenings or a desaturation of 3% or greater.[20] Central apneas may develop after brief arousals when the CO_2 levels abruptly decrease less than a threshold essential to trigger respiration. In others, the end tidal CO_2 level may remain increased. The cause of central apneas in childhood is varied. NREM sleep can sometimes unmask an overly sensitive P_{CO_2} (partial pressure of CO_2) apneic threshold. Central apneas could also be a component of apnea of prematurity, a condition in which they are caused by immature respiratory control. They may also develop in heart failure and brainstem lesions such as trauma, syringobulbia, encephalitis, or neurodegeneration. Patients with Chiari malformation type I may manifest central sleep apnea if there is significant compression of the cervicomedullary junction. Treatment emergent central sleep apnea (ie, complex sleep apnea) that has been observed in adults with OSA who are given PAP therapy has not been reported in childhood.

The treatment of central sleep apnea when it is a component of apnea of prematurity is generally caffeine and watchful waiting because there is spontaneous resolution over time.[39] Congestive heart failure, when present, needs its specific treatment. Magnetic resonance imaging of the head is indicated in children with central apnea who are older than 1 to 2 years in order to exclude Chiari malformation type I or structural lower brainstem lesions. Patients with Chiari malformation may need neurosurgical consultation in order to assess the need for surgical decompression.[40] There is anecdotal evidence of the efficacy of topiramate in adults with central sleep apnea, related perhaps to its tendency to lead to mild metabolic acidosis.[41] It can, perhaps, also be used similarly in children.

Special syndromes

Children with spastic quadriparetic cerebral palsy may show daytime irritability in conjunction with fragmented sleep with frequent nighttime awakenings, and oxygen desaturation from OSA caused by upper airway collapse or adenotonsillar hypertrophy.[42] They may also have impaired central arousal mechanisms and be unable to compensate for apnea by changes in body position, making OSA especially problematic for them. Patients with Leigh syndrome (subacute necrotizing encephalomyelopathy) manifest recurrent central apneas or hypoventilation as a consequence of brainstem involvement.[43] Joubert syndrome may be associated with periods of hyperpnea and panting respiration or central sleep apnea.[44] Rett syndrome is characterized by deep, sighing respiration during wakefulness and normal breathing patterns during sleep, consistent with impairment of the voluntary, cortical control of breathing, and a normal automatic or brainstem control of respiration.[45,46] Patients with Down syndrome may develop OSA from the combination of macroglossia, midface hypoplasia, and hypotonic upper airway musculature.[45,46] Superimposed on this may be an element of hypoventilation and consequent retention of CO_2 caused by decreased contraction of intercostal and diaphragm muscles. Sleep architecture is disrupted, with decreased sleep efficiency, increased arousals, suppression of N3, and REM sleep. Patients with achondroplasia may have OSA during infancy as a result of macroglossia and midface hypoplasia.[47] They may also have central sleep apnea as a consequence of cervicomedullary compression. There is no correlation between the diameter of the foramen magnum and severity of the sleep apnea, but patients need close follow-up of their neurologic and respiratory function. Zucconi and colleagues[47] found sleep-related breathing disorders in close to 75% of patients with achondroplasia. Certain lysosomal storage disorders such as the mucopolysaccharidoses such as Hurler syndrome have been associated with severe OSA, which improves with surgical reduction of macroglossia, bone marrow transplantation, or lysosomal enzyme replacement therapy, when appropriate and feasible.[48]

NARCOLEPSY

This disorder is characterized by chronic daytime sleepiness, hypnagogic hallucinations (vivid dreams at sleep onset), sleep-onset paralysis, cataplexy (sudden loss of skeletal muscle tone in response to emotional triggers like laughter, fright, or surprise), and fragmented night sleep. A meta-analysis of 235 pediatric cases derived from 3 studies[49] found that 34% of all patients with narcolepsy experienced onset of symptoms before age 15 years, 16% before the age 10 years, and 4.5% before age 5 years. Sleepy children may show mood swings and inattentiveness as a consequence of sleepiness-related prefrontal cortical dysfunction. Cataplexy is present in about two-thirds of patients with narcolepsy. The muscle weakness in cataplexy generally lasts for a few seconds to minutes and is associated with muscle atonia in the antigravity muscles and absence of muscle stretch reflexes, with full preservation of consciousness. Cataplexy is associated with abrupt hyperpolarization of the spinal α motor neurons. Because cataplexy can be subtle, the examiner might need to ask leading questions about sudden muscle weakness in the lower extremities, neck, facial muscles, or trunk in response to laughter, fright, excitement, anger, or the anticipation of a reward. Children younger than 7 or 8 years generally do not provide a reliable history of cataplexy, hypnagogic hallucinations, or sleep paralysis. Patients with narcolepsy show less circadian clock–dependent alertness during the daytime and also less circadian clock–dependent sleepiness at night.[50] Secondary narcolepsy is a rare entity, but may develop as a sequel to closed head injury and in patients with deep midline brain tumors, lymphomas, and encephalitis.[51] Obesity and precocious puberty may herald the onset of narcolepsy-cataplexy in childhood,[52–54] likely because of hypocretin deficiency. Stores and colleagues[55] assessed the psychosocial difficulties of 42 children with narcolepsy (mean age 12.4 years, range 7.3–17.9 years), 18 patients with excessive daytime sleepiness (EDS) unrelated to narcolepsy (mean age 14.2 years, range 5.1–18.8 years), and 23 unaffected controls (mean age 11.3 years, range 6–16.8 years). These investigators found significantly higher scores on the Strengths and Difficulties Questionnaire in the narcolepsy and EDS groups. The domains of this questionnaire included prosocial, peer problems, hyperactivity, conduct problems, emotional problems, and adverse impact on the family. Compared with healthy controls, both the narcolepsy and the EDS group scored higher on the Child Depression Inventory, with higher scores indicating more impairment.

The presence of the histocompatibility antigen DQB1*0602 in close to 100% of persons with narcolepsy, compared with a 12% to 32% prevalence in the general population, indicates genetic susceptibility, which by itself seems insufficient to precipitate the clinical syndrome. In genetically susceptible individuals, acquired life stresses (like minor head injury), systemic illnesses (such as infectious mononucleosis), and bereavement may play a role in triggering the disorder, and have been reported in close to two-thirds of patients: "the two-hit hypothesis."[56] The result in human narcolepsy-cataplexy is hypocretin ligand deficiency.[57,58] Hypocretin (orexin) is a peptide that is produced by neurons of the dorsolateral hypothalamus, with widespread projections to the forebrain and brainstem. It enhances alertness, motor activity, and the basal metabolic rate.[58,59] The decrease in hypocretin 1 levels that is characteristic of human narcolepsy-cataplexy is reflected in the cerebrospinal fluid (CSF). Using a radioimmunoassay, Nishino and colleagues[57,58] found that the mean CSF level of hypocretin 1 in healthy controls was 280.3 ± 33.0 pg/mL; in neurologic controls, it was 260.5 ± 37.1 pg/mL; and in those with narcolepsy-cataplexy, hypocretin 1 was either undetectable or less than 100 pg/mL. The hypocretin assay is most useful when an HLA DQB1*0602-positive patient with suspected narcolepsy-cataplexy is already receiving central nervous system stimulants at the time of initial presentation, and in whom discontinuation of these medications for the purpose of obtaining polysomnography and MSLT is inconvenient, unsafe, or impractical.

A combined battery of nocturnal polysomnogram and MSLT is still the most widely accepted method to diagnose narcolepsy. The nocturnal polysomnogram shows almost immediate sleep onset, decreased REM latency of less than 70 minutes (time from sleep onset to onset of the first REM sleep epoch; normal value in teenagers is around 140 minutes), increased arousals and periodic limb movements in sleep, and absence of any other significant sleep disorder such as OSA.[60] There might be persistence of tonic electromyographic activity during REM sleep (REM sleep without atonia). When persistence of electromyographic activity occurs in conjunction with physical dream enactment, patients are defined as having an REM sleep behavior disorder. The MSLT in patients with narcolepsy shows a short mean sleep latency of less than 8 minutes (reference value of 16–18 minutes in preadolescents) and 2 or more sleep-onset REM periods (SOREMPs).[16]

Management of narcolepsy requires a combination of lifestyle changes and pharmacotherapy (**Table 1**). A planned daytime nap of 20 to 30 minutes at school and

Table 1
The management of narcolepsy

Nonpharmacologic Measures (for Narcolepsy)	Pharmacologic Measures
Planned naps	Daytime sleepiness
Maintaining regular sleep-wake schedules	Modafinil, armodafinil
Regular physical exercise	Methylphenidate
Avoiding working near sharp or moving objects	Dextroamphetamine
	Amphetamine/dextroamphetamine mixtures
Psychological counseling for anxiety and reactive depression	Lisdexamphetamine
	Cataplexy
Vocational guidance	Sodium oxybate
	Clomipramine
	Imipramine
	Protriptyline
	Venlafaxine
	Restless legs/periodic limb movements
	Oral iron supplementation (for RLS and periodic limb movement disorder)
	Gabapentin (only for RLS)
	Ropinorole (only for RLS)
	Pramipexole (only for RLS)

another one in the afternoon on return home may enhance alertness. The patient should observe regular sleep-onset and morning wake-up times, avoid alcohol, and exercise regularly. To minimize the risk of accidents, the patient should avoid working or playing near sharp, moving objects. Teenagers should be counseled against driving if they have significant sleepiness. They should also avoid work-related and social situations in which they could endanger themselves or others. Medications used to treat daytime sleepiness and cataplexy are listed in **Box 1**. There have been anecdotal reports of improvement in narcolepsy-cataplexy after infusions of intravenous IgG,[61] but randomized controlled studies have not been carried out. The Narcolepsy Network (http://www.narcolepsynetwork.org/) is a private, nonprofit resource for patients, families, and health professionals. There is also a National Narcolepsy Registry, more information on which can be found at http://www.ninds.nih.gov/disorders/narcolepsy. Experimental treatment efforts are focused on hypocretin replacement therapy, gene therapy, and cell transplantation.[62]

IDIOPATHIC HYPERSOMNIA

This condition is associated with EDS, occurring daily for at least 3 months. Nocturnal polysomnography should have excluded other conditions leading to hypersomnia. In contrast to the mean sleep latency on the MSLT of less than 5 minutes that is typical of narcolepsy, in idiopathic hypersomnia, the mean sleep latency is generally in the 5-minute to 10-minute range. SOREMPs are not typically seen on the MSLT in patients with idiopathic hypersomnia and these patients do not typically show cataplexy, hypnagogic hallucinations, or sleep paralysis.[63] Many have periods of sleep drunkenness with periods of automatic behaviors, such as putting milk in a microwave oven. Two subtypes of idiopathic hypersomnia have been identified: in idiopathic hypersomnia with long sleep, there is prolonged nocturnal sleep lasting 10 or more hours; in idiopathic hypersomnia without long sleep, the major nocturnal sleep period is 6 to 10 hours. In a review of 42 patients evaluated at the University of Michigan over a 10-year period, Basetti and Aldrich[64] observed that idiopathic hypersomnia began at a mean age of 19 ± 8 years (range 6–43 years). Almost half of the patients described restless sleep with frequent arousals. Habitual dreaming was present in about 40% of the patients. The treatment of idiopathic hypersomnia requires use of planned naps, regular exercise, and pharmacologic measures that are identical to those used for narcolepsy.

PERIODIC HYPERSOMNIA (KLEINE-LEVIN SYNDROME)

This disorder occurs in adolescents, with a male predominance of 4:1. Patients develop 10 to 14 days of hypersomnolence, during which they sleep 18 to 20 hours per day, in association with feelings of depersonalization, mood disturbance, compulsive hyperphagia, and hypersexual behavior, with an intervening 2 to 4 months of normal alertness and behavior.[65] The binge eating may be associated with a 2-kg to 5-kg increase in body weight. Atypical forms of the syndrome have also been recognized in which there might be anorexia or lack of the sexual disinhibition. Nocturnal polysomnography during the sleepy periods shows decreased sleep efficiency, shortened latency to REM sleep, and decreased percentage of time spent in N3 sleep. The MSLT reveals moderately shortened mean sleep latency in the 5-minute to 10-minute range, but lacks the 2 or more SOREMPs that are typically seen in narcolepsy. The episodes of sleepiness gradually diminish over time, generally resolving over 5 to 7 years or evolving into classic depression, thus bringing up the issue of whether the disorder might be a variant of depression. A disturbance of hypothalamic function has been hypothesized but not established. The association of Kleine-Levin syndrome with histocompatibility antigen DQB1*0201 and the occasional precipitation after systemic infections, as well as the relapsing and remitting nature, are suspicious for an autoimmune cause.[66] There is no satisfactory treatment, although lithium has been reported to be effective in a case report.[67] Modafinil may reduce the duration of the symptomatic episodes.[68]

RLS

RLS is an autosomal-dominant, sensorimotor disorder in which the patient complains of a peculiar creepy or crawling feeling in the extremities.[69] The discomfort appears in the evening or at night, is exacerbated by keeping the limbs still, and is momentarily relieved by their movement.[70] There is also an urge to move the limbs. The symptoms interfere with sleep initiation and maintenance. Consequences of RLS include fatigue, inattentiveness, or sleepiness. A large population-based survey of more than 10,000 families in the United Kingdom and the United States found a prevalence of definite RLS in 1.9% of 8-year-olds to 11-year-olds and 2% in 12-year-olds to 17-year-olds.[71] Childhood RLS may be synonymous with growing pains in some children.[72] On nocturnal polysomnography, patients with RLS may show periodic limb movements, which are defined as a series of 4 or more rhythmic, electromyographically recorded movements of the legs lasting 0.5 to 10 seconds that occur 5 to 90 seconds apart, generally during stages N1 or N2 of sleep.

The favorable response of RLS in adults to dopamine receptor agonists like pramipexole and carbidopa-levodopa suggests an underlying central nervous system dopamine deficiency. There may be an associated systemic iron deficiency in the form of low levels of serum ferritin.[73] Iron is a cofactor for tyrosine hydroxylase, which is essential for dopamine synthesis. There also seems to be an association between childhood RLS and attention-deficit disorder.[22,74] In a community-based questionnaire survey of 866 children aged 2 to 13.9 years, Lumeng and Chervin[22] found an odds ratio for significant hyperactivity in RLS of 1:9. Besides dopamine agonists, oral iron, clonazepam, and gabapentin, gabapentin enacarbil[75] and pregabalin[76] have also been used to treat RLS, but there has been no randomized controlled trial in childhood.

DELAYED SLEEP PHASE DISORDER

The basis for circadian rhythm disorders is abnormal functioning of a molecular feedback loop between time-keeping genes CLOCK and BMAL1 (transcription regulating proteins) and the expression of *Period* genes *Per1, Per2, Per3*, and *Cryptochrome* genes *Cry1 and Cry2*.[77] Delayed sleep phase syndrome (DSPS) was described initially in a medical student who was unable to wake up in time to attend his morning classes.[78] Despite hypnotic use, the patient was unable to fall asleep before the early morning hours and was mistaken initially to have insomnia. However, sleep in the laboratory was quantitatively and qualitatively normal. The delay in the timing of occurrence of the sleeping phase of the 24-hour sleep-wake cycle was caused by a constitutional inability to prepone sleep, which in turn is secondary to altered function of the circadian timekeeper (ie, the suprachiasmatic nucleus). The disorder typically has onset in adolescence, with a male predominance. Sleep logs and wrist actigraphy for 1 to 2 weeks are helpful in establishing the diagnosis. Bright light therapy is helpful in advancing the sleep-onset time to an earlier hour.[79] It consists of the provision of 2700 to 10,000 lux of bright light via a light box for 20 to 30 minutes immediately on awakening in the morning. The light box is kept at a distance of 18 to 24 inches from the face. The phototherapy leads to a gradual advancement (shifting back) of the sleep-onset time at night. Bright light therapy may be combined with melatonin that is administered about 5 to 5.5 hours before the required bedtime in a dose of 0.5 to 1 mg. Another therapeutic option is one of progressively delaying bedtime by 3 to 4 hours per day until it becomes aligned with socially acceptable sleep-wake hours (chronotherapy), and then adhering to this schedule. However, over time, all patients with DSPS remain at risk for drifting to progressively later and later bedtimes. Daytime stimulants such as modafinil (100–400 mg/d in 2 divided doses) may improve daytime alertness.

PARASOMNIAS

Parasomnias are unpleasant or undesirable events that intrude onto sleep, without altering sleep quality or quantity. These events may occur at the transition to sleep, during REM sleep, or at the time of shifting from N3 sleep into the lighter N2/N1 sleep.[80] The incidence of parasomnias is variable, although 30% of children have at least 1 episode of sleepwalking, and sleeptalking has been noted in about half the population.[81] Frequently, the patient is unaware of the events, but medical attention is sought because of disruption of the sleep of other family members or concerns about injury to the patient.

NREM parasomnias such as confusional arousals, sleepwalking, and sleep terrors occur during N3 sleep, and are thus prevalent in the first third of night, when this type of sleep is most abundant. Confusional arousals are seen most often in toddlers, whereas sleepwalking and sleep terrors may occur throughout the first decade. Children with confusional arousals may sit up in bed, moan or whimper inconsolably, and utter words like "no" or "go away." Autonomic activation characterized by flushing, sweating, and piloerection is minimal to absent. The events generally last 5 to 30 minutes, after which the patient goes back to sleep and has no recollection of the events on awakening the following morning. Patients with night terrors and sleepwalking may show flushing of the face, increased sweating, inconsolability, and agitation, but again with complete amnesia for the event in the morning. In all of the 3 NREM parasomnias, a concurrently obtained EEG shows rhythmic activity in the 2 to 6 Hz range, consistent with partial arousal from slow-wave sleep. A low dose of imipramine or clonazepam (0.25–0.5 mg at bedtime) is helpful in preventing most NREM parasomnias.[82] In some NREM parasomnias, the partial arousals may be triggered by underlying sleep apnea, RLS, or gastroesophageal reflux. If so, treatment of this underlying disorder helps alleviate the parasomnia. Environmental safety measures such as installing a deadbolt lock on the door may be necessary in patients with habitual sleepwalking. NREM parasomnias can be confused with nocturnal seizures, especially those with frontal lobe onset.[83] Features distinguishing NREM arousal parasomnias (confusional arousals, sleepwalking, and sleep terrors) from nocturnal partial seizures are listed in **Table 2**. Most NREM parasomnias subside spontaneously by 10 to 12 years of age.

Common REM sleep parasomnias include nightmares (scary dreams), terrifying hypnagogic hallucinations, and the REM sleep behavior disorder. Because REM sleep is most abundant during the final third of night sleep, nightmares and REM sleep behavior disorder tend to occur during the early morning hours.[80] REM sleep behavior disorder is characterized by motoric dream enactment, during which the patient might kick, jump, or struggle against an imaginary assailant as a result of failure of the customary inhibition of skeletal muscle activity in REM sleep by the medullary nucleus reticularis gigantocellularis. Narcolepsy, autism spectrum disorder, anatomic brainstem abnormalities such as neoplasms, and the use of selective serotonin reuptake inhibitor agents have been associated with childhood-onset REM sleep behavior

Table 2
Differentiating NREM arousal parasomnias from nocturnal partial seizures

Feature	NREM Arousal Parasomnia	Nocturnal Partial Seizure
Time of onset	Generally within 2–3 h of initial sleep onset	Randomly, at any time of the night
Duration of event	5–10 min	1–2 min
Sleep stage	Generally during N3 stage of sleep	Generally during N1 or N2 stage of sleep
Ictal EEG	Rhythmic generalized θ or δ activity	Focal spike or sharp wave discharges
Subsequent recall of event	Impaired	Preserved

disorder.[84] The nocturnal polysomnogram shows increased phasic electromyographic activity during REM sleep. Treatment with clonazepam (0.25–0.5 mg at bedtime) is effective in preventing most REM parasomnias.

SLEEP, BEHAVIORAL, AND PSYCHIATRIC DISORDERS

Higher prevalence of sleep complaints has been noted in children with psychiatric conditions compared with nonpsychiatric controls.[85] Sleep symptoms including restless sleep, long sleep latency, short sleep duration, and frequent nocturnal awakenings were noted to occur frequently among pediatric patients with psychiatric conditions, and frequency and severity of sleep symptoms have been linked to the severity of psychiatric symptoms.[85]

Attention-Deficit/Hyperactivity Disorder

Attention-deficit/hyperactivity disorder (ADHD) is characterized by impulsivity, hyperactivity, and inattention. ADHD is estimated to occur in 3% to 7.5% of school-aged children, making it one of the most prevalent childhood psychiatric conditions. Sleep problems have been reported in clinical practice in an estimated 25% to 50% of children and adolescents with ADHD.[86] Medications used to treat ADHD such as stimulants have been associated with sleep problems in these children.[87] Primary sleep disorders such as RLS and OSA can mimic ADHD symptoms, including inattention and hyperactivity in up to one-third of patients.[23] Treatment of OSA has been associated with improvement of ADHD-like symptoms initially resistant to stimulant medications.[18]

Studies in children with ADHD with no comorbid medical or psychiatric problems have shown sleep-onset insomnia, significant decreases in REM sleep, higher numbers of sleep cycles, differences in sleep patterns and sleep motor activity compared with controls.[88] Sleep problems in ADHD may lead to significant stress for the child and family. The sleep problems can potentially interfere with mood, attention, and behavior, all of which are critical for good daytime functioning. According to 1 study,[89] moderate or severe sleep problems in children with ADHD were strongly associated with the mental health of the primary caregivers, their work attendance, and family functioning.

Behavioral interventions including positive bedtime routines, limit setting, sleep hygiene, and cognitive behavioral therapy may be considered to treat insomnia disorders.

Major Depressive Disorder

Major depressive disorder (MDD) is prevalent in 2% of children and 8% of adolescents and often recurrent in nature. Sleep problems occur in about 70% of the depressed children and adolescents, with most common sleep complaints being sleep initiation/maintenance insomnia in 53% and hypersomnia in approximately 10% of the patients.[90] Depressed children with sleep disturbances also have greater severity of depression and higher rates of comorbid anxiety disorders.[90] Polysomnogram studies in prepubertal children have shown inconsistent results, with some studies reporting shortened REM sleep latency in children with MDD compared with controls,[91] whereas others failed to report any significant disturbances.[92] However, there was a subgroup of depressed patients (8/36) in Dahl and colleagues'[92] study who showed reduced REM sleep latency on 2 successive nights of polysomnography, along with decreased stage 4 sleep and increased time in REM sleep. This subgroup had higher severity scores for depression, but did not otherwise differ from other patients with MDD. Abnormalities have also been documented in the EEG sleep microarchitecture using cross-spectral analysis.[93] This finding shows that compared with healthy controls, children with MDD show decreased coherence of left and right temporal β activity and between δ and β. These abnormalities were most striking in girls, even those younger than 13 years.[93] Simultaneous treatment of insomnia and depression using behavioral and pharmacologic treatments seems to be a rational approach, with the goal of rapid improvement of depressive symptoms and eventual remission.

Anxiety Disorders

Anxiety disorders are one of the most common psychiatric disorders in children, with prevalence rates between 12% and 20%.[94] Anxiety disorders in children include separation anxiety disorder, generalized anxiety disorder, social phobia, specific phobias, obsessive compulsive disorder, posttraumatic stress disorder, and panic disorder with or without agoraphobia. Internalizing symptoms of anxiety correlate with sleep disturbance in all youth.[95] Parenting style, family dynamics, parental psychopathology, trauma, and abuse have been associated with sleep disturbances in anxious children. The common sleep complaints in children with anxiety disorders include sleep initiation and maintenance problems, frequent nocturnal awakenings, bedtime refusal, cosleeping with parents, nightmares, and nocturnal fears.[85] Polysomnography studies in children with anxiety disorders have shown increased sleep latency, increased number of awakenings, and less slow-wave sleep.[96] Successful treatment of anxiety disorders, including behavioral and pharmacologic interventions, is usually associated with improvement in sleep disturbances in children.

Behavioral Insomnia of Childhood

Bedtime resistance and night awakenings are common, affecting 20% to 30% of infants and toddlers.[97] Based on the International Classification of Sleep Disorders 2, there are 2 subtypes of behavioral insomnia syndromes: the sleep-onset association type and the limit-setting type. For both entities, the sleep disruption must not be better explained from another sleep disorder, medical, neurologic, or psychiatric disorder, or medication use.[98,99]

In the sleep-onset association disorder type of behavioral insomnia, the act of falling asleep becomes an extended process that requires special conditions, such as being held by the parent, rocked, or patted. In the absence of these associated conditions, sleep onset is significantly delayed or sleep is otherwise disrupted.[98,99] When the child awakens at night, there is once again a need for caregiver intervention in order for the child to fall back to sleep. This disorder is managed by initially reassuring the parents that there is no underlying medical disorder. Daytime naps are kept to the minimum. At bedtime, the parent is allowed to sit next to the infant or toddler, but not to hold them. The parent should leave the room before the patient falls asleep.

In case of a night awakening, the same process is repeated. The parents are taught to progressively delay the period between the onset of the infant's crying and their intervention.[98,99]

In the limit-setting disorder, the child has difficulty initiating or maintaining sleep, may stall or refuse to go to bed at an appropriate time, or refuse to go back to bed after a night awakening. The caregiver shows insufficient or inappropriate limit setting for establishing appropriate sleeping behavior in the child.[98,99] This disorder is managed by restricting the duration of the daytime nap to the essential (in order to increase the sleep pressure), and by implementing graduated extinction.[98,99] The latter technique involves teaching the parents to consistently ignore bedtime tantrums for specified periods. This period varies with the temperament of the infant and the coping skills of the parent. For the management of both types of behavioral insomnia syndromes, periodic contact of the provider with the parent is essential in order to provide encouragement and implement consistent behavioral reinforcement.

FUTURE CONSIDERATIONS

- There are few satisfactory management options for OSA of infancy. Supraglottoplasty is used in those with laryngomalacia, but rigorous evidence concerning its efficacy is not available. Infants are also not amenable to nonsurgical treatment measures like PAP breathing.
- Adherence to PAP breathing remains a challenge. Techniques to improve adherence are indicated.
- Drugs used to treat narcolepsy-cataplexy and RLS remain off-label. Development of safe and effective drugs for children is a priority.
- The efficacy of oral appliances needs further study.
- Longitudinal studies are needed in childhood headache syndromes to document that improvement is sleep quantity and quality improves the headache symptoms.
- The early recognition of insomnia and hypersomnia in children with major depression and anxiety might open up opportunities for early intervention. Will enhancing sleep in these children have a salutory effect on mood and emotions? This issue needs further exploration.

Case Report

An 8-year-old boy with trisomy 21 presented with increasing irritability, difficulty in school, and difficulty awakening in the morning. On questioning, the child went to bed relatively easily at 8:00 PM, slept in a quiet and comfortable environment, and had no caffeine. The parents noted noisy breathing with witnessed apneas at night. Over the last year, the child screamed out and was inconsolable after approximately 45 minutes of sleep approximately twice per week. He appeared confused and frightened but with gentle coaching returned to bed. His examination showed typical features of trisomy 21, but he also had large tonsils, and poor nasal airflow. Also his behavior was slightly aggressive and he was irritable. A full night polysomnogram showed an obstructive AHI of 17.6, with increase of the end tidal CO_2 to 56 torr. The child underwent tonsillectomy and adenoidectomy and was observed overnight in the step-down unit for postoperative complications. Although the snoring resolved, a follow-up polysomnography at 3 months showed an obstructive AHI of 6.2. The patient had partial improvement in symptoms but still had some irritability and confusional arousals approximately once every 3 weeks. The child underwent a CPAP titration and was found to have resolution of apnea with 6 cm H_2O. In the ensuing clinic visit, the clinician and parents discussed the importance of the use of the CPAP therapy and strategies to ensure compliance. After use of behavioral therapies to positively reinforce the use of the CPAP, the patient returned to his usual happy behavior and had only rare confusional arousals.

This case exemplifies several important points. Children frequently present with symptoms that may not initially seem related to sleep. In this patient, the clues for nighttime disturbance included the daytime irritability, difficulty in school, and trouble awakening in the morning. These daytime manifestations may be nonspecific; however, children who do not get enough sleep or have disturbed sleep often present with behavioral issues. For this child, observant parents recognized noisy breathing and apneas at night. In addition, this child had recurrent sleep terrors or confusional arousals. A progressive increase in these types of events is commonly associated with sleep-disordered breathing. This child proved to have severe OSA, another common disturbance in children with trisomy 21. Given the severity, the child was monitored in the hospital because of the higher risk of postoperative complications. As common in children with severe apnea, but more frequently in disabled children, surgery did not completely resolve the apnea, which shows the importance of follow-up polysomnography. This child was treated with PAP. This treatment requires diligence from the parents and the use of positive reinforcement to help with compliance.

REFERENCES

1. Ipsiroglu OS, Fatemi A, Werner I, et al. Prevalence of sleep disorders in school children between 11 and 15 years of age. Wien Klin Wochenschr 2001;113: 235–44 [in German].
2. Byars KC, Yolton K, Rausch J, et al. Prevalence, patterns and persistence of sleep problems in the first 3 years of life. Pediatrics 2012;129:e276–84.
3. Scher MS. Ontogenesis of EEG-sleep from neonatal through infancy periods. Sleep Med 2008;9:615–36.
4. Van Cauter E, Spiegel K, Tasali E, et al. Metabolic consequences of sleep and sleep loss. Sleep Med 2008;9(Suppl 1):S23–8.
5. Carskadon MA, Wolfson AR, Acebo C, et al. Adolescent sleep patterns, circadian timing, and sleepiness at a transition to early school days. Sleep 1998;21:871–81.
6. Drake C, Nickel C, Burduvali E, et al. The Pediatric Daytime Sleepiness Scale (PDSS): sleep habits and school outcomes in middle school children. Sleep 2003;26:455–8.
7. Owens JA, Spirito A, McGuinn M. The Children's Sleep Habits Questionnaire (CHSQ): psychometric properties of a survey instrument for school-aged children. Sleep 2000;23:1043–51.
8. Arens R, Mazumdar H. Childhood obesity and obstructive sleep apnea syndrome. J Appl Physiol 2010;108:436–44.
9. Kim JH, Guilleminault C. The nasomaxillary complex, the mandible and sleep-disordered breathing. Sleep Breath 2011;15:185–93.
10. Hoban TF, Chervin RD. Sleep-related breathing disorders of childhood: description, and clinical picture, diagnosis and treatment approaches. Sleep Med Clin 2007;2:445–62.
11. Katz ES, D'Ambrosio CM. Management of sleep disordered breathing in children with neuromuscular disease. In: Kothare S, Kotagal S, editors. Sleep in childhood neurological disorders. New York: Demos Medical; 2011. p. 275–94.
12. Misuri G, Lanini B, Gigliotti F, et al. Mechanisms of CO_2 retention in patients with neuromuscular disease. Chest 2000;117:447–53.
13. Aurora RN, Zak RS, Karippot A, et al. Practice parameters for the respiratory indications for polysomnography in children. Sleep 2011;34:379–88.
14. Wise MS, Nichols CD, Grigg-Damberger MM, et al. Executive summary for respiratory indications for polysomnography in children: an evidence based review. Sleep 2011;34:389–98.

15. Morgenthaler T, Alessi C, Friedman L, et al. Practice parameters for the use of actigraphy in the assessment of sleep and sleep disorders: an update for 2007. Sleep 2007;30:519–29.
16. Littner MR, Kushida C, Wise M, et al. Practice parameters for clinical use of the multiple sleep latency test and the maintenance of wakefulness test. Sleep 2005;28:113–21.
17. Iber C, Ancoli-Israel S, Chesson A, et al. The AASM Manual for the Scoring of Sleep and Associated Events: Rules, Terminology and Technical Specifications. 1st edition. Westchester (IL): American Academy of Sleep Medicine; 2007.
18. O'Brien LM, Holbrook CR, Mervis CB, et al. Sleep and neurobehavioral characteristics in 5–7 year old hyperactive children. Pediatrics 2003;111:554–63.
19. O'Brien LM, Mervis CB, Holbrook CR, et al. Neurobehavioral implications of habitual snoring in children. Pediatrics 2004;114:44–9.
20. Goldstein NA, Stefanov DG, Graw-Panzer GD, et al. Validation of a clinical assessment score for pediatric sleep-disordered breathing. The Laryngoscope 2012;122:2096–104.
21. Brunetti L, Rana S, Losppalluti ML, et al. Prevalence of obstructive sleep apnea syndrome in a cohort of 1207 children of Southern Italy. Chest 2001;120:1930–5.
22. Lumeng JC, Chervin RD. Epidemiology of pediatric obstructive sleep apnea. Proc Am Thorac Soc 2008;5:242–52.
23. Chervin RD, Archbold KH, Dillon JE, et al. Associations between symptoms of inattention, hyperactivity, restless legs, and periodic leg movements. Sleep 2002;25:213–8.
24. Gozal D. Obstructive sleep apnea in children: implications for the developing central nervous system. Semin Pediatr Neurol 2008;15:100–6.
25. Guilleminault C, Pelayo R, Leger D, et al. Recognition of sleep-disordered breathing in children. Pediatrics 1996;98:871–82.
26. Brouillette RT, Morielli A, Leimanis A, et al. Nocturnal pulse oximetry as an abbreviated testing modality for pediatric obstructive sleep apnea. Pediatrics 2000; 105:405–12.
27. Kheirandish-Gozal L, Gozal D. Intranasal budesonide treatment for children with mild obstructive sleep apnea syndrome. Pediatrics 2008;122:e149–55.
28. Ambrosio A, Brigger MT. Pediatric supraglottoplasty. Adv Otorhinolaryngol 2012; 73:101–4.
29. Marcus CL, Beck SE, Traylor J, et al. Randomized, double-blind trial of two different modes of positive airway pressure therapy on adherence and efficacy in children. J Clin Sleep Med 2012;8:37–42.
30. Rondeau BH. Dentist's role in the treatment of snoring and sleep apnea. Funct Orthod 1998;15:4–6.
31. Abad VC, Guilleminault C. Treatment options for obstructive sleep apnea. Curr Treat Options Neurol 2009;11:358–67.
32. Zolty P, Sanders MH, Pollack IF. Chiari malformation and sleep-disordered breathing: a review of diagnostic and management issues. Sleep 2000;23: 637–43.
33. Gozal D. New concepts in abnormalities of respiratory control in children. Curr Opin Pediatr 2004;16:305–8.
34. Gozal D, Harper RM. Novel insights into congenital hypoventilation syndrome. Curr Opin Pulm Med 1999;5:335–8.
35. Roshkow JE, Haller JO, Berdon WE, et al. Hirschsprung's disease, Ondine's curse, and neuroblastoma–manifestations of neurocristopathy. Pediatr Radiol 1988;19:45–9.

36. Swaminathan S, Gilsanz V, Atkinson J, et al. Congenital central hypoventilation syndrome associated with multiple ganglioneuromas. Chest 1989;96: 423–4.
37. Trochet D, O'Brien LM, Gozal D, et al. PHOX2B genotype allows for prediction of tumor risk in congenital central hypoventilation syndrome. Am J Hum Genet 2005;76: 421–6.
38. Weese-Mayer DE, Berry-Kravis EM, Ceccherini I, et al. An official ATS clinical policy statement: congenital central hypoventilation syndrome: genetic basis, diagnosis, and management. Am J Respir Crit Care Med 2010;181: 626–44.
39. Spitzer AR. Evidence-based methylxanthine use in the NICU. Clin Perinatol 2012; 39:137–48.
40. Spence J, Pasterkamp H, McDonald PJ. Isolated central sleep apnea in type I Chiari malformation: improvement after surgery. Pediatr Pulmonol 2010;45: 1141–4.
41. Westwood AJ, Vendrame M, Montouris G, et al. Pearls and oysters: treatment of central sleep apnea with topiramate. Neurology 2012;78:e97–9.
42. Kotagal S, Gibbons VP, Stith J. Sleep abnormalities in patients with severe cerebral palsy. Dev Med Child Neurol 1994;36:304–11.
43. Cummiskey J, Guilleminault C, Davis R, et al. Automatic respiratory failure: sleep studies and Leigh's disease. Neurology 1987;37:1876–8.
44. Wolfe L, Lakadamyali H, Mutlu GM. Joubert syndrome associated with severe central sleep apnea. J Clin Sleep Med 2010;6:384–8.
45. Zucconi M. Sleep disorders in children with neurological disease. In: Loughlin GM, Carroll JL, Marcus CL, editors. Sleep and breathing in children. A developmental approach. New York: Marcel Dekker; 2000. p. 363–83.
46. Kotagal S. Sleep in children at risk. Sleep Med Clin 2007;2:477–90.
47. Zucconi M, Weber G, Castronovo V, et al. Sleep and upper airway obstruction in children with achondroplasia. J Pediatr 1996;129:743–9.
48. Valayannopoulos V, de Blic J, Mahalaoui N, et al. Laronidase for cardiopulmonary disease in Hurler syndrome 12 years after bone marrow transplantation. Pediatrics 2010;126:e1242–7.
49. Challamel MJ, Mazzola ME, Nevsimalova S, et al. Narcolepsy in children. Sleep 1994;17:S17–20.
50. Broughton R, Krupa S, Boucher B, et al. Impaired circadian waking arousal in narcolepsy-cataplexy. Sleep Res Online 1998;1:159–65.
51. Autret A, Lucas F, Henry-Lebras F, et al. Symptomatic narcolepsies. Sleep 1994; 17(Suppl 1):21–4.
52. Perriol MP, Cartigny M, Lamblin MD, et al. Childhood-onset narcolepsy, obesity and puberty in four consecutive children: a close temporal link. J Pediatr Endocrinol Metab 2010;23:257–65.
53. Kotagal S, Krahn LE, Slocumb N. A putative link between childhood narcolepsy and obesity. Sleep Med 2004;5:147–50.
54. Plazzi G, Parmeggiani A, Mignot E, et al. Narcolepsy-cataplexy associated with precocious puberty. Neurology 2006;66:1577–9.
55. Stores G, Montgomery P, Wiggs L. The psychosocial problems of children with narcolepsy and those with excessive daytime sleepiness of uncertain origin. Pediatrics 2006;118:1116–23.
56. Billiard M, Seignalet J, Besset A, et al. HLA DR2 and narcolepsy. Sleep 1986;9:149–52.
57. Nishino S, Ripley B, Overeem S, et al. Hypocretin (orexin) deficiency in human narcolepsy. Lancet 2000;355:39–40.

58. Nishino S, Ripley B, Overeem S, et al. Low cerebrospinal fluid hypocretin (orexin) and altered energy homeostasis in human narcolepsy. Ann Neurol 2001;50:381–8.

59. John J, Wu MF, Siegel JM. Systemic administration of hypocretin-1 reduces cataplexy and normalizes sleep and waking durations in narcoleptic dogs. Sleep Res Online 2000;3:23–8.

60. Mason TB 2nd, Teoh L, Calabro K, et al. Rapid eye movement latency in children and adolescents. Pediatr Neurol 2008;39:162–9.

61. Dauvilliers Y, Abril B, Mas E, et al. Normalization of hypocretin-1 in narcolepsy after immunoglobulin G treatment. Neurology 2009;73:1333–4.

62. Ritchie C, Okuro M, Kanbayashi T, et al. Hypocretin ligand deficiency in narcolepsy: recent basic and clinical insights. Curr Neurol Neurosci Rep 2010;10:180–9.

63. Frenette E, Kushida CA. Primary hypersomnias of central origin. Semin Neurol 2009;29:354–67.

64. Basetti C, Aldrich MS. Idiopathic hypersomnia: a series of 42 patients. Brain 1997;120:1423.

65. Arnulf I, Lin L, Gadoth N, et al. Kleine Levin syndrome: a systematic study of 108 patients. Ann Neurol 2008;63:482–93.

66. Dauvilliers Y, Mayer G, Lecendreux M, et al. Kleine Levin syndrome. An autoimmune hypothesis based on clinical and genetic analyses. Neurology 2002;59: 1739–45.

67. Poppe M, Friebel D, Reuner U, et al. The Kleine-Levin syndrome—effects of treatment with lithium. Neuropediatrics 2003;34:113–9.

68. Huang YS, Lakkis C, Guilleminault C. Kleine Levin syndrome: current status. Med Clin North Am 2010;94:557–62.

69. Picchietti MA, Picchietti DL. Restless legs syndrome and periodic limb movement disorder in children and adolescents. Semin Pediatr Neurol 2008;15:91–9.

70. Allen RP, Picchietti D, Hening WA, et al. Restless legs syndrome: diagnostic criteria, special considerations, and epidemiology. A report from the restless legs syndrome diagnosis and epidemiology workshop at the National Institutes of Health. Sleep Med 2003;4:101–19.

71. Picchietti DL, Allen RP, Walters AS, et al. Restless legs syndrome: prevalence and impact in childhood and adolescence–The Peds REST study. Pediatrics 2007; 120:253–66.

72. Walters AS. Is there a subpopulation of children with growing pains who really have restless legs syndrome? A review of the literature. Sleep Med 2002;3:93–8.

73. Kotagal S, Silber MH. Childhood-onset restless legs syndrome. Ann Neurol 2004; 56:803–7.

74. Picchietti DL, Underwood DJ, Farris WA, et al. Further studies on periodic limb movement disorder and restless legs syndrome in children with attention deficit-hyperactivity disorder. Mov Disord 1999;14:1000–7.

75. Bogan RK, Cramer Borneman MA, Kushida CA, et al. Long-term maintenance treatment of restless legs syndrome with gabapentin enacarbil: a randomized controlled study. Mayo Clin Proc 2010;85:512–21.

76. Allen R, Chen C, Soalta A, et al. A randomized, double-blind, 6-week dose-ranging study of pregabalin in patients with restless legs syndrome. Sleep Med 2010;11:512–9.

77. Wulff K, Porcheret K, Cussans E, et al. Sleep and circadian rhythm disturbances: multiple genes and multiple phenotypes. Curr Opin Genet Dev 2009;19:237–46.

78. Weitzman ED, Czeisler CA, Coleman RM, et al. Delayed sleep phase syndrome. A chronobiological disorder with sleep-onset insomnia. Arch Gen Psychiatry 1981;38:737.

79. Morgenthaler TE, Lee-Chiong T, Alessi C, et al. Practice parameters for the clinical evaluation and treatment of circadian rhythm sleep disorders. Sleep 2007;30:1445–59.
80. Kotagal S. Parasomnias in childhood. Sleep Med Rev 2009;13:157–68.
81. D'Cruz FO, Vaughn BV. Parasomnias: an update. Semin Pediatr Neurol 2001;8:251–7.
82. Provini F, Tinuper P, Bisulli F, et al. Arousal disorders. Sleep Med 2011;12(Suppl 2): S22–6.
83. Bisulli F, Vignatelli F, Provini F, et al. Parasomnias and nocturnal frontal lobe epilepsy (NFLE): lights and shadows–controversial points in the differential diagnosis. Sleep Med 2011;12(Suppl 2):S27–32.
84. Lloyd R, Tippman-Peikert M, Slocumb N, et al. Characteristics of REM sleep behavior disorder in childhood. J Clin Sleep Med 2012;8:127–31.
85. Ivanenko A, Johnson K. Sleep disturbances in children with psychiatric disorders. Semin Pediatr Neurol 2008;15:70–80.
86. Weiss MD, Salpekar J. Sleep problems in the child with attention deficit-hyperactivity disorder: defining etiology and appropriate treatments. CNS Drugs 2010;24:811–28.
87. Cohen-Zion M, Ancoli Israel S. Sleep in children with attention deficit hyperactivity disorder (ADHD): a review of naturalistic and stimulant intervention studies. Sleep Med Rev 2004;8:379–402.
88. Gruber R, Xi T, Robert M, et al. Sleep disturbances in prepubertal children with attention deficit hyperactivity disorder: a home polysomnography study. Sleep 2009;32(3):343–50.
89. Sung V, Hiscock H, Sciberras E, et al. Sleep problems in children with attention deficit hyperactivity disorder: prevalence, and the effect on the child and family. Arch Pediatr Adolesc Med 2008;162:336–42.
90. Liu X, Buysse DJ, Gentzler AL, et al. Insomnia and hypersomnia associated with depressive phenomenology and comorbidity in childhood depression. Sleep 2007;30:83–90.
91. Emslie GJ, Rush AJ, Weinberg WA, et al. Children with major depression show reduced rapid eye movement latencies. Arch Gen Psychiatry 1990;47:119–24.
92. Dahl RE, Ryan ND, Birmaher B, et al. Electroencephalographic sleep measures in prepubertal depression. Psychiatry Res 1991;38:201–14.
93. Armitage R, Hoffman R, Emslie G, et al. Sleep microarchitecture in childhood and adolescent depression: temporal coherence. Clin EEG Neurosci 2006;37:1–9.
94. Costello EJ, Egger HL, Angold A. The developmental epidemiology of anxiety disorders: phenomenology, prevalence and comorbidity. Child Adolesc Psychiatr Clin North Am 2005;14:631–48.
95. Alfano CA, Zakem AH, Costa NM, et al. Sleep problems and their relation to cognitive factors, anxiety, and depressive symptoms in children and adolescents. Depress Anxiety 2009;26:503–12.
96. Forbes EE, Bertocci MA, Gregory AM, et al. Objective sleep in pediatric anxiety disorders and major depressive disorder. J Am Acad Child Adolesc Psychiatry 2008;47:148–55.
97. Goodlin-Jones BL, Burnham MM, Gaylor EE, et al. Night waking, sleep-wake organization, and self-soothing in the first year of life. J Dev Behav Pediatr 2001;22:226–33.
98. Mindell AJ, Kuhn B, Lewin DS, et al. Behavioral treatment of bedtime problems and night wakings in infants and young children. Sleep 2006;29:1263–76.
99. Morgenthaler TJ, Owens J, Alessi C, et al. Practice parameters for behavioral treatment of bedtime problems and night wakings in infants and young children. Sleep 2006;29:1277–81.

Sleep in Neurological Disorders

Dementia and Sleep

Heidi L. Roth, MD

KEYWORDS

- Dementia • Sleep • REM sleep behavior disorder (RBD)
- Irregular sleep-wake rhythm (ISWR) • Sundowning • Insomnia • Hypersomnia
- Sleep-disordered breathing

KEY POINTS

- Sleep disorders are common in patients with dementia and are a primary trigger for institutionalization.
- Treatment of sleep disorders in patients with dementia can produce improved cognitive function and reduce caregiver distress.
- Treatment of sleep disorders in patients with dementia should include consideration of a broad spectrum of factors that can affect sleep and wake cycles, including caffeine consumption, the effect of medications, and mood.
- Agitation and delirium can be a sign of obstructive sleep apnea (OSA) and treatment of OSA can produce complete resolution of symptoms in some cases.
- Dementia associated with synuclein disorders (including Lewy body dementia, Parkinson's disease with dementia, and multisystem atrophy) is associated with rapid eye movement sleep behavior disorder (RBD). RBD-like symptoms can also be seen in sleep-disordered breathing, and a polysomnogram study is necessary to exclude OSA as a cause or contributor to symptoms.
- Irregular sleep-wake rhythm is common in Alzheimer's dementia and treatment should focus on behavioral interventions rather than pharmacologic management.
- Sundowning is a nonspecific descriptor. The possibility that pacing and wandering may represent forms of restless leg syndrome should be considered.
- Whether sleep-disordered breathing and/or sleep deprivation is a risk for dementia is controversial and is an active area of investigation.

INTRODUCTION

Sleep disturbances are common in patients with dementia, affecting from 25% to 80% of patients depending on the dementia subtype.[1] Although sleep disturbances are also common in the elderly in general, the impact of sleep disorders in dementia can be greater. Sleep disturbances can magnify the cognitive impairments and mood

Department of Neurology, Cognitive Neurology and Sleep Medicine, University of North Carolina, 170 Manning Drive, CB # 7025, Chapel Hill, NC 27599-7025, USA
E-mail address: hroth@neurology.unc.edu

Neurol Clin 30 (2012) 1213–1248
http://dx.doi.org/10.1016/j.ncl.2012.08.013
0733-8619/12/$ – see front matter © 2012 Elsevier Inc. All rights reserved.

neurologic.theclinics.com

dysregulation that patients with dementia already face, and can be a major reason for loss of function.[2,3] Sleep disturbances also create psychological, physical, and financial burdens for caregivers.[4-7] In addition, sleep disturbances a primary reason for the institutionalization of patients with dementia, and can be a more common trigger for institutionalization than even the cognitive problems.[3,8-11]

Degenerative dementias affect brain systems that are critical for regulation of the sleep-wake cycle. Depending on the areas of the brain affected in a specific dementia, different patterns of sleep disorder can result. Recognizing which specific sleep disorder might be occurring in a patient, based on a recognition of how particular dementias affect sleep systems, can lead to better targeting and treatment of sleep disorders. This article reviews specific sleep disorders that are seen more commonly in specific types of dementia, and the treatment of these disorders. It also offers a practical approach to addressing other external factors that may be affecting patients with sleep-wake problems and dementia, and how these factors should be addressed with the vulnerabilities of the patient with dementia in mind. When evaluating a new patient with apparent cognitive problems, the impact of a sleep disturbance on the presentation needs to be inquired about carefully. In rare, but important, cases, a sleep disturbance such as obstructive sleep apnea (OSA) can lead to agitation, cognitive impairment, and delirium that is completely reversible with treatment. Evaluation and treatment of sleep and wake disturbances in patients with all forms of cognitive impairment and dementia can improve patient function and, in many cases, address a major cause of distress for caregivers and families.

DEMENTIA, DEMENTIA SUBTYPES, AND ASSOCIATION WITH SLEEP DISORDERS

Dementia is common and increasing in prevalence. The prevalence and incidence of dementia is age related and doubles with approximately every 5 years after the age of 65 years. Estimates based on a number of studies generally suggest that approximately 2% of the population has dementia between the ages of 65 and 75 years, 10% between 75 and 85 years, and 35% of people older than 85 years. The prevalence of dementia is increasing as the general population ages and lives longer. In the World Health Organization 2012 report,[12] it was estimated that the number of people with dementia in America, Europe, Asia, and worldwide would nearly double by 2030 and triple by 2050. Approximately 4 million people have dementia in North America and this is expected to nearly triple to 12 million by 2050. An increasing number of dementia subtypes have been recognized in recent years. Alzheimer's disease (AD) is the most common dementia, especially in old age. However, in patients younger than 60 years, frontal temporal lobe dementia (FTLD) is the most common, and, in patients from the ages of 60 to 70 years, it can be as common as AD. Dementia with Lewy Bodies (DLB) is thought to account for about 20% of all dementia. Approximately 40% of patients with Parkinson disease (PD) have dementia, and 80% of patients with PD develop dementia before death. Vascular cognitive impairment is sometimes cited as the second most common cause for dementia overall. It comprises a significant proportion of dementia, given that the lifetime risk for stroke is equal to that of AD, and about one-third of elderly individuals have silent cerebrovascular disease.[13]

As the underlying genetics and neuropathology of dementia-related diseases have become better known, there has been a move toward classification based on the underlying disorder (**Table 1**). The underlying neuropathologic process can be relevant to understanding some of the sleep problems associated with dementia, and knowledge of these associations can help to raise awareness of specific sleep-related

Basic dementia subtypes: overview

Dementias associated with parkinsonism

- **DLB**
  ○ Synuclein neural inclusions (more cortical vs PDD)
- **PDD**
  ○ Synuclein neural inclusions (less cortical vs DLB)
- **Multisystem atrophy**
  ○ Synuclein glial inclusions
- **PSP**
  ○ Tau neural inclusions in 4-repeat form, especially affecting brainstem
- **CBD/CBS**
  ○ Tau inclusions in 4-repeat form, with astrocytic plaques, oligodendroglial coiled bodies, threadlike lesions, achromatic neurons
  ○ Syndrome is also seen with PSP and C17-TDP43 progranulin deficiency
- **FTD-parkinsonism**
  ○ PD with FTD most commonly seen in familial genetic forms of FTD: FTD17-Tau, C17-TDP43 progranulin deficiency, C9orf72
- **Vascular dementia with parkinsonism**
  ○ Typically crural parkinsonism, gait apraxia, no tremor

Vascular dementia

- **Multi-infarct dementia**
  ○ Large complete infarcts in cortex, subcortical areas
- **Strategic infarct dementia**
  ○ Infarct of angular gyrus, thalamus, hippocampal branch PCA artery, anterior choroidal artery
- **Subcortical ischemic vascular dementia**
  ○ Leukoencephalopathy, should also have at least 1 lacune

ALS-associated dementia

- **15% patients with FTD develop ALS; many with ALS develop FTD**
  ○ Familial ALS-FTD most commonly caused by C9orf72-TDP43
  ○ 50% of ALS have dysexecutive syndrome, may not have FTD

FTLD

- **Behavioral variant FTLD**
  ○ 48% Tau inclusions (sometimes Pick bodies, occasional CBD)
  ○ 48% TDP43 (Tar DNA binding protein), ubiquitin positive inclusions. Hippocampal sclerosis common
  ○ 5% fused in sarcoma protein RNA binding protein, ubiquitin positive inclusions, onset usually early before age 50 y (30s–40s)
  ○ 10%–20% of FTLD is autosomal dominantly inherited. Each of the following account for 5%–10% of familial cases:
    ■ FTLD17-Tau; 100% penetrance; early onset (30–60 y)
    ■ C17-TDP43 with progranulin deficiency; lens-shaped neural inclusions, variable penetrance, mean onset age 62 y
    ■ C9orf72-TDP43; hexanucleotide repeat with RNA, can have ALS or family history of ALS
- **Language variant: progressive nonfluent aphasia**
  ○ Tau in most, TDP43 in 20%. Can be seen with PSP, CBD, FTLD-TDP 43 progranulin, and ALS
- **Language variant: semantic dementia**
  ○ TDP43

Dementia with Alzheimer's features

- **Alzheimer's dementia**
  ○ Tau in 3-repeat form causing inclusions (neurofibrillary tangles) and amyloid accumulation causing β-amyloid plaques
- **Language variant: logopenic progressive aphasia**
  ○ Alzheimer's features most common, occasionally TDP-43
- **Posterior cortical atrophy**
  ○ Alzheimer's features most common, occasionally CBD
- **Mixed dementia**
  ○ Alzheimer's features and vascular disease

Abbreviations: ALS, amyotrophic lateral sclerosis; CBD, corticobasal degeneration; CBS, corticobasal syndrome; FTLD, frontal temporal lobe dementia; FTD, frontotemporal dementia; PSP, progressive supranuclear palsy.

issues that may be more common in particular dementia syndromes. In later sections each sleep disorder type will be considered individually in more depth. But here a few of the most prominent sleep problems and the associations of these sleep problems with particular types of dementia are noted. Dementias that have synuclein inclusions, sometimes also referred to as synucleinoptahies, are associated with REM behavior disorder. Synucleinopathies include, DLB, Parkinson's disease with dementia (PDD), and multisystem atrophy. Rapid eye movement (REM) behavior disorder is commonly associated with dementias that have synuclein inclusions, sometimes also referred to as synucleinopathies. These synucleinopathies include LBD, Parkinson's disease with dementia (PDD), and multisystem atrophy. The synucleinopathies are also more often associated with disorders of arousal, and can more commonly have reduced responsiveness periods, and hypersomnia. Parkinson-related dementias have an increased prevalence of restless leg syndrome (RLS) and periodic limb movements. Progressive supranuclear palsy is associated with particularly prominent insomnia, likely caused by several factors including difficulties with swallowing, rigidity, and nocturia, as well as underlying changes in brain-related sleep mechanisms that are more affected in that disease process. Alzheimer's dementia is the prototype dementia affected by an irregular sleep-wake rhythm, and this is thought to be caused by dysfunction and lack of coordination of the circadian rhythm mechanisms of the brain. Vascular dementia is associated with obstructive sleep-disordered breathing (SDB). Although SDB may be more common in vascular dementia, SDB is generally common in elderly patients, and can be seen across all patients with dementia. Patients with dementia of the moderate to severe stage may be more susceptible to the phenomenon commonly described as sundowning, characterized by increased agitation and sometimes even hallucinations that occur in the late afternoon or evening periods. A variety of factors can contribute to this phenomenon in the specific dementias. Dementia subtypes such as AD, vascular dementia, and DLB/PDD are associated with more significant deficiency in cholinergic systems that can contribute to anxiety and agitation, and cholinesterase inhibitor agents can be helpful for neuropsychiatric symptoms in those patients. FTLD is often associated with a more marked deficiency of the presynaptic serotonergic systems, and medications that increase serotonin may be especially effective in improving neuropsychiatric symptoms in these patients, but sometimes cholinergic medications make them worse. Changes in electroencephalography (EEG) and sleep architecture have been studied in relation to specific dementias. For example, progressive supranuclear palsy (PSP) is associated with the most marked loss of REM sleep compared with other dementias. In AD, sleep spindles and K complexes deteriorate more than in other dementias.

Table 2 summarizes the specific sleep-related symptoms that may be most prevalent with particular dementia types and the major changes in sleep architecture that have been observed. In the sections that follow the individual sleep disorders including RBD, Irregular sleep wake rhythm (ISWR), Sundowning, SDB, hypersomnia, restless leg syndrome (RLS)/periodic Limb movements of Sleep (PLMS), and issues of sleep encountered in nursing homes are discussed.

SPECIFIC SLEEP DISORDERS AND DEMENTIA
REM Sleep Behavior Disorder

In REM sleep behavior disorder (RBD), patients briefly act out their dreams because of the loss of normal musculoskeletal inhibition during REM sleep. Dream content is often altered and patients report dreams in which they are being chased by people they do not know or attacked by animals. The patients may act out dreams with fighting or running away, and injuries to self or bedpartners frequently occur. To diagnose RBD definitively, an overnight polysomnogram with video recording is necessary. This can be important to rule out other underlying disorders that can mimic RBD, such as parasomnias or vivid dreams caused by OSA that would require different treatment. During the polysomnogram, patients with RBD may have episodes of complex motor activities in phasic REM or loss of REM atonia.

The full pathophysiology underlying RBD is not completely understood,[14] but it is likely caused by loss of the normal inhibitory mechanisms in REM sleep and excessive motor drive during REM. In animal models, lesions to the perilocus coeruleus region of the cat, and the sublateral dorsal nucleus in the rat, can result in complex behaviors in REM, and it is thought that in humans most RBD is likely to be related to disease affecting the analogous pericoeruleus region located in the human pontine tegmentum. RBD has been found to occur commonly in association with degenerative diseases that have synuclein disorders, in particular when that disorder affects the pontine region. The pericoeruleus region sends glutaminergic projections to the medullary magnocellular reticular nucleus, and this in turn activates glycinergic neuron projections that inhibit anterior horn cell spinal neurons. When pericoeruleus regions are affected by synuclein disease, it is thought that the spinal neurons could become less inhibited, and allow patients to act out their dreams.

In a series of patients with RBD who had dementia and/or parkinsonism, 97% (35/36) had an underlying synucleinopathy. In contrast, in 300 cases of autopsy confirmed non–synuclein-based neurodegenerative disorders, performed by the same group, none had a history of dream reenactment.[14] RBD can therefore sometimes be helpful in the differential diagnosis of dementia disorders. If patients with dementia have RBD, they are more likely to have a synucleinopathy, such as DLB, compared with another dementia such as AD, or those in the FTLD category. The frequency of RBD in the various types of synucleinopathies has been estimated to range from 50% to 80% for DLB,[15] 30% to 60% for PD,[16,17] and 80% to 95% for multisystem atrophy.[18,19] It has been suggested that DLB affects the lower brainstem structures earlier in the disease compared with PD, and this may account for RBD being more prevalent in DLB compared with PD. However, when PD is associated with dementia, there is higher likelihood of RBD than when it is not. Approximately 25% of patients with PD had RBD in 1 series of 65 patients, but, if they had PD and dementia, 77% had RBD.[20] With respect to onset of dementia, those with RBD had earlier onset of dementia compared with patients with PD without dementia. RBD can also be the first manifestation of a synucleinopathy-based degenerative disease and precede the onset of dementia or other manifestations of the disease. Thus, its presence may provide an early indication of a future neurodegenerative disease, and, if early treatments become available for these diseases, the presence of RBD may allow identification of patients at risk when early interventions could be initiated. In the earliest report of RBD as a predictor of neurodegenerative disease, 38% of male patients developed a degenerative disorder associated with parkinsonism 5 years after diagnosis of idiopathic RBD, which was typically 13 years after onset of symptoms.[21] In another longitudinal series of 93 patients older than 50 years diagnosed with RBD without a neurodegenerative disease, the estimated 5-year risk of development of a degenerative disease was about 20%, 10-year risk was 40%, and 12-year risk was 52%.[22] RBD is also more often diagnosed in male patients, although there has been some suggestion that women may have as much REM sleep without atonia (RWSA) in sleep in association with synucleinopathies, but be less likely to manifest it with more active behaviors. In some cases of RBD associated with degenerative disease symptoms can subside as the disease becomes more advanced.[23]

Table 2
Sleep-related symptoms and major changes in sleep architecture associated with dementia types

Dementia Type	Prominent Signs	Associated Sleep Disorders	Highlights Wake/Sleep EEG Changes
Alzheimer's dementia 25%–50% have sleep problems	Early memory loss, early difficulty with naming and word finding, early preservation of social comportment	**ISWR:** chronobiological changes, among others caused by SCN degeneration and pineal/melatonin dysregulation **Sundowning** Possible more OSA (OSA associated with APOE4)	Increased stage I sleep NREM dedifferentiation in later stages → poorly formed K complexes/spindles, poorly formed true δ waves, indeterminate NREM sleep Late stages → reduced REM quantity
DLB Up to 85% have sleep problems	Executive/attentional dysfunction occurring before or at the same time as parkinsonism. Visual hallucinations, sensitivity to neuroleptics, fluctuations in arousal	**RBD** (50%–80% of patients with DLB) **Hypersomnia** (changes in lateral hypothalamus) **PLMS** (high index in up to 74% of DLB) **ISWR** (phenotypically like ISWR in AD, unlikely to be caused by same changes as in AD)	REM without atonia
PDD 60%–90% have sleep problems	Parkinson's (asymmetric resting tremor, bradykinesia, akinesia, rigidity) responsive to Sinemet. PD at least 1 y before any cognitive symptoms. Cognitive symptoms primarily dysexecutive	**RBD** (30%–60% of patients with PD) **Sleep maintenance insomnia** **Hypersomnia** **RLS/PLMS**	Rapid blinking at sleep onset REM intrusion in NREM sleep EEG dedifferentiation in later stages in some cases → indeterminate REM and NREM with wake interspersed. Rapid and slow eye movements throughout sleep

Multisystem atrophy Includes former entities: Shy-Drager, olivopontocerebellar atrophy, and striatonigral degeneration	Axial parkinsonism, less common tremor, variable cerebellar (OPCA), variable autonomic symptoms (Shy-Drager). Dysexecutive cognitive syndromes	**RBD** (70% dream reenactment, 90% REM without atonia) **Nocturnal stridor** (vocal cord abductor paralysis can lead to sudden death at night. Treatment: tracheostomy) **Autonomic dysregulation** (may contribute to sudden risk sudden cardiac death at night)	REM without atonia
Progressive supranuclear palsy	Early falls, vertical eye movement paresis. Pseudobulbar affect. Can have aphasia and frontal cognitive syndromes	**Insomnia** **Hypersomnia** (patients can have low hypocretin) RBD is uncommon (except in the Guadalupean form)	Complete absence or large reduction of REM sleep No vertical eye movements in REM
Vascular dementia	History of vascular disease, stroke	**OSA** (possibly more frequent than in AD)	
FTLD	Early social comportment problems in behavioral variant	No characteristic disorders, can be phase advanced	
ALS dementia	Behavioral change in social comportment, dysexecutive syndrome with fasciculations and motor signs of ALS	**OSA in bulbar ALS**	

Abbreviations: ISWR, irregular sleep-wake rhythm; NREM, non-REM; OPCA, olivopontocerebellar atrophy; PLMS, periodic limb movements with sleep.

Certain medications can worsen RBD when patients have underlying susceptibility to it, or even trigger RBD. Tricyclic antidepressants, selective serotonin reuptake inhibitors (SSRIs), venlafaxine, mirtazapine, excessive caffeine or chocolate intake, and alcohol withdrawal can produce an acute RBD syndrome. It is likely that patients with underlying synucleinopathies or mild RBD would be susceptible to aggravation of their symptoms with these medications and substances. Thus it might be prudent to ensure that none of the medications or substances are exacerbating symptoms in patients with dementia and RBD.

The main treatments that have been shown to be effective for RBD are clonazepam and melatonin. Clonazepam does not reduce the loss of motor atonia in REM, but seems to reduce the impulse to have complex motor activity during phasic REM. Clonazepam at a dose of 0.5 to 2.0 mg at bedtime is approximately 90% effective. Melatonin can also be effective[24,25] and in one series 87% of patients responded.[25] Melatonin can be used alone or in combination with clonazepam. In the setting of dementia, it might be best to start with melatonin because it is likely to have fewer effects on cognition. Starting doses are 1 to 3 mg, which can be increased to 6 and 9 mg if necessary. High doses of melatonin may be associated with headache or gastrointestinal (GI) symptoms. Other treatments that have been tried have variable efficacy. Quetiapine can be helpful in some patients. Pramipexole and carbamazepine can improve RBD, possibly by reducing the amount of REM sleep. Cholinesterase inhibitor agents have variable effects on RBD, and can sometimes exacerbate symptoms. For a summary of a practical approach to evaluation and treatment of RBD in dementia, see the box which summarizes the practical assessment and treatment of sleep disorder in patients with dementia at the end of the article.

Irregular Sleep-Wake Rhythm

Irregular sleep-wake rhythm (ISWR) is a circadian rhythm disorder and is the most common sleep disturbance in AD. Patients with ISWR lack a well-defined sleep period. They may only sleep for 2 to 3 hours at a time, and then be awake for 2 to 3 hours, and continue this pattern throughout the 24-hour light and dark cycle, irrespective of day and night. At night, therefore, when more sleep is expected, they are noted to have lengthy wake periods, and in the day, when more wake is expected, they are noted to have repeated long naps. Typical complaints of the patient or the caregiver relate to issues of insomnia at night, and hypersomnia or sleepiness during the day.

The changes in the circadian rhythm seen in AD are more profound and different than those seen in normal aging, and may underlie in part the symptoms of ISWR. In normal aging there is a reduction of the amplitude of the core body temperature rhythm as well as changes in other circadian rhythm markers that indicate that the rhythm is not as robust. Elderly people also tend to wake about 1 hour before what would be expected based on their circadian period, a possible sign that the circadian rhythm has become less synchronized with wake-sleep cycles. In AD, the suprachiasmatic nucleus (SCN), which is the master biologic clock in the hypothalamus that regulates and coordinates all circadian rhythms, is affected by the disease process. The SCN of patients with AD has been shown to have tangles,[26] and has neuronal cell loss with reactive gliosis.[26,27] Vasopressin, one of the main peptides produced by SCN cells, has been found to be produced at one-third the normal rate, and its production no longer has a normal rhythmicity.[28] The pineal gland and melatonin systems are also affected in AD.[29] Melatonin is usually secreted from the pineal gland at the transition from daylight to evening. It acts on the SCN, and may play a role in resetting the phase of the circadian clock. Patients with AD have melatonin levels lower than age–matched controls, with some studies finding levels one-fifth that of age-matched normals. There is also a reversal of the relationship between night and day, such that nighttime levels are lower than normals, and daytime levels are higher. The pineal gland has several changes in AD that may alter its function. The adrenergic axons that synapse on the pineal gland are abnormal and swollen, the clock-related genes, per 1 and cry 2 genes, no longer oscillate normally, and monoamine oxidase (MAO) levels are increased. Increased MAO levels could deplete serotonin, which is a precursor to melatonin. Patients with AD with E4/E4 alleles, which predisposes to early-onset AD, have been shown to have greater reductions in melatonin levels compared with those with E3/E4 alleles. Some of the dysfunction in the pineal gland may be related to a functional disconnection between the SCN and pineal gland.[29]

Melatonin levels, and the loss of rhythmicity in the per1 and cry2 genes can be apparent early in AD, even before there are clinical symptoms in patients (in pathologic Braak stages I and II).[29] Even when asymptomatic, and when patients have no cognitive decline, cerebrospinal fluid levels of melatonin in these patients are also lower than in aged-matched controls.

The early loss in melatonin seen in patients with AD has stimulated consideration with regard to how this might play a role in the pathophysiology of the underlying degenerative disease. Melatonin has been shown to have neuroprotective and antioxidant properties, as well as reducing hyperphosphorylation of tau and neurofilaments, one of the abnormal processes that occurs in AD. Thus, it has been suggested that the low melatonin levels found in early AD might facilitate the disease process, which has led some to suggest that supplementation with melatonin might warrant study with respect to whether it might alter the course and progression of the disease in the earliest stages.[30]

Besides the SCN and the pineal gland/melatonin systems, patients with AD have changes in the zeitgebers that are critical for reinforcing and entraining regular circadian rhythm patterns. Zeitgebers are environmental cues that include social and physical activities, eating patterns, and light/dark environment cycles. The strongest zeitgeber for circadian rhythmicity is light, and patients with dementia often have disturbed patterns of light exposure, which can be a consequence of the nursing home environment, or caused by inactivity during the day, including sleeping during the day. Even patients with AD living at home may be exposed to only half the bright light stimulation ($\geq$2000 lux) of young adults and normal healthy elderly.[31,32] Light exposure may also not reach brain centers in AD as effectively because of disruption of the visual system. Cataracts and macular degeneration are common in elderly people and can interfere with the light signal reaching the brain, as well as retinal and optic nerve degeneration.

The circadian rhythm disturbances in AD have been found to worsen cognition and strongly affect function in patients with AD in several studies.[2,3] The sleep-related issues associated with it can also be a major cause for caregiver stress.[4,5]

ISWR treatment
The recommended approach to treatment of ISWR currently involves nonpharmacologic measures designed to strengthen zeitgebers and reduce factors that cause disruption of sleep at night. These approaches typically involve efforts to promote stimulation, activity, and light during the day, while reducing stimulation at night and trying to produce a more consolidated quiet period. Various specific types of interventions have been evaluated, including social activity programs, daytime exercise, daytime bright light therapy, and sleep hygiene recommendations (such as setting more regular bedtimes and reducing arousal factors at night). Approaches that implement multiple interventions simultaneously have been called mixed modality treatments and may be the most effective, although more evidence is still needed.[31]

Bright light therapy is one of the most studied therapies for treatment of ISWR. It makes sense that increasing light exposure could be helpful, because in healthy people it is one of the strongest zeitgebers, and light exposure is known to be suboptimal in many patients with dementia. In general, daytime bright light therapy seems to offer some benefit for patients with dementia and for patients in nursing homes, although there are mixed results. In one study, when high-intensity light wall fixtures were installed in a nursing home, sleep time improved by 15 minutes.[33] In another study, when morning outdoor light exposure was combined with physical exercise, reduction of daytime in bed, and reduction of noise and light at night, daytime sleep time was reduced, but there were minimal changes in nighttime sleep continuity and duration measured by actigraphy.[34]

A social intervention study also found promising effects on ISWR.[35] The social intervention program was provided for 1 hour daily for 3 weeks to 137 institutionalized patients with dementia. Sleep-wake rhythms were improved in those patients who had been poor sleepers at the beginning of the study. In poor sleepers with a baseline sleep efficiency of less than 50%, the intervention increased sleep time at night by about 40 minutes, reduced nighttime sleep latency by 40 minutes, and reduced daytime napping by about 40 minutes.

A mixed modality approach to treatment was tried in a randomized controlled study of community-dwelling patients with AD who had mean mini mental state evaluation scores of 12.[36] The treatment included a systematic sleep hygiene program including setting individualized rise times and wake times and reducing nighttime arousal factors in the first week, the addition of daily exercise of 30 minutes in the second week, and the addition of 1 hour of daily light therapy in the third week. Sleep parameters were measured by actigraphy at 6 weeks and 6 months later. Benefits were seen at 6 weeks with a 32% reduction in nighttime wakenings, as well as reduction in daytime sleepiness and depression. The benefits also persisted for 6 months. A larger mixed modality treatment study of 132 community-dwelling patient with AD examined the effects of light therapy, walking therapy, and individualized education regarding nighttime bedtime/rise time and arousal reduction.[37] Light therapy and walking therapy were tested alone and in combination with individualized education. All groups had improvements with therapy compared with a control group provided with only sleep hygiene information that was not individualized. Those who adhered more to therapy had greater gains. At 6 months, the gains did not persist, but there was variability in adherence.

Given that changes in melatonin are postulated to underlie some of the circadian rhythm disturbance in AD, melatonin might be expected to benefit treatment of ISWR in dementia. However, several carefully designed randomized trials with melatonin have been generally disappointing. These trials have included both large-scale multisite studies and smaller randomized studies.[38,39] An exception was the study by Dowling and colleagues[40] (2008) who found that melatonin and light therapy together seemed to produce benefit in reduction in daytime sleep and rest-activity rhythm, even when light therapy alone did not. Thus it might be that melatonin is only effective when used in combination with light therapy in patients with dementia. Differences with respect to the benefits of melatonin may also reflect heterogeneity in patient populations. It is known that later in the course of AD there is loss of melatonin receptors on the SCN (MT1 receptors), and it is possible that this might reduce benefits in that population.[41] Melatonin has occasionally been reported to cause some negative mood-related side effects, but that was not seen in one of the best controlled studies.[38] In one large study of dementia that examined the effects of light therapy and melatonin, benefits were seen for therapy with melatonin and for light, but some patients with melatonin had a deterioration in mood.[42]

Use of medications for treatment of ISWR: potential for harm

Another approach taken to treat the disrupted sleep at night in patients with ISWR is to use standard hypnotic medications. This approach might seem easier to implement from the perspective of caregivers or institutions, relative to the multimodal behavioral strategies described earlier. In general, there is no evidence that pharmacotherapy can help ISWR, and because hypnotics can have adverse effects, especially in dementia, the recent American Academy of Sleep Medicine guideline for treatment of ISWR does not recommend their use.[43]

Several studies have indicated that the use of sedative hypnotics in elderly patients may not alleviate sleep complaints in the chronic state.[44–46] Side effects such as increased sleepiness, sedation, forgetfulness, confusion, or rebound insomnia can occur and worsen overall status and satisfaction about sleep. In a meta-analysis of 24 studies of hypnotic use for treating insomnia in the elderly,[47] hypnotics had a 4.78 odds ratio (OR) for altered cognition and a 3.82 OR for daytime fatigue and sleepiness. The benefit for sleep was only small in this general elderly population, such that the overall risk/benefit ratio was considered unfavorable. The meta-analysis, did not target patients with dementia, only elderly patients, but it might be expected that the risk/benefit ratio for patients with dementia would be even poorer, because of being more vulnerable to the negative cognitive and sedating side effects.

The Beers list was recently updated and identifies medications that are associated with higher risks of side effects in elderly patients.[48] This list contains several medications that have been used for treatment of sleep, and these should be used cautiously in patients with dementia, who are even more likely than the general elderly to have adverse side effects. Included on this list is diphenhydramine (contained in Benadryl, Tylenol PM, and Advil PM), which has a strong anticholinergic profile and potential to cause delirium, as well as other anticholinergic medications including hydroxyzine (Visteril), promethazine (Phenergan), chlorpheniramine (Trimetron), and tricyclic antidepressants like amitriptyline (Elavil). Other medications to be avoided include the long-acting benzodiazepines (eg, flurazepam [Dalmane], diazepam [Valium], clorazepate [Tanxene], chlordiazepoxide [Librium], clidinium-chlordiazepoxide [Librax]), and the muscle relaxants and antispasmodics. It is recommended that the shorter acting benzodiazepines be only used at the smallest doses. Some argue that it is even reasonable to avoid these (eg, temazepam (Restoril), and oxazepam (Serax)) in patients with dementia.

There have been no placebo-controlled trials of newer hypnotics such as zolpidem (Ambien), zaleplon (Sonata), and eszopiclone (Lunesta) in patients with dementia. One study implicated zolpidem as causing a fall risk in an elderly group of patients hospitalized for hip fractures. One of the problems with the studies of fracture risk is that patients who have greater degrees of insomnia might be those who are more likely to get up during the night and are at higher risk of falls independent of taking the medication. One retrospective study showed that fall risk seemed to be higher in patients with insomnia who were not taking sedatives, compared with those on sedatives who did not have any complaints of insomnia.[49] One open-label study reported that trazodone was effective in treating sleep disturbance in two-thirds of patients with dementia with minimal adverse side effects.[50] With respect to other medications, there have been few systematic studies in dementia. Sedating antidepressants, including mirtazapine (Remeron), are sometimes used, but mirtazapine can exacerbate RLS/periodic leg movements syndrome (PLMS) and RBD, and therefore has the potential to worsen nighttime sleep, and can also be associated with morning sedation in some patients. Sedating antipsychotic medications are sometimes used for treatment of nighttime sleep in dementia, but a new black box warning has been added to these medications indicating that they are associated with an increased risk for sudden death in dementia. In general, for agitation, other measures to reduce agitation and hallucinations should be tried first. These alternatives can also include pharmacologic therapy with cholinesterase inhibitor agents, or with antidepressants such as SSRIs for treatment of anxiety (discussed later).

Although ISWR has been examined most extensively in AD and is the prototypical dementia associated with ISWR, other dementia subtypes may exhibit similar dissolution of the circadian rhythm. Although the underlying pathophysiology may be different from that of AD, DLB and PDD can have marked disruption of sleep at night with greater amounts of sleepiness during the day leading to the picture of ISWR. Patients with vascular dementia can also develop highly fragmented sleep at night, and sleepiness in the day. All institutionalized patients with dementia are likely to have reduced strength of zeitgebers that are likely to lead to deterioration of the regular circadian rhythm, independent of dementia subtype.

Sundowning

Sundowning is a term used broadly to refer to agitated neuropsychiatric behaviors in patients with dementia that first appear, or become evident, in the late afternoon or evening. Typical sundowning symptoms include delirium, physical combativeness, loud vocalizations, and wandering. In individual patients, symptoms can occur regularly beginning at a certain time, often between 4 and 11 PM. The prevalence of sundowning in institutionalized patients with AD ranges from 10% to 25%,[51,52] but, in community-dwelling patients, it may be as high as 66%.[6] It is hypothesized that sundowning may in part be related to the alterations in underlying chronobiological rhythms in patients with dementia, although there is little direct evidence for this. Changes in melatonin secretion, delay in the body temperature rhythm, alterations in the cholinergic projections from the nucleus basalis of Meynert, and the dysfunction of the SCN could all contribute to altered brain processing capacities or mood changes in the evening hours. Klaffke and Staedt[53] (2006) proposed that sundowning could be caused by a mismatch in the arousal signals that have to be processed around the evening hours, and the capacity of the neocortex to process these signals when the cortex is becoming deactivated and preparing to sleep. Factors that can worsen sundowning include exhaustion, reduced lighting, increased shadows, new environments, changes in caregivers, or changes of shifts in nursing homes.

Some investigators have questioned the legitimacy of the concept of sundowning, partly because the term is so nonspecific and includes so many different behaviors.[54] A few studies have also found that agitation is sometimes worse in the daytime than in the evening.[52] Investigators have suggested that sundowning might partly be caused by the perception of caregivers and staff who are more fatigued or understaffed in the evening and thus are less able to redirect or offer support to the patient with dementia, which results in increased agitation.[55] In contrast, one study of institutionalized patients found that there were individualized patterns of peak agitation, even when all residents were exposed to the same environment, which argues for a biologic basis for the agitation.[56]

It might be best to understand sundowning as an underlying vulnerability to having increased symptoms around a certain time of day, usually in the evening hours, which can be triggered by environmental circumstances or other individual intrinsic biologic conditions around that time. Thus, factors in the environment such as poor lighting, unfamiliar circumstances, and changes in staff might trigger increased agitation especially around the vulnerable time, and factors related to the patient's underlying biologic state, including a patient's underlying anxiety, sleepiness from sleep disorders, or the side effects of medications, could become more apparent and trigger agitation during the vulnerable period.

Treatment of sundowning

Interventions in the environment to reduce sundowning can include ensuring that lights are bright in the evenings to reduce the likelihood of misperceiving stimuli because of poor visual processing; arranging schedules so that patients are not exposed to unfamiliar environments in the evening; and, in institutions, being careful to minimize disruption and noise associated with staffing changes while offering greater reassurances to the patient around the time that sundowning occurs. Addressing the underlying biologic predispositions of patients to agitation and confusion includes treatment of any underlying anxiety (first-line pharmacologic treatment in patients with dementia might be a morning dose of an acetylcholinesterase inhibitor agent and/or an SSRI) and reduction of medications that could increase the likelihood of development of confusion. Medications that might be used to calm the patient down might be counterproductive if they cause more prolonged changes in arousal that could contribute to confusion (eg, muscle relaxants or diphenhydramine [Benadryl]). Medications that could directly induce a higher likelihood of having hallucinations need to be carefully reviewed and preferably eliminated or used at the lowest necessary doses (eg, amantadine, MAO inhibitors, selegiline). Caffeine can promote a mismatch between processing of information and fatigue as well as contributing to disrupted sleep at night, and therefore might be best carefully controlled or eliminated. If the patient is not getting enough sleep at night, this could lead to increased sleepiness and fatigue at the end of the day, making the patient more vulnerable to confusion. Thus, further factors that cause sleep disruption at night might be carefully reviewed and treated accordingly, see the box "Hallucinations-agitation in evening or night: treatment algorithm" at the end of the article. Several case reports describe resolution of delirium and agitated states after treatment of OSA, showing that disrupted sleep patterns at night can contribute to agitation.

In some cases, especially in patients with more severe dementia, patients may have difficulty communicating their physical needs, and agitation might be related to underlying physical needs that have not been met, such as hunger, pain, or needing to use the bathroom. In individual cases, especially when communication is poor, it might be important to determine whether these issues could be contributing to the agitation. To reduce the likelihood that these factors are playing a role in such patients, such patients could be tried on a scheduled snack before the time that they typically develop agitation, or be scheduled for regular bathroom breaks. If the problem is worse acutely, or the sundowning is of recent onset, the possibility that there might be an acute delirium also needs to be considered. Acute delirium could be caused by underlying infection or drug toxicity and, if the agitation is of recent onset, these possibilities need to be evaluated. Also, symptoms of wandering and pacing, which is often included as one of the symptoms seen with sundowning, may be a presentation of RLS. The symptoms of RLS, like sundowning, occur according to a circadian schedule, and are worse in the evenings (further discussion in section on RLS later).

Various interventions to treat sundowning have been evaluated and investigated in the literature, but there have been no studies of mixed modality approaches, which target a combined group of possible contributors in a specific case, like any combination of those discussed earlier. When isolated interventions for sundowning have been evaluated alone, there have been mixed results. One study evaluated the effect of increasing lighting in the 19:00 to 21:00 period. In this small study, 8 of 10 patients had improved sundowning symptoms, and those who benefitted most had the worst symptoms.[57] However, a review of 8 trials did not find evidence of overall benefit for lighting.[58] As discussed in the context of ISWR, melatonin has been tried for treatment of sleep disturbances, but most trials have not specified the impact on sundowning in particular. Small case reports and open-label studies have found some benefit in afternoon agitation.[59–61] Neuroleptic agents are perhaps the most prescribed medications for agitation and delirium or disruptive behaviors, but the evidence that they help with sundowning is limited.[62] In addition, these agents can worsen confusion, cause sedation, and impair cognition of patients with dementia[63,64] and may contribute to the problems of patients with dementia or even perpetuate agitation.[65] A meta-analysis found that patients with dementia have a higher risk of sudden death with the use of antipsychotics[66] and, as previously mentioned, a black box warning has been added specifically for the use of these agents in patients with dementia because of this risk. Cholinesterase inhibitor agents have consistently been shown to reduce neuropsychiatric symptoms, including hallucinations in patients with dementia,[67] and the evidence suggests that they therefore might be useful in sundowning. One case report found sundowning symptoms to be decreased in a patient with DLB after starting donepezil.[68] Because donepezil can cause increased vivid dreaming, this might not be the first choice of medication to try, and galantamine and rivastigmine might be better. All cholinesterase inhibitor agents should be dosed in the morning, despite package insert instructions, because they can cause insomnia.

Since sundowning includes so many varied behaviors, and treatment often depends on the symptoms in the individual case, including the factors that could be promoting the syndrome in a particular case, and the patient's underlying biologic issues (pain, anxiety, and so forth); some investigators have suggested that it is better to speak to caregivers in terms of the individual symptoms rather than refer to the problem as sundowning. The use of the term sundowning might imply a more unitary concept that would be expected to be treated with a unitary solution. Emphasizing the particular symptoms of the patient may help the caregiver to recognize that there can be varied approaches to treatment depending on the person's symptoms. This approach might also help to facilitate acceptance of a multifactorial approach to treatment that targets environmental as well as intrinsic biologic factors.

Sleep Disordered Breathing (SDB)

Prevalence and association of cognitive impairment and dementia with SDB

Dementia is common in elderly people, with estimates of a prevalence of up to 60%.[69,70] Because dementia is a disease affecting mostly elderly people, SDB would be expected to be common in patients with dementia on that basis. However, dementia may also confer a further risk for having sleep apnea. In institutionalized patients with dementia, one study found that 70% to 80% had an apnea hypopnea index (AHI) of greater than 5 events per hour.[71] SDB has also been reported to be particulary common in patients with vascular dementia. New studies have been indicating that SDB may be an independent risk factor for stroke and cerebrovascular disease, thus it might be expected that patients with vascular disease should have an increased risk for SDB.[72] There have also been studies suggesting that SDB may be more common in AD than in the general population.[73,74] The APO E4, lipoprotein allele, which is linked with a higher risk for AD, has been associated with an increased risk for OSA in some studies,[75,76] although other studies did not find this association.[77,78] Why AD should be associated with an increased risk for SDB is unknown, but some have speculated that it might be because of degeneration of respiratory nuclei in the brainstem. Another possibility is that the hypoxia of apnea in some manner increases the risk for dementia or accelerates manifestation of AD in those who are vulnerable to it.

Signs that a patient might have SDB include snoring, witnessed apneas, and restless behaviors at night that do not respond to usual therapy. If apnea is suspected, then a sleep study can be obtained. A particularly high suspicion for apnea may need to be maintained for patients with vascular dementia, because they may not have the same symptoms as the general population with apnea. Patients with cerebrovascular disease and SDB are less obese and are less likely to be sleepy than other SDB populations.[79,80]

Relationship of SDB to cognition and delirium

The relationship between cognitive impairments and SDB is complex, and variable from individual to individual. At the extreme, there are cases in which SDB can be responsible for severe cognitive impairment and even delirium, which can be completely reversed by continuous positive airway pressure (CPAP) therapy.[81–84] Such cases serve as a reminder that it is important to consider SDB in all patients presenting with cognitive dysfunction and concern for dementia, because, if found, treatment might completely restore normal function.

In most cases of SDB, the impact of OSA on cognition may be less severe. Meta-analyses that have examined nondemented patients indicate that SDB most often affects measures of vigilance, attention, and possibly psychomotor function, whereas its impact on language and memory performance is less consistent.[85,86] Studies that include elderly populations and might be expected to show a stronger relationship between cognitive impairment and apnea have not always found consistent associations between apnea and cognition.[70,87,88] One large study of community-dwelling healthy elderly patients, including 827 subjects with an average age of 68 years, found no relationships between apnea and cognitive measures, despite the use of a sophisticated neuropsychological battery.[70]

However, other studies show associations between SDB or symptoms of SDB and dementia or cognitive impairment.[71,89–91] One recent study followed an elderly group of women with an average of age 82 years and found that those who had an AHI greater than 15 had an increased risk of dementia compared with those of the same age without apnea, when adjusted for a variety of other comorbidities.[91] The adjusted OR was 1.85 for being diagnosed with mild cognitive impairment or dementia when tested 5 years after the initial sleep study.

Discrepancies in the results of studies examining the relationship between cognitive impairment and apnea in the elderly could be caused by differences in the age of patients included, and whether the study was more or less likely to include patients with dementia. Studies including higher age groups, and those with known cognitive problems, might be expected to increase the ability to examine the relationship between cognition and apnea. There may also be a subpopulation of people who are more vulnerable to the cognitive impact of sleep apnea in the elderly, which could vary from study to study. Two recent studies examining cognition in elderly patients found that only those who were APO E4 positive, and not those who were APO E4 negative, had impairment on memory tests that correlated with apnea.[92,93] Thus, the carrier status of the APO E allele might be a marker for patients more vulnerable to the effects of apnea.

The mechanisms by which apnea might impair cognitive function or directly affect dementia include the potentially negative effects of intermittent hypoxia on neuron health, or the effects of chronic sleep deprivation or sleep fragmentation. Sleep may protect against the development of degenerative processes and poor sleep may make the brain more vulnerable. Animal models have suggested that cell death and even amyloid deposition may both be furthered by sleep deprivation.[94,95] However, it should be noted that insomnia in humans has not been shown to be associated with increased risk for dementia.

Treatment of SDB in the setting of cognitive impairment and dementia

With regard to whether apnea treatment improves symptoms of patients with dementia, there are reports of those who do extremely well and can have remarkable improvements (discussed earlier). Other studies have shown generally positive effects, although these are not usually as marked as in the case reports with instances of great improvements. In one small sham-CPAP controlled randomized 6-week cross-over study of 52 patients with mild Alzheimer's dementia, PAP therapy resulted in improvements in sleepiness and mood and had a small positive impact on neuro-psychological test performance.[96] A further small continuation study compared the profile of patients with AD who were able to sustain CPAP use over 1 year versus patients with AD who discontinued use.[97] Although not randomized, the 5 patients who remained compliant on CPAP showed less cognitive decline, had stabilization of depressive symptoms and sleepiness, and had subjectively improved sleep quality compared with those who discontinued use.

In patients with vascular dementia, CPAP therapy may have a particular role in reducing progression of disease, because apnea treatment may reduce the risk for vascular events.[98,99] In this population of patients with stroke or vascular disease, the symptoms and signs that increase suspicion for apnea may not be present, because patients with apnea and stroke are less often obese, and less often sleepy.[79,80] Thus, a high index of suspicion for apnea should be maintained in these patients.

Patients with dementia are generally able to tolerate PAP therapy at about the same rate as healthy individuals.[96,100] Therefore, it should not be assumed that the presence of dementia will present an insurmountable barrier to CPAP adherence. The caregiver may have to be more involved in ensuring that the patient uses PAP therapy and provide reminders to continue to use it. CPAP therapy has been reported to help with the sleep of caregivers because it can reduce nighttime awakenings.[96,97] This benefit to caregivers should also be taken into account when considering recommending PAP treatment, because patients with dementia are reliant on caregivers and caregiver distress is one of the main reasons for institutionalization of patients with dementia.

When CPAP is not tolerated, alternative therapies can be considered. In elderly patients apnea is sometimes highly positional, and positional therapy with a strict lateral sleep positioner may treat apnea. Other alternatives to PAP therapy include dental appliances. In cases of complex apnea that are more difficulty to treat with PAP therapy, positional therapy might be an alternative option. ASV PAP devices can also be tried and can be well accepted in patients with dementia.

Hypersomnia

Hypersomnia can be the consequence of poor sleep at night, ISWR, as well as other factors. Refer Box "Excessive daytime sleepiness and napping: treatment algorithm", addresses factors that should considered in the assessment of hypersomnia in the patient with dementia.

However, hypersomnia can also be the result of an intrinsic disorder affecting the sleep-wake cycle that is specific to certain types of dementia. For example, in DLB, reduction of arousal during the day is a prominent symptom. In one small study of 31 patients with DLB who were not selected for sleepiness, the average latency to fall asleep on the Multiple Sleep Latency Test was markedly abnormal at 5 minutes, compared with more than 10 minutes in patients with AD.[101] The fluctuations in arousal in DLB can cause large fluctuations in attention and cognitive capacity. These fluctuations are different from the cognitive impairments seen with sundowning, because they are not associated with agitation or active behaviors. Instead they are associated with a tendency to be sleepy and a failure to communicate or engage in activities. In the case of DLB, the arousal dysfunction can be variable from day to day and from hour to hour, and does not occur with a circadian pattern. This distinctive arousal fluctuation has been recognized as prominent and specific to DLB, such that it is currently included as one of the 3 core features in the diagnostic criteria used to make the diagnosis (along with visual hallucinations and extrapyramidal/parkinsonism symptoms). Patients with Parkinson-related dementia, like DLB, can similarly descend into somnolent states from which they can be difficult to arouse. Dopaminergic agents such as pramipexole (Mirapex), ropinarole (Requip), or bromocriptine, which are often used in these patients, can induce sleep attacks and sleepiness, but the arousal dysfunction seen in the cases of DLB and PDD is not completely attributable to medications and can occur independently of them.

The pathophysiology underlying the loss of alertness and arousal in PDD and DLB is not fully understood but may have something to do with dysfunction of the lateral hypothalamus, which contains histamine and orexin/hypocretin cells that are important for maintaining alertness during the day. Initial studies failed to show changes in hypocretin/orexin levels in patients with DLB, but recent studies have shown that some DLB and patients with PD have neuropathologic evidence of loss of hypocretin/orexin cells.[102,103] DLB shares some features of narcolepsy, which is also characterized by sleepiness in the day. Patients with DLB can have hallucinations that can occur when they are awakened out of sleep like in narcolepsy.[104] Narcoleptic patients have an increased risk of RBD, which is also seen in patients with DLB. The sleepiness of PD-related diseases is less dependent on nighttime sleep quality.[105,106] Patients who sleep longer at night can still have increased daytime sleepiness, which suggests that the sleepiness is caused by a central mechanism rather than sleep deprivation. Although nighttime sleep in patients with PD can be disrupted for a variety of reasons, the presence of PLMS, sleep apnea, and sleep fragmentation does not necessarily correlate with the degree of daytime symptoms in PD and DLB.

Stimulants like those used in narcolepsy, such as modafinil (Provigil) and armodafanil (Nuvigil), might be helpful for treatment of symptoms in DLB and PDD. One open-label pilot drug sponsored trial showed that armodafanil (Nuvigil), which started with a dose of 150 mg and was titrated to 250 mg after 30 days, caused marked improvement in alertness in patients with DLB, and also improved quality of life for both patient and caregivers.[107]

RLS and Periodic Limb Movements of Sleep

RLS

RLS is an important diagnosis to consider in dementia because it can manifest as increased agitation or wandering and pacing in the evenings, as well as insomnia. RLS may be the underlying disorder responsible for symptoms in some cases described as sundowning if wandering and pacing are prominent symptoms. More than 80% of patients with RLS have problems either falling asleep or getting back to sleep during the night because of their symptoms, and, if RLS is present, this could also be a major cause for sleep disturbance during the night. If the patient has RLS, targeted treatment of RLS may resolve these symptoms. RLS is more common in patients with renal disease, iron deficiency anemia, neuropathy, rheumatoid arthritis, and Crohn's disease, among other conditions, and, if a patient with dementia has any of these conditions, the possibility of this condition should be considered with even more care.

To make the diagnosis of RLS, the patient must endorse 4 essential clinical features of the syndrome: (1) the presence of an urge to move the legs that may or may not be accompanied by uncomfortable sensations; (2) the urge to move or sensations is partially or totally relieved by movement such as walking or stretching as long as the activity continues; (3) the urge to move or sensation has a circadian pattern and occurs more in the evening or at night; and (4) the urge to move or sensation is worsened with rest, inactivity, lying down, or immobility (eg, in a car, airplane, train). Because the diagnosis is based on subjective features, it can be challenging to know whether someone has this syndrome when they are not able to answer questions for themselves reliably, as occurs in some patients with dementia. Supportive information that might help to make the diagnosis in patients with dementia can include a positive family history and a high Periodic Limb Movement Index (PLMI) on a polysomnogram. The caregiver input can also be useful for making the diagnosis. RLS is typically more common in women, and can peak in elderly people. One study showed that 16% of women aged 60 to 69 years met criteria for the syndrome, and up to 10% of people between 65 and 85 years have been reported to have RLS.[108,109] The percentages of patients with RLS in dementia is not known, but RLS may be more common in Parkinson dementia compared with other dementia subtypes. If it seems possible that the patient has the condition, it can be worthwhile trying interventions that might help the condition and evaluate for any benefits.

A few common look-alike conditions in the elderly should be distinguished from RLS. Akathisia may be mistaken for RLS, but akathisia has some different characteristics. It does not vary according to a circadian pattern and gets better when lying down. Pain syndromes caused by arthritis or joint symptoms should be distinguished from RLS as well. In the case of joint pain syndromes, pain relief may be achieved by repositioning, but continued movement is not required for resolution of symptoms once a better position is found. Leg cramps should also not be mistaken for RLS. Leg cramps affect a single muscle suddenly, and are not associated with a general feeling of discomfort or need for continuous movement other than the movement to relieve the cramp.

RLS treatment

RLS can be worsened by a variety of medications, and the first consideration with regard to intervention should be to review whether any medication might be worsening symptoms. Diphenhydramine (in Benadryl, Tylenol PM, and Advil PM) or other centrally acting antihistamines like hydroxyzine (Visteril) can strongly aggravate symptoms and cause markedly increased agitation, which is the opposite to the response that is typically desired when these medications are being used. Other medications and substances that worsen RLS include tricyclic antidepressants, lithium, dopamine blocking agents (including all the antipsychotic medications), and alcohol. Antipsychotic agents are often tried in an attempt to treat agitation or sundowning in patients with dementia, but, if there is a component of RLS, these may provoke greater agitation. SSRI and SNRI medications should preferably be dosed only in the morning because these can also aggravate symptoms. If the patient is not already on an antidepressant, and one is being considered, bupropion might be a best choice, because it can be associated with less of an impact on RLS. Substances such as caffeine and chocolate can aggravate RLS symptoms and should be eliminated. Structured daytime exercise can be helpful, as can massage of the legs, both of which have been shown to lessen RLS symptoms. RLS has been associated with low iron stores, and iron supplementation is another therapeutic approach to treatment. Patients should always have iron stores checked, and iron should be supplemented if it is in the lower end of normal range. Iron supplementation can be helpful for any patients with ferritin less than 45 to 50 ng/ml). Supplementation is typically started orally, although iron infusions can also be considered. Oral iron should be dosed with vitamin C to improve absorption. If iron deficiency is present, the patient should also be evaluated for any causes of iron loss that might need further evaluation.

Pharmacologic management of RLS symptoms has typically included dopaminergic agonists as first-line agents (eg, pramipexole, ropinirole); in patients with dementia, gabapentin and gabapentoid agents are better first-line agents because of their better side effect profile and lower risk of hallucinations. Doses of 100 to 600 mg of gabapentin may be helpful, and can be dosed 1 hour before symptoms and again before sleep at night to help with sleep onset.

Periodic limb movements of sleep

Periodic limb movements of sleep are common in the elderly and may affect up to 50% of people older than 65 years.[110,111] These movements typically consist in dorsiflexion of the foot, but may involve upper limbs as well; and they occur in repeated sequences at regular intervals while a person is sleep and unconscious (typically at intervals of 20–60 seconds). The vigor of the movements and whether they cause arousals from sleep varies from individual to individual. Although the RLS syndrome is more common in women, PLMS are typically present equally commonly in men and women. In the case of dementia, and dementia subtypes, the prevalence PLMS is not known, but PLMS may be especially common in dementia associated with parkinsonism, including PDD, and DLB. Depending on the vigor of the movements and the depth of the patient's sleep, as well as the patient's underlying arousal threshold, the movements may or may not induce arousals from sleep. Patients with RLS typically have periodic limb movements (>80% of patients with RLS have PLMS), but it is only a minority of patients with PLMS who have RLS (<20%).

Periodic limb movements in adults are usually considered clinically significant when they occur at a rate of at least 15 movements per hour (PLMI >15) and result in a daytime symptom. Patients who are elderly, especially in the setting of Parkinson-related disorders, commonly have PLM indices ranging from 50 to 150 per hour. But even in the setting of these high indices, patients may be unaware of the movements. It is sometimes difficult to know how clinically significant the PLMS symptoms might be in a particular patient. When there are symptoms such as disrupted sleep or unrefreshing sleep that are associated with PLMS, the condition is sometimes referred to as PLM disorder (PLMD). In the setting of a patient with dementia, if the PLMI is greater than 20 per hour, and if they are also often associated with arousals, it might be prudent to consider the possibility that these movements could be contributing to sleep disruption.

PLMS treatment

There has been considerable controversy and debate with regard to whether PLMS needs to be treated. If a patient is not symptomatic and does not have a sleep disturbance, then there is little need for treatment or interventions. In contrast, in patients with dementia, who often have problems with sleep-related symptoms, it may be worth targeting treatment to the possibility that the limb movement disturbance is clinically significant. Treatment approaches for high PLM indices typically parallel those of RLS. Most medications that aggravate RLS can aggravate PLMS. Caffeine, chocolate, and alcohol should also be avoided, and daily exercise can be helpful. Oral iron supplementation with vitamin C should be tried if ferritin is less than 45 ng/ml. If pharmacotherapy is desired, gabapentin might be tried as a first-line option, due to the undesirable side effects of dopamine agonists in dementia. However, if gabapentin, or gabapentoid agents, are not effective, then agents such as ropinirole or pramipexole could be tried.

The Nursing Home and Institutional Environment: Specific Considerations

Certain circumstances in nursing homes and institutions can specifically disrupt sleep-wake rhythms in patients with dementia. When reviewing the environment in a nursing home or hospital, the clinician should consider how often residents might be awakened at night by nurses entering their rooms, whether they have a well-matched roommate who is quiet at night, and whether the nighttime bedroom environment is quiet and dark from the perspective of nursing stations and light that might be present in the room. In the daytime, it is preferable that the institution be brightly lit and that there are opportunities to go outside in the natural sunlight. Daytime activities are important to enhance wakefulness during the day. Ample opportunity for walking and aerobic exercise as part of structured physical activity programs is especially important for patients with RLS, but can also be helpful for mood and the circadian rhythm in all patients with dementia. In patients with nighttime sleep disruption, caffeine (including so-called decaffeinated drinks) should be eliminated, including in the morning (see the case example in this article). In patients with insomnia and sleep disruption at night, it is important to review whether patients are being provided too many napping opportunities during the day. Some nursing homes implement structured bedroom rest schedules during the day. If this is the case, consider having these shortened for patients with nighttime sleep difficulties.

PRACTICAL ASSESSMENT AND TREATMENT OF SLEEP DISORDER IN PATIENTS WITH DEMENTIA

A practical approach to treatment of patients with dementia includes identification of general factors in addition to those that might be recognized as reflecting primary sleep disorders. Patients with dementia are more vulnerable to the effects of any external factors on their physiology and sleep, and thus the factors that are known to affect sleep at all ages and under all circumstances need to be scrutinized carefully. A sample initial interview inventory is provided in **Box 1**, which covers some of the most important information needed to identify general factors that might need to addressed to best treat sleep problems. Although OSA, or periodic limb movements of sleep, or REM behavior disorder may be causing sleep disruption in a specific patient, the patients with these specific primary sleep disorders will not have their sleep problems fully addressed even if these specific issues are treated unless other general factors that can have magnified effects in patients with dementia are also considered.

Boxes 2.1, 2.2 and **2.3** provide guidelines for how to use the information gathered in the general inventory when addressing the main complaint of the patient with dementia. These tables are divided into 3 main categories of sleep complaint: (1) insomnia, cannot sleep at night; (2) hallucinations and agitation, in the evening or night; and (3) hypersomnia, including excessive daytime sleepiness and napping. As can be seen in these tables, each of these complaints can be caused by multiple factors, and all these factors need to be considered to best address the underlying sleep problem. For example, if someone is not sleeping well at night and a complete caffeine inventory is not taken and considered, it is unlikely that many other interventions will be fully effective unless caffeine is also eliminated. It is common to see

---

Box 1
Practical guide to evaluating sleep in dementia: individualized assessment sleep inventory

---

Initial interview questions

1. Main complaint (identify what concerns or bothers the patient most without the help of the caregiver first; then from the caregiver perspective). Identify targets/main goals for treatment.

2. After listening to the patients/caregiver, review 3 major categories of sleep related symptoms, and identify which are affected. (1) Insomnia – cannot sleep at night, (2) Hallucinations/anxiety at night, (3) Excessive daytime sleepiness.

3. Perform an inventory of symptoms associated with primary sleep disorders: (1) OSA (loud snoring, witnessed apneas), (2) RLS (discomfort in limbs, worse in evening, relieved by movement, worsened when confined or still), (3) RBD (acting out dreams). Any history of premorbid sleep disorders (prior history of insomnia, hypersomnia; prior concern for OSA).

Amount, timing, and quantity of sleep inventory (gives more objective overview of sleep time and pattern, and can also request sleep log or obtain actigraphy for additional information)

1. Bedtime, wake time.

2. Time to fall asleep: if not falling asleep, any activities (TV, getting up to eat, and so forth)?

3. Waking up at night: number of times, how long each time, any activities associated with wake episodes (eg, bathroom, TV, eating).

4. Daytime naps and dozing: what times, how long.

General intake information related to individual habits, history (these can be major targets for intervention)

1. Caffeine: specifically ask about tea, sweet tea, iced tea, soda, diet soda, coffee, decaffeinated coffee, and chocolate.

2. Alcohol.

3. Detailed and accurate review of all medications.

4. Detailed review of all over-the-counter medication including Tylenol PM, Advil PM, diphenhydramine.

5. Reflux, nasal congestion, coughing at night, pain at night?

6. Temperature at night?

7. Dark at night, light in day? Quiet environment at night, active environment in day?

8. Mood: depression, anxiety?

9. Nocturia?

10. Habits before bedtime? Dinner time, eating after dinner, dozing before bedtime, TV in BR, TV/computer before bedtime.

Epworth Sleepiness Scale (ESS; a useful inventory for comparing treatment efficacy for future; may need caregiver responses if patient is not reliable). How likely are you to doze off or fall asleep in these conditions? 0, never; 1, slight chance; 2, moderate chance; 3, high chance. Reading, watching TV, talking to someone, lying down in the afternoon if circumstances permit, sitting in public place, sitting after lunch, passenger in a car for an hour, driver in traffic a few minutes. Total possible = 24; ESS ≥10 is sleepy. (Johns MW. A new method for measuring daytime sleepiness: the Epworth sleepiness scale. Sleep 1991;14:540–5.)

---

a patient in clinic with dementia on a sleep aid at the same time that the patient is drinking excessive amounts of caffeine. It would be preferable to eliminate all caffeine, and be able to avoid using the sleep aid, which has the potential for negatively affecting the patient's cognition. In part because of their age, patients with

Box 2.1
Insomnia - cannot sleep: treatment algorithm

1. Eliminate all forms of caffeine, including hidden forms, based on careful interview. Inform that caffeine can have effects for more than 24 hours and affect sleep at night even if taken in the morning.

2. Attempt to eliminate alcohol. In patients with dementia, this may require removal from premises or limiting amount provided to patient.

3. If suspicion of reflux (major cause for arousals at night; can be silent or with cough): avoid food and fluids 3 hours before bedtime, consider raising head of bed, consider trial of PPI or other antacid).

4. If any suspicion of allergic rhinitis (a cause for worsening of snoring/apnea, increased arousals at night, postnasal drip, and coughing): trial of nasal steroid spray at bedtime, if more persistent, consider adding daytime antihistamine such as fexofenadine or loratadine.

5. If any suspicion of chronic pain at night, consider scheduled acetaminophen dosing; if not effective, consider gabapentin at night (starting dose 100–300 mg, may increase to 600–900 mg). Avoid opiates. May need mattress foam topper if there are joint difficulties. Ensure firm bed (with or without mattress topper) if there is back pain.

6. Address circadian rhythm factors/ISWR: avoid or time daytime naps, eliminate opportunities for daytime dozing (hard-back chair for TV in living room, no recliners during the day, and so forth), attempt to offer stimulating activities in the day especially at times when the patient might take naps or doze, ensure bright light in day, lower lights in evening and night, consider nighttime melatonin in combination with morning light and strict wake time. Avoid overstimulating activities at night, and eating at night.

7. Try to dose medication with sleep-disrupting effects earlier in the day (β-blockers, cholinesterase inhibitor agents, SSRIs, venlafaxine, bupropion). Consider alternatives to activating antidepressants if insomnia seems related. Donepezil (Aricept) is associated with more sleep disruption than other cholinesterase agents in some studies. Consider trial of switching to alternative galantamine or rivastigmine. Try always dosing cholinesterase inhibitor agents in the morning.

8. Remove TV from the bedroom.

9. Ensure that hands and feet are not cold before bed; if so, suggest feet soaks, warm socks, bath before bedtime. Then ensure that bedroom is not overly hot during the night.

10. If patient is worried about sleep and worries in bed when not able to sleep, review sleep time versus time in bed and consider setting later bedtime, and strict wake time for mild sleep restriction. Make clock not visible in bedroom.

11. Ensure that environment is free of noise and is dark at night (this can be of particular concern for patients in nursing homes).

12. Ensure that patient does not have other primary sleep conditions that affect sleep, like RLS (can cause sleep onset insomnia and arousals and awakenings) and OSA (can cause nighttime sleep disruption and maintenance insomnia). See text for discussion.

13. Nocturia: eliminate all access to fluids in 3 hours before bedtime. Consider taking twice daily medications at dinner rather than immediately before bed to reduce fluid load. Have routine in place to void immediately before bed. Dose diuretics earlier in the day if possible. Recognize that nocturia can be a symptom of OSA, and consider obtaining PSG.

14. Appropriate treatment of anxiety and depression: the cholinesterase inhibitor agents can help neuropsychiatric symptoms in dementia and may be particularly effective in AD and DLB. SSRI agents are first-line mood medication treatment. Both should be dosed in the morning.

15. Avoid use of sleep aids unless all other possible factors that might eliminate the problem without requiring medication have been addressed. Patients with dementia medications have more potential for side effects that can worsen cognition. If a sleep aid is used, target temporary use.

Box 2.2
Hallucinations-agitation in evening or night: treatment algorithm

1. Are the hallucinations benign? As long as they do not worry the patient, do not have paranoid or scary content, or interfere too much with activities, these are not necessary to treat; just educate the caregivers. Benign visual hallucinations/illusions are common with DLB.

2. Ensure that the patient is not taking medications that increase vivid dreams that might be interpreted as hallucinations or cause confusion in patients with dementia. If on donepezil, try alternative such as galantamine or rivastigmine. β-Blockers might be dosed in the morning. Tricyclics might be used at the lowest doses and, if possible, completely avoided because they also typically are anticholinergic. Zolpidem can cause vivid dreams and confusional arousals. If on this medication, then consider alternatives including reevaluation of factors causing sleep disruption that might be addressed without use of medications.

3. Can be secondary in part to sensory deprivation, especially in elderly patients with additional confusion from dementia. Ensure that hearing is good (ears cleaned), cataracts removed, using glasses if needed, good lighting before bedtime and in evening, bathroom lighting.

4. If it is possible that anxiety/depression is fueling hallucinations, consider cholinesterase inhibitor agents in AD, DLB (less so in FTLD) because these can sometimes reduce hallucinations. Rivastigmine or galantamine might be preferred for nighttime hallucinations because donepezil can cause vivid dreams. Could also consider SSRIs. Typical SSRIs: sertraline (Zoloft), escitalopram (Lexapro), citalopram (Celexa). Paroxetine (Paxil) has a more anticholinergic profile and is generally not as good a choice in patients with dementia. Fluoxetine (Prozac) is typically more activating and is not optimal for use in patients with dementia with nighttime sleep disruption. Other agents for mood regulation in dementia include venlafaxine and buproprion. Both these are activating and should be dosed in the morning. bupropion has less effect on PLMS/RLS than SSRIs and serotonin norepinephrine reuptake inhibitors (SNRIs).

5. Reduce use of medications that can increase confusion or cause sedation. These medications can lead to greater misinterpretation of sensory stimuli at night. If the patient is on a chronic benzodiazepine, consider tapering (should taper slowly to avoid withdrawal symptoms and increased anxiety). Should also avoid medications such as opiates, muscle relaxants, and all medicines with anticholinergic side effects (especially in AD and DLB) that might worsen confusion. Amantadine, which is anticholinergic, can cause hallucinations. Any medication being used as a sleep aid might exacerbate the confusion and it can be worth a trial of tapering off that medication while considering alternative behavioral interventions.

6. Reduce factors that cause arousals at night (see **Box 2.1**; eg, any caffeine, reflux, nasal, medications). Arousals in patients with dementia may be associated with more confusion than simply arousals, as might be seen in patients without dementia.

7. Consider basic needs as a cause for arousals and agitation in patients who cannot communicate well. Patients may be trying to communicate needs such as hunger, thirst, urination, pain.

8. If agitation occurs at a regular time every day, this could be sundowning. Consider possible environmental triggers (see text).

9. Is it RBD? Could the agitation or hallucinatory activity be related to brief acting out of dream content? Ensure safety in the environment. Start with trial of melatonin and use PSG to ensure that there is no other cause like OSA for acting out confused.

10. Agitation, delirium, and excessive dreaming can be caused by OSA. Consider evaluation for OSA.

11. Periodic limb movements of sleep and RLS can cause wandering and pacing.

Box 2.3
Excessive daytime sleepiness and napping: treatment algorithm

1. Ensure adequate nighttime sleep. Patients with dementia may not be reliable reporters of nighttime sleep quality or duration. Maintain high suspicion for (1) inadequate or disrupted sleep at night as a cause for daytime sleepiness, and attempt to address factors that might be causing arousals at night (See **Box 2.1**). (2) OSA or PLMS/RLS in selected cases. (3) insufficient sleep time (going to bed late, waking up too early). Inadequate nighttime sleep may be the most common cause of sleepiness during the day, and all the factors noted in **Box 2.1** should be reviewed.

2. Reduce or remove medications causing sedation. Rule out the possibility that hypersomnia might be induced by the use of sedating medications and remove any possible offending agents. Such agents might include muscle relaxants, benzodiazepines, and opiate medications. In the case of opiate medications, these can be slowly tapered, and, if patient had both day and nighttime pain, dose gabapentin generously throughout the day (eg, 300–600 mg 4 times a day and 600–900 mg at bedtime). Other medications that can cause sedation include tricyclic antidepressants; sedating neuroleptic medications, including olanzapine (Zyprexa), quetiapine (Seroquel), and clozapine (Clozaril); hydroxyzine (Atarax); clonidine; cetirizine (Zyrtec); diphenhydramine (Benadryl); and lyrica (Pregabalin). Medications previously well tolerated in middle age, or before dementia, may have more sedating side effects when taken with dementia. Dopamine agonist agents can cause sleepiness and sleep attacks (eg, carbidopa/levodopa (Sinemet), ropinarole (Requip), pramipexole (Mirapex). All nighttime sleep aids can cause residual daytime sleepiness. Need to be suspicious and aware of side effects of sleepiness with all psychoactive medications. Patients with dementia are more likely to be living with the side effects of medications, because they are less likely to report them.

3. Daytime increased sleepiness caused DLB and PD. In a patient with DLB or PDD, hypersomnia may be caused by the underlying physiologic disorder as well as use of dopamine agonist medications. Even in DLB and PDD, consider other possible contributors to hypersomnia that may respond to other interventions. These patients may be especially vulnerable to the effects of other sleep disrupters or factors that produce sleepiness that can be addressed.

4. Daytime sleepiness caused by circadian rhythm disruption (see discussion on ISWR in text earlier, and in **Box 3.1**) is especially common in AD. Treatment is directed at consolidating nighttime sleep and reinforcing activity and stimulation in the day. Treatment suggestions include increased bright lighting in the daytime, increased daytime stimulation and exercise, ensuring quiet nighttime environment, avoiding situations in the daytime that are conducive to dozing (eg, sitting in recliner in front of TV after lunch or in evenings), trial of melatonin at night given at same time every night (0.5–3 mg), and setting a regular sleep-wake cycle with the same bedtime and same wake time. Eliminate caffeine, which can cause nighttime sleep disruption resulting in increased daytime sequelae of sleepiness.

5. Consider the possibility of depression. Depression can be associated with lowered activity levels and increased sleepiness. Such patients may benefit from a trial with an activating antidepressant, such as bupropion or venlafaxine.

6. Consider thyroid screening because it is readily treatable and levothyroxine may have a role in treatment of hypersomnia.

---

dementia may also be on multiple medications. It would similarly be desirable to eliminate certain medications or change to alternatives that might have less impact on sleep if these could be affecting the main sleep complaint, rather than simply adding medications that would be more likely to have a negative impact on cognition. Patients with dementia also often have anxiety or mild mood-related issues. These issues should be addressed with appropriate medications that can result in a positive benefit for both daytime alertness and nighttime sleep. Typical first-line choices are

Box 3.1
Treatment algorithm: SDB, ISWR in dementia

SDB

1. Obtain polysomnogram (PSG) to diagnose and characterize disorder. PSG determines presence and severity of SDB, Cheyne-Stokes breathing, and whether positional therapy is an option for patient.

2. Always maximally treat nasal congestion/allergic rhinitis in the setting of SDB, usually with nightly steroid spray with or without daytime antihistamine such as loratadine because this can worsen obstructive breathing and interfere with treatment, and is treatable.

3. If a patient is taking opiate medications, attempt to taper and substitute with high-dose gabapentin and/or scheduled Tylenol, because opiate medications worsen SDB. For example, if patient has pain in the day, add gabapentin and work up to 300 to 600 mg 4 times a day with 600 mg at bedtime, and taper off opiate medications.

4. If patients have Cheyne-Stokes breathing, ensure that heart failure is not present and, if it is, ensure that it is maximally medically treated.

5. After initiating treatment of rhinitis, and tapering off opiates if present and possible, obtain trial for positive airway pressure (PAP) therapy. In patients with dementia who are elderly with more comorbidities, this is usually best done in an attended PSG study setting. Patients with Cheyne-Stokes breathing or central components to apnea may be more comfortably and effectively treated with adaptive servoventilation (ASV) PAP therapy.

6. Elderly patients may be more likely to have mouth breathing and jaw laxity and may be more comfortably treated with masks that cover both mouth and nose.

7. If starting PAP therapy, it is essential to have good follow-up to work on mask fit issues, and to motivate for treatment adherence. This work can be provided by sleep specialists, or by informed primary physicians, or allied personnel. In follow-up, remind patients that adherence can help sleep continuity, reduce nocturia, reduce arousals with agitation at night, improve daytime alertness, and emphasize any gains to help motivate adherence. PAP may also reduce stroke risk.

8. If a strong positional component is present and REM sleep was evaluated in the lateral position in the diagnostic study, clinicians can consider strict lateral positional therapy as an alternative to PAP. Strict lateral sleep positioners need to be used (eg, commercial vendors are sometimes easier for patients to use and adhere to and include Rematee [www.rematee.com] and zzomaosa [www.zzomaosa.com]). Homemade lateral positional devices (eg, tennis balls in a sock attached to the back of a t-shirt with safety pins) can be used, but elderly patients are sometimes more compliant with commercial options.

9. Patients who are intolerant of PAP therapy, or not candidates for lateral positional therapy alone, can be treated with dental appliances. These can also be used adjunctively with lateral positional therapy if apnea is still present in a lateral position. Sleep studies should ideally be obtained after adjustment of dental appliances to ensure adequate treatment.

Irregular sleep-wake rhythm

1. Review all the factors in **Boxes 2.1** and **2.3** that can be affecting sleep at night or arousal level during the day.

2. Increase bright light exposure throughout the day, reduce ambient light and noise at night.

3. Increase stimulation and activity during the day if possible (scheduled walks, social activities), reduce exposure to environments conducive to sleep during the day (recliners, quiet TV watching).

4. Consider removal of cataracts that reduce light exposure to brain during the day, ensure glasses are provided if necessary, ensure ears are clean and hearing aids provided if necessary.

5. Trial of melatonin at night (0.5–3 mg) before bedtime (in conjunction with bright lights during the day).

6. Eliminate all caffeine except in early morning.

Box 3.2
Treatment algorithm: RBD, RLS/PLMS in dementia

RBD

1. Obtain PSG to ensure diagnosis is accurate and reported activity is not caused by underlying OSA causing arousals and confusion. If OSA present, treatment of OSA, as described later.

2. Immediately on considering diagnosis, advise measures to help ensure safety of patient and bed partner. RBD can be associated with sudden violent activity and lead to serious harm of patient or bed partner. Advise bed partner to sleep in another room until condition is treated. Remove all sharp objects, night stands, and lamps from immediate bedside environment. Consider advising use of light sleeping bag to restrict movements if acting out during sleep.

3. Remove or change dosing of medications/substances that may precipitate activity: MAO inhibitors, tricyclic antidepressants, SSRI, SNRI, alcohol, caffeine, chocolate. In the case of caffeine and chocolate, eliminate all consumption, including in the morning.

4. See **Box 2.2** regarding other causes of hallucinations and agitation at night to ensure that these factors have also been addressed.

5. Consider initiating pharmacologic treatment of RBD. If RBD is not confirmed on PSG, but OSA is found, consider treatment of OSA first.

6. If advice has been given on behavioral therapies, pharmacologic therapy can simultaneously be started. First-line pharmacologic treatment is not necessarily clonazepam in patients with dementia because of cognitive side effects. Instead, recommend first-line trial of melatonin (1 mg and increase to 3 mg, may increase to 6 mg, can increase to 9 mg, but high doses produce more headache and GI side effects). If melatonin not fully effective alone, may add adjunctive clonazepam, starting at lowest necessary adjunctive doses (0.5 mg). Temazepam may also be effective, but has more potential side effects than melatonin.

RLS/PLMS

1. Remove all medications and substances that could be worsening RLS/PLMS. These substances include all caffeine, chocolate, alcohol, tricyclic antidepressants (including amitriptyline), dopamine blocking medications (including antipsychotics, promethazine (Phenergan), metoclopramide (Reglan), prochlorperazine (Compazine), and diphenhydramine (Benadryl, Advil PM, Tylenol PM). SSRI and SNRIs can worsen RLS/PLMS and should be dosed away from bedtime, and, if necessary, an alternative medication for depression such as buproprion (Wellbutrin) might be used that has less effect on RLS/PLMS.

2. Behavioral measures can be helpful including daily aerobic activity, stretching exercises (especially of the legs), and massage of legs.

3. Obtain iron levels and supplement accordingly (for ferritin less than 45 ng/ml, advise supplemental iron every day dosed with tablet of vitamin C to help with absorption). Consider obtaining vitamin B_{12} level, treat if less than 350 pg/ml.

4. Consider initiate pharmacologic treatment of RLS/PLMS. See table.

5. First-line pharmacologic treatment with fewest side effects on cognition is supplemental iron in patients with low iron status (ferritin <45 ng/ml). In elderly patients with systemic disease, ferritin may be falsely increased and may need full iron panel. Iron treatment may be helpful in these cases if there is percent iron saturation <16%, total iron binding capacity >400 Mcg/dl, or total iron <60 Mcg/dl. Advise taking iron with vitamin C to increase absorption. If iron is in clinically deficient range, may also need work-up for sources of iron loss. If additional therapy is needed, try gabapentin at night 1 to 2 hours before bedtime or symptom onset (100–600 mg). Third-line therapy: dopamine agonists (ropinarole, pramixole) but these may cause more confusion. Fourth-line therapy: opiate analgesics (eg, tramadol, but ideally should avoid in patients with dementia).

Box 4
Medication strategies for non-specific sleep problems in dementia (see also discussion in text for specific cautionary information about use of medications (in "Use of medications for treatment of ISWR"))

Rules to remember prior to considering use of medications

1. Always remove medications that cause problems first.
2. Always implement behavioral measures first.
3. Always attempt to identify underlying problems and target specific issues before treating general symptoms.

Insomnia – cannot sleep: pharmacological approaches

Target temporary use, only if removal of agents, changing habits, and addressing other issues has failed (See **Box 2.1**).

First line: gabapentin at low dose can improve sleep symptoms and continuity (100–600 mg at bedtime). Melatonin is helpful in some patients.

Second line: trazadone and mirtazapine (Remeron) can worsen autonomic issues, and are typically associated with more daytime effects than gabapentin or melatonin. Zolpidem (Ambien) and eszopiclone (Lunesta) are also associated with more side effects than gabapentin and melatonin, and should be used at the lowest possible doses (Ambien, half a 5-mg tablet, or one 5-mg tablet; Lunesta, 1 mg). Sedating antipsychotic medications such as quetiapine (Seroquel) can worsen PLMS/RLS (but may help RBD) and are best used in patients with paranoia that is not responsive to cholinesterase inhibitor agents and used at lowest necessary doses (start with half of a 25-mg tablet). Use of benzodiazepines (e.g., lorazepam, diazepam) are not routinely recommended for sleep disruption in dementia, and, if being used chronically, should be tapered off slowly. Temazepam (Restoril) is the benzodiazepine with shortest half-life. Clonazepam is likely to be more effective for sleep than other benzodiazepines and helps RBD (but use at lowest possible doses). Zaleplon (Sonata) has the shortest half-life of newest generation sleep aids and may be useful for sleep-onset insomnia or waking in the middle of the night, but can have more side effects than gabapentin or melatonin. Diphenhydramine (Benadryl), Tylenol PM, and Advil PM have anticholinergic side effects that can worsen confusion/memory and PLMS/RLS.

Escessive daytime sleepiness and napping: pharmacological approaches

If other measures fail (See **Box 2.3**), pharmacologic therapy can be considered. First line, modafinil (Provigil), armodafinil (Nuvigil). Second line, methylphenidate (Ritalin) or other amphetamines can be used but have more side effects. Could also consider low-dose Synthroid (25 μg each morning) to boost wakefulness, especially if the patient has subclinical hypothyroidism (one study showed benefit with use of Synthroid in idiopathic hypersomnia, but this has not been studied in dementia). Consider use of activating antidepressants if there is comorbid mood difficulty: venlafaxine, bupropion.

Agitation in evening or night: pharmacological approaches

If other measures fail (See **Box 2.2**), pharmacologic approaches to treatment can be considered. Cholinesterase inhibitors in DLB, PDD, and AD can improve neuropsychiatric symptoms and should be tried, but dosed in the morning. Donepezil can be associated with causing vivid dreams, and thus galantamine or rivastigmine might be preferable in the setting of hallucinations. Should also address anxiety and depression, which can worsen at night. Use of SSRIs dosed in the morning may help with anxiety. Generally, avoid paroxetine (Paxil) because of anticholinergic side effects and fluoxetine (Prozac) because of activating profile, but can consider sertraline (Zoloft), citalopram (Celexa), escitalopram (Lexapro). Gabapentin (Neurontin) can be helpful at night to reduce arousal tendencies that can be associated with confusion, and typically is not associated with as much sedation as other sleep aids (doses might range from 100–600 mg). Melatonin can be tried. If paranoid content, can consider trials of low-dose antipsychotics (except in the setting of patients with DLB, in whom these should be carefully avoided because they can precipitate more rigidity that may not be reversible). Can consider Seroquel 25 mg tablets, starting with half a tablet at night. If agitation is also present in the day, can add half a tablet in morning. May titrate up to

1 tablet twice a day or higher doses if necessary. Need to be aware that antipsychotics increase risk of death in patients with dementia. Other sleep aids are also often used at night to reduce agitation episodes, including trazodone, but this can cause residual daytime effects and negatively impact cognition. Mirtazapine (Remeron) is sometimes used to help with sleep at night, as noted earlier, and may be helpful in depression or in the setting of weight loss, but can worsen PLMS/RLS, and may be associated with more confusion than gabapentin or melatonin. Typical mirtazapine doses start with 7.5 mg, and may be increased to 15 mg; higher doses are less sedating. See section on Insomnia, above, for other pharmacological approaches to improving sleep continuity which may also reduce agitation at night.

sertraline (Zoloft), escitalopram (Lexapro), or citalopram (Celexa) dosed in the morning.

Primary underlying sleep disorders including sleep apnea, RLS/PLMS, REM behavioral disorder, and ISWR should also be addressed in patients with dementia. Details of the treatment approach to these issues in the setting of dementia are provided in **Boxes 3.1** and **3.2.** It is also important to note that OSA can present as simply sleep maintenance insomnia in some patients, or restless movements at night.

Box 4 addresses the use of medications for the treatment of symptoms in patients with dementia having sleep-related problems. As emphasized, medications

---

General rules for treatment of sleep in patients with dementia

1. When using medications, only start one medication at a time.

2. Always write down the list of recommended interventions at each visit, so the caregiver/patient has a copy for their reference. This list is especially important because of the complex nature of patient care with dementia, in which the patient is not always able to be fully responsible, and the caregiver may be overburdened. In addition, comprehensive behavioral recommendations for sleep health can include many components, which are best written down for reference and can be reviewed specifically at follow-up (eg, recommendations of new set wake-up times, lighting, and reduction of medications).

3. Encourage the caregiver/patient to keep a binder with an accurate list of all medications, and lists from prior visits regarding recommendations.

4. Ensure that medications are being taken reliably. Patients with dementia might be taking repeated doses mistakenly, forgetting doses, or taking them at the wrong times. Pill boxes with structured checking to ensure accurate dosing is important for all medications (even if not prescribing sleep-specific medications, mistakes with regard to other medications can affect arousal, sleep, confusion, and agitation).

5. At clinic visits, first ask patients to provide their perspective on issues while caregivers are quiet for at least 5 minutes to allow patients the opportunity to show knowledge of their condition and their perspective. This opportunity helps clinicians to be able to later explain treatment goals to patients from the perspective of the patient's concerns. Having caregiver input throughout the interview can increase efficiency, but listening to the patient without caregiver input initially, even if information is not always accurate, shows respect for the patient and can help to build a stronger clinical relationship and rapport with the patient.

6. Although a comprehensive review of symptoms and treatment is essential, always target primary underlying sleep disorders such as OSA, RLS/PLMS, or RBD. These primary sleep issues can have as much, if not more, impact on patients with dementia than on patients without dementia. In the absence of targeted treatment of specific underlying sleep disorders, patients may not improve.

When to get a PSG in a patient with dementia and sleep problems

1. In the setting of sleep difficulties, first advise removal of all potentially offending agents and habits as per **Boxes 2.1, 2.2** and **2.3**.

2. Obtain PSG if:

   a. Has symptoms of OSA

   b. Has symptoms of acting out dreams at night (to evaluate for RBD and OSA, which can mimic RBD)

   c. Has nighttime sleep disruption that has not been responsive to other interventions (eg, treatment-resistant sleep maintenance insomnia, agitation, or hypersomnia that may be related to OSA in the absence of snoring)

---

for improving nighttime sleep are typically used as a last resort because they are more likely to be associated with side effects in the patient with dementia, and the effects of performing the general overall sleep assessment and addressing the underlying factors can be effective, and sometimes obviate the use of additional medications. An exception is the case of RBD when medications, starting with the type that is least likely to have side effects in dementia (melatonin), are likely to be needed. Activating medications such as armodafinil and modafinil can also be well tolerated in dementia, but other causes for hypersomnia should be addressed first. Studies examining the effects of newer sleep aid medications in patients with dementia are few, or are not designed to compare treatment with best alternative practice assessments for addressing sleep problems. Because of the lack of high-level evidence that compares the use of different types of sleep aids, the discussion in the table with respect to sleep aids to some degree reflects institutional practice habits.

SUMMARY

Dementia is common and increasing in prevalence worldwide. Sleep-related problems are a major source of caregiver distress and cause for nursing home placement. A practical knowledge of how to assess the patient with regard to whether they have (1) problems with sleep at night, (2) sleepiness during the day, or (3) agitation episodes is provided in this article. Although there are specific types of sleep problems that occur more commonly in patients with dementia and in patients with particular types of dementia, it is still essential at the initial evaluation to address first the common basic factors that might also be affecting sleep disruption, sleepiness, or agitation, because patients with dementia are often vulnerable to these factors. New knowledge has allowed clinicians to understand more directly the reasons why certain types of dementia are more often associated with certain types of symptoms, and it is expected that as knowledge of the underlying pathophysiology of dementias increase these will be refined further and may help in the selection of appropriate treatments. Whether sleep-related disorders including OSA, or limited sleep time, predisposes to the development of dementia is another area that is being explored. Comprehensive sleep evaluation is essential in the treatment of dementia, given that sleep-related issues are common, often treatable, affect patient function, and are a major cause of caregiver distress.

Case example

A 72-year-old woman presented to a sleep clinic with a complaint of sleep onset and maintenance insomnia. She had recently been diagnosed with probable mild dementia of the mixed type (AD and vascular dementia), and had been moved to a nursing facility. She reported having had problems with insomnia throughout her life, but that these had become worse recently. Bedtime was 10 PM and it would take hours to fall asleep. She also had difficulty staying asleep, awakening multiple times, and it was hard for her to get back to sleep. She estimated she would get only about 3 hours of sleep and would leave the bed for the day about 5:30 AM to get ready for breakfast. She also reported a history of snoring at night, chronic nasal congestion, leg jerks at night, leg discomfort at night possibly related to diabetic neuropathy, and nocturia (3–4 times per night). In the facility, she had been paired with a roommate with AD who would yell loudly for about an hour after she was awakened by staff at 2 AM most nights. Caffeine included 1 to 3 cups of half decaffeinated and half caffeinated coffee in the morning, and occasional additional coffee in the afternoon. Donepezil (Aricept) had been started around the time that the sleep problems worsened and she had been taking it at night before bedtime.

Initial recommendations to improve sleep were the following: she was advised to switch donepezil (Aricept) 10 mg to an alternative acetylcholinesterase inhibitor agent, galantamine ER (Razadyne) 16 mg, and to take this in the morning instead of at night. She was advised to discontinue caffeine, she was advised to limit all fluids 3 hours before bedtime, and she was referred for a sleep study.

At a return clinic visit, sleep had improved. She thought that the change was primarily caused by changing the donepezil medication. She now thought she was sleeping about 5 to 6 hours per night. She was still waking up during the night, but could fall sleep a little more easily. She expressed concerns about the facility environment. She continued to have difficulty with her roommate's agitation and she was worried people were stealing her possessions. The sleep study showed mild OSA with an AHI of 9, periodic limb movements of sleep (PLMS) associated with arousals (PLM Index of 15 per hour), increased electromyogram (EMG) in REM with arousals and disruption, and nasal stuffiness with mouth breathing.

During the course of subsequent follow-up visits, a variety of additional sleep-related interventions were implemented. She was treated for nasal stuffiness, underwent a PAP trial, and was started on PAP therapy. She was started on a low dose of gabapentin (200–300 mg at night) for limb movements and nighttime pain, and started on melatonin to help improve REM sleep continuity. Gabapentin and melatonin were started in a staggered fashion so that side effects and benefits could be monitored.

After all interventions had been implemented, sleep was improved. She was falling asleep immediately, and waking up only to go to the bathroom, after which she was readily able to fall back to sleep. She also reported less fatigue in the day when using CPAP therapy. Even though she still had a roommate with agitation, it did not bother her as much. She was generally sleeping well from 11 PM to 7 AM.

Three years later, the patient returned to clinic with new problems with sleep. She again was not able to fall asleep or stay asleep. She had moved to a new facility, where her environment was better, even though sleep onset and maintenance insomnia were worse. All environmental factors and medications were reviewed. The patient reported drinking only decaffeinated beverages, but the facility was contacted and it was determined that they were providing her with regular caffeinated beverages, which she had not realized. She was advised to discontinue drinking all tea and coffee. Sleep once again improved.

Case example comment

This case of insomnia in a patient with mild dementia highlights how many factors can simultaneously affect sleep in patients with dementia. It also highlights some of the special challenges faced when treating patients in the nursing home setting. Although this patient had OSA, it was also critical to consider how to adjust medications that could contribute to insomnia (in this case donepezil) and later to carefully inquire about a caffeine history. Additional interventions included limiting fluids 3 hours before bedtime and treating nasal stuffiness. The choice of sleep aids (gabapentin and melatonin) were made based on a consideration of the presence of periodic limb movements and comorbid pain problems, as well as the finding of increased EMG activity in REM with REM sleep disruption. Patients with vascular dementia are reported to have a higher risk for apnea. In addition to the benefits that apnea treatment may offer for sleep continuity and function, treatment might reduce risk of future strokes.

REFERENCES

1. Bliwise DL, Mercaldo ND, Avidan AY, et al. Sleep disturbance in dementia with Lewy bodies and Alzheimer's disease: a multicenter analysis. Dement Geriatr Cogn Disord 2011;31:239–46.
2. Bonanni E, Maestri M, Tognoni G, et al. Daytime sleepiness in mild and moderate Alzheimer's disease and its relationship with cognitive impairment. J Sleep Res 2005;14(3):311–7.
3. Moe KE, Vitiello MV, Larsen LH, et al. Sleep/wake patterns in Alzheimer's disease: relationships with cognition and function. J Sleep Res 1995;4(1):15–20.
4. Ballard CG, Eastwood C, Gahir M, et al. A follow up study of depression in the carers of dementia sufferers. BMJ 1996;312(7036):947.
5. McCurry SM, Logsdon RG, Teri L, et al. Sleep disturbances in caregivers of persons with dementia: contributing factors and treatment implications. Sleep Med Rev 2007;11(2):143–53.
6. Gallgher-Thompson D, Brooks JO 3rd, Bliwise D, et al. The relations among caregiver stress, "sundowning" symptoms, and cognitive decline in Alzheimer's disease. J Am Geriatr Soc 1992;40:807–10.
7. Mahoney R, Regan C, Katona C, et al. Anxiety and depression in family caregivers of people with Alzheimer disease: the LASER-AD study. Am J Geriatr Psychiatry 2005;13(9):795–801.
8. Pollack CP, Perlick D. Sleep problems and institutionalization of the elderly. J Geriatr Psychiatry Neurol 1991;4:204–10.
9. Bianchetti A, Scuratti A, Zanetti O, et al. Predictors of mortality and institutionalization of in Alzheimer disease patients 1 year after discharge from an Alzheimer dementia unit. Dementia 1995;6:108–12.
10. Gaugler JE, Edwards AB, Femia EE, et al. Predictors of institutionalization of cognitively impaired elders. J Gerontol B Psychol Sci Soc Sci 2000;55(4):247–55.
11. Hope T, Keene J, Gedling K, et al. Predictors of institutionalization for people with dementia living at home with a carer. Int J Geriatr Psychiatry 1998;13:682–90.
12. World Health Organization (WHO) and Alzheimer's Disease International (ADI). Dementia: a public health priority. 2012. Available at: http://www.alz.co.uk/WHO-dementia-report. Accessed August 1, 2012.
13. DeCarli C, Massaro J, Harvey D, et al. Meausres of brain morphology and infarction in the Framingham heart study: establishing what is normal. Neurobiol Aging 2005;491–510.

14. Boeve BF, Silver MH, Saper CB, et al. Pathophysiology of REM sleep behaviour disorder and relevance to neurodegenerative disease. Brain 2007;130(11): 1770–2788.
15. Boeve B, Silber M, Ferman T. REM sleep behavior disorder in Parkinson's disease and dementia with Lewy bodies. J Geriatr Psychiatry Neurol 2004;17:146–57.
16. Comella C, Nardine T, Diederich N, et al. Sleep-related violence injury, and REM sleep behavior disorder in Parkinson's disease. Neurology 1998;51:526–9.
17. Gagnon JF, Medard MA, Fantini M, et al. REM sleep behavior disorder and REM sleep without atonia in Parkinson's disease. Neurology 2002;59:585–9.
18. Plazzi G, Corsini R, Provini F, et al. REM sleep behavior disorder in multiple system atrophy. Neurology 1997;48:1094–7.
19. Tachibana N, Oka Y. Longitudinal change in REM sleep components in a patient with multiple system atrophy associated with REM sleep behavior disorder: paradoxical improvement of nocturnal behaviors in a progressive neurodegenerative disease. Sleep Med 2004;5:155–8.
20. Marion MH, Qurashi M, Marshall G, et al. Is REM sleep behavior disorder (RBD) a risk factor of dementia in idiopathic Parkinson's disease? J Neurol 2008;225: 192–6.
21. Schenck CH, Bundlie SR, Mahowald MW. Delayed emergence of a parkinsonian disorder in 38% of 29 older men initially diagnosed with idiopathic rapid eye movement sleep behavior disorder. Neurology 1996;46:388–93.
22. Postuma RB, Gagnon JF, Vendette M, et al. Quantifying the risk of neurodegenerative disease in idiopathic REM sleep behavior disorder. Neurology 2009;72: 1296–300.
23. Olson E, Boeve B, Silber M. Rapid eye movement sleep behavior disorder: demographic, clinical, and laboratory findings in 93 cases. Brain 2000;123:331–9.
24. Kunz D, Bes F. Melatonin as a therapy in REM sleep behavior disorder patients: an open-labeled pilot study on the possible influence of melatonin on REM-sleep regulation. Mov Disord 1999;14:507–11.
25. Takeuchi N, Uchimura N, Hashizume Y, et al. Melatonin therapy for REM sleep behavior disorder. Psychiatry Clin Neurosci 2001;55:267–9.
26. Stopa EG, Volicer L, Kuo-Leblanc V, et al. Pathologic evaluation of the human suprachiasmatic nucleus in severe dementia. J Neuropathol Exp Neurol 1999; 58:29–39.
27. Swaab DF, Fliers E, Pariman TS. The suprachiasmatic nucleus of the human brain in relation to sex, age and senile dementia. Brain Res 1985;342:37–44.
28. Liu RY, Zhou JN, Hoodendijk WJ, et al. Decreased vasopressin gene expression in the biological clock of Alzheimer disease patients with and without depression. J Neuropathol Exp Neurol 2000;59:314–22.
29. Wu YH, Swaab DF. Disturbance and strategies for reactivation of the circadian rhythm system in aging and Alzheimer's disease. Sleep Med 2007;8: 623–36.
30. Srinivasan V, Luaterbach EC, Ahmed AH, et al. Alzheimer's disease: focus on the neuroprotective role of melatonin. J Neurol Res 2012;2(3):69–81.
31. Campbell SS, Kripke DF, Gillin JC, et al. Exposure to light in healthy elderly subjects and Alzheimer's patients. Physiol Behav 1988;42(2):141–4.
32. Espiritu RC, Kripke DF, Ancoli-Israel S, et al. Low illumination experienced by San Diego adults: association with atypical depressive symptoms. Biol Psychiatry 1994;35(6):403–7.
33. Sloane PD, Williams CS, Mithcell M, et al. High-intensity environmental light in dementia" effect on sleep and activity. J Am Geriatr Soc 2007;55:1524–33.

34. Alessi CA, Martin JL, Webber AP, et al. Randomized, controlled trial of a non-pharmacological intervention to improve abnormal sleep/wake patterns in nursing home residents. J Am Geriatr Soc 2005;53:803–10.

35. Richards KC, Beck C, O'Sullivan PS, et al. Effect of individualized social activity on sleep in nursing home residents. J Am Geriatr Soc 2005;53:1510–7.

36. McCurry SM, Gibbons LE, Logsdon RG, et al. Nighttime insomnia treatment and education for Alzheimer's disease: a randomized controlled trial. J Am Geriatr Soc 2005;53:793–802.

37. McCurry SM, Pike KC, Vitiello MV, et al. Increasing walking and bright light exposure to improve sleep in community-dwelling persons with Alzheimer's disease: results of a randomized, controlled trial. J Am Geriatr Soc 2011;59:1393–402.

38. Singer C, Trachtenberg RE, Kaye J, et al. A multicenter, placebo-controlled trial of melatonin for sleep disturbance in Alzheimer's disease. Sleep 2003;26:893–901.

39. Gehrman PR, Connor DJ, Martin JL, et al. Melatonin fails to improve sleep or agitation in double-blind randomized placebo controlled trial of institutionalized patients with Alzheimer's disease. Am J Geriatr Psychiatry 2009;17:166–9.

40. Dowling GA, Burr RL, Van Someren EJ, et al. Melatonin and bright-light treatment for rest-activity disruption in institutionalized patients with Alzheimer's disease. J Am Geriatr Soc 2008;56:239–46.

41. Wu YH, Zhou JN, Van Heerikhuize J, et al. Decreased MT1 melatonin receptor expression in the suprachiasmatic nucleus in aging and Alzheimer's disease. Neurobiol Aging 2007;28(8):1239–47.

42. Riemersma-van der Lek RF, Swaab DF, Twisk J, et al. Effect of bright light and melatonin on cognitive and noncognitive function in elderly residents of group care facilities. A randomized controlled trial. JAMA 2008;299:2642–55.

43. Sack RL, Auckley D, Auger RR, et al. Circadian rhythm sleep disorders: part II, advanced sleep phase disorder, delayed sleep phase disorder, free-running disorder and irregular sleep-wake rhythm. Sleep 2007;30(11):1484–501.

44. Béland SG, Préville M, Doubois MF, et al. Benzodiazepine use and quality of sleep in the community-dwelling elderly population. Aging Ment Health 2010; 14(7):843–50.

45. Monane M, Glynn RJ, Avorn J. The impact of sedative-hypnotic use on sleep symptoms in elderly nursing home residents. Clin Pharmacol Ther 1996;59:83–92.

46. Englert S, Linden M. Differences in self-reported sleep complaints in elderly persons living in the community who do or do not take sleep medications. J Clin Psychiatry 1998;59:137–44.

47. Glass J, Lanctot KL, Herrmann N, et al. Sedative hypnotics in older people with insomnia: meta-analysis of risks and benefits. BMJ 2005;331(7526):1169.

48. Fick DM, Cooper JW, Wade WE, et al. Updating the Beers criteria for potentially inappropriate medication use in older adults. Arch Intern Med 2003;163: 2716–24.

49. Avidan AY, Bries BE, James ML, et al. Insomnia and hypnotic use, recorded in the minimum data set as predictors of falls and hip fractures in Michigan nursing homes. J Am Geriatr Soc 2005;53:955–62.

50. Camargos EF, Pandolfi MB, Freita MP, et al. Trazodone for the treatment of sleep disorders in dementia: an open-label, observational and review study. Arq Neuropsiquiatr 2011;69(1):44–9.

51. Evans LK. Sundown syndrome in institutionalized elderly. J Am Geriatr Soc 1987;35:101–8.

52. Martin J, Marler M, Shochat T, et al. Circadian rhythms of agitation in institutionalized patients with Alzheimer's disease. Chronobiol Int 2000;17:405–18.

53. Klaffke S, Staedt J. Sundowning and circadian rhythm disorders in dementia. Acta Neurol Belg 2006;106:168–75.
54. Yesavage JA, Friedman L, Ancoli-Israel S, et al. Development of diagnostic criteria for defining sleep disturbance in Alzheimer's disease. J Geriatr Psychiatry Neurol 2003;16:131–9.
55. Bliwise DL, Carroll JS, Lee KA, et al. Sleep and "sundowning" in nursing home patients with dementia. Psychiatry Res 1993;48:277–92.
56. Cohen-Mansfield J. Temporal patterns of agitation in dementia. Am J Geriatr Psychiatry 2007;15:395–405.
57. Satlin A, Volicer L, Ross V, et al. Bright light treatment of behavioral and sleep disturbances in patients with Alzheimer's disease. Am J Psychiatry 1992;149: 1028–32.
58. Forbes D, Culum I, Lischka AR, et al. Light therapy for managing cognitive, sleep, functional, behavioural, or psychiatric disturbances in dementia. Cochrane Database Syst Rev 2009;(4):CD003946.
59. Cohen-Mansfield J, Garfinkel D, Lipson S. Melatonin for treatment of sundowning in elderly persons with dementia – a preliminary study. Arch Gerontol Geriatr 2000;31:65–76.
60. Mahlberg R, Kunz D, Sutej I, et al. Melatonin treatment of day-night rhythm disturbances and sundowning in Alzheimer disease: an open-label pilot study using actigraphy. J Clin Psychopharmacol 2004;24:456–9.
61. de Jonghe A, Korevaar JC, van Munster BC, et al. Effectiveness of melatonin treatment on circadian rhythm disturbances in dementia. Are there implications for delirium? A systematic review. Int J Geriatr Psychiatry 2010;25(2):1201–8.
62. Greve M, O'Connor D. A survey of Australian and New Zealand old age psychiatrists' preferred medications to treat behavioral and psychological symptoms of dementia (BPSD). Int Psychogeriatr 2005;17:195–205.
63. Ancoli-Israel S, Kripke DF. Now I lay me down to sleep: the problem of sleep fragmentation in the elderly and demented residents of nursing homes. Bull Clin Neurosci 1989;54:127–32.
64. Stoppe G, Brandt CA, Staedt JH. Behavioural problems associated with dementia: the role of the newer anti-psychotics. Drugs Aging 1999;14:41–54.
65. Simpson K, Richards K, Enderlin C, et al. Medications and sleep in nursing home residents with dementia. J Am Psychiatr Nurses Assoc 2006;12(5): 279–85.
66. Schneider LS, Dagerman KS, Insel P. Risk of death with atypical antipsychotic drug treatment for dementia: meta-analysis of randomized placebo-controlled trials. JAMA 2005;294:1934–43.
67. Trinh NH, Hoblyn J, Mohanty S, et al. Efficacy of cholinesterase inhibitors in the treatment of neuropsychiatric symptoms and functional impairment in Alzheimer disease: a meta-analysis. JAMA 2003;289:210–6.
68. Skjerve A, Nygaard HA. Improvement in sundowning in dementia with Lewy bodies after treatment with donepezil. Int J Geriatr Psychiatry 2000;15: 1147–51.
69. Ancoli-Isreael S, Kripke DF, Klauber MR, et al. Sleep-disordered breathing in community-dwelling elderly. Sleep 1991;14(6):486–95.
70. Sforza E, Roche F, Thomas-Anterion C, et al. Cognitive function and sleep related breathing disorders in a healthy elderly population: the SYNAPSE study. Sleep 2010;33(4):515–21.
71. Ancoli-Israel S, Klauber MR, Butters N, et al. Dementia in institutionalized elderly: relation to sleep apnea. J Am Geriatr Soc 1991;39:258–63.

72. Erkinjuntti T, Partinen M, Sulkava R, et al. Sleep apnea in multi-infarct dementia and Alzheimer's disease. Sleep 1987;109:419–25.

73. Bliwise DL. Sleep apnea, ApoE4, and Alzheimer's disease: 20 years and counting? J Psychosom Res 2002;53:539–46.

74. Hoch CC, Reynolds CF 3rd, Kupfer DJ, et al. Sleep-disordered breathing in normal and pathological aging. J Clin Psychiatry 1986;47(10):499–503.

75. Kadotani H, Kadotani T, Young T, et al. Association between apolipoprotein Epsilon4 and sleep-disordered breathing in adults. JAMA 2001;285:2888–90.

76. Gottlieb D, DeStefano A, Foley D, et al. APOE epsilon4 is associated with obstructive sleep apnea/hypopnea: the Sleep Heart Health Study. Neurology 2004;63:664–8.

77. Foley DJ, Masaki K, White L, et al. Relationship between apolipoprotein E epsilon4 and sleep-disordered breathing at different ages. JAMA 2001;286(12):1447–8.

78. Saarelainen S, Lehtimaki T, Kallonen E, et al. No relation between apolipoprotein E alleles and obstructive sleep apnea. Clin Genet 1998;53(2):147–8.

79. Arzt M, Young T, Peppard PE, et al. Dissociation of obstructive sleep apnea from hypersomnolence and obesity in patients with stroke. Stroke 2010;41:e129–34.

80. Bassetti CL, Milanova M, Gugger M. Sleep-disordered breathing and acute ischemic stroke. Stroke 2006;37:967–72.

81. Munoz X, Marti S, Sumalla J, et al. Acute delirium as a manifestation of obstructive sleep apnea syndrome. Am J Respir Crit Care Med 1998;158:1306–7.

82. Lee J. Recurrent delirium associated with obstructive sleep apnea. Gen Hosp Psychiatry 1998;20:120–2.

83. Bliwise D. Is sleep apnea a cause of reversible dementia in old age? J Am Geriatr Soc 1996;44:1407–8.

84. Scheltens P, Visscher F, Van Keimpema A, et al. Sleep apnea syndrome presenting with cognitive impairment. Neurology 1991;14:486–95.

85. Aloia MS, Arnedt JT, Davis JD, et al. Neuropsychological sequelae of obstructive sleep apnea-hypopnea syndrome: a critical review. J Int Neuropsychol Soc 2004;10:772–85.

86. Beebe DW, Groesz L, Wells C, et al. The neuropsychological effects of obstructive sleep apnea: a meta-analysis of norm-referenced and case-controlled data. Sleep 2003;26:298–307.

87. Boland L, Shahar E, Iber C, et al. Measures of cognitive function in persons with varying degrees of sleep-disordered breathing: the Sleep Heart Health Study. J Sleep Res 2002;11:265–72.

88. Mathieu A, Mazza S, Decary A, et al. Effects of obstructive sleep apnea on cognitive function: a comparison between younger and older OSAS patients. Sleep Med 2008;9:112–20.

89. Dealberto MJ, Pajot N, Courbon D, et al. Breathing disorders during sleep and cognitive performance in an older community sample: the EVA study. J Am Geriatr Soc 1996;44:1287–94.

90. Cohen-Zion M, Stepnowsky C, Marler Shochat T, et al. Changes in cognitive function associated with sleep disordered breathing in older people. J Am Geriatr Soc 2001;49:1622–7.

91. Yaffe K, Laffan AM, Harrison SL, et al. Sleep-disordered breathing, hypoxia, and risk of mild cognitive impairment and dementia in older women. JAMA 2011; 306(6):613–9.

92. O'Hara R, Schroeder CM, Kraemer HC, et al. Nocturnal sleep apnea/hypopnea is associated with lower memory performance in APOE epsilon4 carriers. Neurology 2005;65:642–4.

93. Spira AP, Blackwell T, Stone KL, et al. Sleep-disordered breathing and cognition in older women. J Am Geriatr Soc 2008;56:45–50.

94. Naidoo N, Ferber M, Master M, et al. Aging impairs the unfolded protein response to sleep deprivation and leads to proapoptotic signaling. J Neurosci 2008;28(26):6539–48.

95. Kang J-E, Lim MM, Bateman RJ, et al. Amyloid-beta dynamics are regulated by orexin and the sleep-wake cycle. Science 2009;326(5955):1005–7.

96. Ancoli-Israel S, Barton WP, Cooke JR, et al. Cognitive effects of treating obstructive sleep apnea in Alzheimer's disease: a randomized controlled study. J Am Geriatr Soc 2008;56:2076–81.

97. Cooke JR, Ayalon L, Palmer BW, et al. Sustained use of CPAP slows deterioration of cognition, sleep, and mood in patients with Alzheimer's disease and obstructive sleep apnea: a preliminary study. J Clin Sleep Med 2009;5(4):305–9.

98. Marin JM, Carizo SJ, Vicente E, et al. Long-term cardiovascular outcomes in men with obstructive sleep apnoea-hypopnea with or without treatment with continuous positive airway pressure: an observational study. Lancet 2005;365: 1046–53.

99. Martinez-Garcia MÁ, Galiano-Blancart R, Román-Sánchez P, et al. Continuous positive airway pressure treatment in sleep apnea prevents new vascular events after ischemic stroke. Chest 2005;128(4):2123–9.

100. Ayalon L, Ancoli-Israel S, Stepnowsky C, et al. Adherence to continuous positive airway pressure treatment in patients with Alzheimer disease and obstructive sleep apnea. Am J Geriatr Psychiatry 2006;14(2):176–80.

101. Ferman T, et al. Presented at the American Academy of Neurology 62nd Annual Meeting. Toronto (Canada), April 10–16, 2010.

102. Thannickal TC, Lai YY, Siegel JM. Hypocretin(orexin) cell loss in Parkinson's disease. Brain 2007;130(6):1586–95.

103. Fronczek R, Overeem S, Lee SY, et al. Hypocretin (orexin) loss in Parkinson's disease. Brain 2007;130(6):1577–85.

104. Arnulf I, Bonnet AM, Damier P, et al. Hallucinations, REM sleep, and Parkinson's disease. Neurology 2000;55(2):281–8.

105. Arnulf I, Konofal E, Merino-Andreu M, et al. Parkinson's disease and sleepiness" an integral part of PD. Neurology 2002;58:1019–24.

106. Rye DB, Bliwise DL, Dihenia B, et al. FAST TRACK: daytime sleepiness in Parkinson's disease. J Sleep Res 2000;9:63–9.

107. Kuntz K, Boeve B, Drubach D, et al. Safety, tolerability, and efficacy of Armodafinil therapy for hypersomnia associated with dementia with Lewy bodies. Presented at the American Academy of Neurology 64th Annual Meeting. New Orleans, April 21–28, 2012.

108. Berger K, Leudemann J, Trenkwalder C, et al. Sex and the risk of restless legs syndrome in the general population. Arch Intern Med 2004;164(2):196–202.

109. Rothdach A, Trenkwalder C, Haberstock J, et al. Prevalence and risk factors of RLS in an elderly population: the MEMO Study. Neurology 2000;54:1064–8.

110. Youngstedt SD, Kripke DF, Klauber MR. Periodic leg movements during sleep and sleep disturbances in elders. J Gerontol A Biol Sci Med Sci 1998;53A(5): M391–4.

111. Ancoli-Israel S, Kripke DF, Klauber MR, et al. Periodic limb movements in sleep in community dwelling elderly. Sleep 1991;14:496–500.

Sleep and Epilepsy
Opportunities for Diagnosis and Treatment

Bradley V. Vaughn, MD[a],*, Imran Ali, MD[b]

KEYWORDS

- Sleep • Epilepsy • Sleep disorders • Nocturnal seizures

KEY POINTS

- Sleep complaints are common in patients with epilepsy and may be related to their underlying epilepsy, the treatment of epilepsy, or other sleep-related issues.
- Epilepsy can cause sleep disruption, and treatment of epilepsy may also improve sleep.
- Sleep disorders are common in patients with epilepsy.
- Treatment of sleep disorders may help reduce recurrent seizures.
- Nocturnal seizures are associated with stereotypic behavior.

INTRODUCTION

Epilepsy and sleep have a complex bidirectional relationship. The condition of epilepsy and some of its treatments can cause sleep disruption and may exacerbate some sleep disorders. Epileptic seizures and interictal discharges can cause sleep fragmentation and changes in sleep architecture. Sleep, alternatively, provides an opportunity for clinicians to better diagnose and treat epilepsy. For many patients with epilepsy, the interictal and sometimes ictal manifestations are best observed during specific sleep states. The act of sleep deprivation as well as oversleeping for some may increase the likelihood of seizure recurrence. There are considerable data that improvement in sleep hygiene and the treatment of sleep disorders can significantly improve outcomes in epilepsy. Individuals with epilepsy frequently complain of symptoms of disturbed sleep. These complaints may come in the form of easily recognizable symptoms, such as daytime sleepiness or insomnia, or in more subtle complaints, such as loss of quality of life or an increase in seizure frequency.

Patients may have their seizures only associated with sleep. Some epileptic syndromes are defined by their sleep-related association. Clinicians must be able to

[a] Division of Sleep and Epilepsy, Department of Neurology, University of North Carolina School of Medicine, CB #7025, 2122 Physicians Office Building, Chapel Hill, NC 27599-7025, USA; [b] Department of Neurology, University of Toledo, College of Medicine and Life Sciences, MS 1195, Toledo, OH 43614, USA
* Corresponding author.
E-mail address: vaughnb@neurology.unc.edu

Neurol Clin 30 (2012) 1249–1274
http://dx.doi.org/10.1016/j.ncl.2012.08.006
0733-8619/12/$ – see front matter © 2012 Elsevier Inc. All rights reserved.

differentiate between a sleep disorder and/or a problem related to epilepsy and its treatment. Patients with epilepsy may also display unusual nighttime events due to seizures or other nonepileptic events, such as parasomnias. These patients can provide a challenge to even the most astute clinicians. Some specific nocturnal epilepsies, however, have characteristics that help identify these patients. This article explores the interactions of sleep and epilepsy and discusses how these may be useful for clinicians.

SLEEP DISRUPTION IN EPILEPSY
Epidemiology

Patients with epilepsy, as with patients with other neurologic disorders, have a greater prevalence of sleep disturbance than normal subjects. Miller[1] found that more than two-thirds of patients with epilepsy seen at a university epilepsy center have complaints regarding sleep. He found 68% complained of feeling sleepy during the day, and 39% complained of difficulty falling asleep or staying asleep. Approximately 42% believed that their sleep issues interfered with their daytime performance. De Weerd[2] reported in 2004 that 39% of a cohort of 486 adults with partial epilepsy had sleep complaints compared with 19% in the control group. Khatami[3] surveyed 100 patients with epilepsy and found that 30% of epilepsy patients had sleep complaints compared with 10% of their control population and patients with epilepsy also had higher prevalence of sleep maintenance and insomnia symptoms (52% vs 38%). Similarly, Chen[4] found in a survey of 117 patients with epilepsy that 20% had excessive sleepiness (compared with 7% of healthy controls) and elevated scores on the Pittsburgh Sleep Quality Index. Chen was also able to show that poor seizure control was associated with an increased the odds ratio of 2.42 for poor sleep compared with healthy controls. Using the Epworth Sleepiness Scale (ESS), Malow and colleagues[5] similarly reported that 28% of 158 adult epilepsy patients surveyed had an elevated score (>10 points), with 44% of subjects reporting a moderate or high tendency to fall asleep while watching television.[5] Similarly Giorelli[6] found that 47% of their cohort had ESS scores over 10, which were reportedly not related to sleep deprivation. Increase in complaints of excessive daytime sleepiness (EDS) is also seen in children with epilepsy. Using the Pediatric Daytime Sleepiness Scale, Maganti[7] reported that children with epilepsy have a higher prevalence of EDS.

Objective sleep studies of patients with epilepsy suggest that there is an increased prevalence of sleep disorders. Patients with primary and focal onset epilepsy have greater sleep fragmentation and sleep stage shifts compared with nonepileptic controls.[8] Zanzmera,[9] using a case-control cohort format, showed that those with refractory epilepsy have longer sleep latency, delayed rapid eye movement (REM) sleep latency, greater number of arousals, overall less sleep (340.4 min [147–673] vs 450.3 min [330–570]) and lower sleep efficiency (80.45% [40.5–98.0] vs 95.45% [88.4–99.7]). This study also showed that those with refractory epilepsy were more likely to have sleep apnea than those with controlled epilepsy (20% vs 0%) on polysomnography (PSG). Sleep-related respiratory disturbances have been well documented in patients with epilepsy. PSG investigation of individuals with epilepsy by Malow[10] showed that approximately one-third of patients with medically refractory epilepsy had an apnea hypopnea index (AHI) of greater than 5 and approximately 10% of the patients had periodic limb movement index greater than 20 events per hour. Manni[11] screened 283 adults with epilepsy for symptoms of sleep apnea and found 40 at risk and 29 to have an AHI great than 5 events per hour. In a case-control study of 53 older adults, Chihorek[12] found that 52% of patients who had late-onset epilepsy or worsening seizures had an AHI greater than 5, and 33% had an AHI greater than 10. These studies seem to indicate that the prevalence of sleep apnea increases with the presence of refractory epilepsy.

Obstructive sleep apnea (OSA) may also influence the prevalence of epilepsy. Seizures as a direct result of apnea are rare. In one patient, an apnea in sleep reportedly caused a seizure after severe oxygen desaturation and cardiac arrest.[13] Yet, Sonka[14] found in their cohort that 4% of patients with OSA had epilepsy. This prevalence exceeds that of the general population. More than three-fourths of these patients had seizures only during sleep and most of the events were generalized seizures. Although this study may be skewed by variances in referral patterns, the elevated prevalence raises the question of sleep apnea provoking seizures or unmasking an underlying potential for seizures.

Pathophysiology

The dynamic relationship of sleep on epilepsy is evident by the impact of each state on the other. As discussed previously, epilepsy disrupts sleep and sleep influences epilepsy. The epileptic process may directly contribute to the sleep disturbance. In animal studies, discharges from the amygdala or mesiotemporal structures produce arousals. Touchon[8] showed that patients with epilepsy have greater sleep fragmentation and instability on seizure-free nights compared with nonepileptic controls. Touchon[8] reported a decrease in sleep efficiency, increase in sleep stage shifts, and periods of wakefulness in patients with primary generalized epilepsy or complex partial seizures compared with normal controls. Touchon[8] also noted that the disruption was greater in individuals with focal onset seizures. These individuals had more stage shifts, less deep sleep, and sleep fragmentation. Sleep fragmentation by awakenings was greater in untreated, newly diagnosed patients. Touchon reported that after treatment with carbamazepine for 1 month, the newly diagnosed epilepsy patients showed improvement in these parameters. Parrino also found that patients with frontal lobe foci have a distinct appearance to their sleep showing more A1 component of cyclic alternating pattern.[15]

Although this work was in focal onset epilepsy, Peled[16] showed that bursts of generalized spike-wave complexes can appear in stages 2 and 3 of non-REM (NREM) sleep and occur with K complexes and arousals. Some of these bursts produced nonconvulsive body movements, resulting in significant sleep fragmentation and decreased amounts of REM sleep. Three patients treated with antiepileptic medications showed reduced paroxysmal events during sleep, increased REM sleep, increased sleep efficiency, and improvement in daytime sleepiness. Not all interictal discharges, however, result in arousals. In temporal lobe epilepsy, Malow and colleagues[17] found that interictal discharges were rarely associated with arousals from sleep and were most prevalent with the onset of SWS. This study used surface electrodes and did not look at other features, such as autonomic arousals or other physiologic parameter shifts. In humans, interictal activity can be associated with limited physiologic changes. Interictal discharges have been reported to change the cardiac cycle times and, in animals, may produce significant changes in hypothalamic function.[18,19] The relationship of these brief discharges to sleep has yet to be fully defined. The chaotic nature of these discharges, however, may disrupt various neuronal drivers and the microarchitecture involved in the regulation of sleep or its many physiologic features.

Seizures also acutely alter the mechanism involved in sleep-wake state determination (**Table 1**). Frequent nocturnal seizures can also produce significant sleep disturbance as evident in patients with frontal lobe seizures who may experience multiple seizures in a single night.[20] The disruption caused by seizures frequently results in

Table 1	
Effect of epilepsy on sleep	
Type of Discharge	**Effect on Sleep**
Interictal discharge	May cause arousals, sleep stage shifts, or autonomic effects or have no effect
Complex partial seizure	Increase sleep fragmentation, decrease REM sleep
Generalized seizure	Increase sleep fragmentation and decrease REM sleep, decrease wakefulness on the following day

patients having additional postictal somnolence and sleep disruption. Patients with nocturnal seizures are subjectively and objectively sleepy on the day after a seizure.[21] The changes produced by seizures also produce sleep fragmentation and suppression of REM sleep. Touchon[8] showed, in a study of 77 subjects with primary or secondarily generalized tonic-clonic seizures, that subjects had reduced total sleep time, a decreased percentage of REM sleep, increased wake time after sleep onset, and an increased stage 2 sleep on nights after generalized seizures compared with seizure-free nights. They also reported that, in 80 subjects, recurrent partial seizures during sleep decreased the percentage of REM sleep. Similarly, other investigators reported this REM-suppressing effect of seizures as well as other effects on sleep organization. Investigation by Crespel and Baldy-Moulinier[18] reported that individuals with partial or generalized seizures had decreased amounts of REM sleep on nights with seizures. Besset[22] found that patients with seizures had a reduction in total sleep time and REM sleep when compared with patients without seizures. Comparing nights when seizures occurred versus seizure-free nights, Bazil reported that nighttime seizures reduced sleep efficiency and REM and stages 2 and 4 sleep and prolonged REM latency and increased drowsiness as measured by the maintenance of wakefulness test on the following day. Bazil[21] also found by studying patients in an epilepsy monitoring unit that when seizures occurred during the day, REM sleep was significantly decreased the ensuing night, with decreased amount of stage 4 sleep. This finding demonstrates that the effect of seizures to alter the regulation of sleep and wake last into the following day.

Sleep also influences the expression of interictal and ictal discharges. Sleep may activate interictal activity in approximately one-third of epileptic patients and up to 90% of subjects with sleep-related, or state-dependent, epilepsies.[23–25] Findings on electroencephalogram (EEG) recording sleep, however, after the administration of chloral hydrate only changed the clinical management in less than 3% of patients.[26] Degen showed an increase in interictal activity on EEG recordings that included sleep and an even greater number of and locations on recordings after sleep deprivation.[27] Sleep deprivation EEG recordings have interictal spike frequency similar to those found on overnight recording EEG recordings.[28]

Curiously the effect of sleep deprivation activating interictal activity recorded on EEG does not extend to magnetoencephalography as reported by Heers.[29] This may be related to differentiating characteristics of magnetic field potentials. Sleep deprivation has long been an established method used to trigger epileptic-related activity (**Table 2**) and is frequently used in long-term epilepsy monitoring settings to promote seizures. Sleep deprivation exacerbates seizures in some patients with epilepsy whereas other patients have little exacerbation with sleep deprivation.[30–32] Janz noted that sleep deprivation frequently provokes seizures in the awakening epilepsies.[30,31] This also seems true for some focal onset epilepsies. Rajna and

Table 2
Effect of sleep on epilepsy

State	Effect on Epilepsy
NREM sleep	Increase in interictal discharges, frequency, and spatial distribution More common seizures (especially frontal and temporal that occipital or parietal)
REM sleep	More well-localized and less-frequent interictal discharges Fewer seizures
Arousal	May cause more seizures frontal or primary generalized seizures
Sleep deprivation	Increases interictal discharges on EEG even during awake Increases likelihood of recurrent seizures
Oversleeping (>10 h)	Seems to increase likelihood for recurrent seizures

Veres[32] found that in 9 of 14 patients with temporal lobe epilepsy, seizures are more likely to occur on the days after sleep deprivation. The mechanism by which this activation occurs is unresolved but may be related to the change in state or related to a loss of natural suppression of the aberrant activity. Sleep deprivation for these patients may occur from a variety of causes, such as schedule limitations, medication effect, epilepsy, or other dysomnias. No matter the cause, these studies demonstrate the importance of correcting potential causes of sleep deprivation to improve seizure control.

Sleep disorders may also increase the likelihood of recurrent seizures. OSA seems to increase the frequency of seizures. This may be related to the recurrent oxygen desaturation, the sleep fragmentation, or sleep deprivation. Sleep apnea is known to cause sleep deprivation as well as sleep fragmentation. This direct sleep disruption deprives patients from attaining restorative sleep as well as increasing the time spent in stages of sleep vulnerable to seizure induction. Sleep apnea also produces oxygen desaturation and hypoxia. Although there was little correlation between the lowest oxygen desaturation and the improvement of seizure frequency in the reported case series, oxygen desaturation is noted to decrease potential seizure inhibitory mechanisms.[33] Although any of these mechanisms may be relevant, further research has yet to determine this mechanism.

Sleep stage influences the appearance of interictal activity. Recording through the night shows interictal activity increases with entrance into the deeper stages of NREM sleep.[17,28] These interictal discharges are more frequent with the onset of the deeper stages of sleep and show greater spatial variability. Shouse[34] postulated that the availability of neurons to be recruited into the epileptic discharge may be an important factor into the effect of sleep on discharge occurrence. In REM sleep, interictal discharges are less frequent and more focal.[17] In patients with depth electrodes placed in the mesial temporal lobes, Staba showed that single neurons had significantly higher burst rates and synchronous discharges during episodes of slow wave sleep and REM sleep and not wakefulness when compared with nonepileptic hippocampal neurons.[35] Although these findings suggest that the epileptogenic site may be more autonomous than other areas of the brain and thus less influenced by sleep regulation, REM sleep activation may explain the decrease of epileptic activity in REM sleep. Several investigators have postulated the corollary hypothesis that the increased activity in REM sleep leaves fewer neurons available for recruitment into an epileptic discharge. Yet, REM sleep has antiepileptogenic effect beyond temporal activation of the neurons. Animal models have also shown that REM-NREM sleep stages to have complex influences on seizure activity. As in humans, NREM sleep and slow wave sleep have been associated in animals to promote the propensity of interictal discharges and REM sleep to suppress seizure discharges. In the kindling model, animals kindled in NREM sleep require fewer overall current and sessions than those kindled in REM sleep. Selective deprivation of REM sleep in animals reduces the required current to elicit seizure activity in other stages of sleep and awake. The converse of this is also true. Kumar increased REM sleep through microinjection of cholinergic agonist and demonstrated significant increase in threshold to produce after discharges in the amygdala during the subsequent period of wakefulness.[36] These findings suggest that REM sleep has broader reaching antiseizure effect than immediate activation of the cortex.

Sleep also has a significant impact on seizures. Most seizures occur out of NREM sleep, with the highest rate per hour occurring from stage 2 sleep.[37,38] Seizures are also noted to frequently occur in relationship to an awakening. This finding has raised significant debate if the seizure caused the arousal or the arousal promoted the seizure. REM sleep has the lowest rate of seizures. This antiseizure property seems to hold true for both the overall sleep time and the seizure rate per hour of REM sleep when compared with other states.[38]

Key Clinical Features and Diagnosis

Patients with sleep complaints typically present as 1 of 3 major categories: EDS, insomnia, or unusual nocturnal events. Clinicians faced with caring for patients with epilepsy should be aware that patients may complain of sleep or may assume that their symptoms are normal for an individual with epilepsy. In addition, patients may not have the ability to perceive nor report sleep-related symptoms. Thus, clinicians must look for other clues of sleep disorders, such as change in daily activities, behavioral issues, or increase in seizure frequency. For patients with epilepsy who present with a sleep issue, clinicians can use a standard clinical approach with several key points. General categories of causes, include circadian rhythm issues, intrinsic and extrinsic sleep disturbances, substances or disorders altering the brain's sleep-wake networks, other medical and psychiatric disorders. The clinician should also search for behaviors that interfere with sleep while also being aware that epilepsy and its treatment may also be partly responsible (**Fig. 1**). Clinicians need to obtain a typical detailed history, including information regarding the clinical course, the degree of impact on the patient, the sleep-wake pattern, report from bed partner or caretaker on sleep activities, dietary and activity schedule, medications (including timing and dosage schedule, over-the-counter agents, and herbs), seizure frequency intensity, and timing. Circadian rhythm disorders should be considered in patients with epilepsy. Many of these patients have sedentary lifestyles, take a variety of supplements, and may have limited exposure to circadian time clues.[39] In addition, these patients may experience brief shifts or attenuations in the circadian rhythms from seizures or medications.[40] Some of the circadian rhythm issues may be related to lower melatonin levels. In one study in children, Paprocka[41] found that those with refractory epilepsy had lower melatonin compared with those with controlled epilepsy. Similarly patients with epilepsy may also have other sleep disorders, such as sleep apnea, periodic limb movements, or restless legs syndrome (RLS), which disturb their sleep and produce daytime sequelae. Patients should be questioned regarding presence of snoring, witnessed apnea, excessive movements at night, and presence of unrefreshing sleep. The presence of these symptoms should trigger consideration of overnight PSG. Intrinsic dysfunction in the regulation of sleep, such as narcolepsy or idiopathic hypersomnia, can also produce significant daytime sleepiness and patients may require

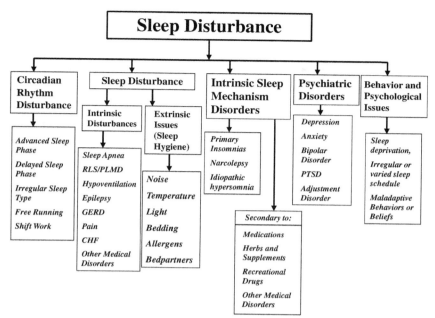

Fig. 1. This figure shows the major groups of causes of sleep disturbance, frequently seen in patients with and without epilepsy. CHF, congested heart failure; GERD, gastroesophageal reflux; PLMD, periodic limb movement disorder; PSTD, post traumatic stress disorder.

overnight PSG and a multiple sleep latency study. Affective disorders are also common in patients with epilepsy and may account for some of the symptoms of insomnia, fatigue, and sleepiness. Lastly, patients with epilepsy are also treated with centrally acting medications to control their seizures. These medications can influence the sleep-wake control mechanisms. Many of these medications produce side effects, which include somnolence or insomnia (**Table 3**). Most of the traditional anticonvulsants have sleepiness as a side effect.[42] Although this is most notable for the barbiturates and benzodiazepines, others, such as carbamazepine, phenytoin, valproate, gabapentin, topiramate, vigabatrin, levetiracetam, oxcarbazepine, and clozabam, can produce complaints of somnolence or fatigue.[43] Medications, such as felbamate, ethosuximide, lamotrigine, and zonisamide, may induce insomnia. Some medications, such as gabapentin, pregabalin, and tiagabine, increase slow wave sleep.[44,45] Drugs may also produce metabolic and endocrine changes that promote appropriate sleep and wakefulness. Enzyme-inducing medications may increase the metabolism of medications used to treat hypersomnolence or insomnia.

Approach to the Epilepsy Patient with Daytime Sleepiness

EDS should be approached by clinicians considering a variety of causes (**Fig. 2**). Daytime sleepiness is common in epilepsy patients, but this symptom is frequently dismissed as an acceptable side effect of therapy.[1,5] For many of these patients, the authors' clinical experience has shown that multiple factors contribute to this symptom (**Box 1**). Patients should be questioned regarding their daily habits, total time dedicated to sleep, wake and sleep schedule, timing of medication, factors that disrupt sleep, and symptoms of other sleep disorders. Many times a sleep diary combined with a seizure diary may provide clues to the impact of schedule on symptoms. Although the ESS has

Table 3
Antiepileptic medication effects on sleep

Drug	Sleep Complaint	Sleep Efficiency	Total Sleep Time	Sleep Latency	Arousals	Stage 1	Stage 2	Stages 3 and 4	REM Sleep
Phenobarbital	Sleepiness	↓	No change	↓	↓	↑	↑	No change	↓
Phenytoin	Sleepiness	↓	No Change	↓	↓	↑	↑	↓	No change
Carbamazepine	Sleepiness	↑	No change	↓	↓	No change	No change	↑	?
Valproate	Sleepiness	No change	No change	No change	↑	↓	No change	↑	No change
Ethosuximide	Insomnia	↓	?	?	↑	↑	No change	↑	↑
Felbamate	Insomnia	↓			↑				
Gabapentin	Sleepiness	↑	↑		↓	↑		↑	↑
Lamotrigine	Insomnia	No change	No change	No change	No change	No change	No change	↑	↑
Topiramate	Sleepiness	?	?	?	?	?	?	?	?
Vigabatrin	Sleepiness	?	No change	No change	?	?	?	?	?
Tiagabine	Varies	No change	No change	No change	–	→	No change	↑	No change?
Levitiracetam	Sleepiness	↑	↑	No change	→	No change	↑	?	No change
Zonisamide	Insomnia	?	?	?	?	?	?	?	?
Pregabalin	Sleepiness	↑	↑	→	↑	–	–	↑	–
Oxcarbazepine	Sleepiness	?	?	?	?	?	?	?	?
Lacosamide	Varies	?	?	?	?	?	?	?	?
Rufinimide	Sleepiness	?	?	?	?	?	?	?	?
Clobazam	Sleepiness	?	?	?	?	?	?	?	?
Retigabine	Varies	?	?	?	?	?	?	?	?

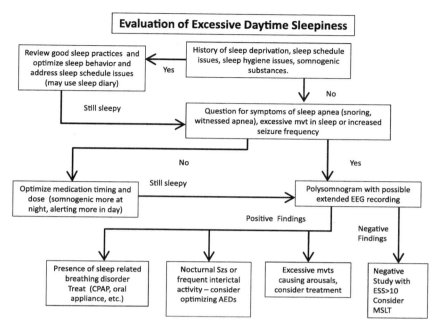

Fig. 2. This algorithm shows the clinical approach to EDS in a patient with epilepsy starts with a detailed history focusing on the possible causes outline in **Fig. 1** and **Box 1**. AED, anti-epileptic drugs; CPAP, continuous positive airway pressure; MSLT, multiple sleep latency test; MVTS, movements; SZS, seizures.

never been validated in patients with epilepsy, useful information can aid clinicians. Individuals with a score of 10 or greater are considered to have excessive sleepiness. Malow showed that elevated scores on the ESS in epilepsy patients were more commonly associated with symptoms of OSA and RLS than the number or type of anti-epileptic medication or seizure frequency.[5] Patients with symptoms, such as snoring, witnessed apnea, or unrefreshing sleep, which suggest nocturnal disturbance, should have an overnight in-laboratory PSG. For some patients, frequent nocturnal interictal discharges and nocturnal seizures may also cause significant sleep disruption and result in daytime sleepiness of patients with epilepsy.[5] Extended EEG montage or video-EEG with PSG may be extremely valuable to elucidate the extent of the sleep disruption. For other complex patients, multiple sleep latency testing may also quantitate the degree of daytime sleepiness and the occurrence of inappropriate REM sleep.[46] This testing paradigm is specifically helpful for evaluating the presence of narcolepsy but may also provide helpful information for idiopathic insomnia.

Approach to the Patient with Epilepsy and Insomnia

Insomnia seems to disrupt sleep in approximately 40% of individuals with epilepsy.[1,2] Patients with insomnia and epilepsy can be approached using a standard sleep medicine paradigm aimed at identifying potential contributing factors (**Box 2, Fig. 3**). At first glance, the issues of sleep schedule, sleep hygiene, and stimulus control need to be addressed. Additionally, patients need to be questioned regarding issues of sleep disruption, snoring, apnea, depression or anxiety, and psychological stressors. Patients with epilepsy may also have a reclusive or sedentary lifestyle, which is a contributor to nocturnal sleep disruption. Some patients use caffeine or other

---

Box 1
Differential diagnosis for hypersomnia

Sleep deprivation

Total sleep time

Sleep disruption—intrinsic

OSA

Periodic limb movements

Sleep disruption—extrinsic

Inadequate sleep environment

Circadian rhythm disorder

Delayed sleep phase

Advanced sleep phase

Irregular sleep pattern

Intrinsic brain sleep regulation disorder

Narcolepsy

Idiopathic hypersomnia

Kleine-Levine syndrome

Menstrual-related hypersomnia

Medications

Affective disorders

Endocrine or metabolic disorders

Nocturnal seizures and epileptic disturbance

---

over-the-counter stimulants to counteract the sedating symptoms of the antiepileptic medications. Patients should be warned not to consume caffeine or other stimulants in the late afternoon and evening hours. Patients may have schedule limitations due to medications or work or driving restrictions; thus, timing of exercise and meals needs to be reviewed. Sleep environment may also play a role. Patients with seizures may have anxiety regarding issues of their epilepsy or fear of recurrence of seizures during their sleep. These fears may be expressed by maladaptive behaviors, such sleeping with the television or light on or sleep in settings where other individuals can observe them. These individuals may benefit from education, reassurance, and counseling. For some patients, relaxation techniques, biofeedback, and stimulus control may also be helpful. The authors have not used sleep restriction, one of the most effective cognitive behavioral therapies for insomnia, for fear of increasing seizures. Insomnia may occur on the basis of frequent arousals caused by epileptic activity. For these patients, higher doses of antiepileptic medication at night and optimization of seizure control may improve symptoms. Patients should be queried about symptoms suggesting RLS or excessive movement in sleep or sleep apnea and referred for PSG when these diagnoses are suspected. Patients with vagus nerve stimulators may also be a greater risk for sleep apnea. Depression or anxiety occurs in more than 40% of patients with epilepsy and may contribute to the complaint of insomnia.[47] In such cases, patients can be treated with antidepressant and antianxiety medications to benefit both the affective and sleep disorder.[48]

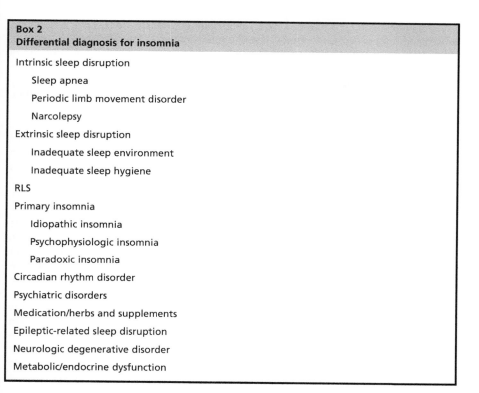

Box 2
Differential diagnosis for insomnia

Intrinsic sleep disruption

    Sleep apnea

    Periodic limb movement disorder

    Narcolepsy

Extrinsic sleep disruption

    Inadequate sleep environment

    Inadequate sleep hygiene

RLS

Primary insomnia

    Idiopathic insomnia

    Psychophysiologic insomnia

    Paradoxic insomnia

Circadian rhythm disorder

Psychiatric disorders

Medication/herbs and supplements

Epileptic-related sleep disruption

Neurologic degenerative disorder

Metabolic/endocrine dysfunction

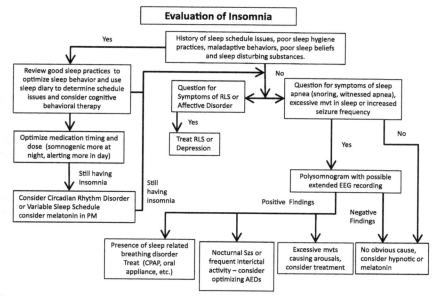

Fig. 3. This algorithm shows the clinical approach to insomnia in a patient with epilepsy starts with a detailed history focusing on the possible causes (outlined in **Fig. 1** and **Box 2**). AED, antiepileptic drugs; CPAP, continuous positive airway pressure; MSLT, multiple sleep latency test; MVTS, movements; SZS, seizures.

Some antiepileptic medications, such as felbamate, ethosuximide, zonisamide, and lamotrigine, can provoke insomnia. These medications may be necessary for control of the seizures but may be given earlier in the evening or doses spread out through the day. Alternatively, a more sedating medication may be substituted or if the insomnia-producing antiepileptic medication is required for seizure control. Patients undergoing medication tapers may also experience insomnia due to removal of sedating medication.

Treatment

Treatment of sleep symptoms in patients with epilepsy should be directed toward 3 primary components. Patients should have the epilepsy optimally treated, the sleep schedule and hygiene should be optimized, and any underlying sleep disorder should be directly treated. With this 3-pronged approach, patients gain the mutual benefit of improving sleep and epilepsy. Optimizing the treatment of epilepsy can improve sleep. Touchon[7] showed in some patients that epileptic discharges can cause sleep disruption; the use of carbamazepine decreased arousals and fragmentation. For these patients, sleep disruption may be treated with higher doses of antiepileptic medication before the sleep period. Yegnanran[49] showed that dividing doses so that two-thirds or greater of the total carbamazepine or phenytoin dose was in the evening was associated with fewer side effects, better compliance, and improved seizure control. Anticonvulsants can produce both symptoms of daytime sleepiness and insomnia. These medications are frequently considered by patients and their physicians the cause of their sleep complaints,[50] yet appropriate timing of doses may improve these symptoms. Traditional anticonvulsants are more commonly associated with somnolence, although some of the newer agents also produce similar effects (see **Table 3**). The course of antiepileptic medication use in patients with epilepsy should be for clinicians to start one medication at a low dose and titrate the dosage until either the patient is seizure-free or develops intolerable side effects. When antiepileptic medications are suspected of causing the daytime sleepiness, the medication dosage may be shifted to more at night or substituted with a less sedating medication. Considering the potential for enhancement of sleep, sedating medications may be dosed so that the peak effect is during the usual sleep period. This technique is also helpful in the treatment of nocturnal seizures when patients can tolerate higher drug levels during sleep.[51] Patients also may choose the time they take their medications based on their own circadian preference.[52] Therefore, patients who are night owls may elect to stay up later and take the medications to promote late night alertness and cause more nighttime sleep disturbance.

Patients may have a variety of opportunities to improve sleep. Patients with chronic conditions frequently have maladaptive behaviors that have a negative impact on their sleep. These factors should be addressed with education regarding sleep hygiene. Patients should be counseled to have a regular sleep routine that persists 7 days per week, avoid caffeine and other stimulants, exercise regularly, and eat meals on a regular basis. Late night activities andinteraction with electronics that produce light, social interaction, or are stimulating may disturb sleep and should be avoided. Some patients may not be willing to make these types of long-term life style changes. The authors have found that making deals for trial periods, tracking symptoms and seizures, documenting the instructions on written materials, and explaining the treatment plan to both patient and a family member is a valuable method to circumvent lapses in memory. Additionally, melatonin may provide some benefit for help reinforce a sleep-wake schedule by having patients take exogenous melatonin 1 hour to 2 hours before the set bed time. This therapy seems to help with schedule and may reduce seizure frequency.[53]

Sleep disorders may influence the frequency of seizures and treatment of disorders, such as sleep apnea, may improve a patient's sleep symptoms and seizure frequency. This is best demonstrated in the relationship between OSA and epilepsy. Several investigators have shown in a significant proportion of patients that treatment of the OSA improved their seizure control. The first report of treatment of sleep apnea in a patient with epilepsy was in 1981, by Wyler and Weymuller.[54] Their patient underwent tracheostomy and attained control of the generalized seizures and improvement in partial seizures. Investigators have found a range of benefits for patients with epilepsy once the sleep apnea is treated.[55–58] The authors' original report showed that 40% of the cohort attained seizure freedom and another 10% had greater than 95% reduction in seizures with treatment of the OSA alone.[49] In a pilot randomized controlled study, Malow showed trends toward seizure reduction in a group of patients with intractable epilepsy.[59] The observations have been extended into the pediatric population.[60] Patients with epilepsy can be effectively treated with continuous positive airway pressure positional therapy and surgery. Continuous positive airway pressure masks need to be fitted appropriately but also designed to easily disconnect to avoid patients becoming entangled during a seizure. In the authors' center, the use of full-face masks is avoided if a patient has a history of postictal vomiting. Similarly, dental devices may be used if a patient does not have a history of ictal or postictal vomiting and the device is tightly fitted to avoid aspiration.

Antiepileptic medications may be chosen to aid with both the epilepsy and sleep disorder. Topiramate has been suggested to aid in the treatment of apnea based on its carbonic anhydrase inhibitor property and the potential for causing weight loss.[61] Additionally, topiramate is used in the treatment of nocturnal eating syndrome and in one case of exploding head syndrome.[62,63] Gabapentin, pregabalin, and carbamazepine have been reported as beneficial in RLS and neuropathic pain disorders.[64–66] Gabapentin and pregabalin also increase slow wave sleep and some investigators have hypothesized the use of these medications may influence daytime attention by improving sleep quality.[67] In addition, clonazepam has been the mainstay of therapy for patients with REM sleep behavior disorder (RBD).[68] As discussed previously, the side effects of certain antiepileptic medications may be used to counter the complaints of insomnia or EDS. Patients with significant sleepiness but without an identifiable cause may be potential candidates for stimulant therapy. Amphetamines may increase frequency of seizures and should be used with extreme caution. With any stimulant use, clinicians should carefully monitor patients to assess the impact both on the epileptic seizures and potential for drug interactions. Whatever the cause, improving the sleep and daytime alertness of individuals with epilepsy may have benefits reaching beyond traditional symptoms of sleep disorders.

Prognosis

Patients with epilepsy and sleep complaints have an overall good prognosis of being helped if the underlying sleep dysfunction can be identified. This requires diligent investigation on the part of clinicians and significant participation on the part of patients and caretakers. Optimization of the treatment of epilepsy and sleep are the keys to improvement.

NOCTURNAL SEIZURES
Introduction

Approximately 20% of patients seen in the epilepsy clinics have seizures or ictal events that occur predominantly or exclusively at night. Most of these patients have focal-onset seizures emanating from frontal or temporal lobes, but some patients, including those with frontal or temporal lobe epilepsy, have identifiable nocturnal epilepsy syndromes.[31] Some of these syndromes are associated with exclusive nocturnal seizure activity, such as benign childhood epilepsy with centrotemporal spikes that does not seem to produce daytime sequelea, whereas others, such as Landau-Kleffner syndrome (LKS) or continuous spike and wave during sleep, can produce devastating daytime cognitive dysfunction without clear nighttime seizures. Similarly, in autosomal dominant nocturnal frontal lobe epilepsy (ADNFLE), a nicotinic receptor abnormality is intimately associated with sleep-related seizures. In benign nocturnal childhood epilepsy (Panayiotopoulos syndrome), sleep-related seizures are accompanied with a variety of autonomic symptoms, such as nocturnal vomiting. Generalized epilepsies, such as juvenile myoclonic epilepsy, are typically associated with seizures on awakening. Myoclonus, absence seizures, and generalized tonic-clonic seizures are all more likely to occur within 1 hour to 2 hours of awakening and are exacerbated by sleep deprivation. Other generalized epilepsies, such as infantile spasms, may also cluster in the morning hours after arousal. These variety of behaviors associated with seizures can make identification of epilepsy a challenge for clinicians.

Epidemiology

In the 1800s, Gower[69] found 21% of the institutionalized epilepsy patients to have seizures strictly when asleep and 42% to have seizures strictly when awake. These results are similar to Janz's and Billiard's studies of epileptic patients one century later.[30,31,70] Patients with frequent nocturnal seizures more often are found to have frontal lobe epilepsy, although this pattern has also been noted in temporal lobe epilepsy.[69] Some sleep-related epilepsy disorders are common, such as benign childhood epilepsy with central temporal spikes, which comprises approximately 15% to 25% of all childhood epilepsy,[71] whereas other sleep-related epilepsy syndromes, such as ADNFLE, are rare. Seizures on awakening are common and can be a useful diagnostic clue in some patients. Primary generalized epilepsy accounts for approximately 15% of all epilepsy, and juvenile myoclonic epilepsy, the classic awakening epilepsy, accounts for approximately 20% of idiopathic primary generalized epilepsy.[72]

More than 3% of adults and 10% to 30% of children have nocturnal events (epileptic and nonepileptic) and some classical symptoms can be easily confused (**Table 4**). The prevalence of nonepileptic parasomnias in patients with epilepsy is not well known. Khatami[3] found in their survey the prevalence of parasomnias in epilepsy patients was no greater than that of their control group. Approximately 30% of children have disorders of arousal, such as sleepwalking or sleep terror events, and the reported prevalence in adults ranges from 2% to 5%.[73,74] Violence can occur in many of these types of nocturnal events.[75]

Pathophysiology

Sleep seems to be a vulnerable state for seizures and, as discussed previously, this may be related to greater neuronal synchronization during sleep state. REM sleep seems protective against epileptic seizures.[37] For some distinct forms of nocturnal epilepsy, sleep and arousals may demonstrate the state dependent receptor abnormality. The Italian form of ADNFLE, originally described by Lugaresi,[76–78] is an example of this vulnerability. Passed in an autosomal dominant pattern, patients have recurrent nocturnal events characterized by brief tonic movements, nocturnal dystonia, paroxysmal arousals, and nocturnal wandering. Patients may demonstrate any combination of these behaviors with few EEG changes and normal daytime EEGs. The genetics of this disorder was originally described in Australia and,

Table 4
Distinguishing features of nocturnal events

Feature	Disorders of Arousal (Sleepwalking, Sleep Terrors, Confusional Arousals)	REM Behavior Disorder	Nocturnal Seizures	Behavioral Events	Rhythmic Movement Disorder
Time of occurrence	First third of night	During REM	Anytime	Anytime	Start of sleep
Memory of event	Usually none	Dream recall	Usually none	None	Variable
Stereotypical movements	No	No	Yes	No	Yes
Eyes open	Yes	No	Yes	Variable	Variable
PSG findings	Arousals from stage N3 sleep	Excessive EMG tone during REM	Potentially epileptiform activity	Occur from awake state	Rhythmic movement artifact

subsequently, in Italy.[79–81] These patients frequently respond to anticonvulsant therapy. The Australian form of ADNFLE has been linked to chromosome 20q 13.2 to the CHRNA4 gene.[80,81] An abnormality of the neuronal nicotinic acetylcholine receptor subunits have been found in association with this disorder. Although augmentation of acetylcholine does not seem to alter the frequency or intensity of the seizures, nicotine may influence some function of select receptor abnormalities.[82,83] The mechanism for other nocturnal epilepsy syndromes has yet to be determined. The benign childhood epilepsies seem to have a combination of multiple genes influence the presence of the EEG findings and the seizures.

CLINICAL SYMPTOMS
Seizure-Related Behavior

Nocturnal seizures can produce a wide range of behaviors depending on the location of the seizure discharge. Nearly any behavior that can be produced by the brain can be exhibited as a seizure, but the hallmark of seizures is their stereotypic nature of the behavior. Frontal and temporal lobes are the most common sites for seizure foci, and these are areas more commonly involved in sleep-related epilepsies. Seizures involving the frontal lobes may evoke tonic posturing, complex bizarre motor activity, thrashing, and even violent behavior other characteristics that may suggest nonepileptic events or parasomnias. These events can be abrupt and involve unilateral and bilateral movements.[84] Temporal lobe seizures usually produce episodes of staring, psychic phenomena, and occasionally complex behaviors. Temporal and frontal lobe seizures can also evoke a wide range of autonomic symptoms, such as bradycardia, asystole, tachycardia, and emesis, and respiratory disturbances, such as central apnea and irregular breathing. Parietal-onset seizures are more likely to evoke disturbances or distortion of sensory perception. Occipital lobe-onset seizures are usually associated with visual phenomena, visual distortion, or eye movement.

After a seizure, patients are frequently confused and disoriented. The authors have recorded wandering behavior, pronounced violence, rhythmic movement, snoring, and even psychosis as postictal events. The confusion may resolve over minutes or may only improve after a patient sleeps. Postictal somnolence is common and can make differentiating seizures from parasomnia difficult. Memory loss is a frequent feature of complex partial or generalized seizures. Patients without bilateral temporal lobe involvement during the seizures can retain memory for the events and, therefore, may have complex behaviors with retained memory. These patients are frequently misdiagnosed as having psychogenic disorders. Seizures may be influenced by the time of day or underlying circadian rhythm. Quigg[85,86] demonstrated that temporal lobe seizures are more common in the afternoon for both humans and rats, but extratemporal seizures did not have a circadian pattern. Quigg[86] also found that seizures produce phase shifts in the circadian rhythm of animals. Loddenkemper[51] reports slightly different findings in the relationship of time to seizure type in children, showing an increase in generalized seizures after awakening and more frontal lobe seizures at night. Although it is difficult to separate, seizures may be influenced by both circadian and sleep-wake states, and some epilepsies are recognized to produce seizures predominantly at a particular time of day (**Table 5**). Some of these seizure types are distinct epileptic syndromes.

Autosomal Dominant Nocturnal Frontal Lobe Epilepsy

ADNFLE is a well-recognized genetic syndrome related to a defect of the neuronal nicotinic acetylcholine receptor subunit. ADNFLE is characterized by a triad of

Table 5
State-dependent epileptic syndromes

Epilepsy	Time of Occurrence
ADNFLE	Nocturnal
BECTS	Nocturnal (more likely first half of night)
Benign nocturnal childhood occiptal epilepsy Panayiotopoulos syndrome	Nocturnal
Continuous spike and wave during sleep or electrical status during sleep	Discharge during sleep
LKS	Interictal discharge in sleep
Primary generalized seizures with awakening/ juvenile myoclonic epilepsy (awakening)	On awakening (more common in morning)

paroxysmal arousals, episodic nocturnal wandering, and paroxysmal dystonic posturing.[76–82] Previously known as hypnogenic paroxysmal dystonia or nocturnal paroxysmal dystonia, this is characterized by repeated dystonic or dyskinetic episodes occurring at night. The dystonic movements can involve a single extremity or up to all 4 extremities and neck and occasionally involve vocalization. Patients may frequently recall portions of the event. They typically occur out of NREM sleep and demonstrate in 2 major forms: short duration (15–60 seconds) and long duration (up to 60 minutes). Patients may have multiple spells per night or may have clusters of spells with quiescent periods. Nocturnal paroxysmal dystonia is considered a form of frontal lobe epilepsy. These events may have no or subtle EEG-associated changes. Some patients may note less frequent events with the use of nicotine.[87] The family history can be difficult to obtain, because the spells may not be recognized by or acknowledged to other family members. Approximately 1 in 2 of these individuals has daytime seizures. Most patients respond to anticonvulsant medication, with carbamazepine, oxcarbazepine, and lamotrigine as likely agents given their propensity for interaction and stabilize the nicotinic receptor.[88,89]

Benign focal epilepsy with centrotemporal spikes (BECTS) or benign rolandic epilepsy is another form of inherited epilepsy with nocturnal seizures. BECTS commonly occurs in children between 5 and 12 years of age.[71] Patients typically present with episodes of hemifacial and body tonic activity, drooling, and speech impairment. These events occur approximately 20 minutes to 2 hours after going to bed. EEG usually demonstrates a high-amplitude centrotemporal spike and wave discharge associated with bifrontal positivity. Patients are often treated with anticonvulsant medications (valproate and carbamazepine), which are highly efficacious; typically the seizures diminish with age. Although clinicians debate who needs treatment, most agree children with generalized tonic-clonic seizures should be treated. The prognosis of this form of epilepsy is good, with or without medications. Some research suggests that children with this syndrome have partial speech and language impairment, yet the effect of treatment on the ultimate outcome is still unknown.[90] There are some data that suggest cognitive impairment is associated with frequency of interictal nocturnal spikes and suppression of those may improve outcome, although this approach is debatable.[90]

Landau-Kleffner Syndrome and Continuous Spike and Wave During Sleep or Electrical Status During Sleep

LKS is an acquired disorder characterized by decline in verbal fluency and centrotemporal spike in sleep.[90–92] These patients may not have frank seizures but are noted to have expressive and receptive language difficulties. This syndrome is potentially a more focal form of continuous spike and wave during sleep. This syndrome is associated with seizure-like electrical activity that replaces the normal features of sleep on EEG. Patry[92] described 6 children in whom the background electrical activity was replaced with slow 1-Hz to 2.5-Hz generalized spike and wave discharges in sleep. These children also may not have significant nocturnal behavioral manifestations, but they have cognitive and psychological deficits. Many of these children have nocturnal and diurnal absence, focal motor, and generalized tonic-clonic seizures.

Both LKS and ESES are associated with childhood onset; progressive cognitive decline in associated with focal (LKS) or generalized (ESES) discharges during NREM sleep.[92] Response to standard antiepileptic medications is usually poor and, in cases of LKS, steroids or intravenous immunoglobulin as well as novel surgical therapy, such as multiple subpial transections, may improve outcome. Patients have been reported to respond to levetiracetam, intravenous immunoglobulin, or corticosteroids.[91–95]

Benign Nocturnal Childhood Occipital Epilepsy (Panayiotopoulos Syndrome)

This syndrome, first described in 1989, was originally characterized by the constellation of nocturnal seizures, tonic eye deviation, and nocturnal vomiting, typically starting in childhood and ending in early adolescence.[96] The EEG demonstrated epileptiform discharges in the occipital region. Further descriptions have expanded the spectrum of clinical manifestations demonstrating cases in which there is overlap with other focal idiopathic epilepsies, such as benign rolandic epilepsy and other generalized epilepsy syndromes. This syndrome is noted to respond well to medications and seems a self-limited form of epilepsy. Benign occipital epilepsy of childhood is frequently confused with nocturnal migraine. With the complexity of these behaviors, an overlap in presentation among patients with seizures and parasomnias can easily be seen.[96]

Primary Generalized Seizures on Awakening/Juvenile Myoclonic Epilepsy

Patients with Primary Generalized Seizures upon Awakening or Juvenile Myoclonic Epilepsy have seizures frequently within 1 hour to 2 hours after awakening.[97] The seizures may be simple myoclonic jerks or include generalized tonic-clonic seizures. Epileptic-based myoclonus usually occurs in clusters soon after awakening. The rapid jerk of myoclonus can involve any portion of the body.[14] Myoclonus associated with the awakening epilepsies frequently occurs soon after arousal. The jerks can occur in a rapid succession or as single events and may lead into a generalized tonic-clonic seizure. Sleep deprivation exacerbates seizures significantly in this form of epilepsy. They should be differentiated from hypnic jerks, which occur at sleep onset, and periodic limb movements, which occur mostly during NREM sleep. These types of seizures are more likely to respond to first line agents such as valproate, topiramate, levetiracetam, and lamotrigine, whereas zonisamide, clonazepam, and phenobarbital, which are helpful second-line agents.[98]

Approach to Nocturnal Events and Epilepsy

The cornerstone of any evaluation of nocturnal events is the history and physical examination. Although there are no absolutes, the foundation of the evaluation is based on the accurate description of the behaviors. Key is the account of the events from witnesses who may give cardinal clues to the cause. Features of stereotypic behavior and a repetitive nature of the events point to a possible underlying epileptic disorder. Patients usually do not have memory for the seizures, and the seizures can occur at any time in the sleep period (day or night). Features in the history, such as frequency of events, time of events in the sleep period, family history of nocturnal events, seizures or parasomnias, and a history of recent stressors or spells during wakefulness are also important. Most nocturnal seizures occur in NREM sleep, whether they are of temporal or frontal onset.[99] Rare REM-related seizures have been described involving recurrent dreams and dreams, similarly to RBD.[100] Other investigators have described seizures involving recurrent dreams.[101] Patients can have a variety of nocturnal behaviors, such as ambulation, confused wandering, or screaming, which seem similar to events of sleepwalking or sleep terrors. Some seizures have a repetitive nature that can be easily confused with rhythmic movement disorder. The overlap of these symptoms can make classification of these extraordinary events difficult.

The physical examination may provide clues to focal neurologic lesions that may increase the likelihood of certain disorders. Focal lesions in the cerebrum increase the risk epileptic seizures, whereas findings indicative of Parkinson disease suggest the possibility of RBD. For epilepsy, historic features, such as stereotyped events, the occurrence of a seizure while awake, or family history of seizures, add to the evidence supporting a diagnosis of nocturnal seizures.

Many times, distinguishing NREM parasomnias from frontal lobe seizures can be difficult, especially because there is significant overlap in PSG features. Derry and colleagues[102] found seizures more likely to come out of stages 1 and 2 sleep whereas parasomnias were from stages 3 and 4 sleep. They also found the captured seizures events were concordant with the historical features of the events, but the parasomnias varied. The prevalence of REM sleep–related parasomnias, such as RBD, is unknown but seems to increase with age.[103] Zacconi[20] proposed that multiple events per night and a continuum of minor to major behaviors was more frequently seen in nocturnal frontal lobe epilepsy than NREM parasomnias. The physical examination is frequently normal, but findings may indicate cerebral insults or other evidence of potential increased risk for seizures. Many clinicians consider a response to anticonvulsant therapy supporting evidence of the diagnosis of epilepsy. In the authors' opinion, the response to anticonvulsant therapy should not be considered supportive evidence, because anticonvulsants have diverse neuropharmacologic effects.

Traditional analog PSG has several technical disadvantages. The limited encephalographic electrode placement decreases the likelihood of capturing an epileptiform discharge. The common paper speed of 10 mm per second is also inadequate for observing many ictal epileptic events and does not allow identifying interictal abnormalities. For PSG evaluation of these patients, the display windows should show 10 seconds of data and the array of cephalic electrodes increased. The display of the EEG data can be easily performed with current digital equipment the display window; however, greater coverage with cephalic electrodes requires more channels of EEG displayed and comfort of the reader in detecting epileptiform activity. Incorporation of a full 10-electrode to 20-electrode array and paper speed of 30 mm per second are helpful in evaluating for seizures. Foldvary[104] found that a 7-channel EEG montage and increasing paper speed to 30 mm per second improved the detection epileptic events to greater than 80%. These settings and expanded electrode array allow for better differentiation of the epileptiform discharges from potential normal variants or artifacts.

Patients suspected of having epilepsy are typically studied with routine EEG. EEG is frequently normal in individuals with sleep-related epilepsies and the absence of an epileptiform discharge does not rule out the possibility of epilepsy. Sleep also plays a significant role in the prevalence, morphology, and location of interictal discharges. Interictal discharges are more common in NREM sleep, whereas REM sleep demonstrates some antiepileptic qualities.[105]

Patients who continue to have events despite multiple medication trials may be considered for further evaluation. Capturing multiple events on video-EEG recording and comparing behaviors, EEG, and other measures, such as postictal prolactin levels, can lead to a greater chance of obtaining an accurate diagnosis.

Treatment

Treatment of nocturnal seizures may be challenging. Even in the best of circumstances, seizures are frequently missed, but seizures during the night are typically not witnessed unless they involve significant motor components. If patients are having seizures only at night, clinicians should strive to use medications that can achieve drug levels in the brain quickly and avoid daytime side effects. Alterations in medication dosing may be used to control daytime seizures. These typically come in the form of standard release forms, because extended-release medications may outlast the sleep period. Clinicians may need to use multiple medications if patients fail monotherapy trials. Patients with ADNFLE are more likely to respond to lamotrigine or carbamazepine, whereas patients with benign childhood epilepsy with centrotemporal spikes seem to respond well to carbamazepine or levetiracetam.[71] Individuals with nocturnal occipital lobe seizures are also likely to respond to carbamazepine, and those with awakening primary generalized seizures respond well to valproate or topiramate.

Patients and families should be cautioned regarding the safety of the patients who have nocturnal seizures. Patients may have wandering as part of the postictal confusion; thus, safety guards and removal of potential hazards may be helpful. Additionally, patients' families should be advised on first aid for seizures, a protocol for when to use emergent intranasal or rectal medication, and when to contact emergency services. More recently, circadian rhythm influence on pharmacokinetics has been suggested in a small study examining phenytoin.[49] The circadian rhythm influences drug absorption, protein binding, distribution, clinical effect, and metabolism and excretion. Two studies suggest that epilepsy patients may have more favorable seizure control and less side effects with chronopharmacology two-thirds or greater of their traditional mediation (phenytoin or carbamazepine) given in the evening.[106,107] Although these studies are preliminary, they do open an area of interaction of the circadian rhythm, pharmacokinetics, and brain response that may prove fruitful in the treatment of epilepsy.

Prognosis

Most patients with nocturnal seizures or awakening epilepsy seem to respond to medication. This condition may be more refractive to therapy especially for those individuals with complex epilepsies, underlying neurologic deficits, and frontal lobe seizures. Attention to type and timing of medication may influence the outcome.

FUTURE DIRECTION

The complexity of the interaction of sleep and epilepsy demands further research dedicated to delineating the mechanisms of both sleep regulation and the development of epilepsy. Each type of epilepsy may have its own vulnerabilities and interaction with the sleep-wake regulatory processes. Further work is also needed to fully determine which patients are most likely to benefit to improvement in sleep and if improvement in sleep should be included in a package of therapies to prevent the development of intractable epilepsy.

Case report

A 24 year old male with a history of generalized tonic-clonic seizures, presumed from a primary generalized epilepsy, presents with an increase in seizures over the past two years. The patient noted that although his seizures were previously controlled with valproate, and now were averaging one to three seizures per week. The patient noted most of his seizures occurred in morning, but rarely during the night. In recounting the evolution of his seizures, the patient noted after he finished college, he gained approximately 40 lbs. He also noted that he was more tired during the day and he suffered from morning headaches. Upon questioning his family complained about his snoring, but no one witnessed apneas. His Epworth Sleepiness Scale total score was 9 and his STOPBANG score was 5. Physical exam showed a mild elevated heart rate of 84 bpm, blood pressure of 123/82 mm Hg, BMI 32, clear oral pharynx and trace pretibial edema. The patient underwent overnight polysomnography which showed an apnea hypopnea index of 15.6 events per hour with desaturation to 85%. The patient had frequent generalized spike and wave discharges, especially with arousals.

The patient subsequently completed a positive airway pressure titration showing resolution of the obstruction at 10 cm H2O. The patient started CPAP and within the first week noted resolution of the morning seizures. At his 1 month follow-up clinic visit, the patient had an Epworth Sleepiness Scale total score of 8, and only one recurrent seizure after he fell asleep without the CPAP. The patient was counseled about weight control, diet and exercise. One year later, the patient was converted from valproate to lamotrigine, and subsequently had 25 lb weight loss. A repeat sleep study showed an apnea hypopnea index of 6.8 and the patient elected to continue the CPAP therapy.

This case demonstrates that sleep may impact epilepsy. For this patient recurrent seizures were the chief complaint but further investigation revealed the underlying provocative factor was the sleep apnea. The associated symptoms of sleepiness, morning headache and weight gain are important clues. The patient's Epworth Sleepiness Scale total score was below the typical threshold of 10 for sleepiness but the STOPBANG score of 5 is very suggestive of sleep apnea. Although most patients will have some symptoms of sleep apnea, the clinician should be cognizant that these patients may not have typical features of sleep apnea. For this patient the weight gain was most likely a combination of medication effect, valproate, and lifestyle. The clinician needs to be aware that medications to treat seizures can improve sleep by decreasing nighttime seizure activity, but also may interfere directly or as in this case indirectly. The case also demonstrates that the treatment of the sleep disorder can improve the epilepsy and sleep symptoms. These patients can tolerate CPAP but close follow up to ensure compliance is key.

REFERENCES

1. Miller MT, Vaughn BV, Messenheimer JA, et al. Subjective sleep quality in patients with epilepsy. Epilepsia 1996;36(Suppl 4):43.
2. de Weerd A, de Haas S, Otte A, et al. Subjective sleep disturbance in patients with partial epilepsy: a questionnaire-based study on prevalence and impact on quality of life. Epilepsia 2004;45(11):1397–404.
3. Khatami R, Zutter D, Siegel A, et al. Sleep-wake habits and disorders in a series of 100 adult epilepsy patients–a prospective study. Seizure 2006;15:299–306.
4. Chen NC, Tsai MH, Chang CC, et al. Sleep quality and daytime sleepiness in patients with epilepsy. Acta Neurol Taiwan 2011;20:249–56.
5. Malow BA, Bowes RJ, Lin X. Predictors of sleepiness in epilepsy patients. Sleep 1997;20(12):1105–10.
6. Giorelli AS, Neves GS, Venturi M, et al. Excessive daytime sleepiness in patients with epilepsy: a subjective evaluation. Epilepsy Behav 2011;21(4):449–52.
7. Maganti R, Hausman N, Koehn M, et al. Excessive daytime sleepiness and sleep complaints among children with epilepsy. Epilepsy Behav 2006;8(1):272–7. Erratum in: Epilepsy Behav 2006;9:216–7.

8. Touchon J, Baldy-Moulinier M, Billiard M, et al. Sleep organization and epilepsy. Epilepsia 1991;2:73–81.

9. Zanzmera P, Shukla G, Gupta A, et al. Markedly disturbed sleep in medically refractory compared to controlled epilepsy - A clinical and polysomnography study. Seizure 2012 May 24. [Epub ahead of print].

10. Malow BA, Fromes GA, Aldrich MS. Usefulness of polysomnography in epilepsy patients. Neurology 1997;48(5):1389–94.

11. Manni R, Terzaghi M, Arbasino C, et al. Obstructive sleep apnea in a clinical series of adult epilepsy patients: frequency and features of the comorbidity. Epilepsia 2003;44(6):836–40.

12. Chihorek AM, Abou-Khalil B, Malow BA. Obstructive sleep apnea is associated with seizure occurrence in older adults with epilepsy. Neurology 2007;69(19): 1823–7.

13. Kryer M, Quesney LF, Holder D, et al. The sleep deprivation syndrome of the obese patient, a problem with periodic nocturnal upper airway obstruction. Amer J Med 1974;56:531–8.

14. Sonka K, Juklichova M, Pretl M, et al. Seizures in sleep apnea patients: Occurrence and time distribution. Sb Lekarsky 2000;1(3):229–32.

15. Parrino L, De Paolis F, Milioli G, et al. Distinctive polysomnographic traits in nocturnal frontal lobe epilepsy. Epilepsia 2012 May 11. [Epub ahead of print].

16. Peled R, Lavie P. Paroxysmal awakenings from sleep associated with excessive daytime somnolence a form of nocturnal epilepsy. Neurology 1986;36(1):95–8.

17. Malow BA, Lin X, Kushwaha R, et al. Interictal spiking increases with sleep depth in temporal lobe epilepsy. Epilepsia 1998;39(12):1309–16.

18. Crespel A, Baldy-Moulinier M, Coubes P. The relationship between sleep and epilepsy in frontal and temporal lobe epilepsies: practical and physiopathologic considerations. Epilepsia 1998;39:150–7.

19. Zaatreh MM, Quint SR, Tennison MB, et al. Heart rate variability during interictal epileptiform discharges. Epilepsy Res 2003;54:85–90.

20. Zacconi M, Ferini-Strambi L. NREM parasomnias: arousals and differentiation from nocturnal frontal lobe epilepsy. Clin Neurophysiol 2000;111(Suppl. 2): S129–35.

21. Bazil CW, Walczak TS. Effect of sleep and sleep stage on epileptic and nonepileptic seizures. Epilepsia 1997;38:56–62.

22. Besset A. Influence of generalized seizures on sleep organization. In: Stermna MB, Shouse MN, Passouant P, editors. Sleep and Epilepsy. New York: Academic Press; 1982. p. p.339–46.

23. Dinner DS. Effect of sleep on epilepsy. J Clin Neurophysiol 2002;19(6):504–13.

24. Ellinson RJ, Wilkin K, Bennett DR. Efficacy of sleep deprivation as an activation procedure in epilepsy patients. J Clin Neurophysiol 1984;1:83–101.

25. Thomaides TN, Kerezoudi EP, Chaudhuri LR, et al. Study of EEG's following 24 hour sleep deprivation in patients with post traumatic epilepsy. Eur Neurol 1992; 32:79–82.

26. Britton JW, Kosa SC. The clinical value of choral hydrate in the routine electroencephalogram. Epilepsy Res 2010;88:215–20.

27. Degen R, Degen HE, Reker M. Sleep EEG with or without sleep deprivation? Does sleep deprivation activate more epileptic activity in patients suffering from different types of epilepsy? Eur Neurol 1987;26(1):51–9.

28. Larsson PG, Evsiukova T, Brockmeier F, et al. Do sleep-deprived EEG recordings reflect spike index as found in full-night EEG recordings? Epilepsy Behav 2010;19(3):348–51.

29. Heers M, Rampp S, Kaltenhauser M, et al. Detection of epileptic spikes by magnetoencephalography and electroencephaolgraphy after sleep deprivation. Seizure 2010;19:397–403.

30. Janz D. The grand mal epilepsies and the sleep waking cycle. Epilepsia 1962;3: 69–109.

31. Janz D. Epilepsy and the sleep-waking cycle. In: Vinken PJ, Bruyn GW, editors. The epilepsias, handbook of clinical neurology, Vol 15. Amsterdam: North Holland; 1974. p. 457–90.

32. Rajna P, Veres J. Correlations between night sleep duration and seizure frequency in temporal lobe epilepsy. Epilepsia 1993;343(3):574–9.

33. Vaughn BV, D'Cruz OF. Obstructive sleep apnea in epilepsy. In: Lee-Chiong T, Mohsenin V, editors. Clinics in chest medicine. Philadelphia: Elsevier Science; 2003. p. 239–48.

34. Shouse MN, Farber PR, Staba RJ. Physiological basis: how NREM sleep components can promote and REM sleep components can suppress seizure discharge propagation. Clin Neurophysiol 2000;111(suppl 2):S9–18.

35. Staba RJ, Wilson CL, Bragin A, et al. Sleep states differentiate single neuron activity recorded from human epileptic hippocampus, entorhinal cortex and subiculum. Jo Neuroscience 2002;22:5694–704.

36. Kumar P, Raju TR. Seizure susceptibility decreases with enhancement of rapid eye movement sleep. Brain Research 2001;922:299–304.

37. Herman ST, Walczak TS, Bazil CW. Distribution of partial seizures during the sleep–wake cycle: differences by seizure onset site. Neurology 2001;56(11):1453–9.

38. Minecan D, Natarajan A, Marzec M, et al. Relationship of epileptic seizures to sleep stage and sleep depth. Sleep 2002;25(8):899–904.

39. Liow K, Ablah E, Nguyen JC, et al. Pattern and frequency of use of complementary and alternative medicine among patients with epilepsy in the midwestern United States. Epilepsy Behav 2007;10(4):576–82.

40. Quigg M. Seizures and circadian rhythms. Sleep and epilepsy: the clinical spectrum. 1st edition. Amsterdam: Elsevier Science; 2002. p.127–p.142.

41. Paprocka J, Dec R, Jamroz E, et al. Melatonin and childhood refractory epilepsy – a pilot study. Med Sci Monit 2010;16:CR389–96.

42. Sammarintino M, Sherwin A. Effect of anticonvulsants on sleep. Neurology 2000; 54(1):S16–24.

43. Brogden RN, Heel RC, Speight TM, et al. Clobazam: a review of its pharmacological properties and therapeutic use in anxiety. Drugs 1980;20(3):161–78.

44. Bazil CW, Dave J, Cole J, et al. Pregabalin increases slow-wave sleep and may improve attention in patients with partial epilepsy and insomnia. Epilepsy Behav 2012;23(4):422–5.

45. Walsh JK, Perlis M, Rosenthal M, et al. Tiagabine increases slow-wave sleep in a dose-dependent fashion without affecting traditional efficacy measures in adults with primary insomnia. J Clin Sleep Med 2006;2(1):35–41.

46. Manni R, Tartara A. Evaluation of sleepiness in epilepsy. Clin Neurophysiol 2000; 111(Suppl. 2):S111–4.

47. Kanner AM, Palac S. Neuropsychiatric complications of epilepsy. Curr Neurol Neurosci Rep 2002;2(4):365–72.

48. Dailey JW, Naritoku DK. Antidepressants and seizures: Clinical anecdotes overshadow neuroscience. Biochem Pharmacol 1996;52(9):1323–9.

49. Yegnanarayan R, Mahesh SD, Sangle S. Chronotherapeutic dose schedule of phenytoin and carbamazepine in epileptic patients. Chronobiol Int 2006;23(5): 1035–46.

50. Salinski MC, Oken BS, Binder LM. Assessment of drowsiness in epilepsy patients receiving chronic antiepileptic drug therapy. Epilepsia 1996;37(2): 181–7.

51. Loddenkemper T, Lockley SW, Kaleyias J, et al. Chronobiology of epilepsy: diagnostic and therapeutic implications of chrono-epileptology. J Clin Neurophysiol 2011;28(2):146–53.

52. Hofstra WA, van der Palen J, de Weerd AW. Morningness and eveningness: when do patients take their antiepileptic drugs? Eur J Pediatr 2012;171(4): 675–9.

53. Goldberg-Stern H, Oren H, Peled N, et al. Effect of Melatonin on Seizure Frequency in Intractable Epilepsy: A Pilot Study. J Child Neurol 2012.

54. Wyler AR, Weymuller EA. Epilepsy complicated by sleep apnea. Ann Neurol 1981;9:403–4.

55. Devinsky O, Ehrenberg B, Bathlen GM, et al. Epilepsy and sleep apnea syndrome. Neurology 1994;44:2060–4.

56. Vaughn BV, D'Cruz OF, Beach R, et al. Improvement of epileptic seizure control with treatment of obstructive sleep apnea. Seizure 1996;5:73–8.

57. Ezpeleta D, Garcia-Penna A, Peraita-Adrados R. Epilepsia y sindrome de apnea del sueno. Rev Neurol 1998;26(151):389–92.

58. Koh S, Ward SL, Lin M, et al. Sleep apnea treatment improves seizure control in children with neurodevelopmental disorders. Pediatr Neurol 2000;22:36–9.

59. Malow BA, Foldvary-Schaefer N, Vaughn BV, et al. Treating obstructive sleep apnea in adults with epilepsy: a randomized pilot trial. Neurology 2008;71(8): 572–7.

60. Segal E, Vendrame M, Gregas M, et al. Effect of treatment of obstructive sleep apnea on seizure outcomes in children with epilepsy. Pediatr Neurol 2012;46(6): 359–62.

61. Westwood AJ, Vendrame M, Montouris G, et al. Pearls & Oysters: treatment of central sleep apnea with topiramate. Neurology 2012;78(16):e97–9.

62. Cooper-Kazaz R. Treatment of night eating syndrome with topiramate: dawn of a new day. J Clin Psychopharmacol 2012;32(1):143–5.

63. Palikh GM, Vaughn BV. Topiramate responsive exploding head syndrome. J Clin Sleep Med 2010;6(4):382–3.

64. Ehrenberg B. Importance of sleep restoration in co-morbid disease: Effect of anticonvulsants. Neurology 2000;54(Suppl. 1):S33–7.

65. Lee DO, Ziman RB, Perkins AT, et al. A randomized, double-blind, placebo-controlled study to assess the efficacy and tolerability of gabapentin enacarbil in subjects with restless legs syndrome. J Clin Sleep Med 2011;7(3):282–92.

66. Misra UK, Kalita J, Kumar B, et al. Treatment of restless legs syndrome with pregabalin: a double-blind, placebo-controlled study. Neurology 2011;76(4):408.

67. Bazil CW, Dave J, Cole J, et al. Pregabalin increases slow-wave sleep and may improve attention in patients with partial epilepsy and insomnia. Epilepsy Behav 2012;23(4):422–5.

68. Mahowald MW, Schenck CH. REM Sleep Parasomnias. Section xi, chapter 75. In: Kryger MH, Roth T, Dement WC, editors. Principles and practice of sleep medicine. 4th edition. Philadelphia: W.B. Saunders; 2003. p. 897–916.

69. Passouant P. Historical aspects of sleep and epilepsy. Epilepsy Res 1991;2: 19–30.

70. Billiard M. Epilepsies and the sleep–wake. In: Sterman MB, Shouse MN, Passouant P, editors. Sleep and epilepsy. New York: Academic Press; 1982. p. 269–86.

71. Shields WD, Snead OC. Benign epilepsy with centrotemporal spikes. Epilepsia 2009;50(Suppl 8):10–5.
72. Mullins GM, O'sullivan SS, Neligan A, et al. A study of idiopathic generalised epilepsy in an Irish population. Seizure 2007;16(3):204–10.
73. Bixler EO, Kales A, Soldatos CR, et al. Prevalence of sleep disorders in the Los Angeles Metropolitan Area. Amer J Psych 1979;136:1257–62.
74. Klackenberg G. Incidence of parasomnias in children in a general population. In: Guilleminault C, editor. Sleep and its disorders in children. New York: Raven Press; 1987. p. 99–113.
75. Siclari F, Khatami R, Urbaniok F, et al. Violence in. Sleep Brain 2010;133: 3494–509.
76. Lugaresi E, Cirigonotta F. Nocturnal paroxysmal dystonia. In: Sternman MB, Shouse MN, Passouant P, editors. Sleep and epilepsy. New York: Academic Press; 1982. p. 507–11.
77. Montplaisir J, Godbout R, Rouleau I. Hypnogenic paroxysmal dystonia: Nocturnal epilepsy or sleep disorder? Sleep Res 1985;14:193.
78. Silvestri R, De Domenico P, Raffaele M, et al. Hypnogenic paroxysmal dystonia: a new type of parasomnia? Functional Neurol 1988;3:95–103.
79. Phillips HA, Scheffer IE, Berkovic SF, et al. Localization of a gene for autosomal dominant nocturnal frontal lobe epilepsy to chromosome 20q 13.2 Nature Genet 1995;10(1):117–8.
80. Steinlein OK, Mulley JC, Propping P, et al. A missense mutation in the neuronal nicotinic acetylcholine receptor alpha 4 subunit is associated with autosomal dominant nocturnal frontal lobe epilepsy. Nature Genet 1995;11(2):201–3.
81. Steinlein OK, Magnusson A, Stoodt J, et al. An insertion mutation of the CHRNA4 gene in a family with autosomal dominant nocturnal frontal lobe epilepsy. Human Mol Genet 1997;6(6):943–7.
82. Oldani A, Zucconi M, Asselta R, et al. Autosomal dominant nocturnal frontal lobe epilepsy. A video-polysomnographic and genetic appraisal of 40 patients and delineation of the epileptic syndrome. Brain 1998;121:205–23.
83. Son CD, Moss FJ, Cohen BN, et al. Nicotine normalizes intracellular subunit stoichiometry of nicotinic receptors carrying mutations linked to autosomal dominant nocturnal frontal lobe epilepsy. Mol Pharmacol 2009;75:1137–48.
84. Ryvlin P, Rheims S, Risse G. Nocturnal frontal lobe epilepsy. Epilepsia 2006; 47(Suppl 2):83–6.
85. Quigg M, Straume M, Menaker M, et al. 3rd Temporal distribution of partial seizures: comparison of an animal model with human partial epilepsy. Ann Neurol 1998;43(6):748–55.
86. Quigg M, Straume M, Smith T, et al. Seizures induce phase shifts of rat circadian rhythms. Brain Res 2001;913(2):165–9.
87. Son CD, Moss FJ, Cohen BN, et al. Nicotine normalizes intracellular subunit stoichiometry of nicotinic receptors carrying mutations linked to autosomal dominant nocturnal frontal lobe epilepsy. Mol Pharmacol 2009;75:1137–48.
88. Di Resta C, Ambrosi P, Curia G, et al. Effect of carbamazepine and oxcarbazepine on wild-type and mutant neuronal nicotinic acetylcholine receptors linked to nocturnal frontal lobe epilepsy. Eur J Pharmacol 2010;643(1):13–20.
89. Zheng C, Yang K, Liu Q, et al. The anticonvulsive drug lamotrigine blocks neuronal {alpha}4{beta}2 nicotinic acetylcholine receptors. J Pharmacol Exp Ther 2010;335(2):401–8.
90. Baglietto MG, Battaglia FM, Nobili L, et al. Neuropsychological disorders related to interictal epileptic discharges during sleep in benign epilepsy of childhood

with centrotemporal or Rolandic spikes. Dev Med Child Neurol 2001;43(6): 407–12.

91. Kothare SV, Kaleyias J. Sleep and epilepsy in children and adolescents. Sleep Med 2010;11(7):674–85.

92. Patry G, Lyagoubi S, Tassinari A. A subclinical "electrical status epilepticus" induced by sleep in children. Arch Neurol 1971;24:242–52.

93. Buzatu M, et al. Corticosteroids as treatment of epileptic syndromes with continuous spike-waves during slow-wave sleep. Epilepsia 2009;50(Suppl 7):68–72.

94. Sinclair DB, et al. Corticosteroids for the treatment of Landau-kleffner syndrome and continuous spike-wave discharge during sleep. Pediatr Neurol 2005;32(5): 300–6.

95. Hoppen T, et al. Successful treatment of pharmacoresistent continuous spike wave activity during slow sleep with levetiracetam. Eur J Pediatr 2003;162(1): 59–61.

96. Capovilla G, Striano P, Beccaria F. Changes in Panayiotopoulos syndrome over time. Epilepsia 2009;50(Suppl 5):45–8.

97. Reutens DC, Berkovic SF. Idiopathic generalized epilepsy of adolescence: are the syndromes clinically distinct? Neurology 1995;45(8):1469–76.

98. Mantoan L, Walker M. Treatment options in juvenile myoclonic epilepsy. Curr Treat Options Neurol 2011;13(4):355–70.

99. Malow BA, Bowes RJ, Ross D. Relationship of temporal lobe seizures to sleep and arousal: A combined scalp-intracranial electrode study. Sleep 2000;23: 231–4.

100. D'Cruz OF, Vaughn BV. Nocturnal seizures mimic REM behavior disorder. Amer J Electro-Neurodiagnosis Technol 1997;37:258–64.

101. Epstein AR, Hill W. Ictal phenomena during REM sleep of a temporal lobe epileptic. Arch Neurol 1966;15:367–75.

102. Derry CP, Harvey AS, Walker MC, et al. NREM Arousal Parasomnia and their distinction from Nocturnal Frontal Lobe Epilepsy: A video EEG Analysis. Sleep 2009;32:1637–44.

103. Schenck CH, Mahowald MW. Polysomnographic, neurologic, psychiatric, and clinical outcome report on 70 consecutive cases with the REM Sleep Behavior Disorder (RBD): sustained clonazepam efficacy in 89.5% of 57 treated patients. Cleveland Clin J Med 1990;57:S10–24.

104. Foldvary N, Caruso AC, Mascha E, et al. Identifying montages that best detect electrographic seizure activity during polysomnography. Sleep 2000;23:221–9.

105. Shouse MN, Siegel JM, Wu MF, et al. Mechanisms of seizure suppression during rapid eye movement (REM) sleep in cats. Brain Res 1989;505:271–82.

106. Yegnanarayan R, Kulkarni HG, Wadia RS. The Effect of Time of Administration of Phenytoin on its Serum Levels and Pharmacodynamic Parameters in Patients of Generalised Tonic Clonic Seizures Biological Rhythm Research 1999;30: 321–31.

107. Guilhoto LM, Loddenkemper T, Vendrame M, et al. Higher evening antiepileptic drug dose for nocturnal and early-morning seizures. Epilepsy Behav 2011; 20(2):334–7.

Sleep, Stroke and Poststroke

Antonio Culebras, MD

KEYWORDS

- Sleep apnea • Stroke • Arousal • Periodic limb movement disorder
- Continuous positive airway pressure • Hypertension • Atrial fibrillation

KEY POINTS

- Sleep apnea, in particular the obstructive form, has been identified as an independent risk factor for cardiovascular and cerebrovascular morbidity.
- Sleep apnea is a modifiable risk factor and efforts to control the condition should be pursued vigorously, particularly in patients at risk of vascular disease.
- Application of nocturnal positive airway pressure (CPAP and variants) is the gold standard treatment of sleep apnea.
- Controlled trials have established that CPAP treatment of patients with moderate to severe sleep apnea lowers blood pressure levels.
- Further clinical research is warranted to determine whether other forms of sleep disruption (PLMS, insomnia, circadian dysrhythmia) are risk factors for vascular disease.

INTRODUCTION

Sleep is one of the pillars of health along with diet and exercise. When sleep is fragmented, not deep enough, or short in duration, a chain of events is released that leads to failing health. Among the most notable offenders is sleep apnea,[1] a highly prevalent disorder that has only been known for just a few decades. There are several forms of sleep apnea (obstructive, nonobstructive or central, and hypopnea) encompassed in the all-inclusive term sleep-related respiratory events. Sleep apnea is the expression used in this article for the generic denomination of all forms of sleep-related disturbance.

Sleep apnea, in particular the obstructive form, has been identified as an independent risk factor for cardiovascular and cerebrovascular morbidity. Sleep apnea alters sleep, night after night, releasing a spectrum of adverse reactions that affect the physical and mental health of the individual and can lead to death. The sleep apnea syndrome refers to sleep apnea with clinical symptoms. It occurs in 4% of adult men and 2% of adult women.[2] The prevalence of sleep apnea without specific complaints might be as high as 24% in men and 9% in women in the general population.[2] In selected populations, such as the obese and the elderly, sleep apnea may occur in as many as 60% of individuals.[3] Although sleep apnea is pre-eminent in

Department of Neurology, Upstate Medical University, 750 East Adams Street, Syracuse, NY 13210, USA
E-mail address: aculebras@aol.com

Neurol Clin 30 (2012) 1275–1284
http://dx.doi.org/10.1016/j.ncl.2012.08.017   neurologic.theclinics.com
0733-8619/12/$ – see front matter © 2012 Elsevier Inc. All rights reserved.

causing vascular disease, recent clinical investigations have unveiled other conditions, such as restless legs syndrome, circadian dysrhythmias, and primary insomnias, as potential additional causes of vascular disease.

AUTONOMIC ALTERATIONS IN SLEEP APNEA

Sleep apnea may provoke a significant increase in sympathetic activity during sleep, which in turn influences heart rate and blood pressure. Increased sympathetic activity seems to be induced through a variety of different mechanisms, including chemoreflex stimulation by hypoxia and hypercapnia, baroreflexes, pulmonary afferents, the Müeller maneuver, impairment in venous return to the heart, alterations in cardiac output, and the arousal response.[4] Sympathetic overactivity seems to be the critical link between sleep apnea and the pathogenesis of hypertension. Sleep apnea influences heart rate variability, not only during sleep but also during wakefulness. Cortelli and colleagues[5] showed that normotensive patients with sleep apnea have higher heart rate at rest during wakefulness and a higher blood pressure response to head-up tilt than control subjects, suggesting sympathetic overactivity. When performing cardiovascular reflex tests, patients with sleep apnea show significantly lower values of respiratory arrhythmia and greater decrease in heart rate induced by cold face testing, indicating normal or increased cardiac vagal efferent activity. Increase in sympathetic activity and autonomic imbalance are possible determinants of cardiovascular comorbidity and increased mortality risk in patients with sleep apnea.[5,6] Treatment of sleep apnea with continuous positive airway pressure (CPAP) leads to a significant improvement of autonomic modulation and cardiovascular variability.[7]

AROUSAL RESPONSE

There is strong evidence indicating that untreated obstructive sleep apnea is a significant risk factor for development of hypertension, cardiovascular disease, and stroke. The pathophysiologic pathway is multifactorial and includes hypoxemia, hypercapnia, and simultaneous elevations in sympathetic and parasympathetic activity, with significant variations in blood pressure and heart rhythm. The arousal response at the termination of untreated sleep apnea events conjugates many of these phenomena and emerges as a principal link in the chain of events that lead to stroke.[8,9] The arousal response is characterized polygraphically by a change in electroencephalogram morphology and an enhancement of muscle tone that facilitates oropharyngeal dilator muscle function, a phenomenon responsible for overcoming the obstruction to air flow. Microneurography, a technique that evaluates autonomic discharges in nerves, has shown surges in sympathetic activity in association with arousals explaining the occurrence of blood pressure elevations and acceleration of the heart rate. Repeated bouts of hypertension night after night in patients with untreated sleep apnea may eventually lead to sustained hypertension through unknown mechanisms.[10]

PROINFLAMMATORY RISK FACTORS

Proinflammatory vascular risk factors, oxidative stress, and endothelial disease may be enhanced by sleep apnea. Inflammation and hypoxia are intertwined at the molecular, cellular, and clinical levels.[11] Repeated hypoxia may damage the endothelium and trigger the release of proinflammatory factors, such as plasma cytokines, tumor necrosis factor-α, and interleukin-6. Chronic intermittent hypoxia causes vascular dysfunction by increasing endothelin, augmenting neurovascular oxidative stress, decreasing vascular neuromuscular reserve, reducing vascular reactivity, and increasing susceptibility to injury.[12] A state of inflammation may be related to gestational hypertension[13,14] and to an increased risk for development of preeclampsia.[15]

BLOOD PRESSURE

Blood pressure values normally drop by 10% to 20% during sleep relative to daytime values, a phenomenon known as "dipping."[16] Nondipping, defined as less than a 10% drop in blood pressure during the night, is common in sleep apnea, increasing in prevalence as the severity of sleep apnea augments.[17] Nondipping has been associated with a higher prevalence of small vessel disease and stroke.[18] Blood pressure tends to increase during daytime hours in patients with sleep apnea, along with variability in blood pressure values.[19] Data from various large-scale population studies clearly demonstrate a dose-dependent relationship between sleep apnea and hypertension,[20,21] particularly when the blood pressure fails to respond optimally to at least three antihypertensive medications. Refractory hypertension is a well-known comorbidity of uncontrolled sleep apnea[22]; it may respond favorably to the successful application of CPAP.[23] Children with sleep apnea may also have abnormal blood pressure levels compared with children without sleep apnea,[24] as noted by signs of cardiac remodeling on echocardiography proportionate to the degree of hypertension.[25]

ATRIAL FIBRILLATION

Atrial fibrillation is another vascular factor increasing the risk of stroke that has been associated with sleep apnea. The prevalence of atrial fibrillation in the United States has been estimated at 3.03 million persons in 2005[26]; it has been increasing as more individuals survive into old age.[27] Clinical data have shown a strong relationship between sleep apnea and atrial fibrillation and epidemiologic studies suggest that sleep apnea is a risk factor for new-onset atrial fibrillation. A large study evaluated 3542 patients without atrial fibrillation who underwent polysomnography and were followed for an average of 5 years.[28] In patients less than 65 years old, nocturnal oxygen desaturation predicted new-onset atrial fibrillation. Furthermore, sleep apnea may confer a poorer prognosis for recovery after atrial fibrillation interventions. In a study of 424 patients undergoing ablation, sleep apnea more than doubled the risk of acute intraprocedural failure.[29] The effects of sleep apnea therapy on atrial fibrillation outcomes are largely unknown and prospective randomized controlled trials are necessary to clarify this issue. There is some indication that in patients with atrial fibrillation undergoing ablation, procedural failure may be predicted by sleep apnea and noncompliance with CPAP.[30]

PATENT FORAMEN OVALE

Patent foramen ovale (PFO) has been estimated to occur with a range of 10% to 30% in the general population,[31] with prevalence dependent on the diagnostic method. The association between PFO and sleep apnea was described in one study where 27% of patients with sleep apnea and 15% of control subjects had PFO ($P<.05$).[32] This association suggests that nocturnal apneic-related shunting could augment the risk of paradoxic embolism and stroke, a risk that increases further should pulmonary hypertension develop as a result of nocturnal hypoxemia.[33] In one study of 339 consecutive patients with stroke,[34] stroke on awakening was found in 39% of patients with sleep apnea and PFO; conversely, stroke on awakening occurred in only 26% of patients with no association, leading to the notion that the association of sleep apnea and PFO might be a risk factor for stroke on awakening (odds ratio [OR], 2.2; 95% confidence interval [CI], 1.2–3.9; $P = .01$). Further studies are warranted.

CEREBRAL HEMODYNAMIC CHANGES

In regions with poor hemodynamic reserve where cerebral circulation is compromised, hemodynamic alterations may act as triggers of irreversible ischemic changes, particularly in borderzone areas and terminal artery territories. Preliminary studies of auditory event-related potentials in patients with treated sleep apnea[35] have found no improvement in abnormal P3 wave latencies, suggesting permanent structural changes in the white matter of the hemispheres, likely as a result of ischemia. Conversely, healthy children with mild sleep-disordered breathing[36] exhibit cerebral hemodynamic and neurobehavioral changes that are potentially reversible after adenotonsillectomy, suggesting normalization of middle cerebral artery blood flow as measured with transcranial Doppler techniques.[37]

During the apnea event there is significant reduction in middle cerebral artery blood flow velocity, according to some cerebral blood flow studies.[38,39] The drop correlates with duration of the apnea event rather than with depth of oxyhemoglobin desaturation. Intracranial hemodynamic changes occurring repeatedly night after night in patients with marginal circulatory reserve may contribute to the risk of stroke, in particular in patients with clinically significant sleep apnea disorder.[40] The phenomenon suggests that hemodynamic disturbances caused by profound intrathoracic negative pressures during obstructive apneas determine a reduction of cerebral blood flow. Furthermore, studies with near-infrared spectroscopy[41] have noted that cerebral hemodynamic autoregulatory mechanisms fail in the presence of frequent apneas (apnea-hypopnea index [AHI] >30) and brain hypoxia.

STROKE

The specific risk of stroke or death in sleep apnea was investigated by Yaggi and colleagues.[42] In their study, the risk of stroke or death of any cause in patients with sleep apnea with a mean AHI of 35 per hour was expressed by a hazard ratio of 2.24 (95% CI, 1.30–3.86). The increased risk of stroke was independent of other risk factors including hypertension, whereas increased severity of sleep apnea was associated with an incremental risk of stroke and death.

Muñoz and colleagues[43] found that severe obstructive sleep apnea/hypopnea (defined as an AHI ≥30 per hour) increases the risk of ischemic stroke in an elderly male, noninstitutionalized population, independently of known confounding factors. In another prospective analysis of 1189 subjects from the general population, Arzt and colleagues[44] found that sleep-disordered breathing with an AHI of greater than or equal to 20 per hour was associated with an increased risk of a first-ever stroke over the subsequent 4 years (unadjusted OR, 4.31; 95% CI, 1.31–14.15; $P = .02$). After adjustment for age, gender, and body mass index, the OR was still elevated, but was no longer significant (OR, 3.08; 95% CI, 0.74–12.81; $P = .12$). The same authors found, in a cross-sectional analysis of 1475 individuals, that subjects with an AHI of greater than or equal to 20 per hour had increased odds for stroke (OR, 4.33; 95% CI, 1.32–14.24; $P = .02$) compared with those without sleep apnea (AHI <5) after adjustment for known confounding factors. The authors concluded that there is a strong association between moderate to severe sleep-disordered breathing and stroke, independent of confounding factors. In the Sleep Heart Health Study[45] men in the highest AHI quartile (≥19 events per hour) had an adjusted hazard ratio of stroke of 2.86 (95% CI, 1.1–7.4). In the mild to moderate range (AHI, 5–25 events per hour), each one-unit increase in AHI in men was estimated to increase stroke risk by 6% (95% CI, 2%–10%). In women, stroke risk increased when there was an AHI greater than or equal to 25 events per hour.

ACUTE STROKE

Vasomotor reactivity may be altered in patients with acute stroke. Alexandrov and colleagues[46] have reported the presence of intracranial blood flow steal in response to vasodilatory stimuli, such as carbon dioxide elevations, in patients with sleep apnea and stroke; they term this phenomenon "reversed Robin Hood syndrome." The syndrome might play an important role in clinical deterioration after an acute stroke. Such observations have led to the notion that noninvasive ventilatory correction in patients with acute stroke and sleep apnea might have a beneficial effect on brain perfusion.

SMALL VESSEL DISEASE AND COGNITIVE DYSFUNCTION

Some studies have suggested that sleep apnea may lead to cognitive dysfunction from the effects of chronic hypoxia and sympathetic stress associated with small-vessel disease in the brain, causing white matter ischemia and lacunar strokes. In a recent publication, Yaffe and colleagues[47] reported that elderly women affected by obstructive sleep apnea develop cognitive deficits compared with age-matched controls. The authors concluded that cognitive decline correlated with hypoxemia rather than with fragmentation of sleep architecture caused by apneas and hypopneas. Early recognition and treatment with CPAP may lead to improvement of cognitive function[48] and prevention of dementia in patients with sleep apnea.

CPAP TREATMENT

Clinically significant sleep apnea is best treated with nightly applications of CPAP. CPAP treatment has been shown to decrease the frequency of nocturnal arousals and suppress acute blood pressure fluctuations. Randomized controlled trials have established that CPAP treatment of symptomatic patients with moderate to severe sleep apnea lowers blood pressure levels. There is suggestive evidence that CPAP applications reduce blood pressure primarily by stabilizing the sympathetic-vagal balance. Patients with drug-resistant hypertension, requiring three antihypertensive drugs or more for control of blood pressure, should be screened for sleep apnea, because successful CPAP therapy contributes to blood pressure reductions that are greater than what can be achieved with drugs alone.[49]

CPAP therapy may also have a favorable effect on atrial fibrillation recurrence. Observational studies have shown a reduction in recurrence of atrial fibrillation after therapeutic procedures in patients treated with CPAP.[30,50] Additional research is required to confirm this therapeutic action of CPAP. Preliminary evidence from several studies also suggests a favorable effect of CPAP applications on stroke recurrence.[51,52] The confirmation requires large randomized, controlled, and prospective studies to establish a favorable effect of CPAP on stroke occurrence and recurrence.

POSTSTROKE SLEEP APNEA

Sleep apnea is common in patients after stroke.[53–56] This observation has implications for the rehabilitation of patients after stroke. Depending on the study, the prevalence of sleep apnea poststroke ranges between 50% and 75%. Sleep apnea may precede the occurrence of stroke or appear poststroke. Sleep apnea may worsen the outcome of rehabilitation weeks and months after stroke occurrence. Central sleep apneas predominate initially, giving way to obstructive apneas in the chronic stages after acute stroke.[57]

As noted by various studies, sleep apnea is associated with poor functional outcome, depressed mood, cognitive dysfunction, deteriorated ability to perform activities of daily living, and psychiatric and behavioral symptoms after stroke.[58,59]

Sleep apnea may be even significantly and independently related to length of hospitalization after stroke.[60,61]

Preliminary results with the application of CPAP poststroke[62] have shown a beneficial effect, particularly with the use of auto-CPAP during the acute phases of stroke.[63] A favorable effect has also been shown on neurologic and cognitive functions during the stable phase of stroke in a rehabilitation setting. Compliance with treatment is a challenging issue that needs to be resolved before CPAP treatment becomes generalized poststroke.

RESTLESS LEGS SYNDROME, PERIODIC LIMB MOVEMENTS OF SLEEP, AND RISK OF STROKE

Emerging evidence suggests that restless legs syndrome and its associated condition periodic limb movements of sleep represent risk factors for cardiovascular and cerebrovascular disease.[64–66] Common factors prevalent in both conditions, such as smoking, the metabolic syndrome, and diabetes, may predispose individuals to heart disease and stroke, whereas sympathetic activation and metabolic dysregulation may constitute the common pathogenetic pathways. Repeated nocturnal heart rate and blood pressure rises associated with periodic limb movements of sleep and related microarousals[67] may facilitate daytime hypertension and open the way to heart disease and stroke.[68] Further studies are needed to evaluate the role of restless legs syndrome and periodic limb movements of sleep in cardiovascular risk.

Box 1
Case study

A 68-year-old man presented with dysphasia and minimal right hemiparesis. He had a history of hypertension, noninsulin-dependent diabetes mellitus, gout, and depression. He was on multiple cardiovascular medications, glipizide, and fluoxetine. On examination his weight was 100 kg and body mass index was 40. His blood pressure was 170/110 mm Hg. He was talking incomprehensibly, and his family said that he had become more forgetful. There was a predominantly Wernicke-type dysphasia and a right visual field cut. Oropharyngeal examination revealed a Mallampati type IV oropharyngeal opening. Chest radiograph showed moderate congestive heart failure. Computed tomography of the head revealed old lacunae in the left hemisphere along with a new hypodensity in the left temporal-occipital area with obliteration of sulci. There were also periventricular ischemic changes suggestive of small vessel disease. The echocardiogram showed enlargement of the left atrium and dysfunction of the left ventricle. The electrocardiogram revealed sinus rhythm. The hospital course was uneventful and the patient was discharged 6 days later with a recommendation to be tested in the sleep center as an outpatient. In the interim, with the help of speech therapy, his dysphasia markedly improved. He complained of insomnia and fatigue since the stroke. On specific questioning the wife reported loud snoring before and after the stroke. A polysomnogram performed 1 month after discharge from the hospital revealed a sleep efficiency of 75%. There were 151 respiratory events, of which 37 were obstructive apneas and 114 hypopneas. The AHI was 25.6, and the lowest oxygen saturation was 89% in rapid eye movement sleep. A brief episode of atrial fibrillation lasting 90 seconds was observed in rapid eye movement sleep. He spent 72% of sleep time in a supine position. The periodic leg movement index was 20 per hour of sleep.

Comment. The diagnosis was sleep apnea, predominantly obstructive, of moderate severity with associated paroxysmal atrial fibrillation and mild periodic limb movement disorder. It was unclear whether sleep apnea had preceded the stroke or was aggravated by the stroke. A recommendation was made to repeat the polysomnogram with the CPAP protocol and to consider administration of an oral anticoagulant for prevention of cardioembolic events.

REFERENCES

1. Culebras A. Sleep and stroke. Semin Neurol 2009;29:438–45.
2. Young T, Palta M, Dempsey J, et al. The occurrence of sleep-disordered breathing among middle-aged adults. N Engl J Med 1993;328:1230–5.
3. Punjabi NM. The epidemiology of adult obstructive sleep apnea. Proc Am Thorac Soc 2008;5:136–43.
4. Somers VK, Dyken ME, Clary MP, et al. Sympathetic neural mechanisms in obstructive sleep apnea. J Clin Invest 1995;96(4):1897–904.
5. Cortelli P, Parchi P, Sforza E, et al. Cardiovascular autonomic dysfunction in normotensive awake subjects with obstructive sleep apnoea syndrome. Clin Auton Res 1994;4:57–62.
6. Friedman O, Logan AG. The price of obstructive sleep apnea-hypopnea: hypertension and other ill effects. Am J Hypertens 2009;22:474–83.
7. Noda A, Nakata S, Koike Y, et al. Continuous positive airway pressure improves daytime baroreflex sensitivity and nitric oxide production in patients with moderate to severe obstructive sleep apnea syndrome. Hypertens Res 2007; 30:669–76.
8. Somers VK, Dyken ME, Mark AL, et al. Sympathetic nerve activity during sleep in normal humans. N Engl J Med 1993;328:303–7.
9. Thomas RJ. Arousals in sleep-disordered breathing: patterns and implications. Sleep 2003;26:1042–7.
10. Narkiewicz K, Somers VK. The sympathetic nervous system and obstructive sleep apnea: implications for hypertension. J Hypertens 1997;15:1613–9.
11. Eltzschig HK, Carmeliet P. Hypoxia and inflammation. N Engl J Med 2011;364: 656–65.
12. Iadecola C. Cerebrovascular dysfunction in chronic intermittent hypoxia. Presented at International Stroke Conference. Los Angeles, February 11, 2011.
13. Champagne K, Schwartzman K, Opatrny L, et al. Obstructive sleep apnoea and its association with gestational hypertension. Eur Respir J 2009;33(3):559–65.
14. Poyares D, Guilleminault C, Hachul H, et al. Pre-eclampsia and nasal CPAP: part 2. Hypertension during pregnancy, chronic snoring, and early nasal CPAP intervention. Sleep Med 2007;9:15–21.
15. Bourjeily G, Ankner G, Mohsenin V. Sleep-disordered breathing in pregnancy. Clin Chest Med 2011;32(1):175–89.
16. Coccagna G, Mantovani M, Brignani F, et al. Laboratory note. Arterial pressure changes during spontaneous sleep in man. Electroencephalogr Clin Neurophysiol 1971;31(3):277–81.
17. Hla KM, Young T, Finn L, et al. Longitudinal association of sleep-disordered breathing and nondipping of nocturnal blood pressure in the Wisconsin Sleep Cohort Study. Sleep 2008;31(6):795–800.
18. Kario K, Pickering TG, Matsuo T, et al. Stroke prognosis and abnormal nocturnal blood pressure falls in older hypertensives. Hypertension 2001;38(4):852–7.
19. Narkiewicz K, Montano N, Cogliati C, et al. Altered cardiovascular variability in obstructive sleep apnea. Circulation 1998;98(11):1071–7.
20. Nieto FJ, Young TB, Lind BK, et al. Association of sleep-disordered breathing, sleep apnea, and hypertension in a large community-based study. Sleep Heart Health Study. JAMA 2000;283(14):1829–36.
21. Peppard PE, Young T, Palta M, et al. Prospective study of the association between sleep-disordered breathing and hypertension. N Engl J Med 2000; 342(19):1378–84.

22. Logan AG, Perlikowski SM, Mente A, et al. High prevalence of unrecognized sleep apnoea in drug-resistant hypertension. J Hypertens 2001;19(12):2271–7.

23. Dernaika TA, Kinasewitz GT, Tawk MM. Effects of nocturnal continuous positive airway pressure therapy in patients with resistant hypertension and obstructive sleep apnea. J Clin Sleep Med 2009;5(2):103–7.

24. Horne RS, Yang JS, Walter LM, et al. Elevated blood pressure during sleep and wake in children with sleep-disordered breathing. Pediatrics 2011;128(1):e85–92.

25. Amin R, Somers VK, McConnell K, et al. Activity-adjusted 24-hour ambulatory blood pressure and cardiac remodeling in children with sleep disordered breathing. Hypertension 2008;51(1):84–91.

26. Naccarelli GV, Varker H, Lin J, et al. Increasing prevalence of atrial fibrillation and flutter in the United States. Am J Cardiol 2009;104(11):1534–9.

27. Miyasaka Y, Barnes ME, Gersh BJ, et al. Secular trends in incidence of atrial fibrillation in Olmsted County, Minnesota, 1980 to 2000, and implications on the projections for future prevalence. Circulation 2006;114:119–25.

28. Gami AS, Hodge DO, Herges RM, et al. Obstructive sleep apnea, obesity, and the risk of incident atrial fibrillation. J Am Coll Cardiol 2007;49(5):565–71.

29. Sauer WH, McKernan ML, Lin D, et al. Clinical predictors and outcomes associated with acute return of pulmonary vein conduction during pulmonary vein isolation for treatment of atrial fibrillation. Heart Rhythm 2006;3(9):1024–8.

30. Patel D, Mohanty P, Di Biase L, et al. Safety and efficacy of pulmonary vein antral isolation in patients with obstructive sleep apnea: the impact of continuous positive airway pressure. Circ Arrhythm Electrophysiol 2010;3(5):445–51.

31. Lynch JJ, Schuchard GH, Gross CM, et al. Prevalence of right-to-left atrial shunting in a healthy population: detection by Valsalva maneuver contrast echocardiography. Am J Cardiol 1984;53:1478–80.

32. Beelke M, Angeli S, Del Sette M, et al. Prevalence of patent foramen ovale in subjects with obstructive sleep apnea: a transcranial Doppler ultrasound study. Sleep Med 2003;4(3):219–23.

33. Sanner BM, Doberauer C, Konermann M, et al. Pulmonary hypertension in patients with obstructive sleep apnea syndrome. Arch Intern Med 1997;157(21):2483–7.

34. Ciccone A, Nobili L, Roccatagliata DV, et al. Causal role of sleep apnea and patent foramen ovale in wake-up stroke. Neurology 2011;76(Suppl 4):A170.

35. Neau JP, Paquereau J, Meurice JC, et al. Auditory event-related potentials before and after treatment with nasal continuous positive airway pressure in sleep apnea syndrome. Eur J Neurol 1996;3:29–35.

36. Hill CM, Hogan AM, Onugha N, et al. Increased cerebral blood flow velocity in children with mild sleep-disordered breathing: a possible association with abnormal neuropsychological function. Pediatrics 2006;118:e1100–8.

37. Hogan AM, Hill CM, Harrison D, et al. Cerebral blood flow velocity and cognition in children before and after adenotonsillectomy. Pediatrics 2008;122:75–82.

38. Netzer N, Werner P, Jochums I, et al. Blood flow of the middle cerebral artery with sleep-disordered breathing. Correlation with obstructive hypopneas. Stroke 1998;29:87–93.

39. Netzer NC. Impaired nocturnal cerebral hemodynamics during long obstructive apneas: the key to understanding stroke in OSAS patients? Sleep 2010;33(2):146–7.

40. Jiménez PE, Coloma R, Segura T. Brain haemodynamics in obstructive sleep apnea syndrome. Rev Neurol 2005;41(Suppl 3):S21–4 [in Spanish].

41. Pizza F, Biallas M, Wolf M, et al. Nocturnal cerebral hemodynamics in snorers and in patients with obstructive sleep apnea: a near-infrared spectroscopy study. Sleep 2010;33:205–10.

42. Yaggi HK, Concato J, Kernan WN, et al. Obstructive sleep apnea as a risk factor for stroke and death. N Engl J Med 2005;353:2034–41.
43. Muñoz R, Durán-Cantolla J, Martínez-Vila E, et al. Severe sleep apnea and risk of ischemic stroke in the elderly. Stroke 2006;37:2317–21.
44. Arzt M, Young T, Finn L, et al. Association of sleep-disordered breathing and the occurrence of stroke. Am J Respir Crit Care Med 2005;172:1447–51.
45. Redline S, Yenokyan G, Gottlieb DJ, et al. Obstructive sleep apnea-hypopnea and incident stroke: the sleep heart health study. Am J Respir Crit Care Med 2010;182:269–77.
46. Alexandrov AV, Nguyen HT, Rubiera M, et al. Prevalence and risk factors associated with reversed Robin Hood syndrome in acute ischemic stroke. Stroke 2009; 40:2738–42.
47. Yaffe K, Laffan AM, Harrison SL, et al. Sleep-disordered breathing, hypoxia, and risk of mild cognitive impairment and dementia in older women. JAMA 2011;306:613–9.
48. Matthews EE, Aloia MS. Cognitive recovery following positive airway pressure (PAP) in sleep apnea. Prog Brain Res 2011;190:71–88.
49. Lozano L, Tovar JL, Sampol G, et al. Continuous positive airway pressure treatment in sleep apnea patients with resistant hypertension: a randomized, controlled trial. J Hypertens 2010;28:2161–8.
50. Kanagala R, Murali NS, Friedman PA, et al. Obstructive sleep apnea and the recurrence of atrial fibrillation. Circulation 2003;107:2589–94.
51. Parra O, Sánchez-Armengol A, Bonnin M, et al. Early treatment of obstructive apnoea and stroke outcome: a randomised controlled trial. Eur Respir J 2011;37: 1128–36.
52. Bravata DM, Concato J, Fried T, et al. Continuous positive airway pressure: evaluation of a novel therapy for patients with acute ischemic stroke. Sleep 2011;34: 1271–7.
53. Dyken ME, Im KB. Obstructive sleep apnea and stroke. Chest 2009;136(6): 1668–77.
54. Yaggi H, Mohsenin V. Obstructive sleep apnoea and stroke. Lancet Neurol 2004; 3(6):333–42.
55. Hudgel DW, Devadatta P, Quadri M, et al. Mechanism of sleep-induced periodic breathing in convalescing stroke patients and healthy elderly subjects. Chest 1993;104(5):1503–10.
56. Mohsenin V, Valor R. Sleep apnea in patients with hemispheric stroke. Arch Phys Med Rehabil 1995;76(1):71–6.
57. Parra O, Arboix A, Bechich S, et al. Time course of sleep-related breathing disorders in first-ever stroke or transient ischemic attack. Am J Respir Crit Care Med 2000;161(2 Pt 1):375–80.
58. Good DC, Henkle JQ, Gelber D, et al. Sleep-disordered breathing and poor functional outcome after stroke. Stroke 1996;27(2):252–9.
59. Sandberg O, Franklin KA, Bucht G, et al. Sleep apnea, delirium, depressed mood, cognition, and ADL ability after stroke. J Am Geriatr Soc 2001;49(4):391–7.
60. Kaneko Y, Hajek VE, Zivanovic V, et al. Relationship of sleep apnea to functional capacity and length of hospitalization following stroke. Sleep 2003;26(3):293–7.
61. Cherkassky T, Oksenberg A, Froom P, et al. Sleep-related breathing disorders and rehabilitation outcome of stroke patients: a prospective study. Am J Phys Med Rehabil 2003;82(6):452–5.
62. Ryan CM, Bayley M, Green R, et al. Influence of continuous positive airway pressure on outcomes of rehabilitation in stroke patients with obstructive sleep apnea. Stroke 2011;42(4):1062–7.

63. Bravata DM, Concato J, Fried T, et al. Auto-titrating continuous positive airway pressure for patients with acute transient ischemic attack: a randomized feasibility trial. Stroke 2010;41:1464–70.

64. Portaluppi F, Cortelli P, Buonaura GC, et al. Do restless legs syndrome (RLS) and periodic limb movements of sleep (PLMS) play a role in nocturnal hypertension and increased cardiovascular risk of renally impaired patients? Chronobiol Int 2009;26:1206–21.

65. Lindner A, Fornadi K, Lazar AS, et al. Periodic limb movements in sleep are associated with stroke and cardiovascular risk factors in patients with renal failure. J Sleep Res 2012;21(3):297–307.

66. La Manna G, Pizza F, Persici E, et al. Restless legs syndrome enhances cardiovascular risk and mortality in patients with end-stage kidney disease undergoing long-term haemodialysis treatment. Nephrol Dial Transplant 2011;26:1976–83.

67. Pennestri MH, Montplaisir J, Colombo R, et al. Nocturnal blood pressure changes in patients with restless legs syndrome. Neurology 2007;68:1213–8.

68. Walters AS, Rye DB. Review of the relationship of restless legs syndrome and periodic limb movements in sleep to hypertension, heart disease, and stroke. Sleep 2009;32:589–97.

Sleep-Related Headaches

Jeanetta C. Rains, PhD[a],*, J. Steven Poceta, MD[b]

KEYWORDS

- Sleep apnea headache • Insomnia • Migraine • Cluster • Hypnic headache
- Psychiatric comorbidity • Treatment algorithm

KEY POINTS

- Irrespective of diagnosis, chronic daily, morning, or "awakening" headache patterns are soft signs of a sleep disorder.
- Sleep apnea headache may emerge de novo or may present as an exacerbation of cluster, migraine, tension-type, or other headache.
- Insomnia is the most prevalent sleep disorder in chronic migraine and tension-type headache, and increases risk for depression and anxiety.
- Sleep disturbance (eg, sleep loss, oversleeping, schedule shift) is an acute headache trigger for migraine and tension-type headache.
- Snoring and sleep disturbance are independent risk factors for progression from episodic to chronic headache.

INTRODUCTION

Epidemiologic and clinical studies have associated sleep disorders with specific headache diagnoses (ie, migraine, tension-type, cluster, hypnic) and nonspecific headache patterns (ie, chronic daily, "awakening," or morning headache). Irrespective of sleep disorders, acute sleep dysregulation is one of the most commonly reported headache triggers for episodic migraine and tension-type headache. Chronobiologic patterns have been identified in hypnic, cluster, and migraine headaches. Common neuroanatomic regulatory brain systems, mostly in the hypothalamus, help account for the interplay of sleep and headache.

Headache has been associated with a wide range of respiratory and nonrespiratory sleep disorders.[1,2] Most epidemiologic studies characterized headache according to frequency or proximity to sleep (ie, chronic daily, awakening, or morning headache) rather than formal diagnoses per the *International Classification of Headache*

Conflicts of interest: The authors have nothing to disclose.
[a] Center for Sleep Evaluation, Elliot Hospital, 185 Queen City Avenue, Manchester, NH 03102, USA; [b] Division of Neurology, Sleep Center, Scripps Clinic, 10666 North Torrey Pines Road, La Jolla, CA 92037, USA
* Corresponding author.
E-mail address: jrains@elliot-hs.org

Neurol Clin 30 (2012) 1285–1298
http://dx.doi.org/10.1016/j.ncl.2012.08.014   **neurologic.theclinics.com**

Disorders, 2nd Edition (ICHD-II).[3] Awakening headache has been most often studied and robustly linked to obstructive sleep apnea (OSA). The relative risk for chronic headache was shown to be increased at least 2- to 3-fold by sleep apnea; the odds ratio (OR) increased at least 8-fold in the case of cluster headache. Thus, although the average headache sufferer probably would not be diagnosed with OSA, patients with cluster and chronic headache not otherwise specified are 2 distinct subgroups at significant risk for OSA.

Insomnia, circadian rhythm disorders, parasomnias, and daytime sleepiness were also shown to increase risk for chronic headache. Insomnia is the most common sleep disorder associated with migraine and tension-type headache. Insomnia (and to a lesser degree hypersomnia) is also a hallmark symptom of mood and anxiety disorders. Patients with migraine and chronic tension-type headache are 2- to 5-fold more likely than controls to experience depression or anxiety.[4] Specifically, in migraineurs the lifetime incidence for major depression is 22% to 32% and for an anxiety disorder is 51% to 58%. Psychiatric comorbidity portends poorer long-term headache outcomes. Thus, the presence of insomnia in a patient experiencing chronic headaches warrants screening for psychiatric comorbidity.

Notwithstanding sleep disorders, sleep loss and oversleeping are acute headache triggers. Stress, menstruation, and fasting are other common triggers. A literature review identified lack of sleep as a trigger in 48% to 74% of migraineurs (5 studies) and 26% to 72% of patients with tension-type headache (2 studies), and oversleeping as a trigger in 25% to 32% (3 studies) of migraineurs and 13% (1 study) of those with tension-type headache.[5] The relationship between sleep duration and headache was confirmed prospectively in time series research by Houle and colleagues[6] and found to be nonlinear, with the extreme ends of the sleep distribution (ie, short [<6 hours] and long sleep duration [>8.5 hours]) associated with increased headache intensity, whereas average sleep duration (7–8 hours) was associated with reduced headache. An interaction effect with stress was noted, suggesting sleep may be a moderating variable in the stress/headache relationship.

EPIDEMIOLOGY AND RISK FACTORS

Chronic daily or awakening headache patterns have been shown to occur in 4% to 6% of the general population compared with 18% to 60% of obstructive sleep apneics and 18% of insomniacs.[2] Epidemiologic research has shown that snorers and apneics exhibit headache, especially daily headache, more frequently than controls in cross-sectional studies, with the relative risk increased at least 2- to 3-fold. Two specific subgroups seem to be at highest risk for OSA: patients with cluster and those with chronic headache patterns. A study of 37 patients with cluster headache who underwent polysomnography identified an 8.4-fold increase in the incidence of OSA relative to age- and gender-matched controls (58% vs 14%, respectively), and this risk increased more than 24-fold among patients with a body mass index (BMI) greater than 25 kg/m²[.7] Likewise, Mitsikostas and colleagues[8] identified OSA in 29% (21/72) of patients with severe headache who were refractory to standard treatments and were diagnosed with medication overuse and cluster and chronic tension-type headache.

Insomnia occurs in half to two-thirds of migraineurs typically seen in neurology or specialty headache practices. In a cross-sectional study, Boardman and colleagues[9] identified a dose–response relationship between headache and sleep (eg, trouble falling or staying asleep, feeling tired or worn out); among 2662 respondents, headache frequency increased with mild (age/gender-adjusted OR, 2.4 [1.7–3.2]), moderate (OR,

3.6 [2.6–5.0]), and severe (OR, 7.5 [4.2–13.4]) sleep complaints. A relationship between insomnia and migraine persists after controlling for depression and anxiety.[10]

Circadian rhythm disorders and parasomnias (eg, nightmares, bruxism, sleepwalking) are at least 2-fold more frequent among individuals with daily headache compared with controls.[11] Likewise, excessive daytime sleepiness seems to be increased in patients with migraine. A case-control study showed a 3-fold increase in pathologic daytime sleepiness based on questionnaires among migraineurs (14%) compared with controls (5%).[12]

DIFFERENTIAL DIAGNOSIS

Several diagnoses should be considered in cases of headache that emerge preferentially during or after sleep (**Box 1**).

Sleep Apnea Headache

Sleep apnea headache is the only headache secondary to a sleep disorder recognized by the ICHD-II, coded under the major classification "headache attributed to disorder of homeostasis" and the subclassification of "headache attributed to hypoxia or hypercapnia." Although OSA would account for most cases, diagnosis includes central sleep apnea, Cheyne-Stokes respiration, obesity hypoventilation syndrome, and mixed and complex sleep apnea syndromes. The diagnostic criteria and presumed mechanisms have yet to be validated and a sizable proportion of cases do not fulfill the criteria. Empirically, sleep apnea headache may present as migraine, tension, cluster, or unclassifiable; as bilateral (53%) or unilateral (47%); located frontal (33%), frontotemporal (28%), or temporal (16%); with pressing/tightening pain in most patients (79%); and with mild (47%), moderate (37%), or severe (16%) intensity.[13] Headaches remit within 30 minutes of waking (criterion A.3) in only 40% of cases.

Hypnic Headache

By definition, hypnic headache is confined to sleep and is known to occur in the mid to latter portion of the night, often between 1:00 and 3:00 AM, and less commonly during daytime naps. Because of the regularity of onset, it has been called "alarm clock" headache. Pain is usually mild to moderate, but may be severe.[14] Hypnic headache is rare (only 174 cases were reported in the literature by 2011; <0.1% of specialty headache clinic cases). A meta-analysis of data pooled from 71 cases of hypnic headache published in the medical literature revealed an average duration of 67 ± 44 minutes, a frequency of 1.2 ± 0.9 per each 24 hours, and that 60% were bilateral and usually moderate in severity.[15] Polysomnography has not isolated hypnic headache to a specific sleep stage, although anecdotal reports have suggested an association between hypnic headaches and OSA or rapid eye movement (REM)–related oxygen desaturations.[14]

Cluster Headache

Characterized by distinct circadian and, in some cases, circannual patterns, cluster headaches occur in series for weeks or months, separated by remissions of several months or years. Most headaches occur between 9:00 PM and 10:00 AM. OSA is prevalent among patients with cluster headache, especially those who are overweight and obese.

Exploding Head Syndrome

Classified under parasomnias by the *International Classification of Sleep Disorders, 2nd Edition* [ICSD-2],[16] criteria for exploding head syndrome include waking from

Box 1
ICHD-II diagnostic criteria for sleep apnea, hypnic, and cluster headaches[3]

10.1.3 SLEEP APNEA HEADACHE

A. Recurrent headache with at least one of the following characteristics and fulfilling criteria C and D:

1. Occurs on more than 15 days per month

2. Bilateral, pressing quality and not accompanied by nausea, photophobia, or phonophobia

3. Each headache resolves within 30 minutes

B. Sleep apnea (respiratory disturbance index ≥5) shown on overnight polysomnography

C. Headache is present on awakening

D. Headache ceases within 72 hours and does not recur after effective treatment of sleep apnea

4.5 HYPNIC HEADACHE

Attacks of dull headache that always awaken the patient from asleep.

A. Dull headache fulfilling criteria B through D

B. Develops only during sleep and awakens patient

C. At least 2 of the following characteristics:

1. Occurs on more than 15 times per month

2. Lasts 15 minutes or longer after waking

3. First occurs after 50 years of age

D. No autonomic symptoms and no more than one of nausea, photophobia, or phonophobia

E. Not attributed to another disorder

3.1 CLUSTER HEADACHE[a]

A. At least 5 attacks fulfilling criteria B through D

B. Severe or very severe unilateral orbital, supraorbital, and/or temporal pain lasting 15 to 180 minutes if untreated

C. Headache is accompanied by at least one of the following:

1. Ipsilateral conjunctival injection and/or lacrimation

2. Ipsilateral nasal congestion and/or rhinorrhea

3. Ipsilateral eyelid edema

4. Ipsilateral forehead and facial sweating

5. Ipsilateral miosis and/or ptosis

6. A sense of restlessness or agitation

D. Attacks have a frequency from 1 every other day to 8 per day

E. Not attributed to another disorder

---

[a] Cluster headache is subclassified as 3.1.1 episodic (at least 2 cluster periods lasting 7–365 days and separated by pain-free remission periods of ≥1 month) or 3.1.2 chronic (attacks recur over >1 year without remission periods or with remission periods lasting <1 month).

Modified from Headache Classification Subcommittee of the International Headache Society. The International Classification of Headache Disorders. 2nd edition. Cephalalgia 2004;24(Suppl 1):1–151; with permission.

sleep or the wake–sleep transition with a sense of noise or explosion that is usually frightening to the patient and is notable for the absence of pain. The syndrome is not included in ICHD-II headache diagnoses because of the absence of pain, but the condition is often described among rare or short-lived headache disorders and may present to headache or sleep specialists.

PATHOPHYSIOLOGY

Brennan and Charles[17] recently described brain mechanisms that may underlie the relationship between sleep and headache. The central nervous system anatomy that generates sleep and alertness is centered in the monoaminergic and cholinergic nuclei in the basal forebrain and the brainstem interacting with the thalamus and the hypothalamus. The arousal-associated tuberomammillary nucleus, locus coeruleus, and dorsal and median raphe are inhibited by the ventrolateral preoptic nucleus of the hypothalamus via γ-aminobutyric acid (GABA) and galanin. Adenosine, considered an endogenous somnogen, activates ventral lateral preoptic neurons in the hypothalamus, which induces sleep and is part of the homeostatic regulation of sleep and wake. In addition to the homeostatic drive for sleep and wake, a circadian mechanism exists to determine the likelihood of sleep at any point in the 24-hour day, and many headache syndromes also demonstrate circadian tendencies.

The anatomy of headache and head pain is even more widespread, involving cervical inputs to the trigeminal nucleus caudalis, hypothalamus, periaqueductal gray (PAG) region, thalamus, cerebral cortex, cranial vessels. Several potential sites of interaction exist between the sleep and pain systems, notably in the hypothalamus and PAG. The ventrolateral portion of the PAG in particular, as mentioned by Brennan, is a region with both sleep and pain functions. Stimulation of this region of the PAG has affected motor behavior (quiescence) and the likelihood of REM sleep, and is also antinociceptive.

The importance of the hypothalamus in the anatomic and physiologic underpinnings of migraine, cluster, and sleep mechanisms has been reviewed.[1] The evidence for involvement of the hypothalamus in headache and sleep is suggested partly by the anatomy. For example, the hypothalamus is the site of the suprachiasmatic nucleus, the major circadian pacemaker in the brain; its nuclei contains hypocretin cells, in which loss of function is pathogenic in narcolepsy. Furthermore, the hypothalamus has extensive connections with the PAG matter, spinal nociceptive neurons, and the reticular system, and hence plays a regulatory role in pain and headache.

Clinical aspects of the headache process also suggest involvement of the hypothalamus, such as the autonomic activation, yawning, and sleepiness associated with migraine. Direct imaging evidence shows hypothalamic activation in cluster headache and brainstem activation in migraine headache.[18,19] A recent study assessed sleep using polysomnography in 3 patients with refractory chronic cluster headache before and after posterior hypothalamic deep brain stimulation.[20] After deep brain stimulation, the expected improvement in headaches was associated with improved sleep efficiency and duration and decreased periodic limb movements in sleep. The timing of the circadian rhythm as measured by the temperature cycle was not altered.

The clinical relationship between sleep and headache is defined by the fact that patients overwhelmingly identify sleep as a trigger for migraine. Several plausible mechanisms explain an effect of sleep on the likelihood of headache occurrence and its severity. For example, assessment of pain response in both humans and animals generally demonstrates a lower threshold after partial or complete sleep deprivation.[21,22] The nature of this link and its underlying mechanisms are not clear.

For example, REM sleep deprivation seems to have different effects from total sleep deprivation. Furthermore, one study suggested that sleep disruption is more likely to affect pain measures than is sleep restriction.[23] In this study, groups of women were randomized to sleep overnight with either hourly interruptions or no interruptions. The interrupted group experienced increased spontaneous bodily pain and a significant loss of pain inhibition compared with the sleep-deprived (but continuous sleep) group. To the extent that headache pain is mediated by the same systems as bodily pain, which is not entirely clear because headache is a unique type of spontaneous pain syndrome, sleep duration and interruption seem to have the potential to alter the headache threshold.

CLINICAL FEATURES AND DIAGNOSIS

Diagnosis begins with a thorough clinical interview, examining the headache history and patterns in relation to the sleep cycle. History may be supplemented by standardized questionnaires, a prospective diary, and objective monitoring.

Headache History

A thorough headache history will obtain information on headache onset and course, chronology, pain characteristics, severity, frequency/duration/intensity, prodromes and auras, associated symptoms, precipitants, and past treatments,[24] and will yield a specific ICHD-II diagnosis.

Sleep History

Headache history may be examined in the context of a 24-hour sleep/wake cycle, considering presleep routine, sleep period (eg, sleep latency, duration of sleep relative to time in bed, mid-cycle and early morning awakenings), nocturnal symptoms (eg, respiratory, movement, waking), daytime functioning (eg, napping, alertness vs sleepiness, fatigue), and behavioral measures or substances to promote sleep or wakefulness. Useful information may be obtained from not only the patient but also the spouse or other observer. Patients who complain of insomnia should be questioned about internal and environmental contributors, such as (1) bedroom not conducive to sleep (eg, light, noise, television, cell phones, or other stimulation), (2) irregular sleep schedule, (3) napping or resting during the day, (4) medications and substances (eg, caffeine, alcohol, nicotine), and (5) emotional or cognitive arousal.

Prediction Equations and Questionnaires

Risk for OSA,[25] insomnia, and other sleep disorders may be assessed with validated tools. The most widely used tool for OSA is the Berlin Sleep Questionnaire, which yields a positive predictive value of 89%, and is based on neck circumference, habitual snoring or witnessed apnea, and hypertension.[26] The STOP-Bang questionnaire was initially developed for screening presurgical patients for sleep apnea risk,[27] but was more recently validated in the general medical population,[28,29] and includes snoring, tiredness/sleepiness, observed apnea, blood pressure, BMI, age, neck circumference, and gender.

Sleep Diary

A comprehensive diary for self-monitoring incidence of headache, sleep patterns, and other triggers of headache, such as stress, mood, and diet, is available elsewhere.[30] Prospective sleep diaries are the most commonly used tool for diagnosing insomnia or circadian rhythm disorders and identifying headache triggers.

Polysomnography

Attended polysomnography provides well-validated objective measures of sleep and wakefulness under standardized conditions, and normative data are available for a variety of sleep-disordered populations and normal controls. Typically, polysomnography is needed to confirm sleep-related breathing disorders, narcolepsy or idiopathic hypersomnia, and potentially injurious parasomnias. In uncomplicated cases in which a high pretest suspicion exists without confounding comorbidities, unattended and abbreviated portable monitoring may be sufficient to confirm OSA.

TREATMENT

The following 6 recommendations follow the proposed headache management algorithm[31] (**Fig. 1**) and the authors' assessment of empiric evidence based on ICHD-II headache diagnoses and diagnosis-specific risk for sleep and psychiatric disorders.

First, headache should be diagnosed according to standard criteria. Consider systematically diagnosing primary and secondary headaches according to ICHD-II criteria. Determine headache frequency (eg, chronic vs episodic).

Second, a sleep history should be obtained. Consider headache symptoms in relation to the 24-hour sleep history; proximity to sleep (awakening headache); snoring; sleep schedule regularity; abnormal sleep duration (especially ≤6 hours or >8 hours); sleep hygiene; insomnia (difficulty initiating or maintaining or nonrestorative sleep); sleepiness; parasomnias and other perturbations of sleep (eg, restless legs, bruxism, nocturia); and daytime sequela, such as emotional and cognitive complaints.

Third, sleep apnea headache should be ruled out in high-risk headache diagnoses. Patients diagnosed with cluster, hypnic, or any headache diagnosis that presents as chronic daily or awakening should be examined for symptoms and risk factors suggestive of sleep apnea (**Box 2**). Sleep apnea headache may represent an exacerbation of preexisting migraine or tension-type headache. STOP-Bang or other screening tools may prompt sleep specialist consultation or polysomnography. Confirmed OSA warrants treatment according to sleep medicine evidence-based guidelines[32] using continuous positive airway pressure (CPAP), oral appliances, surgical intervention, or conservative management calibrated to symptoms. Conservative treatments alone are unlikely to be the preferred treatment for sleep apnea headache.

Although headache would be expected to improve with treatment of sleep apnea, no basis exists to withhold headache treatment during the process of sleep evaluation or treatment. Concurrent headache treatment is usually indicated. Avoiding sedation with hypnotics or opiates is prudent until adherence to CPAP or other effective treatment for OSA is established. Treatment of headache that persists despite treatment of OSA depends on the exact headache diagnosis, but standard headache treatments apply for types such as migraine and cluster. Reevaluation of headache diagnosis and severity is recommended 1 month after sleep apnea treatment. After treatment is established, narcotic and sedative-hypnotics can be considered.

Fourth, the presence of chronic headache and comorbid insomnia should be determined. Patients with chronic migraine and chronic tension-type headache are at particular risk for insomnia. Patients with chronic headache should be screened for insomnia, particularly those who are refractory to standard treatments (eg, receiving prophylaxis, experiencing withdrawal from medication overuse). Patients with

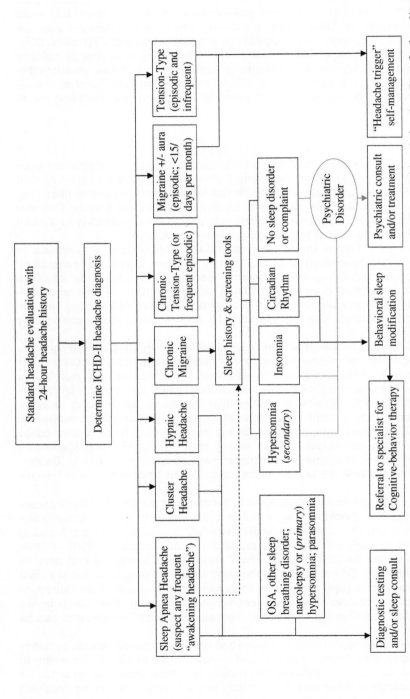

Fig. 1. Algorithm for management of sleep-related headache. (*Adapted from* Rains JC, Poceta JS. Sleep and headache. Curr Treat Options Neurol 2010;12:1–15; with permission.)

Box 2
OSA: symptoms, risk factors, diagnosis, and treatment

Clinical symptoms

- Habitual snoring
- Witnessed apnea
- Wake gasping or choking
- Morning headache
- Hypersomnia (or less often insomnia)
- Night sweats
- Nocturia

Risk factors

- Overweight to obese (increased BMI, neck, chest, hips, and waist measurements)
- Male gender (less after menopause)
- Age (positive correlation)
- Family history
- Craniofacial morphology
- Oral anatomy (increased Mallampati score [Likert scale range, 1–4], tonsillar size [Likert scale range, 0–4])
- Neuromuscular disorders
- Substance use (eg, tobacco, alcohol, sedatives)

Screening procedures

- Questionnaires
- Prediction equations
- Screening overnight airflow, respiratory effort, and/or pulse oximetry

Diagnostic testing

- Attended polysomnography
- Home or portable unattended cardiopulmonary monitoring

Treatment options

- CPAP
- Surgery (eg, uvulopalatopharyngoplasty, tonsillectomy, tracheostomy, maxillomandibular surgery)
- Oral appliances (tongue retaining devices, mandibular advancement)
- Conservative measures
  - Positional therapy to avoid supine sleep
  - Weight loss
  - Avoidance of alcohol, muscle relaxants, anxiolytics, sedatives, hypnotics, narcotics, and other medications that induce respiratory suppression

---

episodic migraine and tension-type headache may also benefit from screening for insomnia and other sleep disorders when their history suggests a significant sleep complaint or daytime sleepiness. Those with insomnia or poor sleep hygiene should be encouraged to undergo behavioral sleep regulation, which has been shown to significantly improve chronic migraine.[33] The 5-component intervention used by Calhoun and Ford[33] instructed patients to (1) schedule consistent bedtime that allows 8 hours in bed; (2) eliminate watching television, reading, or listening to music in bed; (3) use a visualization technique to shorten time to sleep onset; (4) move supper at least 4 hours before bedtime and limit fluids within 2 hours of bedtime; and (5) discontinue naps.

Referral for more-intensive behavioral insomnia treatments may be needed. Although behavioral treatments are considered the preferred treatment for chronic insomnia, pharmacologic treatments may be indicated. No studies show that headache improves solely with pharmacologic treatment for insomnia, but pharmacologic treatment for insomnia may be warranted on a case-by-case basis. Benzodiazepines and nonbenzodiazepine hypnotics are effective, and some evidence shows that antidepressant medications are effective, although benefits must be weighed against potential adverse effects. No data are available to recommend a particular sleep aid for patients with headache among the available hypnotics, anxiolytics, or sedating antidepressants used to manage insomnia, but treatment should be tailored to symptom patterns.

Choice of sedative-hypnotic, if used, depends on the nature of the insomnia, comorbid medical and psychiatric diagnoses, prior experience with hypnotics, substance abuse history, and pharmacokinetic properties of the drug (T_{max}, half-life, side-effect profile, dependency risk). Drug choice also depends on whether the insomnia pattern involves sleep onset, maintenance (frequent awakenings at several time points in the night), or early morning awakening.

Fifth, the presence of psychiatric comorbidities should be determined. Individuals with chronic migraine and tension-type headache are at risk for a psychiatric disorder, and screening for mood and anxiety disorders is warranted, especially when either insomnia or hypersomnia is present. Psychiatric symptoms impact choice of sedating versus alerting versus neutral pharmacologic agents.[4]

Sixth, sleep-related triggers of episodic headache should be identified. All patients with headache, and particularly those with episodic migraine and tension-type headache, may benefit from inclusion of sleep variables in trigger management. Prospective sleep diaries track the regularity, duration, and quality of sleep. The diary is the most commonly used systematic self-report tool for identifying headache triggers.

Steps to manage headache triggers include

1. Prospective self-monitoring using the daily diary to record headache onset (or exacerbation in the case of chronic daily headache) along with common headache precipitants. Sleep variables of importance may be identified initially on interview but often may include daily monitoring of sleep schedule, quality and duration of sleep, daytime sleepiness, and napping.
2. Identifying triggers or events that result in a headache within 24 hours of exposure. Definite triggers cause headache 50% of time, possible triggers 25% to 50% of the time, and unlikely triggers less than 25% of the time.
3. Prioritizing triggers. Patients should be encouraged to address 2 or 3 of the most important triggers rather than undertake major lifestyle changes that often result in nonadherence. Ongoing self-monitoring allows patients to observe the outcome of behavior changes, which provides opportunities for refinement of strategies and reinforcement of self-management skills, and a sense of mastery and self-control of headache (self-efficacy).
4. Self-management skills. Patients may eliminate avoidable triggers, such as diet; modify their sleep environments (eg, light, noise); or predict and prepare for uncontrollable triggers (eg, menstrual).

PROGNOSIS

Sleep regulation may improve headache. In the case of sleep apnea headache, headache improved or resolved in one-third to half of cases based on case series and uncontrolled studies,[34–37] with few controlled trials.[38] Few trials exist, and whether either hypnotics or behavioral insomnia therapies improve headache is unclear. However, a recent randomized controlled trial[33] showed improvement in chronic migraine after a 12-week behavioral sleep intervention compared with a sham intervention; headache change was proportionate to the number of sleep behaviors changed (dose–response relationship). By the sixth week of treatment, 35% of the treatment group reverted from chronic to episodic headache compared with none of the controls. After treatment, the treatment group significantly improved over the control group in headache frequency (39% vs 12%) and index (28% vs –3%).

Case study: sleep apnea headache

A 62-year-old man presented with daily headache that occurred "90% of the time" on awakening from the nocturnal sleep period and "25% to 50%" of the time when awakening from daytime naps. Pain was bilateral and temporal, throbbing, and moderate (5–6 on 10-point pain scale). No nausea or vomiting, aggravation with exertion, or phonophobia were experienced, but he did experience photophobia. Headache improved in 1 to 2 hours after waking with ibuprofen and/or acetaminophen and hydrocodone, or otherwise persisted "all morning" untreated. He had a history of cluster headache, treated prophylactically with verapamil. The most recent cluster phase was 6 months prior.

Past medical history included asthma, hypertension, hyperlipidemia, gastroesophageal reflux, osteoarthritis, sinusitis, above-the-knee amputation for complications of methicillin-resistant *Staphylococcus aureus* after knee replacement in 2001 (without his prosthesis on motorized scooter). Medications included Symbicort, albuterol, furosemide, omeprazole, simvastatin, verapamil, isosorbide mononitrate, Losartan, and labetalol. His BMI was 42 kg/m^2 (height, 69 in; weight, 285 lb); neck circumference was 20 in; and Mallampati score was 3 to 4. He wore dentures. His blood pressure was 150/84 mm Hg. He had no edema or clubbing and no focal neurologic deficits.

He described his sleep history as "no trouble falling asleep, but my problem is staying asleep." His presleep routine included dozing on the couch while watching television. He was in bed from 10:00 PM until 6:00 or 7:00 AM. His sleep latency was estimated at 2 minutes. His wife slept in a separate room because of his snoring. His family witnessed heroic snoring and apparent apneic events. His sleep was interrupted by nocturia 3 times per night, nightmares, sipping water for dry mouth, waking self from snoring, and pain awakenings. He denied worry or anticipation of poor sleep. He denied engaging in alerting activities in bed. He estimated sleeping only 3 to 4 hours net per night, although he was in bed 8 to 9 hours. He would awaken unrefreshed and would be dozing in the chair within 1 hour of waking. He napped ad-lib, falling to sleep during periods of inactivity, including while "holding my grandchild" and in social settings. He had a history of drowsy driving, which included a single-car, probably sleepiness-related motor vehicle accident 12 years ago at 4 PM while driving home from work. His score on the Epworth Sleepiness Scale was 17 (out of a maximum 24 possible), which was indicative of hypersomnia. His family history of sleep disorders included a son who was treated with CPAP for sleep apnea.

Headache diagnoses included probable sleep apnea headache versus chronic tension-type headache versus medication overuse headache and history for episodic cluster headache. Polysomnography indicated OSA, he met all criteria on the STOP-Bang (+snoring, +tiredness, +observed apnea, +hypertension, +BMI, +age, +neck circumference >17 in, +male gender), and he was diagnosed with nocturia. A split-night sleep study was conducted after OSA was diagnosed and deemed severe. During the initial approximately 3.5 hours of testing, the patient showed an apnea-hypopnea index of 65 events per hour, with oxygen desaturation to 66% and respiratory-related arousals. His CPAP was titrated to 14 cm H$_2$O, with normalization of respiratory parameters in REM and non-REM sleep while supine. Sleep architecture included 5.3 hours net sleep, 71% of which occurred in bed, with 21% slow wave or stage 3 sleep and an extended REM cycle after CPAP, suggesting REM rebound. His arousal index was 38.3 and was mostly associated with pre-CPAP respiratory events. No periodic limb movements or other abnormalities were observed.

He was prescribed CPAP at 14 cm H_2O. At 30-day follow-up, his daily headaches were resolved and his subjective sleep and nocturia were improved. His objective CPAP adherence was 100% (30 of 30 days), with a mean daily use of 4 hours and 40 minutes per night. Daytime sleepiness was improved but not resolved, with a score on the Epworth Sleepiness Scale of 12 of 24. His treatment plan included long-term CPAP use, monitoring of mild persistent sleepiness, weight management, and determining whether treatment of apnea impacted cluster recurrence.

Current controversies and future considerations

Sleep has been identified among risk factors for transformation from episodic to chronic headache in a sort of "disease progression" model. Lipton and Pan[39] originally postulated that migraine might be conceptualized as a chronic progressive disorder. The progression or "chronification" of headache from episodic to "chronic daily headache" is a well-described clinical phenomenon, in which episodic migraine transforms to chronic daily headache over the span of months or years. Potential mechanisms for headache chronification have been described elsewhere,[40] but progression is thought to be a consequence of the cortical spreading depression mechanisms that generate the migraine attacks; a function of the activations generated by the attacks, such as lesions in the periaqueductal gray area; and genetic and/or environmental risk factors.

Snoring and sleep disturbance specifically were identified among risk factors for progression. Scher and colleagues[41] found that patients with chronic daily headache were 3.3-fold more likely to be daily snorers than controls; the association was independent of headache type, gender, or age; and obesity was an independent risk factor for progression. These investigators and Wiendels and colleagues[42] have also identified sleep disturbance as a significant risk factor for progression. Other risk factors included medication overuse, stress, psychiatric comorbidity, and obesity.

Understanding the link between risk factors and headache may yield novel preventive and therapeutic approaches in the management of headache. Sleep and other modifiable risk factors may be potential targets for primary or secondary headache prevention rather than solely variables for management. Although yet untested in patients with headache, snoring interventions and sleep regulation strategies could be considered for prevention. The natural history of sleep-disordered breathing indicates a progression of simple snoring to OSA, influenced by aging and weight gain. Interventions aimed at weight loss, conservative measures for snoring, and basic sleep regulation warrant consideration. Longitudinal studies in the future would help determine if sleep regulation can reduce the risk of headache progression, but a fundamental shift from management to prevention could be realized currently.

REFERENCES

1. Poceta JS, Rains JC. Sleep and headache syndromes. Sleep Med Clin 2008;3(3): 427–41.
2. Rains JC, Poceta JS, Penzien DB. Sleep and headaches. Curr Neurol Neurosci Rep 2008;8:167–75.
3. Headache Classification Subcommittee of the International Headache Society. The international classification of headache disorders, second edition. Cephalalgia 2004;24(Suppl 1):1–151.
4. Smitherman TA, Maizels M, Penzien DB. Headache chronification: screening and behavioral management of comorbid depressive and anxiety disorders. Headache 2008;48:45–50.

5. Martin PR, MacLeod C. Behavioral management of headache triggers: avoidance of triggers is an inadequate strategy. Clin Psychol Rev 2009;29:483–95.

6. Houle TT, Butschek RA, Turner DP. Stress and sleep predict headache severity in chronic headache sufferers. Pain, in press.

7. Nobre ME, Leal AJ, Filho PM. Investigation into sleep disturbance of patients suffering from cluster headache. Cephalalgia 2005;25(7):488–92.

8. Mitsikostas DD, Vikelis M, Viskos A. Refractory chronic headache associated with obstructive sleep apnoea syndrome. Cephalalgia 2007;28(2):139–43.

9. Boardman HF, Thomas E, Millson DS, et al. Psychological, sleep, lifestyle, and co-morbid associations with headache. Headache 2005;45(6):657–69.

10. Vgontzas A, Lihong C, Merikangas KR. Are sleep difficulties associated with migraine attributable to anxiety and depression? Headache 2008;48(10):1451–9.

11. Ohayon MM. Prevalence and risk factors of morning headaches in the general population. Arch Intern Med 2004;164(1):97–102.

12. Barbanti P, Fabbrini G, Aurilia C, et al. A case-control study on excessive daytime sleepiness in episodic migraine. Cephalalgia 2007;27(10):1115–9.

13. Alberti A, Mazzotta G, Gallinella E, et al. Headache characteristics in obstructive sleep apnea and insomnia. Acta Neurol Scand 2005;111:309–16.

14. Holle D, Wessendorf TE, Zaremba S, et al. Serial polysomnography in hypnic headache. Cephalalgia 2011;31(3):286–90.

15. Evers S, Goadsby PJ. Hypnic headache: clinical features, pathophysiology, and treatment. Neurology 2003;60(6):905–9.

16. American Academy of Sleep Medicine. The International classification of sleep disorders. diagnostic and coding manual. 2nd edition. Westchester (IL): American Academy of Sleep Medicine; 2005.

17. Brennan KC, Charles A. Sleep and headaches. Semin Neurol 2009;29(4):406–18.

18. Aurora SK, Barrodale PM, Tipton RL, et al. Brainstem dysfunction in chronic migraine as evidenced by neurophysiological and positron emission tomography studies. Headache 2007;47(7):996–1003 [discussion: 1004–7].

19. May A, Matharu M. New insights into migraine: application of functional and structural imaging. Curr Opin Neurol 2007;20(3):306–9.

20. Vetrugno R, Pierangeli G, Leone M, et al. Effect on sleep of posterior hypothalamus stimulation in cluster headache. Headache 2007;47(7):1085–90.

21. Wei H, Zhao W, Wang YX, et al. Pain-related behavior following REM sleep deprivation in the rat: influence of peripheral nerve injury, spinal glutamatergic receptors and nitric oxide. Brain Res 2007;1148:105–12.

22. Roehrs T, Hyde M, Blaisdell B, et al. Sleep loss and REM sleep loss are hyperalgesic. Sleep 2006;29(2):145–51.

23. Smith MT, Edwards RR, McCann UD, et al. The effects of sleep deprivation on pain inhibition and spontaneous pain in women. Sleep 2007;30(4):494–505.

24. Silberstein SD, Lipton RB, Dalessio DJ. Overview, diagnosis, and classification of headache. In: Silberstein SD, Lipton RB, Dodick DW, editors. Wolff's headache and other head pain. 8th edition. Oxford University Press; 2007.

25. Abrishami A, Khajehdehi A, Chung F. A systematic review of screening questionnaires for obstructive sleep apnea. Can J Anaesth 2010;57(5):423–38.

26. Flemons WW, Whitelaw WA, Brant R, et al. Likelihood ratios for a sleep apnea clinical prediction rule. Am J Respir Crit Care Med 1994;150(5 Pt 1):1279–85.

27. Chung F, Yegneswaran B, Liao P, et al. STOP questionnaire: a tool to screen patients for obstructive sleep apnea. Anesthesiology 2008;108:812–21.

28. Ong TH, Raudha S, Fook-Chong S, et al. Simplifying STOP-Bang: use of a simple questionnaire to screen for OSA in an Asian population. Sleep Breath 2010;14:371–6.

29. Silva GE, Vana KD, Goodwin JL, et al. Identification of patients with sleep disordered breathing: comparing the Four-Variable screening tool, STOP, STOP-Bang, and Epworth Sleepiness Scales. J Clin Sleep Med 2011;7(5):467–72.

30. Rains JC, Poceta JS. Headache and sleep disorders: review and clinical implications for headache management. Headache 2006;46(9):1344–61.

31. Rains JC, Poceta JS. Sleep and headache. Curr Treat Options Neurol 2010;12:1–15.

32. Morgenthaler TI, Kapen S, Lee-Chiong T, et al. Practice parameters for the medical therapy of obstructive sleep apnea. Sleep 2006;29(8):1031–5.

33. Calhoun AH, Ford S. Behavioral sleep modification may revert transformed migraine to episodic migraine. Headache 2007;47(8):1178–83.

34. Barloese M, Jennum P, Knudsen S, et al. Cluster headache and sleep, is there a connection? A review. Cephalalgia 2012;32(6):481–91.

35. Nath Zallek S, Chervin RD. Improvement in cluster headache after treatment for obstructive sleep apnea. Sleep Med 2000;1(2):135–8.

36. Paiva T, Farinha A, Martins A, et al. Chronic headaches and sleep disorders. Arch Intern Med 1997;157(15):1701–5.

37. Chervin RD, Zallek SN, Lin X, et al. Sleep disordered breathing in patients with cluster headache. Neurology 2000;54(12):2302–6.

38. Kiely JL, Murphy M, McNicholas WT. Subjective efficacy of nasal CPAP therapy in obstructive sleep apnoea syndrome: a prospective controlled study. Eur Respir J 1999;13(5):1086–90.

39. Lipton RB, Pan J. Is migraine a progressive disease? JAMA 2004;291(4):493–4.

40. Bigal M, Lipton RB. Concepts and mechanisms of migraine chronification. Headache 2008;48:7–15.

41. Scher AI, Lipton RB, Stewart WF. Habitual snoring as a risk factor for chronic daily headache. Neurology 2003;60(8):1366.

42. Wiendels NJ, Neven AK, Rosendaal FR, et al. Chronic frequent headache in the general population: prevalence and associated factors. Cephalalgia 2006; 26(12):1434–42.

Traumatic Brain Injury and Sleep Disorders

Mari Viola-Saltzman, DO[a], Nathaniel F. Watson, MD, MSc[b],*

KEYWORDS

- Traumatic brain injury • Concussion • Insomnia • Fatigue • Hypersomnia
- Sleep apnea • Restless legs syndrome

KEY POINTS

- Sleep disturbances occur in 30% to 70% of individuals with traumatic brain injury.
- Insomnia, fatigue, and sleepiness are the most frequent complaints after head injury.
- The two main types of traumatic brain injuries leading to altered sleep involve contact and acceleration or deceleration injuries.
- Diagnosis of sleep disorders after traumatic brain injury may include polysomnography, multiple sleep latency testing, and actigraphy.
- Treatment is disorder-specific and may include the use of medications, continuous positive airway pressure (or similar device), or behavioral modifications.

INTRODUCTION

Traumatic brain injury (TBI) is a significant cause of disability and death in the United States and worldwide. An estimated 1.6 to 3 million TBIs occur in the United States each year[1] causing more than 1 million emergency department visits, 290,000 hospitalizations, and 51,000 deaths.[2] TBI is classified as mild, moderate, or severe using the Glasgow Coma Scale (mild = 13–15; moderate = 9–12; severe = $\leq$8 out of 15). TBI can result in significant motor, sensory, cognitive, and emotional impairments. Even mild TBI can be associated with headache, dizziness, nausea and vomiting, impaired balance and coordination, vision changes, tinnitus, mood and memory changes, difficulty with memory and attention, and fatigue or sleep disturbances.[3] The relationship between head trauma and impaired consciousness and cognitive disturbance has been well described,[4] but the association between head injury and sleep disturbance has not been extensively studied (**Table 1**).

Disclosure: Drs Viola-Saltzman and Watson have no relevant financial relationships to disclose.
[a] Pritzker School of Medicine, NorthShore University HealthSystem, Department of Neurology, 2650 Ridge Avenue, Evanston, IL 60201, USA; [b] University of Washington Medicine Sleep Center, 325 Ninth Avenue, Box 359803, Seattle, WA 98104–2499, USA
* Corresponding author.
E-mail address: nwatson@uw.edu

Table 1
TBI grading system: Glasgow Coma scale

	1	2	3	4	5	6
Eyes	Do not open	Open to painful stimuli	Open to voice	Open spontaneously	n/a	n/a
Verbal	No sounds	Incomprehensible sounds	Inappropriate words	Confused/disoriented	Normal conversation	n/a
Motor	No movement	Extension to painful stimuli (decerebrate posturing)	Flexion to painful stimuli (decorticate posturing)	Withdrawal to painful stimuli	Localizes painful stimuli	Obeys commands

In the context of sports-related injuries, mild head trauma with an alteration in mental state is referred to as "concussion." The American Academy of Neurology classifies concussion by three grades and provides corresponding activity-limiting recommendations. Grade 1 concussion involves confusion that lasts less than 15 minutes absent loss of consciousness (LOC). In this instance, the athlete may return to activity after 15 minutes if they have a normal sideline neurologic examination with rest and exertion. However, in the presence of a previous grade 1 concussion, the athlete should abstain from play for a week. Grade 2 concussion also does not involve LOC, but here the confusion persists for greater than 15 minutes. In this instance, the athlete should not return to play for 1 week and if the athlete has suffered a previous grade 2 concussion, he or she should refrain from participation for 2 weeks. Any LOC with athletic head injury is a serious grade 3 concussion. If this is the athlete's first high-grade concussion then he or she should not participate in athletics for 1 week if LOC lasted only "seconds"; 2 weeks if LOC lasted "minutes"; or a month (or indefinitely) in the presence of multiple grade 3 concussions (**Table 2**).[5] Although it is known that repetitive head injuries can lead to "chronic traumatic encephalopathy" or "dementia pugilistica," this topic is receiving increasing attention. Recently, congressional hearings focused on the long-term effects of multiple concussions in athletes. The National Football League is paying particular attention to this issue because retired football players, having suffered multiple concussions, later are developing severe cognitive or psychologic issues, such as dementia and depression (**Box 1**).[6]

EPIDEMIOLOGY AND RISK FACTORS

Civilian closed head injuries are typically caused by falls (28%); motor vehicle accidents (20%); impact from an object (19%); and assaults (11%).[7] These injuries often occur in the context of construction or industrial accidents and domestic and child abuse. There is increasing awareness of TBI in military personnel returning from conflicts abroad. Among those deployed, 11% to 23% have suffered mild TBI, often from improvised explosive device blasts.[8] Theodorou and Rice noted that 59% of blast-exposed veterans of the Afghanistan/Iraq conflict had TBI.[9]

Sleep disturbances after TBI are estimated to occur in 30% to 70% of head-injured patients, often impairing the resumption of normal activities.[10] The exact prevalence of individual posttraumatic sleep disorders is unknown for several reasons. First, the actual occurrence of the causative injury is difficult to ascertain on a population scale, with many milder injuries going unreported. Second, even when reported, there is

Table 2
Concussion grading system: American Academy of Neurology

	Confusion?	Loss of Consciousness?	When to Return to Activity?	Previous Same-Grade Concussion?
Grade 1	<15 min	No	After 15 min if normal neurologic examination	Out of play for 1 wk
Grade 2	>15 min	No	Out of play for 1 wk	Out of play for 2 wk
Grade 3	Yes	Yes	Out of play for 1 wk if LOC lasted only "seconds" or out of play for 2 wk if LOC lasted "minutes"	Out of play for 1 mo or more

---

Box 1
Differential diagnosis of sleep disturbance after TBI

Obstructive sleep apnea

Central sleep apnea

Complex sleep apnea

Hypersomnia caused by medical condition

Circadian rhythm sleep disorder

Insomnia

Parasomnias

Periodic limb movement disorder

Posttraumatic stress disorder

Pain

Depression or anxiety

Fatigue

---

substantial variability in gradation of injury along a severity continuum. Lastly, most TBI sufferers are never investigated for sleep disorders. Nevertheless, a few studies provide some insight. In a prospective study, Baumann and colleagues[11] found that approximately three out of four patients who were initially hospitalized for TBI developed sleep-wake disturbances by 6 months after the injury. Most had hypersomnia or fatigue, with insomnia present in only 5%. Other authors have found a higher prevalence of insomnia after TBI.[12] In 200 veterans returning from Operation Enduring Freedom/Operation Iraqi Freedom, those with mild TBI and posttraumatic stress disorder (PTSD) had the greater sleep disturbances compared with those without PTSD.[13] In children, 10% to 38% with TBI experience sleep disturbances, the highest being in the acute period after the injury (**Box 2**).[14–16]

PATHOPHYSIOLOGY

Head injuries are either penetrating (breaching the calvarium) or closed, in which the calvarium remains intact. The injury may be classified by severity (from mild to severe); mechanism; anatomic features; direction; intensity; or duration. Closed head injury

---

Box 2
Causes of TBI

Falls

Motor vehicle accidents

Impact from an object

Assault, violence, abuse

Sports-related injury

Blasts (ie, improvised explosive device)

Firearms

---

may be focal (ie, cerebral contusion, epidural hematoma, or intracerebral hemorrhage directly affecting a particular area of brain tissue) or diffuse leading to more widespread axonal injury. Focal injury can result in a coup-contrecoup TBI mechanism where a coup injury occurs under the site of impact with an object, and a contrecoup injury occurs on the side opposite the impacted area. Brain bruising occurs at both sides of the injury. Diffuse injury typically results from acceleration/deceleration or blast waves (eg, improvised explosive device blast). Axonal injury results from shearing forces causing microhemorrhages, cerebral edema, increased intracranial pressure, or changes in cerebral blood flow leading to hypoxia or anoxia. Diffuse damage may have no magnetic resonance imaging correlate, although white matter changes can be seen in some cases (**Figs. 1–3**).

The type of sleep disturbance resulting from a closed head injury depends on the location of injury within sleep-regulating brain regions. Posttraumatic hypersomnia is seen when areas involving the maintenance of wakefulness are damaged. These regions include the brainstem reticular formation, posterior hypothalamus, and the area surrounding the third ventricle. High cervical cord lesions have also been known to cause sleepiness and obstructive sleep apnea (OSA).[17] In addition, whiplash may cause hypersomnia by precipitating sleep-disordered breathing.[18]

Low cerebral spinal fluid hypocretin-1 levels are found in most cases of narcolepsy with cataplexy, but deficiency of this neuropeptide may not be found in other central hypersomnias.[19] Most patients with moderate-to-severe TBI have low or intermediate hypocretin-1 levels in the acute injury phase.[20] Hypocretin levels tend to normalize (become >200 pg/mL) 6 months after the injury, which may explain why post-TBI sleepiness resolves in many over time.[11,21–24]

Coup-contrecoup brain injury after head trauma occurs most frequently at the base of the skull in areas of bony irregularities (especially the sphenoid ridges), with consequent damage to the inferior frontal and anterior temporal regions, including the basal forebrain (an area involved in sleep initiation). As a result, insomnia is a common symptom after injuries of this mechanism. Closed head injury can involve the suprachiasmatic nucleus or its output tracts leading to disturbance of circadian rhythmicity with concomitant hypersomnia and insomnia.

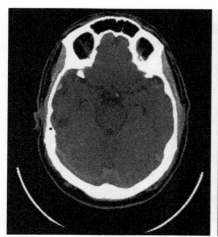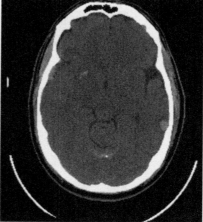

Fig. 1. Coup-contrecoup injury after right temporal TBI with hemorrhagic contusion in the right frontotemporal and left tempooccipital regions, with scattered subarachnoid hemorrhage, and a right occipitoparietal subdural.

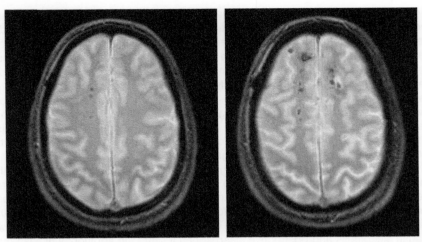

Fig. 2. Axial gradient-recalled echo magnetic resonance image showing multiple punctate microhemorrhages consistent with diffuse axonal injury after a motor vehicle accident.

CLINICAL FEATURES AND DIAGNOSIS

Sleep disturbance is a common complaint after head injury, with milder injuries more likely to disrupt sleep than more severe head trauma.[25–29] Mahmood and colleagues[25] postulate that this may be caused by multiple factors such that those with more severe head injuries are less aware of their deficits and may underreport sleep issues. In addition, those with mild TBI may over-endorse sleep complaints or may have greater pressures to reintegrate into their daily life more quickly leading to increased stress and sleep issues. Lastly, neurobiologic differences between mild and severe injuries may lead to more sleep complaints in mild TBI. A common pattern after TBI includes difficulties initiating and maintaining sleep, with or without concomitant daytime

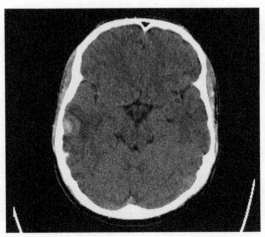

Fig. 3. Computed tomography showing a right temporal epidural hematoma with adjacent contusion and vasogenic edema.

sleepiness. A large epidemiologic study showed that up to half of those suffering TBI endorsed insomnia symptoms of some type.[30] Causation can be the result of diverse clinical and other factors, such as pain; injury to sleep-wake regulatory nuclei and pathways in the brain (eg, ventrolateral preoptic nucleus or its projections); PTSD; maladaptive behaviors; or other factors preventing the occurrence of sleep.

In some cases, the post-TBI insomnia is a manifestation of a circadian rhythm sleep disorder, typically delayed sleep phase or irregular sleep-wake type.[31] In delayed sleep phase, the subject is delayed in relation to naturally occurring light-dark cycles, resulting in early morning bedtimes and late morning-afternoon wake times. When the patient with TBI with this circadian pattern attempts to conform to traditional bedtime and wake times they struggle with sleep-onset insomnia, having gone to bed long before their internal biologic clock would have preferred. In irregular sleep-wake circadian type, the TBI patient has multiple irregular sleep-wake bouts throughout the day and night with seemingly no link to traditional light-dark cycles. The only thing normal about their sleep is the amount they get per 24 hours.

Objective testing with polysomnography (PSG) and multiple sleep latency testing (MSLT) can be helpful in the work-up of these patients. Patients with mild TBI (27.9 months postinjury; SD = 15.5 months) undergoing PSG were found to have less efficient sleep and longer sleep-onset latencies compared with control subjects.[32] Nightmares commonly interrupt sleep in veterans with PTSD and mild TBI.[33] Veterans of the US campaigns in Afghanistan (Operation Enduring Freedom) and Iraq (Operation Iraqi Freedom) complaining of insomnia associated with mild TBI and PSTD were subjectively sleepier compared with veterans with insomnia caused by PTSD alone.[34]

Hypersomnia with or without involuntary sleep attacks may also develop after a head injury, so called "secondary narcolepsy" or "posttraumatic hypersomnia." If hypersomnia persists for 3 months after a head injury (with or without cataplexy) with a mean sleep-onset latency (SOL) of less than 8 minutes and two or more sleep-onset rapid eye movement periods are found on MSLT, the diagnosis is "narcolepsy caused by medical condition." If 3 months of hypersomnia persists after a head injury and MSLT shows a mean SOL of less than 8 minutes with less than two sleep-onset rapid eye movement periods, then the diagnosis is "hypersomnia caused by medical condition" (posttraumatic hypersomnia).[35] Overnight sleep may or may not be prolonged compared with the pretrauma period. Ancillary symptoms attributed to daytime somnolence may also occur, such as difficulty with concentration, memory impairment, and fatigue.

Several other sleep disorders have also been found in patients with head trauma. Masel and colleagues[36] examined a series of 71 patients with brain injury in a residential treatment program, all without a prior history of hypersomnia or sleep disturbances. Among the 33 (46.5%) hypersomnolent patients, four had OSA, seven had periodic limb movement disorder, and one had narcolepsy (in addition to periodic limb movement disorder). The remaining 21 hypersomnolent patients were given a diagnosis of "posttraumatic hypersomnia." In an extensive series of 184 patients with TBI, Guilleminault and colleagues[18] found that most patients admitted to objective sleepiness and only 17% of the patients had a normal mean SOL (>10 minutes) on MSLT. Thirty-two percent of the patients were found to suffer from sleep-disordered breathing (primarily OSA). The authors noted that all 16 whiplash patients were diagnosed with sleep-disordered breathing indicating the importance of considering the mechanism of the injury when evaluating the patient with TBI with a sleep complaint. Pain was also found to be a significant cause of nocturnal sleep disruption and daytime impairment. Castriotta and colleagues[37] prospectively studied 87 adults at least 3 months after TBI. PSG and MSLT were administered to all subjects; 46%

had abnormal sleep studies. The authors diagnosed 23% with OSA, 11% with post-traumatic hypersomnia, 7% with periodic limb movements in sleep, and 6% with narcolepsy. Head trauma has been reported to precipitate a few cases of Kleine-Levin syndrome, a rare disorder consisting of recurrent hypersomnia and cognitive or behavioral disturbances, hypersexuality, and compulsive eating.[38]

Head trauma occasionally triggers parasomnias, including sleepwalking; sleep terrors; rapid eye movement sleep behavior disorder (abnormal dream-enacting behavior during a normally atonic state); and dissociative disorders.[39] These studies indicate that TBI can precipitate almost every sleep disorder, which emphasizes the importance of careful history taking and physical examination when diagnosing sleep disturbance in this patient population.

Fatigue is another complaint associated with TBI with untoward consequences for quality of life. In a study of 119 patients at least 1 year after TBI, up to 53% reported fatigue, which was more prevalent in women or those with symptoms of depression, pain, or sleep disturbances.[40] In another study of individuals with moderate-to-severe TBI, 16% to 32% and 21% to 34% (at years 1 and 2, respectively) reported significant levels of fatigue.[41] Fatigue and sleepiness can be difficult to disentangle by even the most experienced clinician highlighting the importance of objective assessments in these patients of sleepiness, such as the MSLT, and the ability to stay awake, such as the maintenance of wakefulness test.

Depression and anxiety are common after TBI. Patients with mild TBI and sleep complaints reported feeling depressed at 10 days and 6 weeks after their injury.[42] New-onset anxiety after head injury is a significant predictor of sleep disturbance, although the cause-effect relationship is unclear.[43] In addition, pain is a common comorbid condition, contributing to sleep disturbances and also associated with mood issues.

The relationship between sleep disturbance and TBI in children is less well characterized than in adults. Common risk factors for disturbed sleep in children after TBI include mild injury; psychosocial problems (defined by the Pediatric Symptoms Checklist, a one-page questionnaire completed by the parent to assess emotional and behavioral problems in the child); and pain. Children with TBI suffer from a higher severity and more prolonged duration of sleep disturbances compared with children with orthopedic injury. Sleep disturbances are significant predictors of poorer functional outcomes in children with moderate or severe TBI.[44] Other studies in children indicate that mild TBI increases nocturnal waking and reduces sleep efficiency.[45] These sleep disturbances may contribute to psychologic, social, and academic difficulties.

TREATMENT

Post-TBI insomnia is often refractory to conventional treatments. Patients are commonly treated with benzodiazepines, especially in patients with underlying anxiety. The nonbenzodiazepine benzodiazepine receptor agonists zolpidem, zaleplon, and eszopiclone have been extensively used in this population with moderate success. Cognitive behavioral therapy for insomnia including stimulus control, sleep restriction, cognitive restructuring, sleep hygiene education, and fatigue management can improve nocturnal sleep quality and reduce daytime fatigue.[46] In veterans suffering from PTSD and chronic sleep disturbances (TBI not defined), prazosin and cognitive behavioral therapy were found to be effective (compared with placebo) in improving sleep continuity and nightmare frequency.[47] Acupuncture may also be a viable treatment in improving sleep quality after TBI.[48]

Patients with narcolepsy or hypersomnia secondary to a head injury may require stimulant medications, such as modafinil, methylphenidate, or amphetamines, in doses similar to those used for idiopathic narcolepsy. A prospective, double-blind, randomized, placebo-controlled trial found that modafinil (100–200 mg given each morning) significantly improved sleepiness in those with TBI as measured by the Epworth Sleepiness Scale and the maintenance of wakefulness test. However, modafinil was not found to be effective for fatigue in these individuals.[49] In contrast, another study found modafinil to be of limited effectiveness for sleepiness associated with TBI.[50] Clinicians should note that more conservative treatments, such as strategic naps and caffeine use, are quite helpful for those with post-TBI hypersomnolence.

Cases of sleep apnea resulting from head injury are treated with continuous positive airway pressure (CPAP) or bilevel positive airway pressure with or without a backup rate. Sometimes adaptive-servo ventilation is necessary for central sleep apnea or complex sleep apnea (a combination of obstructive and central events). Other treatments for OSA may include mandibular advancement devices; surgical approaches to the proximal airway; and conservative treatments, such as weight loss and body positioning during sleep. Mandibular advancement devices are constructed by a dentist (ideally one with a specialization in sleep medicine) and reposition the lower jaw forward to reduce obstructions in the airway by pulling the tongue away from the posterior pharyngeal wall and tightening up the palate. Surgical approaches are diverse and typically tailored to the individual patient, with common procedures including uvulopalatopharyngopasty, tonsillectomy, and genioglossus advancement (**Flowchart 1**).

Periodic limb movement disorder related to TBI is typically treated with dopamine agonist medications (ie, ropinirole or pramipexole). Importantly, iron storage levels should be investigated in these patients to ensure a ferritin greater than 50. Iron is a cofactor for tyrosine hydroxylase in the production of dopamine in the presynaptic bouton, with low levels thought to compromise dopamine synthesis and precipitate

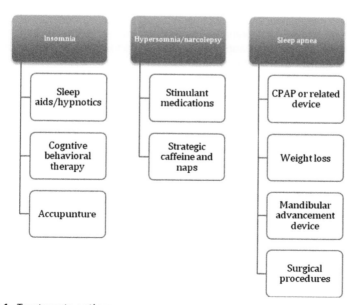

Flowchart 1. Treatments options.

restless legs syndrome and periodic limb movement disorder. In the event of low ferritin, iron supplementation is the treatment of choice.

Parasomnias are often treated with behavioral approaches (ie, relaxation techniques, mental imagery, or anticipatory awakenings) and such medications as benzodiazepines and tricyclic antidepressants. It is pertinent to rule out another sleep disorder (especially OSA) as the cause of the parasomnia. Medications, alcohol use, stress, or illness may contribute to or cause parasomnia symptoms. In those with sleep walking behaviors it is pertinent to ensure a safe sleeping environment by locking doors and windows, moving obstacles, and sleeping on the ground floor. A low dose of clonazepam or melatonin may be used to treat REM sleep behavior disorder. Lastly, prazosin is often used in veterans with PTSD to treat nightmares.

When approaching the patient with post-TBI sleep disorders, the clinician must also attend to underlying pain, depression, and anxiety because these issues can greatly impact sleep. However, avoidance (or minimization) of narcotic medications for pain is prudent if possible because these medications can worsen TBI-related sleep apnea. Tricyclic antidepressants are frequently used to treat chronic pain issues and may also be helpful with insomnia because of their sedating effects. Benzodiazepines used for anxiety or sedation may also worsen sleep apnea and are associated with worse cognitive outcomes. Those "self-medicating" post-TBI symptoms with alcohol risk sleep disruption, nightmares, reduction in rapid eye movement sleep, and worsening sleep apnea. Selective serotonin reuptake inhibitors for depression or anxiety should be taken in the morning because they can induce insomnia when taken at bedtime. Lastly, sedating antidepressants, such as trazodone and mirtazapine, are helpful to treat insomnia, regardless of the presence or absence of comorbid mood issues (**Flowchart 2**).

PROGNOSIS

There are few follow-up studies regarding posttraumatic sleep disorders and therefore the natural history of these disorders is not well known. In general, sleep disruption in TBI may impair rehabilitation participation and delay recovery because of its negative impact on psychologic functioning (ie, depression and anxiety) and pain perception. Once stabilized, sleep disturbances related to TBI show little further change, other than an improvement with treatment. A prospective cohort study examined sleepiness in 514 patients with TBI 1 month after the injury and again at 1 year. At 1 month, 55%

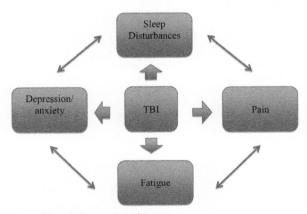

Flowchart 2. Relationship of sleep-related issues.

Box 3
Case presentation

A 42-year-old man suffered closed head and whiplash injuries after a motor vehicle accident. About 1 month after the event he developed symptoms of sleep apnea, including snoring, sleepiness, and witnessed apneas. He denied experiencing these symptoms before the injury. Examination was remarkable for a body mass index of 27, neck circumference of 17 in, and normal oropharyngeal anatomy.

PSG showed an apnea hypopnea index of 65, consisting mainly of obstructive apneas and hypopneas, but also included a moderate number of central and mixed apneas. He was given a diagnosis of "severe sleep apnea, predominantly obstructive but with a central component." He underwent a CPAP titration study and then initiated CPAP therapy. This improved his sleepiness, but he continued to have frequent nocturnal awakenings despite use of eszopiclone. His CPAP download showed persistence of central apneas. He then returned to the laboratory for an adaptive-servo ventilation titration study and reported improved hypersomnia after implementation of this treatment modality.

---

endorsed at least one item on a four-item sleepiness questionnaire. Injury severity was associated with sleepiness endorsement, with the more severely injured indicating greater sleepiness. One year later, although 27% continued to endorse sleepiness on at least one of four items, most subjects had some level of improvement in their sleepiness. This study suggests that, although symptoms persist in many, some patients with TBI can expect their sleepiness to improve or resolve over time.[21] Another prospective study of 51 patients with TBI showed that at 3 years postinjury, 67% of the patients continued to complain of sleep-wake disturbances, especially fatigue and hypersomnia.[51] In a study of 31 patients with closed head injury admitted to a TBI rehabilitation unit, nurses maintained patient sleep logs and disturbed nocturnal sleep was believed to be a marker of more severe injury because these patients had longer stays in the acute trauma center and rehabilitation unit.[52] Lastly, a study of 14 patients in a TBI rehabilitation unit wearing actigraphy, and monitored daily by speech and language therapists using the Orientation Log for assessment of posttraumatic anmnesia, revealed improved sleep efficiency with resolution of posttraumatic amnesia.[53]

In persons with TBI, the presence of OSA is associated with greater impairment of sustained attention and memory than in patients with comparable severity TBI without OSA.[54] Patients with TBI with excessive daytime sleepiness have slower reaction

---

Box 4
Current controversies and future considerations

1. What is the role of potential neuroprotection or immunomodulation (ie, steroids) after TBI and the effect on subsequent development of sleep disorders?

2. Should the timing of assessment of sleep in post-TBI patients be in the acute setting or later? Does intervening sooner improve rehabilitation participation and improve long-term outcomes?

3. What is the neuroanatomic substrate of narcolepsy caused by medical condition in patients with post-TBI sleepiness? Is there a role for serial cerebrospinal fluid hypocretin-1 measurement to assess prognosis in these patients?

4. What is the mechanism for post-TBI OSA? Is whiplash injury the primary mechanism or are there other neuroanatomic causes?

times and poorer performance on the Psychomotor Vigilance Test than nonsleepy patients.[37]

Unfortunately, treatment of sleep disorders associated with TBI often does not improve sleepiness or neuropsychologic function. In an unselected group of 57 patients with TBI, Castriotta and colleagues[55] documented sleep disorders in 22 subjects (39%) by PSG. Treatment did not lead to significant changes in quality of life, mood, or cognitive performance. Treatment of OSA (13 subjects, 23%) with CPAP did not lead to improvement in sleepiness, as measured by the Epworth Sleepiness Scale and MSLT (see the case report in **Box 3** and current controversies in **Box 4**).

REFERENCES

1. Centers for Disease Control, Prevention (CDC). Nonfatal traumatic brain injuries from sports and recreation activities—United States, 2001-2005. MMWR Morb Mortal Wkly Rep 2007;56(29):733–7.
2. Rutland-Brown W, Langlois JA, Thomas KE, et al. Incidence of traumatic brain injury in the United States, 2003. J Head Trauma Rehabil 2006;21(6):544–8.
3. Winston SR. Preliminary communication: EMT and the Glasgow [correction of Glascow] Coma Scale. J Iowa Med Soc 1979;69(10):393, 398.
4. Bricolo A, Gentilomo A, Rosadini G, et al. Long-lasting post-traumatic unconsciousness. A study based on nocturnal EEG and polygraphic recording. Acta Neurol Scand 1968;44(4):513–32.
5. Practice parameter: the management of concussion in sports (summary statement). Report of the Quality Standards Subcommittee. Neurology 1997;48(3): 581–5.
6. DeKosky ST, Ikonomovic MD, Gandy S. Traumatic brain injury: football, warfare, and long-term effects. N Engl J Med 2010;363(14):1293–6.
7. Langlois JA, Rutland-Brown W, Wald MM. The epidemiology and impact of traumatic brain injury: a brief overview. J Head Trauma Rehabil 2006;21(5):375–8.
8. Schultz BA, Cifu DX, McNamee S, et al. Assessment and treatment of common persistent sequelae following blast induced mild traumatic brain injury. NeuroRehabilitation 2011;28(4):309–20.
9. Theodorou AA, Rice SA. Is the silent epidemic keeping patients awake? J Clin Sleep Med 2007;3(4):347–8.
10. Ouellet MC, Savard J, Morin CM. Insomnia following traumatic brain injury: a review. Neurorehabil Neural Repair 2004;18(4):187–98.
11. Baumann CR, Werth E, Stocker R, et al. Sleep-wake disturbances 6 months after traumatic brain injury: a prospective study. Brain 2007;130(Pt 7):1873–83.
12. Verma A, Anand V, Verma NP. Sleep disorders in chronic traumatic brain injury. J Clin Sleep Med 2007;3(4):357–62.
13. Lew HL, Pogoda TK, Hsu PT, et al. Impact of the "polytrauma clinical triad" on sleep disturbance in a Department of Veterans Affairs outpatient rehabilitation setting. Am J Phys Med Rehabil 2010;89(6):437–45.
14. Blinman TA, Houseknecht E, Snyder C, et al. Postconcussive symptoms in hospitalized pediatric patients after mild traumatic brain injury. J Pediatr Surg 2009; 44(6):1223–8.
15. Hawley CA, Ward AB, Magnay AR, et al. Children's brain injury: a postal follow-up of 525 children from one health region in the UK. Brain Inj 2002;16(11):969–85.
16. Kraus J, Hsu P, Schaffer K, et al. Preinjury factors and 3-month outcomes following emergency department diagnosis of mild traumatic brain injury. J Head Trauma Rehabil 2009;24(5):344–54.

17. Leduc BE, Dagher JH, Mayer P, et al. Estimated prevalence of obstructive sleep apnea-hypopnea syndrome after cervical cord injury. Arch Phys Med Rehabil 2007;88(3):333–7.
18. Guilleminault C, Yuen KM, Gulevich MG, et al. Hypersomnia after head-neck trauma: a medicolegal dilemma. Neurology 2000;54(3):653–9.
19. Dauvilliers Y, Baumann CR, Carlander B, et al. CSF hypocretin-1 levels in narcolepsy, Kleine-Levin syndrome, and other hypersomnias and neurological conditions. J Neurol Neurosurg Psychiatry 2003;74(12):1667–73.
20. Baumann CR, Stocker R, Imhof HG, et al. Hypocretin-1 (orexin A) deficiency in acute traumatic brain injury. Neurology 2005;65(1):147–9.
21. Watson NF, Dikmen S, Machamer J, et al. Hypersomnia following traumatic brain injury. J Clin Sleep Med 2007;3(4):363–8.
22. Carter KA, Lettieri CJ, Pena JM. An unusual cause of insomnia following IED-induced traumatic brain injury. J Clin Sleep Med 2010;6(2):205–6.
23. Shekleton JA, Parcell DL, Redman JR, et al. Sleep disturbance and melatonin levels following traumatic brain injury. Neurology 2010;74(21):1732–8.
24. Llompart-Pou JA, Perez G, Raurich JM, et al. Loss of cortisol circadian rhythm in patients with traumatic brain injury: a microdialysis evaluation. Neurocrit Care 2010;13(2):211–6.
25. Mahmood O, Rapport LJ, Hanks RA, et al. Neuropsychological performance and sleep disturbance following traumatic brain injury. J Head Trauma Rehabil 2004; 19(5):378–90.
26. Pillar G, Averbooch E, Katz N, et al. Prevalence and risk of sleep disturbances in adolescents after minor head injury. Pediatr Neurol 2003;29(2):131–5.
27. Clinchot DM, Bogner J, Mysiw WJ, et al. Defining sleep disturbance after brain injury. Am J Phys Med Rehabil 1998;77(4):291–5.
28. Beetar JT, Guilmette TJ, Sparadeo FR. Sleep and pain complaints in symptomatic traumatic brain injury and neurologic populations. Arch Phys Med Rehabil 1996; 77(12):1298–302.
29. Fichtenberg NL, Millis SR, Mann NR, et al. Factors associated with insomnia among post-acute traumatic brain injury survivors. Brain Inj 2000;14(7):659–67.
30. Ouellet MC, Morin CM. Subjective and objective measures of insomnia in the context of traumatic brain injury: a preliminary study. Sleep Med 2006;7(6): 486–97.
31. Ayalon L, Borodkin K, Dishon L, et al. Circadian rhythm sleep disorders following mild traumatic brain injury. Neurology 2007;68(14):1136–40.
32. Williams BR, Lazic SE, Ogilvie RD. Polysomnographic and quantitative EEG analysis of subjects with long-term insomnia complaints associated with mild traumatic brain injury. Clin Neurophysiol 2008;119(2):429–38.
33. Ruff RL, Ruff SS, Wang XF. Improving sleep: initial headache treatment in OIF/OEF veterans with blast-induced mild traumatic brain injury. J Rehabil Res Dev 2009;46(9):1071–84.
34. Wallace DM, Shafazand S, Ramos AR, et al. Insomnia characteristics and clinical correlates in Operation Enduring Freedom/Operation Iraqi Freedom veterans with post-traumatic stress disorder and mild traumatic brain injury: an exploratory study. Sleep Med 2011;12(9):850–9.
35. American Academy of Sleep Medicine. The international classification of sleep disorders: diagnostic and coding manual. 2nd edition. Westchester (IL): American Academy of Sleep Medicine; 2005. p. xviii, 297.
36. Masel BE, Scheibel RS, Kimbark T, et al. Excessive daytime sleepiness in adults with brain injuries. Arch Phys Med Rehabil 2001;82(11):1526–32.

37. Castriotta RJ, Wilde MC, Lai JM, et al. Prevalence and consequences of sleep disorders in traumatic brain injury. J Clin Sleep Med 2007;3(4):349–56.
38. Arnulf I, Zeitzer JM, File J, et al. Kleine-Levin syndrome: a systematic review of 186 cases in the literature. Brain 2005;128(Pt 12):2763–76.
39. Schenck CH, Boyd JL, Mahowald MW. A parasomnia overlap disorder involving sleepwalking, sleep terrors, and REM sleep behavior disorder in 33 polysomnographically confirmed cases. Sleep 1997;20(11):972–81.
40. Englander J, Bushnik T, Oggins J, et al. Fatigue after traumatic brain injury: association with neuroendocrine, sleep, depression and other factors. Brain Inj 2010; 24(12):1379–88.
41. Bushnik T, Englander J, Wright J. Patterns of fatigue and its correlates over the first 2 years after traumatic brain injury. J Head Trauma Rehabil 2008;23(1):25–32.
42. Chaput G, Giguere JF, Chauny JM, et al. Relationship among subjective sleep complaints, headaches, and mood alterations following a mild traumatic brain injury. Sleep Med 2009;10(7):713–6.
43. Rao V, Spiro J, Vaishnavi S, et al. Prevalence and types of sleep disturbances acutely after traumatic brain injury. Brain Inj 2008;22(5):381–6.
44. Tham SW, Palermo TM, Vavilala MS, et al. The longitudinal course, risk factors, and impact of sleep disturbances in children with traumatic brain injury. J Neurotrauma 2012;29(1):154–61.
45. Kaufman Y, Tzischinsky O, Epstein R, et al. Long-term sleep disturbances in adolescents after minor head injury. Pediatr Neurol 2001;24(2):129–34.
46. Ouellet MC, Morin CM. Efficacy of cognitive-behavioral therapy for insomnia associated with traumatic brain injury: a single-case experimental design. Arch Phys Med Rehabil 2007;88(12):1581–92.
47. Germain A, Richardson R, Moul DE, et al. Placebo-controlled comparison of prazosin and cognitive-behavioral treatments for sleep disturbances in US military veterans. J Psychosom Res 2012;72(2):89–96.
48. Zollman FS, Larson EB, Wasek-Throm LK, et al. Acupuncture for treatment of insomnia in patients with traumatic brain injury: a pilot intervention study. J Head Trauma Rehabil 2012;27(2):135–42.
49. Kaiser PR, Valko PO, Werth E, et al. Modafinil ameliorates excessive daytime sleepiness after traumatic brain injury. Neurology 2010;75(20):1780–5.
50. Jha A, Weintraub A, Allshouse A, et al. A randomized trial of modafinil for the treatment of fatigue and excessive daytime sleepiness in individuals with chronic traumatic brain injury. J Head Trauma Rehabil 2008;23(1):52–63.
51. Kempf J, Werth E, Kaiser PR, et al. Sleep-wake disturbances 3 years after traumatic brain injury. J Neurol Neurosurg Psychiatry 2010;81(12):1402–5.
52. Makley MJ, English JB, Drubach DA, et al. Prevalence of sleep disturbance in closed head injury patients in a rehabilitation unit. Neurorehabil Neural Repair 2008;22(4):341–7.
53. Makley MJ, Johnson-Greene L, Tarwater PM, et al. Return of memory and sleep efficiency following moderate to severe closed head injury. Neurorehabil Neural Repair 2009;23(4):320–6.
54. Wilde MC, Castriotta RJ, Lai JM, et al. Cognitive impairment in patients with traumatic brain injury and obstructive sleep apnea. Arch Phys Med Rehabil 2007; 88(10):1284–8.
55. Castriotta RJ, Atanasov S, Wilde MC, et al. Treatment of sleep disorders after traumatic brain injury. J Clin Sleep Med 2009;5(2):137–44.

The Sleep-Immunity Relationship

Charlene E. Gamaldo, MD, FAASM[a],*, Annum K. Shaikh, BS[b],
Justin C. McArthur, MBBS, MPH, FAAN[c]

KEYWORDS

- Sleep • Inflammation • Insomnia • Infectious diseases • Apnea • Immunity
- Interleukins • Cytokines

KEY POINTS

- There is a strong interrelationship between sleep quality and immune function.
- Sleep deprivation can lead to increased risk of immune compromise and increased circulating levels of inflammation markers.
- Several conditions associated with immune dysregulation (eg, human immunodeficiency virus, multiple sclerosis, Lyme disease) have also been associated with increased risk of developing several sleep disorders (eg, insomnia, restless legs syndrome, obstructive sleep apnea [OSA], circadian rhythm disorders).
- Immune system abnormalities have been shown in several primary sleep disorders (shift work disorder, OSA, insomnia), which may help to explain the increased morbidity (eg, malignancy, heart disease, stroke) and mortality risk observed in these conditions.

INTRODUCTION

Evidence in a variety of animal research models suggests a strong symbiotic relationship between sleep and the immune system. Symptoms of sleepiness and fatigue in the face of illness have long been appreciated by patients and their doctors. Scientific investigations uncovering the physiologic basis behind this relationship have only become robust in the last 30 years. The first physiologic support for the relationship came with the identification of factor S, a muramyl peptide extracted from a goat's cerebrospinal fluid (CSF) that was thought to have both immune and sleep-regulatory properties.[1] Since the identification of the factor S peptide, human and various animal research models have uncovered additional proinflammatory cytokines with sleep-regulatory properties (**Box 1** and **Table 1**). All of the substances officially

[a] Neurology, Pulmonary and Critical Care Medicine, Johns Hopkins Sleep Disorders Center, 600 North Wolfe Street, Meyer 6-119, Baltimore, MD 21287, USA; [b] Emory University Rollins School of Public Health, 1518 Clifton Road, NE Atlanta, GA 30322, USA; [c] Department of Neurology, The Johns Hopkins Hospital, Johns Hopkins University School of Medicine, 600 North Wolfe Street, Meyer 6-113, Baltimore, MD 21287-7613, USA
* Corresponding author.
E-mail address: cgamald1@jhmi.edu

Neurol Clin 30 (2012) 1313–1343
http://dx.doi.org/10.1016/j.ncl.2012.08.007
0733-8619/12/$ – see front matter © 2012 Elsevier Inc. All rights reserved.

Box 1
Summary of substances with sleep-regulatory properties

- Substance level or receptor density fluctuate with sleep-wake state
- Support for direct link with substance and sleep-regulatory mechanisms
- Sleep-wake state affected by substance administration
- Agonist or antagonist introduction affects sleep-wake state
- Disease states known to affect sleep also affect substance levels or substance receptor properties

Substances meeting full criteria

- IL-1
- TNF-α/β
- IL-6
- Growth hormone releasing hormone
- Prolactin
- Nitric oxide
- Brain-derived neurotrophic factor

Substances meeting partial criteria

- Natural killer cells
- Cytotoxic tumor-infiltrating lymphocytes
- IL-1β
- IL-2
- IL-4
- IL-8
- IL-10
- IL-12
- IL-13
- IL-15
- IL-18
- TNF-β
- Interferon α/β (IFN-α/β)
- IFN-α
- IFN-γ
- CCL4 (macrophage inflammatory protein)

Data from Krueger JM, Obal FJ, Fang J, et al. The role of cytokines in physiological sleep regulation. Ann N Y Acad Sci 2001;933:211–21; and Obal F Jr, Krueger JM. Biochemical regulation of non-rapid-eye-movement sleep. Front Biosci 2003;8:d520–50.

---

qualifying as a sleep-regulatory substance (SRS) have the ability to affect an organism's sleep requirement (theoretically based on an individual's homeostatic sleep need [process S] and circadian rhythm [process C]), architecture, and subjective sleepiness symptoms (**Table 1**). Of those fulfilling the SRS criteria, interleukin (IL)-1, IL-6, and tumor necrosis factor (TNF)-α (see **Box 1** and **Table 1**) represent the substances with strong roles in both sleep and immune function, although several other immunomodulators and cytokines possess at least some of the SRS properties (see **Box 1**).

Sleepiness with increased sleep duration caused by non–rapid eye movement (NREM) sleep promotion and rapid eye movement (REM) sleep suppression is the most consistent physiologic response observed with the sleep-regulatory cytokines (IL-1, IL-6, and TNF-α). However, this response can vary depending on the dose administered and the species being observed. The neurobiological mechanism behind this somnogenic response has been studied in most depth in IL-1, which has been linked with the regulation of several sleep-related neurotransmitters (**Table 2**).

Sleep and Immune Connection?

Most studies of immune function in the state of normal physiologic sleep patterns have shown that sleep strengthens the immune response, with most immune cells (excluding natural killer cells) showing a peak in their response to immune challenges during the night.[2]

As discussed by Imeri and colleagues,[1] the body is best equipped to thermoregulate during NREM sleep and least equipped during wakefulness or REM sleep. Therefore, the body is most adept to mount a febrile and effective immune response during NREM sleep. Evidence to further support this claim comes with data showing that, at the time of infections, SRSs such as IL-1, IL-6, and TNF-α are at increased levels and result in longer sleep durations and a disproportionately higher percentage of that sleep time spent in NREM sleep. These sleep architectural changes also correlated with higher core body temperatures, greater shivering capabilities, and thus greater capacity to combat illnesses and infection. Moreover, the immune systems' ability to mount this type of response is attenuated in the setting of sleep deprivation. The weakened immune responses seen with sleep deprivation in the form of attenuated T-cell response to antigen challenges and overall attenuated immune response after vaccination parallel a similar response seen as a product of normal aging.[3]

COMMON SLEEP DISORDERS IN CENTRAL NERVOUS SYSTEM INFECTIOUS AND IMMUNOLOGIC DISEASES

Individuals with chronic medical conditions that affect the immune system are at a cumulative risk for sleep disorders and disruption. Sleep disorders currently affect 50 to 70 million Americans.[4] Sleep conditions such as insomnia, obstructive sleep apnea (OSA), and circadian rhythm disorders have been linked to several comorbid health risks. In turn, chronic medical illness has been associated with an increased risk for comorbid sleep complaints. The relationship between sleep and chronic medical conditions becomes even more complicated when discussing sleep complaints in medical conditions that occur as a result of infectious and/or immune system dysregulation/dysfunction. Conditions ranging from autoimmune white matter disease to those with viral, parasitic, or prion origins, which clearly exemplify this interrelationship, are discussed in the following section.

Sleep and White Matter Disease Connection: Multiple Sclerosis

Individuals with multiple sclerosis (MS) are more likely to have sleep disturbances than those without the disease. Evidence also suggests that women with MS are more likely to experience sleep disturbances than their male counterparts.[5] Fatigue can often represent the single most common and disabling symptom, with some studies reporting prevalence as high as 40%.[6] General sleep quality–related complaints have been

Table 1
Substances with immune and sleep-regulatory substance properties

Immune Cell/Cytokine	Immune Function	Clinical Impact on Sleep-Wake State	Physiologic Evidence of Sleep-regulatory Properties
IL-1	Inducer of cytokines[92] such as IL-2, interferons, IL-3, and other bone marrow colony-stimulating factors, B cell-stimulating factor [2] Mediator of inflammation[92] Attracts leukocytes to inflamed tissues Causes degranulation of basophils and eosinophils Stimulates thromboxane synthesis in macrophages and neutrophils Potentiates activation of neutrophils by chemoattractant peptides Osteoclast activation	Sleepiness as NREM sleep inducer at low dose NREM sleep suppression at high dose[93] NREM sleep fragmentation[2,94]	Increases Ca^{2+} flux, critical for transmitter release in hypothalamic neurons[2,95] Decreases suprachiasmatic nucleus synaptic activity Administration into preoptic area/basal forebrain of rats decreases firing rate of serotonergic pathways involved in alertness[94] Administration at sleep onset resulted in 3-h sleep duration increase, increased in NREM sleep but decreased in REM sleep in rabbits[90,94,95] NREM sleep density increased and REM sleep decreased with intraventricular rat administration[97,98] Increased levels noted in sleep-deprived goat brain[99]

TNF-α	Proinflammatory[100] Regulates cell differentiation, proliferation, apoptosis, energy metabolism[100] Regulates production of other proinflammatory cytokines (such as IL-6 and IL-1)[100]	Sleepiness results caused by NREM stage 2 inducer but inhibitor of NREM stage 3 (slow wave sleep)[94]	Administration into preoptic area/basal forebrain of rats decreases firing rate of serotonergic pathways involved in alertness[94] Downregulates expression of clock genes (Per1, Per2, Per3)[101]
IL-6	Proinflammatory T cell–derived lympokine[102,103] Induces final maturation of B cells into antibody-producing cells[102,103] Induction of differentiation of specific gene[102,103] expression Stimulation or inhibition of cell growth[104]	Increased levels associated with reports of sleepiness, fatigue Sleepiness as an NREM stage 3 (slow wave sleep) inducer and a REM sleep inhibitor[98,105] Increased levels associated with excessive daytime sleepiness disorders (narcolepsy, sleep apnea, chronic insomnia)[84,88]	Increased levels noted in plasma of insomniacs Increased levels noted the morning following total sleep deprivation with reduction during the following night of sleep acquisition Increased levels noted the morning following partial sleep deprivation in sleep-deprived individuals[84] 4 h of nightly sleep restriction in healthy subjects resulted in increased levels along with increased TNF-α, TNR-α R1[2] Injection of recombinant human IL-6 in healthy adult resulted in increased fatigue, malaise, changes in sleep architecture alterations[105] Induces fever in rats and alters NREM sleep in a dose-related manner

Abbreviations: IL, interleukin; NREM, non–rapid eye movement; REM, rapid eye movement; TNF, tumor necrosis factor.

reported in as many as 50% of all patients with MS.[5] The various types of sleep disorders affecting patients with MS include restless legs syndrome (RLS), periodic limb movement disorder, chronic insomnia, REM sleep behavioral disorder, narcolepsy, and circadian rhythm disturbances.[7] Various mechanisms have been proposed to explain the increased risk for sleep disruption and related daytime sequelae in individuals with MS. As a result, the MS literature has offered suggestions on various sleep-related and fatigue-related symptoms unique to the MS population that warrant formal sleep evaluation and applicable treatment (**Table 3**).

Sleep and Viral Connection: Rhinovirus, Influenza Virus, Encephalitis Lethargica, and Human Immunodeficiency Virus

Depending on the type of viral infection, there may or may not be an impact on the sleep architecture. For instance, an infection with infectious mononucleosis does not change sleep architecture.[8] In contrast, sleep studies in both humans and rodents exposed to rhinovirus have consistently shown an increase in the percentage of total sleep time spent in NREM sleep, and subsequent reduction in time spent in REM sleep (**Table 4**).

Similar alterations in sleep architecture have also been observed in mice after influenza virus administration. Sleep studies in rabbits have also indicated an increase in the slow wave sleep amplitude as well as the percentage of total sleep time spent in N3 sleep in response to influenza virus exposure.[9] Encephalitis lethargica (von Economo encephalitis) is a meningoencephalitic infection marked by significant sleepiness, fatigue, ophthalmic (oculogyric crisis, ptosis, ophthalmoplegia) and extrapyramidal features, mirroring those seen in Parkinson disease. Residual symptoms in those

Table 2
Sleep-regulatory neurotransmitter and IL-1

Neurotransmitter	CNS Production Location	Sleep-regulatory Role	IL-1 Impact
Serotonin	Dorsal raphe nucleus	Initially increases wakefulness, subsequently increases NREM sleep	Inhibits corresponding neurons
Acetylcholine	Pons, mesencephalon, and basal forebrain	REM sleep generator	Inhibits release
Monoamines	Locus coeruleus, substantia nigra, ventral tegmental area, posterior hypothalamus	Promotes wakefulness	Activates the corresponding neurons and enhances release
Adenosine	Basal forebrain	Promotes sleep	Stimulates production
Glutamate	Diffuse; from brainstem reticular formation to hippocampus	Promotes wakefulness	Activate or inhibit, depending on the specific factor induced, such as nitric oxide synthase, arachidonic acid[106]

Data from Imeri L, Opp MR. How (and why) the immune system makes us sleep. Nat Rev Neurosci 2009;10(3):199–210; and Spath-Schwalbe E, Hansen K, Schmidt F, et al. Acute effects of recombinant human interleukin-6 on endocrine and central nervous sleep functions in healthy men. J Clin Endocrinol Metab 1998;83(5):1573–79.

who survive (estimated 40%) can include profound neuropsychiatric disability including catatonia, mutism, and parkinsonism-type extrapyramidal symptoms. Pandemics occurred in both 1915 and 1927, with documented cases becoming sparse thereafter. The temporal relationship between the influenza epidemic outbreaks and the subsequent meningoencephalitic pandemics led scientists to speculate that influenza was the causative agent for encephalitis lethargica. However, several retrospective studies, including autopsy studies using modern virology techniques, have failed to show a strong link between influenza virus exposure and patients with encephalitis lethargica. Autopsy studies have also shown evidence of neuronal loss and gliosis in several subcortical areas (substantia nigra, dorsal raphe, and locus ceruleus) involved in sleep/wake stability, which may explain the potential neurobiological mechanism for the significant sleep disturbance in these cases.[10] Nonetheless, the direct causative agent and underlying neurodegenerative mechanism of this encephalitic presentation remains unknown.[11-16]

Sleep complaints have been reported to affect between 18% and 73%[17-20] of individuals who are human immunodeficiency virus (HIV) seropositive (see **Table 4**). Several studies have shown that the virus can be associated with sleep architectural changes[21-23] and increased slow wave sleep has been shown to be induced with the introduction of certain HIV viral proteins.[24] Studies using polysomnographic methods have most consistently shown a disproportionately high percentage of total sleep time spent in NREM sleep, prolonged REM sleep latency. and reduced overall time spent in REM sleep in the early stage of the disease. In the more advanced phases of the disease, studies report greater sleep disruption in the form of sleep fragmentation and arousals.[21-23,25-27] However, other studies have failed to find such abnormalities. Variability in sleep architectural findings and sleep disorder prevalence is likely caused by the variety of tools used to assess subjects (validated and unvalidated questionnaires, polysomnogram, actigraphy devices, and so forth) in the different studies.[27] In addition, some studies were conducted before the introduction of combined antiretroviral therapy (cART). In those studies that occurred in the post-cART era, it remains controversial what impact the medications may play in sleep disruption independent of the virus. Mood disorders are prominent in individuals with HIV and thus impart an additional covariable to consider as the investigations into the sleep and HIV relationship evolve.[28] Some studies have shown the presence of a bidirectional relationship between sleep and depression; thus treating depression may improve sleep quality.[29] One study also showed that in HIV-infected patients, depression and increased waist size were significantly associated with insomnia.

Regarding treatment of insomnia in HIV infection, caffeine reduction may lead to an increase in sleep quality.[30] Hypnotics may serve as effective treatment in the short term, but there are concerns of tolerance, rebound insomnia, and impairment in motor function and coordination.[31] Behavioral interventions are effective for persistent primary insomnia, and warrant studies evaluating efficacy based on cognitive behavioral treatment strategies that incorporate common HIV disease–specific comorbidities that are likely to affect alertness, fatigue, and sleep-related complaints.[32] Moreover, nonspecific fatigue is a common complaint in the HIV population, with a prevalence of 20% to 60% in patients with chronic HIV infection and up to 85% in patients with acquired immune deficiency syndrome (AIDS).[33] Studies have reported some therapeutic benefit with modafinil in HCV-positive and HCV-negative patients with AIDS complaining of disabling fatigue.[34]

Studies are limited that distinguish nonspecific fatigue caused by other HIV-related medical, psychiatric, or treatment-related issues as opposed to fatigue resulting from a primary sleep disorder.[35] Thus further studies are warranted to descriptively

Table 3
MS and commonly encountered sleep disorders/complaints

Sleep Disorder/ Complaint	Prevalence	Proposed Mechanism	MS-Specific Signs/Symptoms and Symptoms Requiring Formal Evaluation	Potential Treatment Options
RLS	~3–5 times that of the general population[7] Predictive factors for RLS in patients with MS include older age, longer duration of disease, progressive primary forms of the disease, greater disability (as measured by the EDSS scale), and increased leg movements before sleep onset[107]	Cervical cord involvement increases likelihood of RLS; damage to dopaminergic diencephalospinal and reticulospinal pathways that project to spinal cord in MS can lead to decrease in sensory threshold and increased susceptibility to RLS[108] Decreased dopaminergic activity caused by low dopaminergic (D2) receptor occupancy[109–111]; impaired iron metabolism, indirectly affecting the dopamine system[112,113]	MS-specific sign or symptoms: RLS symptoms more likely to present in an asymmetric pattern. Younger age of onset. Family history of RLS less likely to be present Formal evaluation suggested if symptoms result in significant sleep and associated daytime dysfunction	Therapeutic options similar to those recommended for RLS in Non-MS cases include dopaminergic agents (pramipexole, ropinirole), GABAergic agents (gabapentin, gabapentin encarbil); Benzodiazepines/ benzodiazepine receptor agonists (clonazepam, zolpidem)
Sleep-disordered breathing	Obstructive sleep apnea, central sleep apnea, nocturnal hypoventilation reported in MS cases, although a large-scale prevalence study has yet to be conducted[114]	MS lesions affecting medullary respiratory centers can lead to central sleep apnea, central-acting therapies for pain and spasticity may reduce respiratory drive[7]	MS-specific signs or symptoms: fatigue, inattention, psychomotor slowing, mood instability, nocturia[115] Formal evaluation suggested if symptoms result in significant sleep and associated daytime dysfunction	In the case of central alveolar hypoventilation caused by MS flare affecting bulbar region, corticosteroids may be of benefit. Otherwise, treatment recommendation strategies similar to current guidelines for non-MS cases. Risk factor reduction (weight loss, improved sleep hygiene), oral appliances, positive upper airway pressure (CPAP or BiPAP), positional therapy, diaphragmatic pacer in case of severe central sleep apnea, and upper airway surgery in[115–118]

Excessive daytime sleepiness/fatigue	Prevalence reported to be as high as 80%–90% of patients with MS[5]	Presumably multifactorial to include any 1 or a combination of the following:	MS-specific signs or symptoms:	Evaluate and treat for underlying medical, psychiatric, or iatrogenic causes
		1. Sleep disturbance (PSG findings notable for indices of sleep fragmentation to include increased wake after sleep onset, increased arousal index, decreased sleep efficiency, increased periodic limb movement index, primary sleep disorders such as OSA, RLS, narcolepsy, and RSBD[7]	symptoms of fatigue may worsen with increased temperature	Pharmacologic therapies such as modafinil and amantadine have shown potential benefit in limited trials
		2. Iatrogenic (sedative side effects of medications used to treat MS symptoms related to spasticity, pain, mood instability, and so forth)	Formal evaluation suggested when sleepiness and/or fatigue symptoms linked with increased disability (ie, cognitive function, interpersonal relationship, job performance)	Nonpharmacologic options such as cooling, exercise, and rehabilitation therapy may also be of benefit[115]
		3. Soporific effects of the highly concentrated proinflammatory cells and SRSs (ie, IL-1, IL-2, IL-6, TNF-α)	Differentiating daytime sleepiness from fatigue can be determined subjectively with validated questionnaire such as Epworth Sleepiness Scale vs Fatigue Severity Scale and objectively with procedures such as the MSLT or actigraphy monitoring	
		4. Demyelination of central sleep-wake regulatory pathways in brainstem		
		5. Hypothalamic-pituitary-adrenal axis dysregulation		
		6. Psychiatric comorbidities associated with sleepiness/fatigue (ie, depression, anxiety)		

(continued on next page)

Table 3
(continued)

Sleep Disorder/ Complaint	Prevalence	Proposed Mechanism	MS-Specific Signs/Symptoms and Symptoms Requiring Formal Evaluation	Potential Treatment Options
PLMS	Increased limb movements noted in patients with MS (36%) compared with healthy controls (8%)[7,115]	Increased MS lesion load in cerebellum and brainstem more likely to be present[109–112]	No MS-specific symptoms or signs Formal evaluation suggested when increased limb movement activity along with sleep disturbance and/or associated daytime complaints that cannot be otherwise explained by another sleep or neurologic condition	Therapeutic options similar to those recommended for PLMS associated with or without clinical symptoms of RLS in Non-MS cases to include dopaminergic agents (pramipexole, ropinirole), GABAergic agents (gabapentin, gabapentin encarbil)
CRD	Frequency compared with general population unknown[119]	Demyelination in efferent and afferent suprachiasmatic nucleus (primary circadian rhythm pacemaker) projections; plaques in the periventricular area of hypothalamus (region of SCN or its efferents[119,120])	No MS-specific symptoms or signs Formal evaluation suggested when misalignment between internal sleep-wake cycle and desired sleep-wake cycle that results in sleep (ie, insomnia) and daytime functional complaints (ie, fatigue, sleepiness, mood instability)	Treatment options similar to conventional therapies for CRD including chronotherapy, phototherapy, and melatonin[121]

Chronic insomnia	Increased risk among patients with MS (prevalence reports as high as 40%) compared with general population (reported prevalence rates of 10%–30%)[87,122–124]	Risk is secondary to pain, spasticity, depression, anxiety, nocturia, medication effects, or primary sleep disorders such as RLS or periodic limb movement disorder[87,122–124]	MS-specific symptom: early morning awakening most common symptom reported in more than 50% Formal evaluation suggested if symptoms result in significant sleep and associated daytime dysfunction	Individualized multifaceted approach includes: Optimal treatment of underlying sleep disruptive medical or psychiatric cause Pharmacologic (usually recommended for short-term therapy including benzodiazepine receptor agonists, sedating antidepressants) Cognitive behavior strategies (education on lifestyle changes, stimulus control, sleep restriction, cognitive behavioral therapy[115])
RSBD	Prevalence of RSBD in MS unknown.[115]	Through a destructive inflammatory lesion in brain stem[115]	No MS-specific RSBD features Diagnosis of RSBD requires clinical history of dream enactment along with polysomnographic evidence of abnormally increased muscle tone during REM sleep Formal evaluation suggested if symptoms result in significant sleep and associated daytime dysfunction or history concerning for possible safety risk to patient or bed partner	Corticosteroids may be of benefit if RSBD symptoms occur at the time of MS exacerbation, otherwise clonazepam, melatonin, and strategies to ensure safe sleeping environment for patient and bed partner remains first line. Limit substances and medication known to be associated with triggering RSBD symptoms, such as selective serotonin reuptake inhibitors and alcohol. Treat sleep apnea if present because it may be associated with pseudo-RSBD

(continued on next page)

Table 3
(continued)

Sleep Disorder/ Complaint	Prevalence	Proposed Mechanism	MS-Specific Signs/Symptoms and Symptoms Requiring Formal Evaluation	Potential Treatment Options
Narcolepsy	Prevalence in general population is 0.047%; MS fourth most common cause for secondary narcolepsy caused by an underlying condition Prevalence of narcolepsy among individuals with MS is unknown[115]	Both narcoleptics (95%) and patients with MS (>50%) show positivity for DR2 haplotype Presence of DQB1*0602 human leukocyte antigen associated with increased likelihood of developing narcolepsy with cataplexy and MS MS lesions affecting the hypocretinergic system[115]	No MS-specific features Narcolepsy features include: Excessive daytime sleepiness Automatic behaviors Sleep paralysis Hypnopompic/hypnagogic hallucinations Cataplexy Significant sleep fragmentation Formal evaluation suggested if symptoms result in significant sleep and associated daytime dysfunction	Narcoleptic symptoms in the context of an acute MS flare maybe improved with a course of corticosteroids and lifestyle modifications Modafinil has shown benefit for daytime sleepiness caused by narcolepsy as well as MS-related fatigue Otherwise no MS-specific guidelines; treatment options for narcolepsy include amphetamine classes for excessive daytime sleepiness, and sodium oxybate, tricyclic antidepressant, or selective serotonin inhibitors for cataplexy

Abbreviations: BiPAP, biphasic positive airway pressure; CPAP, continuous positive airway pressure; CRD, circadian rhythm disorder; EDSS, Expanded Disability Status Scale; MSLT, Multiple Sleep Latency Test; OSA, obstructive sleep apnea; PLMS, periodic limb movements; PSG, polysomnography; RSBD, REM sleep behavior disorder; SCN, suprachiasmatic nucleus.

Table 4
Overview of interrelationship of sleep disorders and infectious diseases

Disorder/Infectious Agent (Class)	Sleep-Related and Other Common Symptoms	Sleep/EEG Patterns	Studies in Humans	Studies in Rodents
Sleeping sickness: *Trypanosoma brucei* (protozoan parasite)[125]	Disturbance of sleep-wake cycle[125] Daytime somnolence[126] Insomnia[83] Headache[125] Fever[125] Weakness[125] Joint pain[125] Stiffness[125] Psychiatric disorders[125] Seizures[125] Visual Impairment[125] Coma[125] Ultimately death[125]	Sleep-onset REM episodes[38] Sleep-wake alterations[38] Decrease in non-REM sleep[38]	MRI: lesions to deep white matter[127] Increased levels of TNF-α and IFN-γ in plasma[128] Increased levels of IL-1β in serum of stage 2 patients[129] Numerous trypanosomes with histologic lesions found in pleural, peritoneal, pericardium, and CSF in autopsy studies[130]	Rats infected with *Tb*: alterations in the SCN SCN neurons' response to light stimulation impaired
Fatal familial insomnia: Inherited or sporadic genetic mutation (prion)[131]	Inattention Hypovigilance Sympathetic hyperactivity Dysautonomia Ataxia and dysarthria	Disappearance of sleep spindles and K-complexes in EEG Progressive slowing of EEG background activity Flattening of EEG in terminal disease stage	Episodes of unresponsiveness correlated with subjective dreamlike states Alterations in circadian hormonal secretion Atrophy of the anteroventral and mediodorsal thalamic nuclei Loss of neurons and astrogliosis in thalamus	In strains with a version of the FFI mutation: knockout mice showed an altered motor cortex, atrophied cerebellum, and enlarged ventricles[131] Mice behavior: reduced levels of overall activity, increased measures of sleep interruption, and increased fluctuation of body temperature, suggesting lack of entering deep sleep[131]

(continued on next page)

Table 4
(continued)

Disorder/Infectious Agent (Class)	Sleep-Related and Other Common Symptoms	Sleep/EEG Patterns	Studies in Humans	Studies in Rodents
HIV	Fatigue[132] Insomnia Poor sleep hygiene OSA Fever[133] Muscle soreness[133] Rash[133] Headache[133] Sore throat[133] Mouth or genital ulcers[133] Swollen lymph glands[133] Joint pain[133] Night sweats[133] Diarrhea[133]	Early Stages: Increased occurrence of SWS, delayed REM latency, reduced time spent in REM sleep Later Stages: Increased sleep fragmentation Note: most of these EEG charaterization studies were done prior to cART.	Evidence of circadian rhythm disruption[132,134,135] Evidence that sleep-related symptoms are strongly associated with psychological disturbances, more so than biologic markers of virus[136]	Suggest that transcription factor (Tat; necessary for HIV) does not alter circadian rhythms but does decrease overall locomotor activity[137] TNF-α levels in serum coupled with sleep EEG δ-frequency amplitude[138]
Rhinovirus (virus) Rhinovirus type 23 was used in the cited human study[139]	Insomnia Poor sleep quality Malaise[139] Impaired psychomotor performance[139] Sneezing[139] Runny nose/sore throat[139] Headache[139] Chills[139]	Decrease in stage 1 NREM sleep percentage (during both incubation and active viral periods)[139] Decreased consolidated sleep time and sleep efficiency[139]	Increased levels of IL-1β and TNF in nasal fluids of patients with naturally acquired viral rhinitis[109,140] Increased secretion of TNF-α and IL-1β in primary cultures of human tracheal epithelial cells after exposure to HRV-2 and HRV-14[10]	None identified

CJD: PrP[Sc] (prion)[111] 15% familial	Insomnia (early symptom) Startle myoclonus Rapid dementia associated with hallucinations (visual and auditory) and dream-reality confusion[111] Pyramidal and extrapyramidal signs[141] Incoordination[141] Personality changes[141] Impaired vision[141]	No K-complexes, sleep spindles, or vertex sharp waves in EEG[111] Abnormal architecture and transition of REM/NREM cycles[111]	Spongiform degeneration and gliosis in frontal, parietal, temporal, and occipital areas[111] No significant degeneration in thalamus cited in sporadic form[111] Other studies noted thalamic abnormalities in some patients[142–144]	Mouse model with an expressed homolog mutation associated with CJD showed neurologic, EEG, and sleep abnormalities[145] (specifically reduced REM sleep),[96] and increased IL-1 and TNF levels[91,146]
Lyme disease: Borrelia burgdorferi (spirochete bacteria)	Fatigue[147] Insomnia Nocturnal Awakenings[148] Daytime somnolence[148] Rash[147] Chills[147] Fever[147] Headache[147] Muscle and joint aches[147] Swollen lymph nodes[147] Bell palsy[147]	Increased fragmentation in stage 2 and 3 of NREM sleep[148] Decreased sleep efficiency[148] Prolonged sleep latency[148] Increased arousal index[148]	Consistently high scores on validated fatigue scales[148] Patients complain of difficulty initiating and maintaining sleep, but 1 study showed normal objective sleep latency on MSLT scores[148] Lesions observed predominantly within deep white matter[149]	None identified

Abbreviations: CJD, Creutzfeldt-Jakob disease; EEG, electroencephalography; HIV, human immunodeficiency virus.

characterize these symptoms in order to gain further insight on the potential neurobiological mechanisms and efficacious treatment options.

Sleep and Parasite Connection: Sleeping Sickness

Sleeping sickness, also known as human African trypanosomiasis (HAT), is caused by the *Trypanosoma brucei* (*Tb*) parasite. The infection results in a severe disruption in sleep and wake state stability. Abnormalities in the clinical and physiologic aspects of the sleep and wake state degrade as the infectious process progresses (**Table 5**).

Individuals initially have somnolence that eventually progresses to overt sleep attacks and premature REM periods. The inflammatory cytokines such as IL-1β, TNF-α, and IFN-γ are found in high concentrations peripherally and centrally in the CSF.[36] Affected individuals have shown increased *Fos* expression in orexin-producing neurons, suggesting that their degeneration may be contributing to the sleep-onset REM periods observed in the advanced stages of infection.[37] In studies performed on rats infected with *Tb*, the

Table 5 Two stages of sleeping sickness			
	(1) Hemolymphatic	**Intermediate**	**(2) Meningoencephalitic**
Innoculation stages	Parasites enter from site of innoculation into the lymphatic system and bloodstream of the host, then multiply and lead to waves of parasitemia	No difference noted	Development of neuropsychiatric syndrome
Peripheral immune response	WBC at <5 cells/μL	WBC at 5–20 cells/μL	WBC at 20 cells/μL or more and/or parasites in CSF
Clinical sleep disturbances	Undisturbed sleep-wake distribution sleeping at night and staying awake during the day	Slight disturbances of sleep maintenance	Daytime sleepiness: most reported, alteration of nychthemeral (night and day) alteration of sleep and wakefulness
Physiologic sleep and wake abnormalities	Sleep architecture: 1 or no SOREMP seen in a 48-h recording period Background EEG wake rhythm: normal	Sleep architecture: 3 SOREMPs observed during a 48-h recording Background EEG rhythm: none reported in this study; none identified	Sleep architecture: SOREMPs seen in all patients; altered K-complexes; degraded spindles; slow wave hypersynchrony; and hypnopompic δ bursts Background EEG wake rhythm: overall background slowing with periodic slow waves

Abbreviations: SOREMP, sleep onset rapid eye movement period; WBC, white blood cell.
Data from Buguet A, Bisser S, Josenando T, et al. Sleep structure: a new diagnostic tool for stage determination in sleeping sickness. Acta Trop 2005;93(1):107–17.

response of suprachiasmatic nucleus (SCN) neurons to light stimulation is impaired,[38] with spontaneous firing rate and expression of α-amino-3-hydroxy-5-methyl-4-isoxazo-lepropionic acid (AMPA) receptors in the ventral SCN also reduced, which provides insight regarding the profound circadian rhythm disruption also seen in these cases. Therapeutic guidelines are primarily based on diagnostic stage at presentation of HAT.[36] At times, overt central nervous system (CNS) involvement that differentiates the late encephalitic stage from the earlier stages can be difficult, which makes therapeutic choices difficult. It is important to first know the context of geographic location where HAT is endemic. To identify the nonspecific nature of HAT requires excluding other infections like malaria, tuberculosis, HIV, and viral encephalitis. Serologic tests are crucial in narrowing down the diagnosis; a common one is the antibody-detecting card agglutination trypanosomiasis test (CATT) frequently used in serologic gambiense diagnosis, which is simple, easy to perform, and rapid. Recommended work-up and appropriate treatment are based on the presumed stage of the disease at the time of presentation. In those suspected with late-stage disease and all CATT-positive patients, lumbar puncture has been suggested. These patients show a lymphocytic pleocytosis and increased protein levels typically ranging from 40 to 200 mg/100 mL.[39]

The World Health Organization (WHO) criteria for CNS involvement includes presence of parasites in the CSF or white blood cells (WBC) of more than 5/μL, but this has been challenged in some locations where the measurement of 20 WBC/μL in the CSF has been used instead.[36] Another method for diagnosis is latex agglutination assay for CSF immunoglobulin M quantitation, which can be applied in the field and has shown promise for staging CNS sleeping sickness and monitoring development of treatment relapses.[40] In 2012, the WHO released treatment guidelines that primarily involve the specific timing and administration of the following 4 medications: suramin, pentamidine, melarsoprol, and eflornithine (**Box 2**).

Box 2
WHO treatment overview for sleeping sickness

Pentamidine (introduced 1941): used for the treatment of the first stage of *Trypanosoma brucei gambiense* sleeping sickness. Side effect profile: generally well tolerated by patients.

Suramin (introduced 1921): used for the treatment of the first stage of *Trypanosoma brucei rhodesiense*. Side effect profile: can include significant urinary tract symptoms/involvement and allergic reactions.

Melarsoprol (introduced 1949): used in both forms of infection. Side effect profile: can be significant and severe to include reactive encephalopathy (encephalopathic syndrome), which can be fatal (3%–10%) presumably because of the drug's arsenic derivation. An increase in resistance to the drug has been observed in several regions, particularly in central Africa.

Eflornithine (introduced 1990): only effective against *Tb gambiense*. Side effect profile: less toxic than melarsoprol; however, the regimen is strict and difficult to apply.

Nifurtimox and eflornithine combination treatment (introduced 2009): simplifies the use of eflornithine in monotherapy, but registered as effective treatment of American trypanosomiasis only and not effective for *Tb rhodesiense* or African trypanosomiasis. Because of solid safety and efficacy data, it is provided free of charge for this purpose by WHO.

Side effect profile: fever, seizures, and confusion. Combination therapy with eflornithine and nifurtimox is safer and easier than treatment with eflornithine alone, and seems to be equally or more effective.

Data from World Health Organization. WHO profile on human African trypanosomiasis. World Health Organization Web site. Available at: http://www.who.int/trypanosomiasis_african/diagnosis/en/index.html. Accessed July 5, 2012.

Sleep and PRION Connection: Creutzfeldt-Jakob Disease and Fatal Familial Insomnia

Sleep complaints have been reported in the prion disorders Creutzfeldt-Jakob disease and fatal familial insomnia (FFI), with FFI being linked with the most serious presentation of insomnia in the context of a spongiform encephalopathy (see **Table 4**). FFI is an autosomal dominant prion disease, characterized by inattention, sleep loss, hypovigilance, sympathetic hyperactivity, dysautonomia, and alterations in circadian hormonal secretion.[41] At the molecular level, this disease is linked to a missense mutation at codon 178 of the prion protein gene, PRNP, coupled with a methionine-valine polymorphism at codon 129. On pathology, this disease is characterized by thalamic degeneration and the interruption of thalamocortical limbic circuits, which causes a homeostatic sleep and wake state imbalance. Studies in human patients reveal characterizations such as persistent drowsiness interspersed with episodes of unresponsiveness. During the less responsive periods, individuals report episodic dreamlike sensations both visually and physically, with complex purposeful gestures as they presumably act out their dreams. Electroencephalography (EEG) background and sleep architecture over the course of the infection degrades, with eventual disappearance of sleep spindles and K-complexes that correlates with concurrent atrophy observed in the medial dorsal and reticular thalamic nuclei, which serve as the generator of sleep spindles.[42]

Motor signs such as ataxia and dysarthria appear weeks or months after sleep-wake behavioral disturbances. Hallmarks of this disease are a loss of neurons and astrogliosis in the thalamus. The severe and consistent atrophy of the anteroventral and mediodorsal thalamic nuclei is the only finding shared by all FFI cases. The symptoms distinguishing FFI from other prion disease such as sleep loss, sympathetic hyperactivity, and flattening of circadian oscillations is likely caused by the disconnection between thalamolimbic and more caudal structures in the central network that regulates the sleep-wake cycle and body homeostasis.[43]

Most of the drugs suggested for treatment have yielded mixed results, no significant improvement, serious adverse effects, or even inconclusive results. Hence, there are currently no treatments leading to clinical improvements in human patients with prion diseases.[44] However, preliminary data for doxycycline suggest potential prolongation in survival time based on animal models and observational studies of humans prion cases.[44] Early diagnosis, through biomarkers, could allow treatment introduction before severe brain damage occurs. Another such experimental treatment method is nocturnal noninvasive ventilation (NIV), which may help to improve daytime hypercapnia and subjective sleep quality.[45]

Sleep and Bacterial Connection: Lyme Disease

Alterations in sleep architecture have been noted with exposure to several bacterial antigens. As discussed earlier, sleep disruption and/or restriction have also been associated with attenuated response to bacterial antigen exposure to include endotoxin *Escherichia coli*.[46,47]

Because of significant fatigue often associated with Lyme disease, the responsible bacterial agent (the spirochete *Borrelia burgdorferi*) has been studied regarding its direct impact on symptoms of malaise and sleepiness (see **Table 4**). As shown in **Table 4**, Lyme disease can be linked with several sleep-related clinical and physiologic abnormalities.

Early Lyme disease, without specific neurologic manifestations, can be treated with doxycycline (100 mg twice a day, for 10–21 days), amoxicillin (500 mg 3 times a day, for 14–21 days), and cefuroxime axetil (500 mg twice a day, for 14–21 days). Lyme meningitis, associated with early neurologic manifestations such as meningitis or radiculopathy, can be treated with ceftriaxone (2 g/d intravenously for 14 days). For late neurologic Lyme disease affecting the central or peripheral nervous system, intravenous ceftriaxone treatment for 2 to 4 weeks has been suggested.[48] There are no established treatment guidelines specifically for sleep-related complaints.

IMMUNOLOGIC SEQUELAE SEEN IN PRIMARY SLEEP DISORDERS

Sleep restoration requires that an individual obtains good sleep quality and quantity. Quantity is based on the individual's personal sleep duration requirement, predetermined by the individual's homeostatic drive for sleep commonly referred to as process S, with most studies showing that most adults require between 7 and 8 hours of sleep to function at their best.[49] The increase in process S (sleep drive) directly corresponds with duration of wakefulness, so the longer an individual remains awake, the stronger their process S drive becomes (ie, propensity for sleep). In order to maintain wakefulness throughout the day and to ensure consolidated sleep and wake periods, the homeostatic sleep drive of process S is counteracted by an alerting drive commonly referred to as process C. Unlike process S, process C is neither directly nor linearly related to duration of wakefulness. Instead, process C oscillates independently in a sinusoidal pattern. It represents the circadian component of the sleep and wake state that is slightly longer than the 24-hour day, with a full cycle length reportedly between 24.1 and 24.2 hours in most individuals.[50] When process C enters the natural sinusoidal dip during the late evening hours, then the homeostatic sleep drive is unopposed and thus allows the individual to have proper sleep initiation and sleep consolidation. The 2 processes must be in synchrony in order to achieve maximal sleep restoration. Evidence is now emerging to suggest that the disruption in the sleep-wake cycle through either process can negatively affect immune function. As such, several sleep disorders that occur because of disruption in 1 or both of these processes have also been linked with immune system dysfunction. This section presents the evidence of immune dysregulation in several chronic primary sleep disorders: (1) chronic sleep deprivation, (2) circadian rhythm disorders, (3) RLS, (4) OSA, and (5) insomnia. In many cases, individuals can have more than 1 sleep disorder at a time. For this reason, this section is introduced by the following clinical vignette for the reader to consider as a clinical reference point for the discussion of the impact of sleep disorders on immune function.

Case

A 59-year-old, otherwise healthy woman presents because of concerns regarding the link between shift work disorder and cancer discussed in a television health show she recently viewed. She has worked a rotating shift as an intensive care unit (ICU) nurse for 25 years. She reports obtaining 6 to 7 hours of sleep on average. She easily shifts back and forth between night and day shifts and denies problems with daytime sleepiness, fatigue, or decline in overall function. Her body mass index is 35. She recently underwent a routine physical examination that was normal and she is on no medications. However, she has a strong family history of breast cancer and wants to discuss the evidence regarding shift work status and malignancy.

Chronic Sleep Deprivation and Immune Function

Chronic sleep deprivation has become an epidemic problem in American society. According to the latest National Sleep Foundation (NSF) poll, adults between the ages of 13 and 64 years obtain approximately 6 hours and 55 minutes of sleep on weeknights.[51] Because of familial and work responsibilities (including shift work job requirements, as in the aforementioned vignette), many of these adults can no longer use the weekends to catch up on this lost sleep. Moreover, NSF polls have also shown that adults in America are obtaining at least 30 minutes less sleep per night than even 10 years ago. The increased susceptibility to infection in the face of a sleep-deprived state is confirmed by both human and animal studies.[52]

Studies have indicated that sleep deprivation can lead to increased circulating levels of proinflammatory markers such as IL-6, TNF-α, and C-reactive protein.[2,53,54] It can also lead to decreased number of natural killer cells,[55] lower antibody titers after influenza virus immunization,[46] decreased lymphokine-activated killer activity, and decreased IL-2 production.[56] Their increased levels as a result of sleep deprivation suggest that mild sleep loss may be associated with long-term risks of significant morbidity and mortality and that these increased risks are similar to those associated with obesity or aging.[53,57] The American Academy of Sleep Medicine recommends that the average adult strive to obtain 7.5 to 8.5 hours of sleep per night based on sleep deprivation studies showing that most adults perform optimally if they consistently obtain this amount of sleep nightly on average.[58]

Circadian Rhythm Disorders and Immune Functions

Circadian rhythm sleep disorders all result in symptomatic disruption in the sleep and wake patterns because of misalignment with the inherent circadian rhythm (process C) and the individual's desired sleep schedule that subsequently results in functional complaints. Shift work sleep disorder (SWSD) is one of the most commonly encountered circadian rhythm disorders, affecting more than 6 million Americans. The clinical vignette presented earlier discusses a case of an ICU nurse who is at high risk for both SWSD as well as the potential comorbid health complications linked with a long-term shift work schedule. The potential negative sleep-related problems in SWSD are 2-fold, namely, sleepiness during the time of work and difficulty in maintaining sleep during the daytime, which leads to sleep deprivation. Shift workers tend to revert to a regular schedule on the nonwork days for normal daytime social functions and activities. Surveys done in Europe and in the United States have confirmed that night shift workers get 10 hours less sleep per week than their daytime counterparts.[59] As discussed earlier, chronic sleep deprivation is likely contributing to increased morbidity and mortality in this cohort. In addition, a long-term rotating shift work schedule also involves circadian factors. The immune system also seems to function according to an inherent circadian cycle with most substances showing peak concentrations in the early evening and minimum levels in early morning.[46] Studies have shown that, in a socially isolated environment, approximately 5 to 6 days (roughly 90 minutes per day) are needed to realign the circadian rhythm to night shift work. In some cases, shift workers rotate shift work time schedules weekly, which never allows them to appropriately adjust to the constant shift change. There are zeitgebers (exogenous cues that synchronize the endogenous biologic clock), particularly unconventional exposure times to bright light, which works against the natural sleep-wake alignment in the environment. Timing and concentration of melatonin levels is a prominent factor in the circadian rhythm alignment of sleep and wake consolidation. Release of melatonin from the pineal gland is based on diminution of light received from the melanopsin retinal cells that subsequently project to the SCN (thought to be the master pacemaker of most circadian biorhythms). In addition to increased risk of gastrointestinal and cardiovascular disease, diabetes, and metabolic syndrome, patients with long-term rotating shift work schedule are at increased risk of malignancy (prostate, colorectal, and endometrial cancer),[60–62] with the strongest link being found with breast cancer (**Table 6**).[63] Several studies (see **Table 6**) have investigated the potential role that melatonin disruption may play in the increased risk of malignancy observed in shift workers. The overarching theory is that suppression of melatonin can increase

Table 6
Evidence supporting melatonin and malignancy link

Properties of Melatonin	Studies Supporting Melatonin's Oncostatic Actions[64,150]	Effect of Melatonin on Cytokines and other Proinflammatory Substances[64,151,152]

Acts as free radical scavenger[64]
 	
Indirect actions to detoxify carcinogens via activation of glutathione and related antioxidant pathways[64]
 	
Melatonin suppresses accumulation of DNA adducts formed by carcinogens that lead to DNA damage and neoplastic transformation of cells[64]
 	
Promotes repair of DNA damage after it occurs[64]
	1. Epidemiologic studies show that women working night shifts present with increased risk of breast cancer.[63,150,152] Endometrial[87] and colorectal cancer[61] caused by increased exposure to light at night
	
	2. Tissue-isolated human breast cancer xenografts were placed in immune-deficient nude rats with melatonin-rich blood, which suppressed tumor proliferation activity and linoleic acid uptake (potent promoter of human tumorigenesis), compared with the tissues with melatonin-deficient blood
	
	3. Addition of melatonin-receptor blocker negated the tumor-suppressive effects, indicating that endogenous melatonin was an active factor
	
	4. Surgical removal of pineal gland or exposure to constant light, which suppresses melatonin release, also correlated with mammary tumorigenesis in rodents[57,64]
	
	5. In experimental models of neoplastic cancer cells (in vitro), nocturnal circulating concentrations of melatonin inhibit proliferation of these cancer cells
	
	6. Studies in experimental rat models of chemical carcinogenesis indicate that physiologic melatonin suppresses the initial phase of tumorigenesis[64]
		• Increased T lymphocytes
		• Melatonin dysregulation may cause immune suppression by leading to decreased production of:
		  ○ IL-10
		  ○ Natural killer cells
		  ○ Cytotoxic tumor-infiltrating lymphocytes
		  ○ Cancer-inhibiting cytokines: IL-2, IL-12, INF-γ, TNF-α

cancer risk through direct and indirect physiologic effects such as altering estrogen levels[64] or influencing the circadian gene expression of oncostatic cellular processes (see **Table 6**). Treatment strategies for circadian rhythm disorders are primarily aimed at exogenous techniques to shift the inherent sleep-wake clock to be more in line with the individual's desired sleep-wake schedule. Thus, approaches involving combination therapies that involve chronotherapy, phototherapy, and melatonin administration are usually the mainstay of treatment. In the case of shift work disorder, modafinil also serves as a US Food and Drug Administration–approved pharmacotherapeutic option.[65]

RLS and Immune Function

RLS is a common sensorimotor disorder that can result in significant sleep disruption and sleep loss in severe cases.[66] Prevalence for this disease is 10% in the United States, and it is more prominent in women and increases with age.[67] RLS can also be encountered in the face of other common sleep disorders, namely sleep apnea and shift work disorder.[66,68,69] Iron dysregulation and iron deficiency have been implicated in the neuropathology of RLS based on several neuroimaging studies.[66] A recent study showed an increased prevalence of small intestinal bacterial overgrowth (SIBO) in RLS.[70] Moreover, individuals with HIV infection, systemic lupus, hepatitis C, streptococcus, *Mycoplasma* and *Borrelia* seem to be at higher risk of developing RLS, which suggests a potential role of inflammation and/or immunologic function in this condition.[71–76]

Three theories have been suggested for how inflammation and the alteration of the immune system could cause or exacerbate RLS[77]:

1. Inflammation causes CNS iron deficiency through alterations in hepcidin
2. Humoral or cellular immunologic mechanisms cause direct attack on the central or peripheral nervous system
3. Genetic variants can predispose an individual to immune alterations and/or chronic infections, leading to RLS

In support of these theories, a double-blind, placebo-controlled study showed that treatment of RLS with hydrocortisone leads to a reduction in symptoms.[78] Treatment of small SIBO with nonabsorbed antibiotic alone or with treatment directed at increasing intestinal immune function and permeability led to an improvement in RLS symptoms in 2 open-labeled studies.[70,79]

Other therapeutic options for RLS include FDA-approved pharmacotherapies such as dopaminergic agents (pramipexole, ropinirole) and the GABAergic agent gabapentin encarbil. Other non–FDA-approved pharmacotherapies that have also been used commonly in this patient population include other GABAergic agents (gabapentin, pregabilin), benzodiazepines/benzodiazepine receptor agonists (clonazepam, zolpidem), and opioids (codeine, hydrocodone, methadone).[80] Treatment of other primary sleep disorders that may result in significant sleep fragmentation, such as treatment of OSA with positive airway pressure (PAP) therapy in those individuals with RLS, has also shown direct improvement in RLS symptoms.

OSA and Immune Function

An estimated 5% to 10% of Americans have OSA.[81,82] Untreated sleep apnea increases the risk for developing several conditions, including cardiovascular disease, stroke, metabolic syndromes, glucose intolerance, and cardiac conduction abnormalities.[47] OSA characteristically involves repeated sleep-disordered breathing events that usually result in sleep fragmentations and episodes of intermittent hypoxia.

C-reactive protein levels were significantly increased in individuals with OSA compared with controls, which may help provide a physiologic link between the condition and the increased cardiovascular risk.[83] Other studies have associated OSA with increases in TNF-α, IL-6, and T lymphocytes levels, which are all substances with established atherogenic properties.[84] Patients with OSA, increased TNF-α and IL-6 levels, reported a reduction in subjective sleepiness, and showed reduction in their apnea-hypopnea severity and decreased sleepiness after being given TNF-α and IL-6 inhibitors,[47,85] which provides further evidence of a potential reciprocal relationship. Treatment options for OSA include PAP therapy, which remains the gold standard for mild, moderate, or severe disease. Oral appliance has now been accepted as an appropriate line of therapy for mild to moderate cases of apnea in those unsuited to PAP therapy. Positional therapy may be a treatment option in mild cases that manifest primarily in the supine position. Risk factor reduction must be a primary focus of management that includes, but is not limited to, weight loss management, improved sleep hygiene, and smoking cessation. Surgical options may be considered in individualized cases to include bariatric surgery and otolaryngologic procedures.

Insomnia and Immune Function

Primary insomnia is currently subclassified by the International Classification of Sleep Disorders 2[58] into 3 subcategories: primary idiopathic insomnia, paradoxical insomnia, and psychophysiologic insomnia. Among all of the sleep conditions, insomnia has the greatest lifetime prevalence, affecting 30% of the general population.[86,87] A complaint regarding poor sleep quality caused by an inability to initiate and/or maintain sleep that directly results in reduced daytime function is the core feature of chronic insomnia. Although subjective complaints of reduced daytime function must be apparent (eg, fatigue, irritability, reduced concentration), many people with chronic insomnia do not display overt subjective or objective signs of sleepiness. Nonetheless, 1 study still found that the levels of IL-6 were significantly higher among individuals with insomnia compared with controls and that levels were negatively related to the percentage of total sleep time spent in slow wave sleep. Another study reported a diurnal shift toward a more daytime peak in IL-6 and TNF-α levels in those individuals with insomnia compared with controls.[88] Treatment options for insomnia can include pharmacotherapy, behavioral therapy, or a combination of the two. Several FDA-approved medications are on the market to treat insomnia. Most of these agents are benzodiazepine receptor agonists such as zolpidem, eszoiclone, and zaleplon. An exception is ramelteon, which acts as a central melatonin (MT1 and MT2) receptor agonist. FDA-approved treatment duration for these agents are mainly for short term or transitional insomnia for durations of less than 6 months. Behavioral techniques that involve a variety of sleep-specific cognitive behavioral strategies have shown equivalent and, in some cases, greater long-term efficacy in treating chronic insomnia compared with pharmacotherapy.[89]

SUMMARY

The analysis of epidemiologic and neurobiological studies to date reveals that sleep and immunity have a strong interrelationship. Several immune and proinflammatory cells possess sleep-regulatory properties. In turn, sleep deprivation and sleep disruption can also have deleterious effects on immune system response and functioning. Further studies of this relationship will likely provide greater insight on the association and the potential preventative and therapeutic medical applications that could be derived as more is learned about this interaction.

REFERENCES

1. Imeri L, Opp MR. How (and why) the immune system makes us sleep. Nat Rev Neurosci 2009;10(3):199–210.
2. Shearer WT, Reuben JM, Mullington JM, et al. Soluble TNF-alpha receptor 1 and IL-6 plasma levels in humans subjected to the sleep deprivation model of spaceflight. J Allergy Clin Immunol 2001;107(1):165–70.
3. Perras B, Born J. Sleep associated endocrine and immune changes in the elderly. Adv Cell Aging Gerontol 2005;17:113–54.
4. Sleep Disorders Research Plan Task Force. NHLBI (National Heart, Lung, and Blood Institute); 2003. Available at: http://www.nhlbi.nih.gov/health/prof/sleep/res_plan/sleep-rplan.pdf.
5. Fleming WE, Pollak CP. Sleep disorders in multiple sclerosis. Semin Neurol 2005;25(1):64–8.
6. Bakshi R. Fatigue associated with multiple sclerosis: diagnosis, impact and management. Mult Scler 2003;9(3):219–27.
7. Braley TJ, Chervin RD. Fatigue in multiple sclerosis: mechanisms, evaluation, and treatment. Sleep 2010;33(8):1061–7.
8. Guilleminault C, Mondini S. Mononucleosis and chronic daytime sleepiness. A long-term follow-up study. Arch Intern Med 1986;146(7):1333–5.
9. Majde JA, Krueger JM. Links between the innate immune system and sleep. J Allergy Clin Immunol 2005;116(6):1188–98.
10. Haraguchi T, Ishizu H, Terada S, et al. An autopsy case of postencephalitic parkinsonism of von Economo type: some new observations concerning neurofibrillary tangles and astrocytic tangles. Neuropathology 2000;20(2):143–8.
11. Taubenberger JK, Reid AH, Krafft AE, et al. Initial genetic characterization of the 1918 "Spanish" influenza virus. Science 1997;275(5307):1793–6.
12. McCall S, Henry JM, Reid AH, et al. Influenza RNA not detected in archival brain tissues from acute encephalitis lethargica cases or in postencephalitic Parkinson cases. J Neuropathol Exp Neurol 2001;60(7):696–704.
13. Rail D, Scholtz C, Swash M. Post-encephalitic parkinsonism: current experience. J Neurol Neurosurg Psychiatry 1981;44(8):670–6.
14. Howard RS, Lees AJ. Encephalitis lethargica. A report of four recent cases. Brain 1987;110(Pt 1):19–33.
15. Blunt SB, Lane RJ, Turjanski N, et al. Clinical features and management of two cases of encephalitis lethargica. Mov Disord 1997;12(3):354–9.
16. Kiley M, Esiri MM. A contemporary case of encephalitis lethargica. Clin Neuropathol 2001;20(1):2–7.
17. Rubinstein ML, Selwyn PA. High prevalence of insomnia in an outpatient population with HIV infection. J Acquir Immune Defic Syndr Hum Retrovirol 1998;19(3):260–5.
18. Rothenberg S, Zozula R, Funesti J, et al. Sleep habits in asymptomatic HIV-seropositive individuals. Sleep Res 1990;19:342.
19. Cohen FL, Ferrans CE, Vizgirda V, et al. Sleep in men and women infected with human immunodeficiency virus. Holist Nurs Pract 1996;10(4):33–43.
20. Darko DF, McCutchan JA, Kripke DF, et al. Fatigue, sleep disturbance, disability, and indices of progression of HIV infection. Am J Psychiatry 1992;149(4):514–20.
21. Norman SE, Resnick L, Cohn MA, et al. Sleep disturbances in HIV-seropositive patients. JAMA 1988;260(7):922.
22. Norman SE, Chediak AD, Kiel M, et al. Sleep disturbances in HIV-infected homosexual men. AIDS 1990;4(8):775–81.

23. Wiegand M, Moller AA, Schreiber W, et al. Nocturnal sleep EEG in patients with HIV infection. Eur Arch Psychiatry Clin Neurosci 1991;240(3):153–8.
24. Toth L. Microbial modulation of sleep. In: Lydic R, Baghdoyan HA, editors. Handbook of behavioral state control: cellular and molecular mechanisms. Boca Raton (FL): CRC Press; 1999. p. 641.
25. Moeller AA, Oechsner M, Backmund HC, et al. Self-reported sleep quality in HIV infection: correlation to the stage of infection and zidovudine therapy. J Acquir Immune Defic Syndr 1991;4(10):1000–3.
26. Brown S, Mitler M, Atkinson H. Correlation of subjective sleep complaints, absolute T-4 cell number and anxiety in HIV illness. Sleep Res 1991;20:363.
27. Reid S, Dwyer J. Insomnia in HIV infection: a systematic review of prevalence, correlates, and management. Psychosom Med 2005;67(2):260–9.
28. Cruess DG, Evans DL, Repetto MJ, et al. Prevalence, diagnosis, and pharmacological treatment of mood disorders in HIV disease. Biol Psychiatry 2003;54(3):307–16.
29. Crum-Cianflone NF, Roediger MP, Moore DJ, et al. Prevalence and factors associated with sleep disturbances among early-treated HIV-infected persons. Clin Infect Dis 2012;54(10):1485–94.
30. Dreher HM. The effect of caffeine reduction on sleep quality and well-being in persons with HIV. J Psychosom Res 2003;54(3):191–8.
31. Kupfer DJ, Reynolds CF 3rd. Management of insomnia. N Engl J Med 1997;336(5):341–6.
32. Smith MT, Perlis ML, Park A, et al. Comparative meta-analysis of pharmacotherapy and behavior therapy for persistent insomnia. Am J Psychiatry 2002;159(1):5–11.
33. Jong E, Oudhoff LA, Epskamp C, et al. Predictors and treatment strategies of HIV-related fatigue in the combined antiretroviral therapy era. AIDS 2010;24(10):1387–405.
34. Rabkin JG, McElhiney MC, Rabkin R. Modafinil and armodafinil treatment for fatigue for HIV-positive patients with and without chronic hepatitis C. Int J STD AIDS 2011;22(2):95–101.
35. Gamaldo CE, McArthur JC. The evaluation and diagnosis of "Insomnia" in relation to sleep disturbance prevalence and impact in early-treated HIV-infected persons. [Epub ahead of print].
36. Kennedy PG. Human African trypanosomiasis of the CNS: current issues and challenges. J Clin Invest 2004;113(4):496–504.
37. Mistlberger RE. Circadian regulation of sleep in mammals: role of the suprachiasmatic nucleus. Brain Res Brain Res Rev 2005;49(3):429–54.
38. Bentivoglio M, Kristensson K. Neural-immune interactions in disorders of sleep-wakefulness organization. Trends Neurosci 2007;30(12):645–52.
39. de Atouguia JL, Kennedy PG. Neurological aspects of human African trypanosomiasis. In: Davis LE, Kennedy PG, editors. Infectious diseases of the nervous system. London (UK): Butterworth-Heinemann; 2000. p. 321–72.
40. Lejon V, Legros D, Richer M, et al. IgM quantification in the cerebrospinal fluid of sleeping sickness patients by a latex card agglutination test. Trop Med Int Health 2002;7(8):685–92.
41. Piao YS, Kakita A, Watanabe H, et al. Sporadic fatal insomnia with spongiform degeneration in the thalamus and widespread PrPSc deposits in the brain. Neuropathology 2005;25(2):144–9.
42. Cortelli P, Gambetti P, Montagna P, et al. Fatal familial insomnia: clinical features and molecular genetics. J Sleep Res 1999;8(Suppl 1):23–9.

43. Lugaresi E, Tobler I, Gambetti P, et al. The pathophysiology of fatal familial insomnia. Brain Pathol 1998;8(3):521-6.
44. Appleby BS, Lyketsos CG. Rapidly progressive dementias and the treatment of human prion diseases. Expert Opin Pharmacother 2011;12(1):1-12.
45. Casas-Mendez LF, Lujan M, Vigil L, et al. Biot's breathing in a woman with fatal familial insomnia: is there a role for noninvasive ventilation? J Clin Sleep Med 2011;7(1):89-91.
46. Spiegel K, Sheridan JF, Van Cauter E. Effect of sleep deprivation on response to immunization. JAMA 2002;288(12):1471-2.
47. Balachandran DD, Ewing SB, Murray BJ, et al. Human host response during chronic partial sleep deprivation. Sleep 2002;25:A106-7.
48. Wormser GP, Dattwyler RJ, Shapiro ED, et al. The clinical assessment, treatment, and prevention of Lyme disease, human granulocytic anaplasmosis, and babesiosis: clinical practice guidelines by the Infectious Diseases Society of America. Clin Infect Dis 2006;43(9):1089-134.
49. Balachandran D. Sleep and the immune system: implications for health and mortality. Sleep and Safety 2011;52-9.
50. Czeisler CA, Gooley JJ. Sleep and circadian rhythms in humans. Cold Spring Harb Symp Quant Biol 2007;72:579-97.
51. Sleep in America poll. National Sleep Foundation (NSF); 2011. Available at: http://www.sleepfoundation.org/category/article-type/sleep-america-polls.
52. Bollinger T, Bollinger A, Oster H, et al. Sleep, immunity, and circadian clocks: a mechanistic model. Gerontology 2010;56(6):574-80.
53. Vgontzas AN, Zoumakis E, Bixler EO, et al. Adverse effects of modest sleep restriction on sleepiness, performance, and inflammatory cytokines. J Clin Endocrinol Metab 2004;89(5):2119-26.
54. Meier-Ewert HK, Ridker PM, Rifai N, et al. Effect of sleep loss on C-reactive protein, an inflammatory marker of cardiovascular risk. J Am Coll Cardiol 2004;43(4):678-83.
55. Ozturk L, Pelin Z, Karadeniz D, et al. Effects of 48 hours sleep deprivation on human immune profile. Sleep Res Online 1999;2(4):107-11.
56. Irwin M, McClintick J, Costlow C, et al. Partial night sleep deprivation reduces natural killer and cellular immune responses in humans. FASEB J 1996;10(5):643-53.
57. van Leeuwen WM, Lehto M, Karisola P, et al. Sleep restriction increases the risk of developing cardiovascular diseases by augmenting proinflammatory responses through IL-17 and CRP. PLoS One 2009;4(2):e4589.
58. The International classification of sleep disorder: diagnostic and coding manual. vol. 2. Westchester (IL); American Academy of Sleep Medicine 2005.
59. Gohar A, Adams A, Gertner E, et al. Working memory capacity is decreased in sleep-deprived internal medicine residents. J Clin Sleep Med 2009;5(3):191-7.
60. Viswanathan AN, Hankinson SE, Schernhammer ES. Night shift work and the risk of endometrial cancer. Cancer Res 2007;67:10618-22.
61. Schernhammer ES, Laden F, Speizer FE, et al. Night-shift work and risk of colorectal cancer in the nurses' health study. J Natl Cancer Inst 2003;95(11):825-8.
62. Kubo T, Ozasa K, Mikami K, et al. Prospective cohort study of the risk of prostate cancer among rotating-shift workers: findings from the Japan collaborative cohort study. Am J Epidemiol 2006;164(6):549-55.
63. Chen ST, Choo KB, Hou MF, et al. Deregulated expression of the PER1, PER2 and PER3 genes in breast cancers. Carcinogenesis 2005;26:1241-6.

64. Blask DE. Melatonin, sleep disturbance and cancer risk. Sleep Med Rev 2009; 13(4):257–64.
65. Roth T. Appropriate therapeutic selection for patients with shift work disorder. Sleep Med 2012;13(4):335–41.
66. Gamaldo CE, Earley CJ. Restless legs syndrome: a clinical update. Chest 2006; 130(5):1596–604.
67. Phillips B, Hening W, Britz P, et al. Prevalence and correlates of restless legs syndrome: results from the 2005 National Sleep Foundation Poll. Chest 2006; 129(1):76–80.
68. Natarajan R. Review of periodic limb movement and restless leg syndrome. J Postgrad Med 2010;56(2):157–62.
69. Connor JR, Wang XS, Patton SM, et al. Decreased transferrin receptor expression by neuromelanin cells in restless legs syndrome. Neurology 2004;62(9): 1563–7.
70. Weinstock LB. Antibiotic therapy may improve idiopathic restless legs syndrome: prospective, open-label pilot study of rifaximin, a nonsystemic antibiotic. Sleep Med 2010;11(4):427.
71. Weinstock LB, Walters AS. Restless legs syndrome is associated with irritable bowel syndrome and small intestinal bacterial overgrowth. Sleep Med 2011; 12(6):610–3.
72. Hassan N, Pineau CA, Clarke AE, et al. Systemic lupus and risk of restless legs syndrome. J Rheumatol 2011;38(5):874–6.
73. Happe S, Kundmuller L, Reichelt D, et al. Comorbidity of restless legs syndrome and HIV infection. J Neurol 2007;254(10):1401–6.
74. Matsuo M, Tsuchiya K, Hamasaki Y, et al. Restless legs syndrome: association with streptococcal or mycoplasma infection. Pediatr Neurol 2004;31(2):119–21.
75. Tembl JI, Ferrer JM, Sevilla MT, et al. Neurologic complications associated with hepatitis C virus infection. Neurology 1999;53(4):861–4.
76. Hemmer B, Riemann D, Glocker FX, et al. Restless legs syndrome after a borrelia-induced myelitis. Mov Disord 1995;10(4):521–2.
77. Weinstock LB, Walters AS, Paueksakon P. Restless legs syndrome - theoretical roles of inflammatory and immune mechanisms. Sleep Med Rev 2012;16(4): 341–54.
78. Hornyak M, Rupp A, Riemann D, et al. Low-dose hydrocortisone in the evening modulates symptom severity in restless legs syndrome. Neurology 2008;70(18): 1620–2.
79. Weinstock LB, Fern SE, Duntley SP. Restless legs syndrome in patients with irritable bowel syndrome: response to small intestinal bacterial overgrowth therapy. Dig Dis Sci 2008;53(5):1252–6.
80. Salas RE, Gamaldo CE, Allen RP. Update in restless legs syndrome. Curr Opin Neurol 2010;23(4):401–6.
81. Tishler PV, Larkin EK, Schluchter MD, et al. Incidence of sleep-disordered breathing in an urban adult population: the relative importance of risk factors in the development of sleep-disordered breathing. JAMA 2003;289(17):2230–7.
82. Young T, Peppard PE, Gottlieb DJ. Epidemiology of obstructive sleep apnea: a population health perspective. Am J Respir Crit Care Med 2002;165(9):1217–39.
83. Punjabi NM, Beamer BA. C-reactive protein is associated with sleep disordered breathing independent of adiposity. Sleep 2007;30(1):29–34.
84. Vgontzas AN, Papanicolaou DA, Bixler EO, et al. Elevation of plasma cytokines in disorders of excessive daytime sleepiness: role of sleep disturbance and obesity. J Clin Endocrinol Metab 1997;82(5):1313–6.

85. Vgontzas AN, Zoumakis E, Lin HM, et al. Marked decrease in sleepiness in patients with sleep apnea by etanercept, a tumor necrosis factor-alpha antagonist. J Clin Endocrinol Metab 2004;89(9):4409–13.

86. Roth T. Insomnia: definition, prevalence, etiology, and consequences. J Clin Sleep Med 2007;3(Suppl 5):S7–10.

87. Chesson A Jr, Hartse K, Anderson WM, et al. Practice parameters for the evaluation of chronic insomnia. An American Academy of Sleep Medicine report. Standards of Practice Committee of the American Academy of Sleep Medicine. Sleep 2000;23(2):237–41.

88. Vgontzas AN, Zoumakis M, Papanicolaou DA, et al. Chronic insomnia is associated with a shift of interleukin-6 and tumor necrosis factor secretion from nighttime to daytime. Metabolism 2002;51(7):887–92.

89. Jacobs GD, Pace-Schott EF, Stickgold R, et al. Cognitive behavior therapy and pharmacotherapy for insomnia: a randomized controlled trial and direct comparison. Arch Intern Med 2004;164(17):1888–96.

90. Krueger JM, Obal FJ, Fang J, et al. The role of cytokines in physiological sleep regulation. Ann N Y Acad Sci 2001;933:211–21.

91. Obal F Jr, Krueger JM. Biochemical regulation of non-rapid-eye-movement sleep. Front Biosci 2003;8:d520–50.

92. Dinarello CA. Biology of interleukin 1. FASEB J 1988;2(2):108–15.

93. Opp MR, Obal F Jr, Krueger JM. Interleukin 1 alters rat sleep: temporal and dose-related effects. Am J Physiol 1991;260(1 Pt 2):R52–8.

94. Olivadoti MD, Opp MR. Effects of i.c.v. administration of interleukin-1 on sleep and body temperature of interleukin-6-deficient mice. Neuroscience 2008; 153(1):338–48.

95. Okun ML, Giese S, Lin L, et al. Exploring the cytokine and endocrine involvement in narcolepsy. Brain Behav Immun 2004;18(4):326–32.

96. Krueger JM, Dinaerello CA, Chedid L. Promotion of slow wave sleep (SWS) by a purified interleukin-1 (IL-1) preparation. Fed Proc 1983;42:356.

97. Imeri L, Ceccarelli P, Mariotti M, et al. Sleep, but not febrile responses of Fisher 344 rats to immune challenge are affected by aging. Brain Behav Immun 2004; 18(4):399–404.

98. Hogan D, Morrow JD, Smith EM, et al. Interleukin-6 alters sleep of rats. J Neuroimmunol 2003;137(1–2):59–66.

99. Fencl V, Koski G, Pappenheimer JR. Factors in cerebrospinal fluid from goats that affect sleep and activity in rats. J Physiol 1971;216(3):565–89.

100. Cawthorn WP, Sethi JK. TNF-alpha and adipocyte biology. FEBS Lett 2008; 582(1):117–31.

101. Cavadini G, Petrzilka S, Kohler P, et al. TNF-alpha suppresses the expression of clock genes by interfering with E-box-mediated transcription. Proc Natl Acad Sci U S A 2007;104(31):12843–8.

102. Muraguchi A, Kishimoto T, Miki Y, et al. T cell-replacing factor- (TRF) induced IgG secretion in a human B blastoid cell line and demonstration of acceptors for TRF. J Immunol 1981;127(2):412–6.

103. Hirano T, Taga T, Nakano N, et al. Purification to homogeneity and characterization of human B-cell differentiation factor (BCDF or BSFp-2). Proc Natl Acad Sci U S A 1985;82(16):5490–4.

104. Kishimoto T. The biology of interleukin-6. Blood 1989;74(1):1–10.

105. Spath-Schwalbe E, Hansen K, Schmidt F, et al. Acute effects of recombinant human interleukin-6 on endocrine and central nervous sleep functions in healthy men. J Clin Endocrinol Metab 1998;83(5):1573–9.

106. Fogal B, Hewett SJ. Interleukin-1beta: a bridge between inflammation and exci- totoxicity? J Neurochem 2008;106(1):1–23.
107. Italian REMS Study Group, Manconi M, Ferini-Strambi L, Filippi M, et al. Multi- center case-control study on restless legs syndrome in multiple sclerosis: the REMS study. Sleep 2008;31(7):944–52.
108. Manconi M, Rocca MA, Ferini-Strambi L, et al. Restless legs syndrome is a common finding in multiple sclerosis and correlates with cervical cord damage. Mult Scler 2008;14(1):86–93.
109. Roseler S, Holtappels G, Wagenmann M, et al. Elevated levels of interleukins IL-1 beta, IL-6 and IL-8 in naturally acquired viral rhinitis. Eur Arch Otorhinolar- yngol 1995;252(Suppl 1):S61–3.
110. Staedt J, Stoppe G, Kogler A, et al. Single photon emission tomography (SPET) imaging of dopamine D2 receptors in the course of dopamine replacement therapy in patients with nocturnal myoclonus syndrome (NMS). J Neural Transm Gen Sect 1995;99(1–3):187–93.
111. Landolt HP, Glatzel M, Blattler T, et al. Sleep-wake disturbances in sporadic Creutzfeldt-Jakob disease. Neurology 2006;66(9):1418–24.
112. Allen R. Dopamine and iron in the pathophysiology of restless legs syndrome (RLS). Sleep Med 2004;5(4):385–91.
113. Allen RP, Adler CH, Du W, et al. Clinical efficacy and safety of IV ferric carbox- ymaltose (FCM) treatment of RLS: a multi-centred, placebo-controlled prelimi- nary clinical trial. Sleep Med 2011;12(9):906–13.
114. Trojan DA, Da Costa D, Bar-Or A, et al. Sleep abnormalities in multiple sclerosis patients. Mult Scler 2008;14:S160.
115. Caminero A, Bartolome M. Sleep disturbances in multiple sclerosis. J Neurol Sci 2011;309(1–2):86–91.
116. Howard RS, Wiles CM, Hirsch NP, et al. Respiratory involvement in multiple scle- rosis. Brain 1992;115(Pt 2):479–94.
117. Flemons WW. Clinical practice. Obstructive sleep apnea. N Engl J Med 2002; 347(7):498–504.
118. Fleetham JA. Medical and surgical treatment of obstructive sleep apnea syndrome, including dental appliances. Handb Clin Neurol 2011;98:441–57.
119. Tachibana N, Howard RS, Hirsch NP, et al. Sleep problems in multiple sclerosis. Eur Neurol 1994;34(6):320–3.
120. Taphoorn MJ, van Someren E, Snoek FJ, et al. Fatigue, sleep disturbances and circadian rhythm in multiple sclerosis. J Neurol 1993;240(7):446–8.
121. Baker S, Zee P. Circadian disorders of the sleep-wake cycle. In: Kryger MH, Roth T, Dement WC, editors. Principles and practice of sleep medicine, vol. 3. Philadelphia: WB Saunders; 2000. p. 606–14.
122. Amarenco G, Kerdraon J, Denys P. Bladder and sphincter disorders in multiple sclerosis. Clinical, urodynamic and neurophysiological study of 225 cases. Rev Neurol (Paris) 1995;151(12):722–30.
123. Rae-Grant AD, Eckert NJ, Bartz S, et al. Sensory symptoms of multiple sclerosis: a hidden reservoir of morbidity. Mult Scler 1999;5(3):179–83.
124. Merlino G, Fratticci L, Lenchig C, et al. Prevalence of 'poor sleep' among patients with multiple sclerosis: an independent predictor of mental and phys- ical status. Sleep Med 2009;10(1):26–34.
125. Rodgers J. Trypanosomiasis and the brain. Parasitology 2010;137(14):1995–2006.
126. WHO Profile on Human African trypanosomiasis. World Health Organization Web site. Available at: http://www.who.int/trypanosomiasis_african/diagnosis/ en/index.html. Updated 2012. Accessed April 24, 2012.

127. Sabbah P, Brosset C, Imbert P, et al. Human African trypanosomiasis: MRI. Neuroradiology 1997;39(10):708–10.

128. Courtin D, Jamonneau V, Mathieu JF, et al. Comparison of cytokine plasma levels in human African trypanosomiasis. Trop Med Int Health 2006;11(5): 647–53.

129. Courtioux B, Boda C, Vatunga G, et al. A link between chemokine levels and disease severity in human African trypanosomiasis. Int J Parasitol 2006;36(9): 1057–65.

130. Hawking F, Greenfield JG. Two autopsies on rhodesiense sleeping sickness; visceral lesions and significance of changes in cerebrospinal fluid. Transactions of the Royal Society of Tropical Medicine and Hygiene 1941;35(3):155–6, IN1-IN2, 157–64. Available at: http://www.tropicalmedandhygienejrnl.net/article/PIIS0035920341900494/abstract.

131. Jackson WS, Borkowski AW, Faas H, et al. Spontaneous generation of prion infectivity in fatal familial insomnia knockin mice. Neuron 2009;63(4):438–50.

132. Lerdal A, Gay CL, Aouizerat BE, et al. Patterns of morning and evening fatigue among adults with HIV/AIDS. J Clin Nurs 2011;20(15–16):2204–16.

133. HIV/AIDS: Symptoms Mayo Clinic Web site. Available at: http://www.mayoclinic.com/health/hiv-aids/DS00005/DSECTION=symptoms. Updated 2012. Accessed April 24, 2012.

134. Bourin P, Mansour I, Doinel C, et al. Circadian rhythms of circulating NK cells in healthy and human immunodeficiency virus-infected men. Chronobiol Int 1993; 10(4):298–305.

135. Bhansali A, Dash RJ, Sud A, et al. A preliminary report on basal & stimulated plasma cortisol in patients with acquired immunodeficiency syndrome. Indian J Med Res 2000;112:173–7.

136. Perkins DO, Leserman J, Stern RA, et al. Somatic symptoms and HIV infection: relationship to depressive symptoms and indicators of HIV disease. Am J Psychiatry 1995;152(12):1776–81.

137. Duncan MJ, Bruce-Keller AJ, Conner C, et al. Effects of chronic expression of the HIV-induced protein, transactivator of transcription, on circadian activity rhythms in mice, with or without morphine. Am J Physiol Regul Integr Comp Physiol 2008;295(5):R1680–7.

138. Darko DF, Miller JC, Gallen C, et al. Sleep electroencephalogram delta-frequency amplitude, night plasma levels of tumor necrosis factor alpha, and human immunodeficiency virus infection. Proc Natl Acad Sci U S A 1995; 92(26):12080–4.

139. Drake CL, Roehrs TA, Royer H, et al. Effects of an experimentally induced rhinovirus cold on sleep, performance, and daytime alertness. Physiol Behav 2000; 71(1–2):75–81.

140. Noah TL, Henderson FW, Wortman IA, et al. Nasal cytokine production in viral acute upper respiratory infection of childhood. J Infect Dis 1995;171(3):584–92.

141. Creutzfeldt-Jakob disease fact sheet. National Institute of Neurological Disorders and Stroke Web site. Available at: http://www.ninds.nih.gov/disorders/cjd/detail_cjd.htm. Updated 2012. Accessed April 24, 2012.

142. Schroter A, Zerr I, Henkel K, et al. Magnetic resonance imaging in the clinical diagnosis of Creutzfeldt-Jakob disease. Arch Neurol 2000;57(12):1751–7.

143. Tschampa HJ, Murtz P, Flacke S, et al. Thalamic involvement in sporadic Creutzfeldt-Jakob disease: a diffusion-weighted MR imaging study. AJNR Am J Neuroradiol 2003;24(5):908–15.

144. Fulbright RK, Hoffmann C, Lee H, et al. MR imaging of familial Creutzfeldt-Jakob disease: a blinded and controlled study. AJNR Am J Neuroradiol 2008;29(9): 1638–43.

145. Dossena S, Imeri L, Mangieri M, et al. Mutant prion protein expression causes motor and memory deficits and abnormal sleep patterns in a transgenic mouse model. Neuron 2008;60(4):598–609.

146. Kordek R, Nerurkar VR, Liberski PP, et al. Heightened expression of tumor necrosis factor alpha, interleukin 1 alpha, and glial fibrillary acidic protein in experimental Creutzfeldt-Jakob disease in mice. Proc Natl Acad Sci U S A 1996;93(18):9754–8.

147. Signs and symptoms of Lyme disease. Centers for Disease Control and Prevention Web site. Available at: http://www.cdc.gov/lyme/signs_symptoms/index.html. Updated 2011. Accessed April 24, 2012.

148. Greenberg HE, Ney G, Scharf SM, et al. Sleep quality in Lyme disease. Sleep 1995;18(10):912–6.

149. Belman AL, Coyle PK, Roque C, et al. MRI findings in children infected by *Borrelia burgdorferi*. Pediatr Neurol 1992;8(6):428–31.

150. Blask DE, Dauchy RT, Sauer LA. Putting cancer to sleep at night: the neuroendocrine/circadian melatonin signal. Endocrine 2005;27(2):179–88.

151. Carrillo-Vico A, Guerrero JM, Lardone PJ, et al. A review of the multiple actions of melatonin on the immune system. Endocrine 2005;27(2):189–200.

152. Carrillo-Vico A, Reiter RJ, Lardone PJ, et al. The modulatory role of melatonin on immune responsiveness. Curr Opin Investig Drugs 2006;7(5):423–31.

Movement Disorders and Sleep

Erika D. Driver-Dunckley, MD*, Charles H. Adler, MD, PhD

KEYWORDS

- Restless legs syndrome • Periodic limb movements of sleep • Parkinson disease
- Movement disorders

KEY POINTS

- Sleep disturbances in movement disorders are crucial to recognize and treat.
- Parkinson disease is much more than a disorder characterized by slowness of movement, tremor, rigidity, and postural instability. These patients have multiple nonmotor symptoms that may predate the motor signs (including excessive daytime sleepiness and REM sleep behavior disorder) and increase with advancing disease (including insomnia, excessive daytime sleepiness, periodic leg movements of sleep, and RBD).
- Sleep disorders lead to decreased quality of life by interfering with the ability to carry out daily affairs and by disrupting sleep at night.
- With poor sleep quality and reduced sleep duration patients with movement disorders often suffer reduced cognitive function and depression.

INTRODUCTION

Restless legs syndrome (RLS) and periodic limb movements of sleep (PLMS) affect millions of adults. In addition to these sleep-related disorders, other movement disorders may adversely impact sleep efficiency and lead to daytime fatigue, pain, depression, and reductions to overall quality of life. It is important for clinicians to routinely inquire about daytime somnolence and nocturnal sleep practices to help decipher if a sleep disorder exists so that further investigations may be undertaken. Discovering and treating underlying sleep disturbances impacts and improves patients' quality of life. The following movement disorders and their impact on sleep are discussed further in this article:

- Parkinson disease
- Essential tremor
- Parkinsonism
- Dystonia

Disclosures: Erika D. Driver-Dunckley, MD, none. Charles H. Adler, MD, PhD, consulting for Teva.
Department of Neurology, Movement Disorders Division, Mayo Clinic Arizona, 13400 East Shea Boulevard, Scottsdale, AZ 85259, USA
* Corresponding author.
E-mail address: Driverdunckley.erika@mayo.edu

Neurol Clin 30 (2012) 1345–1358
http://dx.doi.org/10.1016/j.ncl.2012.08.019
0733-8619/12/$ – see front matter © 2012 Elsevier Inc. All rights reserved.

- Huntington disease
- Myoclonus
- Ataxias

PARKINSON DISEASE
Epidemiology

Parkinson's disease (PD) is the second most common neurodegenerative disease. Motor symptoms include rigidity, tremor, and bradykinesia leading to change in gait and difficulties with speech and activities of daily living.[1] Nonmotor symptoms of PD include sleep disturbances, dysautonomia, and cognitive behavioral disorders. These symptoms can severely impact a patient's quality of life. Sleep disturbances can affect as many as 60% to 98% of patients with approximately 40% of patients with PD requiring sleeping pills.[2] Sleep issues may predate motor findings. In the Honolulu-Asia Aging Study investigators found that excessive daytime sleepiness (EDS) was three times more common in subjects who developed PD than in those who did not develop PD.[3] Additionally, there is now significant evidence showing that RBD predates PD and that idiopathic RBD is a synucleinopathy (the pathologic hallmark of PD). Two recent questionnaire studies reveal how significant sleep issues are in PD. In the PRIAMO study of 1072 patients with PD 15% had RLS, 21% had EDS, 30% had RBD, 37% had insomnia, and 58% had fatigue that limited daytime activities.[4] A second questionnaire study of nonmotor symptoms in 411 patients with PD found that 32% had RLS, 47% had daytime sleepiness, 50% had difficulty falling asleep, 66% had fatigue, and 68% had nocturia.[5] Additional studies report that 15% to 57% of patients with PD suffer from EDS, as defined by a score of 10 on the Epworth Sleepiness Scale or a mean sleep latency of less than 5 minutes on the Multiple Sleep Latency Test, whereas daytime fatigue can be 32% to 70%.[6] Other sleep disturbances include insomnia, RBD, rapid eye movement (REM) sleep without atonia, PLMS, RLS, sleep apnea, nocturia, and significant off time impairing movement in bed (**Box 1**).

Pathophysiology

The clinical features of PD develop from neuronal cell loss in the substantia nigra, brainstem nuclei, and cerebral cortex. Lewy bodies are found in the brainstem nuclei, particularly in the REM sleep centers in the pedunculopontine tegmental nucleus in PD and REM sleep behavior disorder (RBD).[2,7] The synuclein pathology of RBD follows the topography and temporal sequence as explained in Braak staging for PD. This explains how RBD can develop in the premotor phase of PD and suggests that patients with "idiopathic" RBD may actually have an early manifestation of a neurodegenerative disease.[8–10]

The known brainstem pathology in PD correlates with patients' significant sleep-wake cycle disturbances. It is this disruption of the circadian rhythm that can produce insomnia and secondary daytime hypersomnia. Dopamine and other neurotransmitters, including acetylcholine, serotonin, and norepinephrine, all play a pivotal role in the sleep-wake cycle. Interference of the dopaminergic pathways along with dopaminergic medications all have an influence on sleep in patients with PD.

The cause of EDS in PD seems to be multifactorial. Poor quality of sleep caused by multiple sleep disorders may play a role. Dopaminergic medications can cause EDS as can other concomitant medications including anxiolytics. One study did not find abnormality in hypocretin-1 levels in lumbar cerebrospinal fluid,[11] whereas another study found that patients with PD had a decreased number of hyporetin neurons in

---

Box 1
Classification of sleep disturbances in PD

PD-related motor symptoms
- Tremor
- Nocturnal akinesia
- Nocturnal dystonia
- Early morning akinesia
- Early morning dystonia

Cognitive-behavioral–related symptoms
- Hallucinations
- Agitation
- Dementia
- Panic attacks
- Depression

Treatment-related symptoms
- Excessive daytime sleepiness
- Sleep-attacks
- Vivid dreams
- Hallucinations
- Insomnia

Other sleep disorders
- REM sleep behavior disorder
- Restless leg syndrome
- PLMS
- Sleep-related breathing disorders
- Parasomnias
- Insomnia

---

the hypothalamus and decreased hypocretin-1 concentration in postmortem ventricular cerebrospinal fluid and prefrontal cortex.[12] A third study found a loss of hypocretin neurons in the hypothalamus that increased with disease severity.[13] Thus, the role for hypocretin-1 in PD is not clear, yet may be important in the sleep disruption in more severe states of the disease.

Another factor in quality of sleep in PD relates to motor problems. Many patients with PD take their last dose of medication in the early evening so that in the middle of the night their slowness, rigidity, and possibly dystonia may result in decreased ability to turn, discomfort, and poor sleep quality. Alternatively, some patients who take their medication in the middle of the night may develop dyskinesias, which disrupt sleep.

Key Clinical Features and Diagnosis

It is important to distinguish between PD-related sleep symptoms and those of normal aging or other age-related illnesses. With increasing age, the prevalence of sleep disorders increases and individuals experience more spontaneous awakenings, daytime sleepiness, and napping.[14] Nocturia is a common complaint among the elderly with many underlying causes. This leads to nocturnal awakenings and frequently difficulty returning to sleep. Patients with PD suffer from overactive bladder and frequent nocturia, hence disruption of their sleep.[15]

The likelihood of a sleep disturbance in PD is directly related to the severity of the disease. Patients with considerable motor dysfunction, wearing off, cognitive changes, and hallucinations have more disruptions of their sleep. The complexity of their disease, multiple symptoms, and drug interactions leads to great difficulty for the clinician to decipher which symptoms are affecting sleep and how sleep is impacting their daytime motor and cognitive functioning.

Clinical Features

PD-related motor symptoms

The impaired mobility that can occur with PD can lead to akinesia and subsequent pain and awakenings. Motor fluctuations can also lead to dystonia and pain and, subsequently, to multiple nocturnal awakenings. Patients may report painful cramps, spasms, or difficulty rolling over in bed. They may describe foot in-turning or toe curling. The akinesia may also lead to discomfort and patients reporting an inability to find a good position to sleep at night. However, some patients are unable to describe why they wake up at night, but on further questioning, comment on their poor motor functioning at night. This may provide a clue that they are experience off time that is leading to nighttime arousals. Questions need to be asked related to how much difficulty the patient is having turning in bed (suggests undermedication); getting out of bed to walk (suggests undermedication); the urge to get out of bed to walk around (may suggest RLS); and whether dyskinesias are present at night (suggesting overmedication). It is also important to ask the bed-partner whether any of these motor findings are present including kicking of the legs at night (suggests PLMS) or dream-enactment behavior (suggests RBD), neither of which would be apparent to the patient themselves.

Cognitive-behavioral–related symptoms

Depression and insomnia are linked, regardless of PD. However, depression is common in PD, affecting up to 45% of patients.[16] Symptoms of depression include psychomotor slowing, anhedonia, and sleep disturbances. Thus, sleep disorders in PD could be attributable, in part, to the high prevalence of depression in these patients. The depression of PD can be intrinsic; reactive (motor or nonmotor symptoms); or a combination of both. Spouses typically report that the patient has become more withdrawn, no longer participating in prior social activities. Patients prefer to be alone, engage less in conversations, and give up previous hobbies. It is important for the clinician to ask not only the patient how they feel their mood is, but also the spouse or family members, because they more likely divulge these personal details. It is often difficult to differentiate between depression and motor slowing (including masked facies), but this is best done by thorough questioning.

Anxiety is also a common occurrence in PD and may affect sleep. The patient may relate difficulty falling asleep, maintaining sleep, or early morning awaking. Patients may also note difficulty letting their mind relax. Questioning the patient and any caregiver may allow for this to be diagnosed and appropriately treated. Special attention to this is needed, however, because most antianxiety agents also can lead to EDS.

Hallucinations occur in up to 40% of patients with PD and are associated with cognitive impairment, age, and disease duration and severity.[16] Hallucinations tend to worsen at night and can be disruptive of sleep. Hallucinations are usually visual and not auditory, and are often patients seeing people or animals that are not there. Sometimes insight is retained, but often as the disease progresses insight is lost. These hallucinations may be accompanied by paranoid delusions, which also may disrupt sleep. Many medications used to treat PD can exacerbate hallucinations and cognitive symptoms. It may be difficult to distinguish the cause of the hallucinations (disease vs medication effect). The only way to try to distinguish between these causes is by reducing the PD medications to see if the hallucinations resolve and sleep improves.

Treatment-related symptoms

Drugs used to treat PD can lead to EDS, and affect sleep architecture and sleep-wake mechanisms.[6] These medications include dopaminergic and anticholinergics. They may affect sleep indirectly by effects on motor symptoms, worsening depression, or causing confusion. Levodopa may have varying effects on sleep depending on the dosage. Smaller doses can improve sleep, whereas larger doses impair sleep. EDS can also be caused by dopaminergic drugs, particularly dopamine agonists. This tends to occur while the dose is being increased, sometimes causing sleep attacks. Studies report these attacks may happen in approximately 7% of patients on these medications.[17,18] It is reported that 15% to 57% of patients with PD suffer from EDS, as defined by a score of 10 on the Epworth Sleepiness Scale or a mean sleep latency of less than 5 minutes on the Multiple Sleep Latency Test. More commonly, however, patients suffer from daytime fatigue, reported to be as high as 32% to 70%.[6]

Other sleep disorders

Insomnia is the most common subjective sleep complaint in PD.[16] Patients experience primary (sleep onset) and secondary (sleep maintenance) insomnia. Primary insomnia is associated with PD directly, whereas secondary insomnia arises from nocturnal motor and nonmotor symptoms. These nighttime awakenings lead to sleep fragmentation and typically occur more frequently in stages 1 or 2 of sleep even though they can occur in any sleep stage. The awakenings can be prolonged and, therefore, reduce total sleep time. The overall reduction in sleep time can then contribute to daytime sleepiness.

Sleep-related breathing disorders are more likely in PD that in the general population.[19] The mechanism of this is thought to be related to diaphragmatic dysfunction, rigidity, or abnormal movements of the upper airways, or autonomic failure of respiratory control mechanisms. Parasomnias involve autonomic, motor, or cognitive activation causing vivid dreams, sleep walking, sleep talking, or sleep terrors. These can be worsened with levodopa therapy.

Diagnosis

Diagnosing a sleep disorder in patients with PD begins with a thorough history and interview of the patient and spouse or caregiver. Patients may be unaware of their sleep movements or behaviors or can underestimate their severity of sleepiness. Important elements of the history to obtain include difficulty falling asleep, nocturnal awakenings, early morning awakenings, morning fatigue, snoring, leg aches or pains, abnormal leg movements, sleep talking, sleep walking, or acting out of dreams. After this information is obtained, patients' symptoms can be divided into one or more of the following categories: hypersomnia, insomnia, parasomnia, or movement related. Further potential evaluations to help with solidifying the diagnosis include sleep diaries, sleep questionnaires, mood assessments, actigraphy, or polysomnography.

The Epworth Sleepiness Scale (although not validated) can help ascertain the degree of daytime sleepiness along with the PD sleep scale.[20] Assessment of depression or other mood disorders is also critical. Referral to a sleep specialist or psychiatrist for more in-depth evaluations may be required, including actigraphy or overnight polysomnography.

Treatment

Pharmacologic and nonpharmacologic measures are helpful for managing sleep disorders in PD.[7,21]

Hypersomnia

In patients with PD, hypersomnia may be related to sleep deprivation, sleep disruption, circadian rhythm disorder, medication effect, or from the primary disease. The clinician should systematically focus the therapy toward these areas. Good activity during the day, adequate sleep time at night, and appropriate timing of stimulating clues (bright light, food, social interactions, or exercise) are essential cornerstones to managing hypersomnia. Dopaminergic medication can produce hypersomnia and temporal relationship to dosing is a good clue that the dose may need to be reduced or spread out. Patients with PD may be more sensitive to sedating medication, over-the-counter medications, or supplements and thus eliminating or focusing these agents toward bedtime may be helpful. However, given the reduced clearance rate of medications in the elderly, even nighttime medications may cause daytime sleepiness. Patients with PD may also have other underlying sleep disorders that may disrupt sleep and contribute to the sleepiness; thus, treatment of these disorders is essential. If hypersomnia continues, modafinil has been shown to improve daytime somnolence and fatigue and to have a beneficial effect on patients with PD.[21]

Insomnia

Treatment of insomnia in most patients is multifactorial and therefore all approaches should include some nonpharmacologic therapies; a focus at the root drivers; and consideration for pharmacologic therapy (discussed in the article on insomnia elsewhere in this issue). Because patients with PD have a variety of causes of insomnia this multipronged approach may be helpful in diminishing the patient's symptoms. There should be a review of the patient's daytime and nighttime activities with an emphasis on timing of stimulating activities (bright light, social interactions, meals, and exercise) and medications during the day and more sleep-inducing agents at night. Other directed nonpharmacologic therapies include sleep restriction, stimulus control therapy, relaxation training, and sleep hygiene education.

Sleep restriction involves limiting the amount of time spent in bed to help improve sleep efficiency. Stimulus control therapy involves removing arousing stimuli from the bedroom including watching television, eating, and reading. Sleep hygiene education teaches patients to create a peaceful and soothing environment in the bedroom while following and maintaining routines. These measures include reducing light and noise in the bedroom, avoiding caffeine and alcohol at night, avoiding heavy meals before bed, regular daily exercise, and establishing regular bedtimes and wake-up times. All of these adjustments are helpful for those patients suffering from insomnia.

Pharmacologic therapies should also be considered for patients with PD with insomnia and include the following:

- Adjusting dopaminergic medications
- Cautious use of benzodiazepines
- Psychiatric medications

- Nonbenzodiazepine agents
- Treatment of other sleep disorders

Although clinicians typically think of adding hypnotics, in these patients taking away a medication or adjusting the dose and timing may provide significant benefit. Patients may also be self-medicating with alcohol, over-the-counter agents, or herbal supplements. Many of these agents may produce other side effects or promote maladaptive behaviors that ultimately promote the insomnia. Although benzodiazepines are generally used for insomnia, they should be used with caution in this elderly population because of significant sedative side effects or paradoxic agitation. Sedating antidepressants can be helpful for managing sleep in patients with PD. However, these medications should be used with caution because of anticholinergic and autonomic side effects. Nonbenzodiazepine agents are useful for managing sleep disorders in PD and have a low risk of hangover side effects.

Parasomnia
Clonazepam has been shown to be very effective for managing RBD.[7] For patients who develop daytime sedation from this long-acting benzodiazepine, melatonin is an excellent substitution. Managing underlying sleep disorders (sleep apnea, RLS, parasomnias, or RBD) is crucial, and is discussed elsewhere in this issue.

Movement related
Patients with PD with nocturnal or early morning "off" time may benefit from longer-acting dopaminergic therapy at night. The contrary is also true for patients experiencing nocturnal dyskinesias; reducing evening and bedtime dopamine medications can be beneficial. Muscle relaxers can also be a helpful adjunct to dopaminergic medications to help with painful leg spasms.

Prognosis
Sleep disturbances are common in PD, but can go untreated if not assessed by the treating physician. A thorough and careful history is required to gain the information necessary to help manage the sleep disorders of PD. After appropriate behavior modifications and pharmacologic adjustments are made, patients can have an improved quality of sleep that leads to improved mood, activities of daily living, and quality of life.

ESSENTIAL TREMOR
Epidemiology

Essential tremor (ET) is a common, familial, and slowly progressive movement disorder that produces a kinetic or postural tremor of the body. The hands, head, and voice are most commonly affected. In addition to the tremor, patients may also suffer from nonmotor manifestations including fatigue, mood disorders, cognitive changes, and sleep disturbances. In the past these nonmotor symptoms went unrecognized in patients.[22] At this time there is no clear-cut evidence that sleep disorders are more common in ET than in the general population. Preliminary evidence from several small studies has revealed sleep dysregulation is present in ET,[22–24] although other studies have not found an increase in RBD or EDS.[7]

Pathophysiology

The cause of ET is not entirely understood. It is apparent that most cases are familial. The pathophysiology of ET is unclear with conflicting data on whether this disorder could be related to PD and some data suggesting there is a cerebellar degenerative process. It is unclear if these cerebellothalamocortical tracts involved in ET could be related to sleep disturbance pathology. Although it is clear that synucleinopathies (PD and dementia with Lewy bodies) are associated with RBD, no association between RBD and ET has yet been found, suggesting that patients with ET are not at risk for developing PD.[7]

Key Clinical Features and Diagnosis

Patients with ET experience poorer sleep quality compared with control subjects and report higher rates of depressive and anxiety symptoms along with fatigue and pain. These factors can significantly affect patients' quality of life. However, there are not enough studies available to ascertain the prevalence of sleep disturbances in this patient population.[7]

Making a diagnosis of a sleep disturbance in ET requires questioning beyond the standard evaluation for tremor, by asking pertinent questions of restorative sleep, daytime fatigue, and associated symptoms of mood or pain disorders. As with PD, a valuable tool to assess daytime fatigue is the Epworth Sleepiness Scale. Also, a thorough review of the patient's medication list can help determine if there are any pharmacologic agents contributing to sleep changes. Many ET medications also cause daytime fatigue or cognitive changes. Propranolol is one of the most frequently prescribed drugs for ET and is known to affect melatonin levels, hence disrupting the circadian rhythm.

Treatment

Pharmacologic and nonpharmacologic measures may be required to help restore sleep in patients with ET. No formal studies have addressed the treatment of sleep disorders in ET. The use of benzodiazepines may be helpful for managing sleep and tremor, along with sedating antiepileptic medications, mysoline and gabapentin. These medications are known to induce daytime fatigue and may contribute to patients' complaints of daytime fatigue. In such cases, nonsedating antitremor medications are warranted or only nocturnal use of the sedating antitremor medications. Stimulants to help improve daytime fatigue should be avoided because these may worsen tremor. Addressing associated mood disorders that could be linked or contributing to the sleep disorder is beneficial for improving patients' overall quality of life.

Prognosis

It is well known that ET is a chronic and progressive condition and likely the nonmotor symptoms progress along with the disease. Further studies are needed to assess the long-term effects of sleep disorders in ET and the efficacy of pharmacologic and nonpharmacolgic treatments in managing the sleep disturbances. If all factors of sleep, mood, and pain are addressed and properly treated, it is assumed that this should improve quality of life, but further studies are needed for validation.

PARKINSONISM
Epidemiology

In addition to PD, patients with progressive supranuclear palsy (PSP) and multiple systems atrophy (MSA) also suffer from sleep-related disorders. MSA is a neurodegenerative disease with a clinical spectrum of dysfunction comprising cerebellar, parkinsonian, and autonomic symptoms. These patients have multiple sleep-related disorders including sleep apnea, RBD, sleep-related stridor, insomnia, and EDS. Sudden death may occur from obstructive sleep apnea or sleep-related stridor.[25]

PSP is a neurodegenerative disease leading to extrapyramidal symptoms, dysphagia, impaired eye movements, and poor balance. Although RBD may occur in patients with PSP, it is not as frequent as seen in PD or MSA.[26] The most common sleep disturbance in PSP is insomnia, and this is related to severe motor impairment and to a lesser degree cognitive dysfunction.[27–29]

Pathophysiology

Although MSA and PSP are neurodegenerative disorders in nature they are very different pathologically. MSA pathology involves Lewy body deposition, whereas PSP is a tauopathy.

MSA may cause sleep-disordered breathing from degeneration of brainstem nuclei in the pontomedullary respiratory centers leading to central sleep apnea. Larynx narrowing from vocal cord abductor paralysis and excessive adductor activation leads to nocturnal stridor and obstructive sleep apnea, and often if untreated, sudden death.

Key Clinical Features and Diagnosis

Because of the potential of severe and underdiagnosed sleep apnea and sleep-related stridor in patients with MSA, all patients should be screened with polysomnography. As the disease progresses patients may require repeat sleep studies.

Treatment

Patients with MSA with sleep apnea or nocturnal stridor require continuous positive airway pressure (CPAP) and often, if not effective, tracheostomy. Insomnia and RBD can be treated medically as outlined in the PD section of this article.

Prognosis

Unfortunately, the prognosis for MSA and PSP is poor. As these diseases progress the motor, cognitive, or autonomic dysfunction may be difficult to manage leading to severe disability. Sleep disorders may confound this and may be difficult to recognize and treat in these complex patients.

DYSTONIA
Epidemiology

Dystonia is defined as an abnormal movement or posture caused by sustained muscle contractions. Dystonias are classified by age of onset, distribution, and cause. Non-motor symptoms have also been reported in dystonia. Similar to PD and ET these symptoms include changes in mood, sleep, cognition, and pain. The symptoms may or may not be secondary to the motor symptoms, but have a significant impact on patients' quality of life.[30]

There are only a few studies that have addressed sleep in patients with dystonia. Conflicting sleep data have been reported in various dystonia populations. One study found EDS in patients suffering from cervical dystonia and another found no significant difference between patients and control subjects.[30] Similarly for blepharospasm and oromandibular dystonia, studies have inconsistent results. One small study with polysomnography revealed that patients suffer from difficulty with sleep initiation and maintenance.[30]

Pathophysiology

The cause of the sleep symptoms in dystonia is not fully understood. Direct sleep disruption from pain or posturing from the dystonia may play a significant role. Additionally, medication effects can induce daytime fatigue and change sleep architecture. The relationship between disease severity and impairment of sleep is not well correlated.[30] Some forms of dystonia, such as blepharospasm and Meige syndrome, may persist into sleep with a decreased frequency and intensity. Further studies are needed to assess motor function, sleep impairment, and daytime fatigue.

Key Clinical Features and Diagnosis

Patients with dystonia may come in for evaluation complaining of twisting, posturing, or difficulty with their activities of daily living; however, they also need to be assessed for sleep dysfunction. A complete history with questions focused at daytime fatigue, sleep complaints, pain, mood changes, or cognitive complaints is pertinent. Next, review their medication history for sedating medications and maximize treatment with newer, nonsedating medications or treatments (ie, botulinum toxins).

Treatment

Recommendations are similar to what has previously been outlined. Attempting to focus sedating drugs to the nighttime, treating associated pain and mood disorders, and treating insomnia when present could all help to improve the patient's quality of life. If patients are still suffering from daytime fatigue or complaints of insomnia after these recommendations have been completed, consider referral to psychiatry or a sleep specialist for further testing.

Prognosis

There are no reported studies on the long-term management of dystonia and sleep disorders. Based on personal experience, most patients with dystonia respond well to therapy with botulinum toxins and this in turn improves their quality of life including mood and sleep.

HUNTINGTON DISEASE
Epidemiology

Huntington's disease (HD) is a chronic, progressive, autosomal-dominant neurodegenerative disorder. Patients develop chorea, cognitive changes, and mood disorders. Sleep disturbances do not correlate to the length of the CAG repeat.[31] Sleep is fragmented and disrupted in patients with HD, often from choreiform movements in lighter stages of sleep.

Pathophysiology

Neurodegeneration in HD likely leads to disruption of the sleep-wake cycle. This can be postulated from the transgenic HD mouse model that shows progressive sleep dysfunction with progression of the disease.[32] These studies suggest treating the sleep-wake cycle disruptions with alprazolam and modafinil.[33]

Key Clinical Features and Diagnosis

A recent questionnaire-based study showed sleep-related difficulties were more common in patients with HD compared with control subjects.[34] This study showed quality and quantity of sleep was affected.

To make a diagnosis of sleep impairment in patients with HD it is crucial to ask the patient or primary caregiver sleep-related symptoms or use a sleep questionnaire, such as the Epworth Sleepiness Scale. A sleep diary can also help provide pertinent information. Actigraphy and polysomnography are useful diagnostic tests to determine if there is an underlying sleep disorder.

Treatment

Treatment begins by reviewing the patient's medication list to determine if any sedating medications may be playing a role in daytime fatigue. By adjusting or eliminating sedating medications or initiating a sleep agent, improvements can be made in sleep quantity and quality. Depression is common in HD and should be addressed with mood stabilizers, because this may have an impact on sleep. Stimulants should be avoided because this may worsen the choreiform movements. Atypical neuroleptics can be beneficial for sleep and chorea. There is no contraindication for the use of CPAP in these patients.

Prognosis

The chronic progressive nature of HD can lead to significant impairment in functioning requiring multiple medications that can induce numerous side effects and subsequently impair sleep or produce daytime fatigue. However, addressing sleep symptoms as part of the comprehensive neurologic evaluation can lead to improvement in the patient's quality of life.

MYOCLONUS
Epidemiology

Myoclonus is defined as a sudden, rapid, involuntary movement that lasts only briefly. It is a descriptive term referring to a symptom or a sign. Myoclonus is rare and can be classified as physiologic, essential, epileptic, or symptomatic. One type of physiologic myoclonus is nocturnal myoclonus, which is also labeled as PLMS. This is discussed elsewhere in this issue. Two types of nonphysiologic myoclonus known to disrupt sleep are propiospinal myoclonus and excessive hypnic fragmentary myoclonus.[35,36]

Pathophysiology

The pathophysiology of myoclonus is complex and depends on the cause. Propiospinal myoclonus most commonly is generated at the thoracic level and leads to myoclonic jerks of the abdominal wall muscles that are worse with lying down. This can disrupt sleep onset and lead to overall poor quality of sleep.[37] Excessive hypnic fragmentary myoclonus is generated from the brainstem and leads to excessive body twitches during non-REM and REM sleep.

Key Clinical Features and Diagnosis

Patients may present with EDS unaware of their nocturnal movements if no bed partner is present. Polysomnography is used to make the diagnosis by characterizing the different pattern and frequency of myoclonic movements.

Treatment

Treatment for propiospinal myoclonus includes clonazepam and zonisamide,[37] whereas dopamine agonists, carbamazepine, or clonazepam are used to treat excessive hypnic fragmentary myoclonus.

Prognosis

After these disorders are recognized, patients respond well to therapy and treatment leads to improved quality of sleep.

ATAXIAS
Epidemiology

Ataxia is defined as an uncoordinated movement of the limbs, torso, or speech. There can be many causes of ataxia, and most are related to cerebellar dysfunction. These include spinocerebellar ataxias (SCA), Friedreich ataxia (FA), and episodic ataxias.

Nonmotor dysfunction has been recognized in the SCAs. Sleep complaints, predominantly RLS and PLMS, have been observed in some forms of SCA, with a higher frequency in SCA1, SCA2, SCA3, and SCA6.[38] Commonly these patients relate sleep issues of insomnia, hypersomnia, circadian rhythm disorders, sleep apnea, and excessive motor activity at night. It has been reported that 20% to 30% of patients with SCA experience RLS.[38] RBD and PLMS have been shown to be linked to an increase in ataxia scores in patients with SCA2. The mechanism for this is not fully understood.[39]

FA is the most common autosomal-recessive ataxia. Data on sleep and FA are lacking. One published case reported mixed apnea in a patient with FA.[38]

Pathophysiology

Although the underling pathophysiology of sleep disorders in cerebellar ataxias has not been fully explained, likely the cause is related to brainstem degeneration and disrupted cerebellar outflow tracts.

Key Clinical Features and Diagnosis

These patients commonly present with the typical sleep-related complaints of insomnia, excessive sleepiness, or nighttime activity. Asking a broad question, such as "are you satisfied with your sleep or do you get sleepy during the day," may help open the dialogue for sleep issues. Clinical screening sleep questionnaires also can help identify patients with sleep issues. A standard approach to each sleep complaint is helpful in identifying the root cause of the complaint. Bedpartner report is also an important part of the history because patients may be unaware of nighttime movements, parasomnias, or snoring. Polysomnography is warranted for those patients who have symptoms of sleep apnea or excessive movement at night.

Treatment

Treatment for these various associated sleep disorders should follow the standard lines of therapy. Currently, there are no large double-blind controlled trials to guide therapy in this group of patients. Therefore, therapies typically involve dopaminergic therapy for RLS or PLMS, benzodiazepines if warranted for PLMS, and treatment of sleep apnea.

Prognosis

After sleep disorders are recognized and treated patients have improved quality of sleep and subsequently quality of life.

Case study

A 65-year-old man with PD returns to the office to be evaluated for daytime fatigue. The patient's wife complains that he is always napping, yet he sleeps for at least 9 hours at night. The patient is not taking any sedating medications and has not been evaluated for a sleep disorder. His wife denies nocturnal leg kicking or dream-enactment behavior; however, he snores incessantly. Polysomnography reveals severe obstructive sleep apnea. After CPAP is initiated the patient reports improved daytime fatigue. The key point here is that multiple sleep-related disorders may occur in PD, and often the only way to identify and treat the issue is to perform a sleep study.

REFERENCES

1. Alvarez M, Evidente V, Driver-Dunckley E. Differentiating Parkinson's disease from other parkinsonian disorders. Semin Neurol 2007;27:356–62.
2. Adler CH, Thorpy MJ. Sleep issues in Parkinson's disease. Neurol Clin 2005;64: S12–20.
3. Abbott RD, Ross GW, White LR, et al. Excessive daytime sleepiness and subsequent development of Parkinson disease. Neurology 2005;65:1442–6.
4. Barone P, Antonini A, Colosimo C, et al. The PRIAMO study: a multicenter assessment of nonmotor symptoms and their impact on quality of life in Parkinson's disease. Mov Disord 2009;24:1641–9.
5. Martinez-Martin P, Rodriguez-Blazquez C, Kurtis MM, et al. The impact of nonmotor symptoms on health-related quality of life of patients with Parkinson's disease. Mov Disord 2011;26:399–406.
6. Kaynak D, Kiziltan G, Kaynak H, et al. Sleep and sleepiness in patients with Parkinson's disease before and after dopaminergic treatment. Eur J Neurol 2005;12:199–207.
7. Adler C, Hentz J, Shill H, et al. Probable RBD is increased in Parkinson's disease but not in essential tremor or restless legs syndrome. Parkinsonism Relat Disord 2011;17:456–8.
8. Claassen DO, Josephs KA, Ahlskog JE, et al. REM sleep behavior disorder preceding other aspects of synucleinopathies by up to half a century. Neurology 2010;75:494–9.
9. Boeve BF, Silber MH, Saper CB, et al. Pathophysiology of REM sleep behaviour disorder and relevance to neurodegenerative disease. Brain 2007;130:2770–88.
10. Postuma RB, Aarsland D, Barone P, et al. Identifying prodromal Parkinson's disease: pre-motor disorders in Parkinson's disease. Mov Disord 2012;27: 617–26.
11. Compta Y, Santamaria J, Ratti L, et al. Cerebrospinal hypocretin, daytime sleepiness and sleep architecture in Parkinson's disease dementia. Brain 2009;132: 3308–17.
12. Fronczek R, Overeem S, Lee SY, et al. Hypocretin (orexin) loss in Parkinson's disease. Brain 2007;130:1577–85.
13. Thannickal TC, Lai YY, Siegel JM. Hypocretin (orexin) cell loss in Parkinson's disease. Brain 2007;130:1586–95.
14. Thorpy MJ, Adler CH. Parkinson's disease and sleep. Neurol Clin 2005;23: 1187–208.
15. Winge K, Nielsen KK. Bladder dysfunction in advanced Parkinson's disease. Neurourol Urodyn 2012. [Epub ahead of print].
16. Schulte E, Winkelmann J. When Parkinson's disease patients go to sleep: specific sleep disturbances related to Parkinson's disease. J Neurol 2011;258:S328–35.
17. Frucht S, Rogers JD, Green PE, et al. Falling asleep at the wheel: motor vehicle mishaps in persons taking pramipexole and ropinirole. Neurology 1999;52: 1908–10.
18. Homann CN, Wenzel K, Suppan K, et al. Sleep attacks in patients taking dopamine agonists: review. BMJ 2002;324:1483–7.
19. Oerlemans W, de Weerd A. The prevalence of sleep disorders in patients with Parkinson's disease. A self-reported, community-based survey. Sleep Med 2002;3:147–9.
20. Dhawan V, Dhoat S, Williams AJ, et al. The range and nature of sleep dysfunction in untreated Parkinson's disease (PD). A comparative controlled clinical study

using the Parkinson's disease sleepscale and selective polysomnography. J Neurol Sci 2006;248:158–62.

21. Barone P, Amboni M, Vitale C, et al. Treatment of nocturnal disturbances and excessive daytime sleepiness in Parkinson's disease. Neurology 2004;63: S35–8.

22. Chandran V, Pal P. Essential tremor: beyond the motor features. Parkinsonism Relat Disord 2012;18(5):407–13.

23. Chandran V, Pal P, Reddy J, et al. Non-motor features in essential tremor. Acta Neurol Scand 2011;125(5):332–7.

24. Gerbin M, Viner A, Louis E. Sleep in essential tremor: a comparison with normal controls and Parkinson's disease patients. Parkinsonism Relat Disord 2012;18: 279–84.

25. Gaig C, Iranzo A. Sleep-disordered breathing in neurodegenerative diseases. Curr Neurol Neurosci Rep 2012;12:205–17.

26. Nomura T, Inoue Y, Takigawa H, et al. Comparison of REM sleep behaviour disorder variables between patients with progressive supranuclear palsy and those with Parkinson's disease. Parkinsonism Relat Disord 2012;18:394–6.

27. Aldrich MS, Foster NL, White RF, et al. Sleep abnormalities in progressive supranuclear palsy. Ann Neurol 1989;25:577–81.

28. Chokrovery S. Sleep and degenerative neurologic disorders. Neurol Clin 1996; 14:807–26.

29. Perret JL, Jouvet M. Sleep study of progressive supranuclear paralysis. Electroencephalogr Clin Neurophysiol 1980;49:323–9 [in French].

30. Kuyper D, Parra V, Aerts S, et al. Nonmotor manifestations of dystonia: a systemic review. Mov Disord 2011;26:1206–17.

31. Hansotia P, Wall R, Berendes J. Sleep disturbances and severity of Huntington's disease. Neurology 1985;35:1672–4.

32. Kudo T, Schroeder A, Loh DH, et al. Dysfunctions in circadian behavior and physiology in mouse models of Huntington's disease. Exp Neurol 2011;228:80–90.

33. Pallier PN, Morton AJ. Management of sleep/wake cycles improves cognitive function in a transgenic mouse model of Huntington's disease. Brain Res 2009; 1279:90–8.

34. Goodman A, Rogers L, Pilsworth S, et al. Asymptomatic sleep abnormalities are a common early feature in patients with Huntington's disease. Curr Neurol Neurosci Rep 2011;11:211–7.

35. Merlino G, Gigli G. Sleep-related movement disorders. Neurol Sci 2011;33(3): 491–513.

36. Frauscher B, Kunz A, Brandauer E, et al. Fragmentary myoclonus in sleep revisited: a polysomnographic study in 62 patients. Sleep Med 2011;12:410–5.

37. Roze E, Bounolleau P, Ducreux D, et al. Propriospinal myoclonus revisited: clinical, neurophysiologic, and neuroradiologic findings. Neurology 2009;72: 1301–9.

38. Pedroso J, Braga-Neto P, Felício A, et al. Sleep disorders in cerebellar ataxias. Arq Neuropsiquiatr 2011;69:253–7.

39. Velázquez-Pérez L, Voss U, Rodríguez-Labrada R, et al. Sleep disorders in spinocerebellar ataxia type 2 patients. Neurodegener Dis 2011;8:447–54.

Sleep Disorders in Neuromuscular Diseases

Sushanth Bhat, MD*, Divya Gupta, MD, Sudhansu Chokroverty, MD

KEYWORDS

- Sleep dysfunction in neuromuscular diseases
- Sleep-disordered breathing in neuromuscular diseases • Obstructive sleep apnea
- Breathing in amyotrophic lateral sclerosis • Sleep complaints in myopathies
- Sleep dysfunction in myotonic dystrophy
- Polysomnography in neuromuscular diseases

KEY POINTS

- Sleep disorders are common in patients with neuromuscular diseases. Sleep complaints may not always be volunteered, requiring the clinician to maintain a high index of suspicion.
- Sleep-disordered breathing (SDB), resulting in nocturnal hypoxia and hypercapnia, is the most common sleep disorder in patients with neuromuscular diseases. SDB is generally due to a combination of (1) alveolar hypoventilation owing to respiratory muscle weakness and (2) increased upper airway resistance secondary to pharyngeal dilator muscle atonia (causing obstructive sleep apnea).
- SDB in the early stages of neuromuscular disorders may occur predominantly in rapid eye movement (REM) sleep because of greater muscle atonia and decreased chemoreceptor responsiveness, but with progression of the disease may appear in non-REM sleep and wakefulness.
- No single diurnal test has been found to be uniformly predictive of nocturnal hypoventilation, and overnight oximetry and capnography have significant limitations. A combination of maximal inspiratory pressure and nasal sniff pressure testing may be most sensitive in this regard, but in-laboratory polysomnography is the recommended diagnostic tool for SDB in patients with neuromuscular diseases.
- Nocturnal upper airway pressurization, particularly with noninvasive positive-pressure ventilation devices providing pressure support, is the mainstay of treatment of SDB in patients with neuromuscular disorders.
- Patients with myotonic dystrophy types 1 and 2 may also exhibit signs of central sleep-wake regulation dysfunction, including excessive daytime sleepiness out of proportion to SDB, and abnormalities of REM sleep.

Disclosures: Dr Chokroverty serves as editor-in-chief of the journal *Sleep Medicine* and has spoken on behalf of Cephalon, Inc. Drs Bhat and Gupta have nothing to disclose.
NJ Neuroscience Institute at JFK Medical Center, Seton Hall University, 65 James Street, Edison, NJ 08818, USA
* Corresponding author.
E-mail address: sbhat2012@yahoo.com

INTRODUCTION

Neuromuscular diseases encompass disorders of the motor unit, which includes the anterior horn cell, the motor root and axon, the peripheral nerve, the neuromuscular junction, and the muscle fibers. A large number of disorders, both hereditary and acquired, fall under this classification. **Fig. 1** is a schematic of the motor unit, with a list of diseases arising from lesions at its various sites. The hallmark of neuromuscular diseases, in general, is motor weakness. When the peripheral nerve or dorsal root ganglion is involved, patients may also experience numbness, paresthesias, and sensory ataxia, along with hyporeflexia on examination, caused by disruption of afferent sensory pathways. **Box 1** lists common neuromuscular diseases in which respiratory dysfunction may be seen.

The presence of sleep dysfunction in patients with neuromuscular disorders is not always obvious, and patients may not volunteer symptoms related to disrupted sleep, often attributing daytime sleepiness and fatigue to their underlying neurologic illness. In addition, symptoms often develop insidiously and may be difficult for patients to discern. Nevertheless, sleep dysfunction, particularly sleep-disordered breathing (SDB), is a major cause of morbidity and mortality in patients with neuromuscular diseases. It is therefore extremely important that practitioners be aware of the manifestations of sleep dysfunction in this population, and maintain a high index of

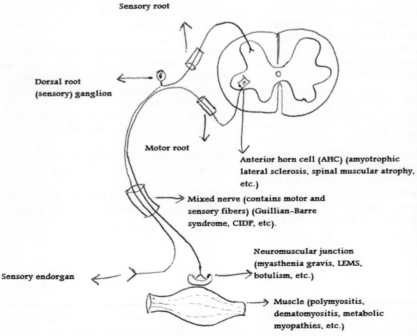

Fig. 1. The motor unit, showing major disorders that can affect each component. The sensory end organ, sensory fibers within the peripheral nerve, and dorsal root ganglion are not part of the motor unit, but are considered part of the peripheral nervous system and may be involved in certain neuromuscular diseases. See text for details. CIDP, chronic inflammatory demyelinating polyradiculoneuropathy; LEMS, Lambert-Eaton myasthenic syndrome. (*Modified from* Chaudhuri A, Behan PO. Fatigue in neurologic disorders. Lancet 2004;363(9413):978–88; with permission.)

Box 1
Common neuromuscular disorders causing sleep-disordered breathing

- Diseases of motor neurons
  - Amyotrophic lateral sclerosis
  - Spinal muscular atrophy
  - Postpolio syndrome
- Diseases of peripheral nerve
  - Guillian-Barré syndrome (acute demyelinating polyradiculoneuropathy, AIDP)
  - Phrenic neuropathies (brachial plexopathies, vasculitis, and so forth)
- Disorders of neuromuscular junctions
  - Myasthenia gravis
- Diseases of muscle
  - Myotonic dystrophy types 1 and 2
  - Muscular dystrophies (Duchenne, limb-girdle, and so forth)
  - Metabolic myopathies (acid-maltase deficiency)
  - Congenital myopathies (nemaline rod, central core disease, centrotubular myopathies)

Data from Chokroverty S. Sleep and breathing in neuromuscular disorders. Handb Clin Neurol 2011;99:1087–108.

---

suspicion. Early identification and treatment of SDB improve the quality of life and prolong survival in patients with neuromuscular diseases.

CLINICAL APPROACH TO SLEEP DYSFUNCTION IN NEUROMUSCULAR DISORDERS

Initial evaluation of these patients usually takes place in an office setting. In a patient with a known neuromuscular condition, it is essential that a detailed sleep history be obtained. The patient's bed partner should be interviewed as well. Obstructive sleep apnea (OSA) may be suspected when there are complaints of sleep initiation or maintenance insomnia and frequent awakenings with choking/gasping in sleep, as well as a history of snoring and witnessed apneas. Nocturnal orthopnea may be a sign of early respiratory compromise and hypoventilation as a result of neuromuscular weakness. However, patients may not manifest any symptoms despite having significant SDB. Patients with SDB may also complain of morning headaches, cognitive impairment, and sleepiness during the day. The occurrence of abnormal behavior in sleep, excessive movements in sleep, and dream-enacting behavior must be carefully elicited. **Box 2** summarizes the symptoms that should alert the clinician to possible underlying SDB.

Excessive daytime sleepiness is often the end result of all of these conditions, and can be assessed using the Epworth Sleepiness Scale (ESS), which measures the propensity to fall asleep during various activities during the day on a scale of 0 to 24. Scores higher than 10 indicate pathologic hypersomnolence.[1] Although there are conflicting reports on the degree of correlation between the ESS and more objective measures of hypersomnolence, such as the Multiple Sleep Latency Test (MSLT),[2,3] the ESS is still a very useful screening tool and has been shown to correlate well with the apnea/hypopnea index (AHI) (see the section Patterns of Sleep-Disordered Breathing in Neuromuscular Diseases) in patients with OSA.[4] Most studies, however, have shown no significant correlation between the ESS and degree

> **Box 2**
> **Symptoms of SDB in neuromuscular diseases**
>
> - Frequent unexplained arousals from sleep
> - Nocturnal restlessness and abnormal movements
> - Excessive daytime sleepiness and fatigue
> - Shortness of breath
> - Orthopnea
> - Morning headache
> - Cognitive deficits and mood disorders
> - Unexplained dependent edema
> - In children, failure to thrive and declining school performance
>
> *Data from* Chokroverty S. Sleep and breathing in neuromuscular disorders. Handb Clin Neurol 2011;99:1087–108.

of nocturnal hypoxia, which is often seen in patients with neuromuscular diseases.[5] Attempts are still being made to identify a simple clinic-based questionnaire that might be useful in predicting the development of sleep dysfunction in patients with neuromuscular disease. A recent example is the Sleep-Disordered Breathing in Neuromuscular Disease Questionnaire (SiNQ)-5, in which a score of 5 or greater had a sensitivity of 86.2%, specificity of 88.5%, positive predictive value of 69.4%, and a negative predictive value of 95.5% in identifying SDB in neuromuscular diseases.[6] More tools of this nature would unquestionably improve the care of patients with neuromuscular disorders.

A thorough physical examination is also an essential component of the initial evaluation of patients with neuromuscular diseases and suspected sleep disorders. The single-breath test can be useful in exploring the extent of impairment of a patient's vital capacity (see later discussion). This test is performed by asking the patient to take a maximal inspiratory breath and begin counting. Normal patients can reach up to 50, but severe impairment of vital capacity is indicated by a single-breath count of less than 15.[7] In addition to typical patterns of weakness seen in specific neuromuscular conditions, the presence of rapid, shallow breathing, use of accessory muscles of respiration, paradoxic breathing, and supine orthopnea suggests weakness of the diaphragm, raising the suspicion for impending nocturnal hypoventilation and possibly respiratory failure.[8] Patients with respiratory insufficiency exhibit tachypnea, inability to complete sentences, use of accessory muscles of inspiration with retraction of intercostal spaces, cyanosis, drowsiness, and lethargy.[9]

Patients with narrow oropharyngeal passages caused by tonsillar hypertrophy, retrognathia/micrognathia, macroglossia or high-arching palates, or increased neck circumferences (greater than 17 inches [43.2 cm] in men and 16 inches [40.6 cm] in women), and those with increased body mass indices (25–29 kg/m^2 being considered overweight, 30 kg/m^2 and greater being considered obese) are at risk for developing OSA.

Patients with significant nocturnal hypoventilation and resultant hypoxemia may show signs of cor pulmonale, with limb edema, hepatosplenomegaly, and elevated jugulovenous pressure. Pulmonary hypertension may be evident on echocardiography or right heart catheterization.[10] As the neuromuscular disease process worsens, alveolar hypoventilation begins to occur during the day as well, resulting in hypercapnia in the awake state.

PATHOPHYSIOLOGY OF SLEEP-DISORDERED BREATHING IN NEUROMUSCULAR DISEASES

SDB remains the most frequent cause of sleep dysfunction in neuromuscular diseases. OSA is a condition characterized by recurrent episodes of partial or complete airway closure in sleep resulting from loss of muscle tone in the upper airway. This loss causes increased upper airway resistance, affecting airflow and resulting in fragmentation of sleep and repeated oxygen desaturations. Respiratory events in sleep, seen on an overnight polysomnogram (PSG), must last at least 10 seconds to be scored in adults. Hypopneas are characterized by diminished airflow in the presence of continued respiratory effort, and require a 50% reduction in airflow with a 3% oxygen desaturation or an arousal, or a 30% reduction in airflow with a 4% oxygen desaturation. Apneas are characterized by complete cessations in airflow. During an obstructive apnea, airflow ceases while respiratory effort persists, whereas during a central apnea both airflow and effort cease. Central apneas generally indicate an absence of the neurologic drive to breathe, as may be seen in narcotic use, in congestive heart failure (CHF) as part of Cheyne-Stokes respirations, or with neurologic conditions such as strokes, multiple sclerosis, or Arnold-Chiari malformations. Mixed apneas begin as central apneas and end as obstructive apneas (**Fig. 2**). The severity of OSA is based on the AHI, which measures the average number of respiratory events per hour of sleep on a PSG (mild between 5/h and 15/h, moderate between 15/h and 30/h, and severe >30/h).[11]

OSA is quite frequent in patients with neuromuscular diseases, although there have not been many studies that compare its prevalence in this group of patients with that in the general population. Although OSA in neuromuscular conditions has been

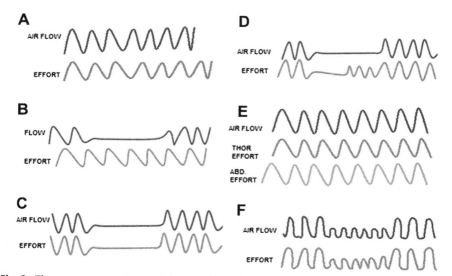

Fig. 2. The most common types of abnormal breathing patterns in sleep in patients with neuromuscular disorders as seen on polysomnography (PSG). (*A*) Normal breathing pattern. (*B*) Upper airway obstructive apnea. (*C*) Central apnea. (*D*) Mixed apnea (initial central following by obstructive apnea). (*E*) Paradoxic breathing. (*F*) Hypopnea. Also commonly seen is alveolar hypoventilation, whereby the breathing pattern may appear normal on PSG, but where hypoxia and hypercapnia are detected. (*Data from* Chokroverty S. Sleep and breathing in neuromuscular disorders. Handb Clin Neurol 2011;99:1087–108.)

traditionally thought to be secondary to a greater degree of muscle atonia in sleep leading to collapse of the upper airway and backward displacement of the tongue in this population, some have suggested that this may not necessarily be true. These investigators point to studies showing that patients with OSA do not have greater tongue-muscle fatigability than do controls, and that tongue strength and fatigability do not worsen in OSA patients after sleep.[12] Other factors, such as weight gain due to inactivity and muscular weakness, state-dependent decrease in neural drive to the upper airway dilators, and vibratory mechanical damage to the upper airway dilators and sensory nerves, may be to blame.[13] OSA leads to a pattern of hypoxemia referred to as event-related hypoxemia, characterized by the occurrence of repeated episodes of arterial oxygen (Sao_2) desaturations resulting from obstruction of airflow as a result of increased upper airway resistance, as is typical in OSA, or as a result of cessation of breathing, as may occur with central sleep apnea. Oxygen resaturation when the event is terminated brings the Sao_2 back to baseline.

More commonly seen in neuromuscular disorders is the phenomenon of nocturnal alveolar hypoventilation. As discussed earlier, in normal subjects ventilation decreases with the onset of sleep, because of progressive atonia of respiratory muscles and decreasing responsiveness of the chemoreceptors to changes in the partial pressures of oxygen and carbon dioxide (Pao_2 and Pco_2), all of which are more marked in rapid eye movement (REM) than in non–rapid eye movement (NREM) sleep. In addition, the wakefulness drive to breathe is lost with the onset of sleep. Respiration is then under purely metabolic control. The end result is a decreased tidal volume, again worse in REM sleep. However, in normal subjects diaphragmatic activity is sufficient, even in REM sleep, to maintain a tidal volume that ensures adequate gas exchange in the lungs. Therefore, significant Sao_2 reduction does not occur. In patients with neuromuscular disease, however, the sleep-related atonia in muscles already weakened by the underlying neurologic process results in profound hypoventilation. For the reasons already described, patients with diaphragmatic weakness exhibit nocturnal hypoventilation that is worst in and may initially present exclusively in REM sleep, when the nondiaphragmatic respiratory muscles are paralyzed and chemoreceptors are at their least sensitive level. This process results in a baseline hypoxemia and hypercapnia in REM sleep. As the disease progresses, this pattern becomes evident in NREM sleep as well. The pattern of hypoxemia seen in this situation is referred to as sleep hypoxemia. Unlike the hypoxemia seen in OSA, whereby there is return of oxygen saturation to the baseline once the respiratory event (apnea or hypopnea) is overcome, baseline oxygen saturation remains low throughout, only falling further transiently if there are superimposed respiratory events (**Fig. 3**).

Box 3 summarizes the factors that predispose patients with neuromuscular diseases to SDB.

LABORATORY INVESTIGATIONS

Once the presence of sleep dysfunction in a patient with neuromuscular disease is suspected, appropriate laboratory investigations can be performed to confirm it and to quantify its severity. One of the most important objectives of such testing is to predict nocturnal hypoventilation with resultant sleep hypoxemia and hypercapnia. To date, no single test has been proved to be sufficient to make this prediction. A large number of diagnostic tests are available (**Box 4**) and are discussed here, but in general daytime pulmonary function testing has proved to be more useful than surrogate markers of nocturnal gas exchange in predicting SDB in neuromuscular patients, and in guiding the treatment of these patients.

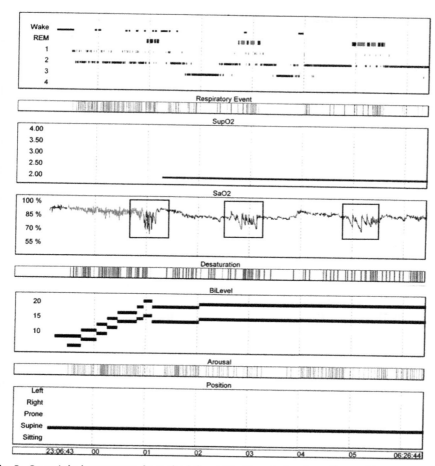

Fig. 3. Overnight hypnogram from the bilevel titration study of a patient with amyotrophic lateral sclerosis and severe obstructive sleep apnea (OSA) diagnosed by previous PSG. Even at the highest pressure tried (20/15 cm H_2O), residual OSA (with respiratory events marked in the hypnogram) accompanied by desaturations occurred in rapid eye movement (REM) sleep, although they were better controlled in non-REM sleep. However, arterial oxygen saturation (Sao_2) remained below 90% even in the absence of OSA and despite the addition of supplemental O_2 at 2 L/min. There is superimposed cyclical worsening of Sao_2 in REM sleep (*boxes*). This pattern was due to sleep hypoxemia, with superimposed event-related hypoxemia in REM sleep caused by OSA. In patients with neuromuscular weakness, this pattern is the result of alveolar hypoventilation caused by diaphragmatic weakness, with superimposed OSA owing to upper airway muscle atonia, both of which are worse in REM sleep. SupO2; supplemental O_2; SaO2, arterial oxygen saturation by pulse oximetry.

Arterial Blood Gases

Hypoxia (Pao_2 <60 mm Hg) and hypercapnia ($Paco_2$ >45 mm Hg) are the end result of respiratory insufficiency, and can be detected by arterial blood gas (ABG) measurements. ABG analysis is usually performed in the acute setting rather than in sleep laboratories or in outpatient clinics because of the invasive nature of the test. Nevertheless, ABG analysis can provide crucial information about a patient's respiratory status.[14,15]

Box 3
Factors promoting SDB in neuromuscular disease

- Respiratory muscle weakness
- Hyporesponsive chemoreceptors
- Sleep-related decreased minute and alveolar ventilation owing to accentuation of above factors in REM sleep initially, then in NREM sleep as disease progresses
- Upper airway muscle atonia
- Skeletal deformities (scoliosis, kyphosis) worsening pulmonary restrictive deficits
- Failure of central mechanisms in many neurologic diseases

Data from Chokroverty S. Sleep and breathing in neuromuscular disorders. Handb Clin Neurol 2011;99:1087–108.

Diurnal ABG abnormalities tend to occur only late in the course of neuromuscular disorders with respiratory involvement, but may be seen when there is a superimposed acute respiratory insult. When present, however, abnormalities of daytime ABGs strongly suggest nocturnal hypoventilation. In a study of patients with Duchenne muscular dystrophy, a $Paco_2$ greater than 45 mm Hg was found to be a 91% sensitive and 75% specific indicator of nocturnal hypoventilation. The researchers found that with the initiation of noninvasive positive-pressure ventilation (NIPPV; see later discussion), wakeful $Paco_2$ values improved despite worsening daytime lung-function test results.[16] Gas-exchange abnormalities limited to sleep is the most common pattern in early SDB. Although in theory continuous measurements of nocturnal Pao_2 and $Paco_2$ provide this crucial information, this is an invasive and impractical method to use in a nonresearch setting. Comparison of a single nocturnal ABG sample (or a sample drawn immediately on awakening) with one drawn during the day may provide evidence of nocturnal hypoventilation. An increase of $Paco_2$ by 10 mm Hg from a diurnal value suggests nocturnal hypoventilation.[11]

Box 4
Common laboratory investigations in neuromuscular patients with suspected SDB (see text for details)

- Arterial blood gases
  - Pao_2 and $Paco_2$
- Pulmonary function testing
  - Forced vital capacity (FVC) sitting and supine, forced expiratory volume in 1 second (FEV_1), FEV_1/FVC ratio
  - Maximal peak inspiratory force (PImax or negative inspiratory force, NIF), Maximal peak expiratory force (PEmax)
- Maximal sniff maneuvers
  - Esophageal, transdiaphragmatic, nasal (Pnsn)
- Overnight pulse oximetry and capnography
- Polysomnography (PSG) and Multiple Sleep Latency Testing (MSLT)

Data from Chokroverty S. Sleep and breathing in neuromuscular disorders. Handb Clin Neurol 2011;99:1087–108.

Pulmonary Function Testing and Measures of Ventilatory Muscle Function

Daytime pulmonary function testing (PFT) using spirometry is used to diagnose and classify disorders of ventilation, whether of intrinsic pulmonary, neurologic, or musculoskeletal etiology. Lung volumes and capacities are measured and compared with expected normal values. **Box 5** defines commonly measured PFT parameters, graphically represented in **Fig. 4**.

Of particular importance to practitioners caring for patients with neuromuscular disorders are the forced vital capacity (FVC) and the forced expiratory volume in 1 second (FEV_1). FVC is defined as the volume of air that can be maximally exhaled after a full inspiration, and FEV_1 is defined as the percentage of the FVC that is expired in the first second of exhalation. The FEV_1/FVC ratio is an extremely important value; in patients with obstructive lung diseases (such as chronic obstructive pulmonary disease [COPD]) whereby there is air trapping and increased end-expiratory volumes, the FEV_1/FVC ratio is less than 80% of the expected value, due to a proportional decrease in both FEV_1 and FVC. On the other hand, in patients with restrictive lung diseases characterized by an inability to fully expand the chest wall owing to intrinsic pulmonary reasons (eg, fibrosis), musculoskeletal reasons (eg, kyphoscoliosis or obesity), or neuromuscular diseases (amyotrophic lateral sclerosis [ALS], myopathies), the FEV_1/FVC ratio is normal or increased, owing to preservation of FEV_1 in the face of absolute reduction of FVC. Lung volumes are low in restrictive lung diseases. Measurement of lung volumes and capacities is highly dependent on patient cooperation, which may be a limiting factor in some cases and may require serial testing for identification.

Once a pattern of restrictive lung disease is detected in a patient with neuromuscular weakness, strength of respiratory muscles can be further assessed by measuring the maximum peak inspiratory force (PImax, also known as negative inspiratory force, NIF), which reflects mainly diaphragmatic function, and the

---

Box 5
Commonly measured PFT parameters

Lung Volumes

- Tidal volume (TV): Volume (ml) of air per normal inspiration or expiration
- Inspiratory reserve volume (IRV): Volume of air during maximal inhalation following a normal breath
- Expiratory reserve volume (ERV): Volume of air during maximal exhalation following a normal breath
- Residual volume (RV): Volume of air remaining after maximal exhalation

Lung Capacities (Derived from Lung Volumes)

- Vital capacity (VC): Volume of air that can be exhaled maximally after maximal inspiration (IRV + TV + ERV)
- Inspiratory capacity (IC): Inspiratory reserve volume plus tidal volume (IRV + TV)
- Functional residual capacity (FRC): Volume of air remaining after a normal expiration (ERV + RV)
- Total lung capacity (TLC): Vital capacity plus residual volume (VC + RV)

Data from Chokroverty S. Sleep and breathing in neuromuscular disorders. Handb Clin Neurol 2011;99:1087–108.

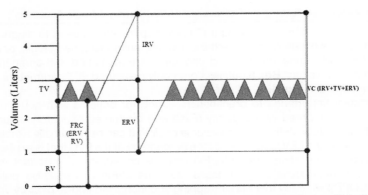

Fig. 4. Lung volumes and capacities. ERV, expiratory reserve volume; FRC, functional residual capacity IRV, inspiratory reserve volume; RV, residual volume; TV, tidal volume; VC, vital capacity. (*From* Chokroverty S, Montagna P. Sleep, breathing and neurological disorders. In: Chokroverty S, editor. Sleep disorders medicine: basic science, technical considerations, and clinical aspects. 2nd edition. Elsevier/Saunders; 2009; with permission.)

maximum peak expiratory force (PEmax), reflecting the function of expiratory muscles. These values are then compared with reference ranges. Normal PImax values in adults (18–65 years old) range from −92 to −121 cm H_2O in men and −68 to −79 cm H_2O in women; mean PEmax value was 140 cm H_2O in men and 95 cm H_2O in women. These ranges are further adjusted for subjects outside this age group. A PImax in the normal range effectively excludes inspiratory muscle weakness. The PImax is useful as a means to serially follow respiratory function in a patient with neuromuscular weakness. However, there are large ranges of published normal values in each category, with the lower limits of normal reflecting a value of 50% of predicted.[17–19] Also, measurement of PImax and PEmax requires the patient to blow into a mouthpiece, which requires both patient cooperation and the ability to form a tight lip seal, which may not be possible in a patient with bulbar and facial weakness. Therefore, PImax values below the normal range need to be interpreted with caution.[20]

Reports of the relative usefulness of PFTs in predicting nocturnal hypoventilation vary widely. Hukins and Hillman[16] reported that in patients with Duchenne muscular dystrophy, an FEV_1 of less than 40% was 91% sensitive but only 50% specific as an indicator of sleep hypoxemia (defined by them as nocturnal Sao_2 <90% for ≥2% of the time). Other investigators have published cutoff values that have high sensitivity and specificity in predicting various degrees of SDB in neuromuscular diseases (FVC <60%, PImax <4.5 kPa predicting hypoventilation limited to REM sleep, FVC <40%, PImax <4.0 kPa predicting hypoventilation also occurring in NREM sleep, and FVC <25%, PImax <3.5 kPa predicting diurnal respiratory failure).[21,22] It has also been suggested that supine FVC measurement may have some value in identifying diaphragmatic weakness and, thus, SDB. Lechtzin and colleagues[23] found that a supine FVC less than 75% was 100% sensitive and specific for predicting an abnormally low transdiaphragmatic pressure. Varrato and colleagues[24] found supine FVC measurements, and the difference between erect and supine FVC values, predictive of orthopnea. Another study found FVC and PImax of equal predictive value in predicting hypercapnia in patients with myotonic dystrophy type 1.[25] On the other hand, Kumar and colleagues[26] found that 33% of patients with myotonic dystrophy type 1 with significant SDB had normal FVC values.

Given the concerns about the sensitivity of standard diurnal respiratory function testing for the presence of nocturnal hypoventilation, especially early in the course of the underlying neuromuscular condition,[27] some laboratories have used maximal sniff maneuvers, which are much easier to perform and are more direct measurements of diaphragmatic functioning. Esophageal and transdiaphragmatic sniff pressures are semi-invasive, but there has been increasing interest in the value of nasal sniff pressure (Pnsn) measurement, a noninvasive technique, in the evaluation of respiratory muscle weakness. Most studies suggest that the Pnsn is a reliable indicator of the strength of inspiratory muscles, comparable with esophageal sniff pressures,[28] and that it may be the main determinant in the generator of FVC.[29] Morgan and colleagues[30] found that a Pnsn of less than -40 cm H_2O was more sensitive than a supine FVC of less than 50% in predicting 6-month mortality in ALS. Lyall and colleagues[31] found that in ALS patients without bulbar weakness, Pnsn was superior to PImax and FVC in predicting both nocturnal hypercapnia and the AHI on subsequent PSG. Similarly, Carratù and colleagues[32] found a negative correlation between a Pnsn of less than 60 cm H_2O and time spent with a nocturnal SaO_2 of less than 90% in ALS patients, whereas the FVC in these patients did not correlate with any nocturnal parameter. More recently, Pnsn was studied in a group of children with a variety of neuromuscular disorders including Duchenne muscular dystrophy and spinal muscular atrophy, and was found to correlate positively with FVC, FEV_1, and PImax.[33]

The use of multiple investigational modalities to evaluate respiratory muscle function increases diagnostic precision and prevents overestimation of inspiratory weakness.[34] A combination of PImax and Pnsn has been recommended to evaluate patients with neuromuscular weakness and suspected respiratory dysfunction.[35]

Overnight Pulse Oximetry and Nocturnal Capnography

Overnight pulse oximetry is considered a relatively inexpensive screening test to look for nocturnal respiratory disturbances. In some patients with neuromuscular diseases and suspected nocturnal hypoventilation, it is often the first test ordered. A typical pattern seen is low baseline oxygen saturations with cyclical worsening, especially early in the course of the illness, suggesting sleep hypoxemia with either superimposed REM-related worsening or significant REM-predominant OSA (see **Fig. 3**). However, a similar pattern may be seen in patients with alveolar or interstitial lung diseases such as COPD, pulmonary fibrosis, or obesity hypoventilation syndrome, and overnight pulse oximetry alone cannot distinguish between these classes of conditions. A recent study of nocturnal pulse oximetry in patients with ALS identified a group of patients with periodic desaturations and normal diaphragm function as measured by diaphragmatic electromyography (EMG) and phrenic nerve response, and central respiratory dysfunction was suspected.[36]

The hyperbolic nature of the oxyhemoglobin dissociation curve (**Fig. 5**) results in a possible underestimation of the degree of alveolar hypoventilation and overestimation of the PaO_2 in arterial blood, especially as SaO_2 falls close to 90%. In addition, there are several technical limitations in the use of pulse oximetry, such as easy dislodgment of the probe and inaccuracy in patients with anemia or hemoglobinopathies.[37]

Overnight oximetry has also been proposed as a method to determine the efficacy of home mechanical ventilation in patients with neuromuscular diseases, but a recent study found that it alone was insufficient in this regard, and recommended a combination of pulse oximetry and end-tidal CO_2 ($EtCO_2$) measurements.[38] On the other hand, a recent study found that nocturnal $EtCO_2$ measurement alone was reliable and strongly correlated with patients' respiratory symptoms, with the duration of nocturnal hypercapnia exhibiting significant predictive power for good compliance with

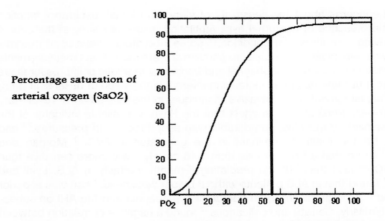

Percentage saturation of arterial oxygen (SaO2)

Partial pressure of arterial oxygen (PaO2) in mm Hg

Fig. 5. The oxyhemoglobin dissociation curve. Note the precipitous fall in partial pressure of arterial oxygen (Pao₂) when arterial oxygen saturation (Sao₂) falls to near and below 90%. This curve illustrates a major limitation in using Sao₂ monitoring alone in screening for nocturnal hypoventilation.

subsequent NIPPV treatment. By contrast, the same group found no significant predictive values for nocturnal pulse oximetry.[39]

Given the significant limitations of surrogate markers of nocturnal gas exchange, it is recommended that suspected sleep dysfunction in neuromuscular disorders be investigated with full-night in-laboratory PSG.

Polysomnography

In-laboratory full-night PSG is the gold standard in diagnosing SDB, as it allows for a detailed analysis of multiple simultaneously recorded parameters. Home sleep studies with limited channels are not recommended in patients with neuromuscular disease.[40] Standard recommended PSG calls for a minimum of 3 channels of electro-encephalography (EEG) (although 4–6 are preferred), 2 electrooculogram (eye) leads, chin EMG, leg EMG, flow channels (oronasal thermistor and nasal pressure transducer), and effort channels (thoracic and abdominal respiratory inductive plethysmography belts).[11] There are also channels for electrocardiography, Sao₂ and snoring. This setup allows the staging of sleep into NREM and REM, scoring of respiratory events, marking of Sao₂ desaturations, and analysis of abnormal movements in sleep (**Fig. 6**). PSG identifies the presence of OSA, central sleep apnea, or Cheyne-Stokes type respirations, identifies periodic limb movements in sleep (PLMS), and assesses REM sleep for the absence of atonia, which is required to diagnose REM behavior disorder (RBD; see later discussion). Etco₂ measurements provide crucial additional information in the identification of nocturnal alveolar hypoventilation; impaired gas exchange caused by underlying neuromuscular weakness results in elevation of Etco₂ values in sleep in comparison with the wakeful state. Analysis of the pattern of Sao₂ abnormalities helps distinguish whether desaturation is due to OSA (event-related hypoxemia), alveolar hypoventilation (sleep hypoxemia), or, as is common in patients with neuromuscular diseases, a combination of both (see section Pathophysiology of Sleep-Disordered Breathing in Neuromuscular Diseases).

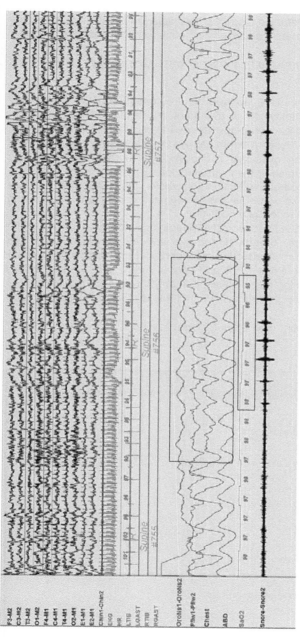

Fig. 6. A representative 90-second epoch of REM sleep from the overnight PSG of an 18-year-old woman with limb-girdle muscular dystrophy. She complained of orthopnea, insomnia due to poor sleep continuity with frequent awakenings, excessive daytime sleepiness, and cognitive concerns. On examination she had generalized, symmetric weakness, rated (right/left) 1/1 deltoids, 1/1 arm extensors, 2/2 elbow flexors, 3/3 elbow extensors, 3/3 wrist and finger extensors, 4/4 finger flexors, 1/1 in the hip flexors, 4/4 knee extensors, 4/4 knee flexors, 0/0 dorsiflexion at the ankles, and 4/4 plantarflexion bilaterally. Reflexes were intact and symmetric throughout. She was nonambulatory and wheelchair bound. Her PSG showed mild OSA, with an apnea-hypopnea index of 10.3/h, and an Sao_2 nadir of 93%. Note the occurrence of paradoxic breathing (*upper box*) in REM sleep, with alternating movements of the chest and abdominal effort belts, accompanied by an Sao_2 desaturation of 3% (*lower box*). A second, shorter event without accompanying Sao_2 desaturation is noted toward the end of the epoch. In non-REM sleep, she had mostly short-cycle central apneas. Top 8 channels: electroencephalography recording with electrodes placed according to the 10-20 international electrode placement system. Chest and ABD, effort belts; Chin1-Chin2, submental electromyogram (EMG); E1-M1 and E2-M1, electrooculogram channels; EKG, electrocardiogram; HR, heart rate; LGAST, left gastrocnemius EMG; LTIB, left tibialis anterior EMG; OroNs1-OroNS2, oronasal airflow; Pflw1-Pflw2, nasopharyngeal pressure transducer recording; RGAST, right gastrocnemius EMG; RTIB, right tibialis anterior EMG; Sao_2, arterial oxygen saturation by finger oximetry. Also included is a snore channel (Snore-Snore2).

Other tests for daytime diaphragmatic dysfunction, such as transdiaphragmatic pressure measurements (involving comparison of esophageal and gastric pressures through balloon techniques), fluoroscopic chest radiography evaluation (involving real-time imaging of diaphragm movements during a supine sniff maneuver), intercostal and phrenic nerve conduction studies, and diaphragmatic EMG are rarely necessary because of their semi-invasive nature and the little additional information they provide.

GENERAL PRINCIPLES IN THE TREATMENT OF SLEEP DYSFUNCTION IN NEUROMUSCULAR DISORDERS

Most neuromuscular diseases have no specific treatment, and care is largely supportive. In addition to optimization of treatment and alleviation of discomfort from symptoms attributable to the neurologic disease itself, the early diagnosis and treatment of SDB is crucial. Persistent nocturnal hypoxemia, the end result of SDB from any cause, results in cardiovascular and pulmonary morbidity and mortality from causes such as lethal cardiac arrhythmias, pulmonary hypertension, right heart failure, and propensity to myocardial infarction and stroke. In addition, SDB causes fragmentation of sleep and excessive daytime sleepiness and fatigue, decreasing the quality of life and affecting mood and cognition.

The goal of treatment of SDB is to support the weakened ventilatory muscles or the motor nerves supplying them, thereby improving alveolar ventilation and gas exchange. In the case of syndromes related to increased nocturnal upper airway resistance or decreased drive to breathe (OSA and central sleep apnea, respectively), treatment is aimed at overcoming these issues, primarily through the use of devices meant to supply upper airway pressurization. In turn, this leads to better sleep continuity.

Box 6 lists available treatment modalities for sleep dysfunction in neuromuscular diseases.

Box 6
Treatment modalities available for sleep dysfunction in neuromuscular diseases

- Upper airway pressurization
  - Continuous positive airway pressure
  - NIPPV
- Supplemental O_2 therapy
- Surgical treatment
  - Tracheostomy
  - Diaphragm pacing
- Pharmacotherapy
  - For excessive daytime sleepiness
    - Wakefulness-promoting agents (modafinil, armodafinil)
    - Stimulants (methylphenidate and amphetamines)
  - For restless legs syndrome
    - Pramipexole, ropinirole, rotigotine; serum ferritin

Data from Chokroverty S. Sleep and breathing in neuromuscular disorders. Handb Clin Neurol 2011;99:1087–108.

All patients should be advised to lose weight, avoid supine sleep, and avoid agents that may increase muscle relaxation (such as alcohol and benzodiazepines) as well as narcotic pain medications that may induce or worsen central sleep apnea.[8]

Upper Airway Pressurization

Devices that provide assistance with ventilation through the means of positive upper airway pressurization have become the mainstay in the treatment of SDB in patients with neuromuscular diseases. These devices have largely replaced ones that provided negative pressure ventilation (eg, "iron lungs"), which are impractical because of their bulk and have been associated with the development of OSA in patients with neuromuscular disease.[41]

For patients with SDB primarily as a result of increased upper airway resistance and collapse (ie, OSA), a continuous positive airway pressure (CPAP) device is usually the first line of treatment. CPAP eliminates obstructive events, normalizes oxygen saturation, and improves sleep continuity. However, it does not provide pressure support. In patients with a combination of OSA and nocturnal hypoventilation, or in those in whom nocturnal hypoventilation is the main pathologic factor, NIPPV is often required.[42]

Noninvasive Intermittent Positive-Pressure Ventilation

It has been well established that NIPPV is beneficial in patients with SDB and neuromuscular disease, with most studies having been conducted in patients with ALS. NIPPV improves survival and slows the rate of decline in pulmonary function.[43,44] Studies have shown that tolerability to NIPPV, which was better in patients with less severe bulbar involvement, slowed the rate of progressive decline of FVC, which in turn improved survival. Survival has a positive correlation with greater than 4 hours of NIPPV use a night.[45] NIPPV enhances the quality of life in patients with ALS,[46] particularly in patients with relatively spared bulbar function and orthopnea.[24] It has been shown to potentially improve cognition,[47] and allows placement of percutaneous endoscopic gastrostomy tubes in patients whose respiratory status may be otherwise deemed to be too risky to allow such a procedure.[48] The benefits of NIPPV seem to persist long term, and one study showed that at the end of the first year, blood gases and a variety of quality-of-life indicators were strikingly better in patients using NIPPV despite progression of ALS, with no significant additional burden on caregivers.[49]

The decision on when to initiate NIPPV in patients with neuromuscular diseases is still being debated. In 1999, the US Consensus Conference Report published guidelines for NIPPV in patients with neuromuscular diseases as well as those with chronic restrictive lung diseases.[50] More recently the American Academy of Neurology reviewed available literature and published updated practice parameters in this regard,[51] with recommendations for more aggressive initiation of NIPPV. These recommendations are summarized in **Box 7**. These guidelines were based in part on a recent study in 20 ALS patients showing that earlier initiation of NIPPV (when nocturnal Sao_2 was cumulatively <90% for >1 minute) resulted in improvement of the vitality subscale of the Short-Form-36 questionnaire,[52] and better compliance with therapy than when the 1999 guidelines were followed. **Box 8** summarizes the consensus recommendations of the NIPPV Titration Task Force of the American Academy of Sleep Medicine (AASM) for titration and determination of the final settings for bilevel devices in the sleep laboratory for patients with chronic alveolar hypoventilation.[53]

<table>
<tr><td>

Box 7
Guidelines on initiation of NIPPV in neuromuscular disorders

1999 US Consensus Conference Report Guidelines

- Appropriate clinical symptoms and signs
- One of the following physiologic criteria:
  - $Paco_2 \geq 45$ mm Hg
  - Nocturnal O_2 desaturation (finger oximetry) $\leq 88\%$ for 5 consecutive minutes
  - PImax <60 cm H_2O or
  - FVC >50% predicted (in cases of progressive disease)

American Academy of Neurology 2009 Practice Parameters Update

- In addition to FVC and PImax cutoffs described above, also recommended consideration for NIPPV with a Pnsn <40 cm H_2O, with nocturnal Sao_2 <90% for a cumulative time of greater than 1 minute, and in the presence of orthopnea

Abbreviations: FVC, forced vital capacity; PImax, maximum inspiratory pressure; Pnsn, nasal sniff pressure.

Data from Chokroverty S. Sleep and breathing in neuromuscular disorders. Handb Clin Neurol 2011;99:1087–108; and Miller RG, Jackson CE, Kasarskis EJ, et al. Practice Parameter update: the care of the patient with amyotrophic lateral sclerosis: drug, nutritional, and respiratory therapies (an evidence-based review). Report of the Quality Standards Subcommittee of the American Academy of Neurology. Neurology 2009;73(15):1218–26.

</td></tr>
</table>

Supplemental Oxygen

In general, supplemental oxygen therapy alone has no role in the treatment of SDB secondary to OSA. Its use in nocturnal hypoventilation is controversial, with studies suggesting that in patients with neuromuscular disease there may be worsening of underlying CO_2 retention.[54] See **Box 8** for recommendations on adding supplemental O_2 while titrating a patient with bilevel devices.

Other Treatment Modalities

Surgical implantation of a diaphragmatic pacing device consisting of a subcutaneous generator and electrodes that stimulate the phrenic nerve was recently approved by the Food and Drug Administration (FDA) for ALS patients under the Humanitarian Device Exemption.[55] Its role in treating SDB in these patients remains to be elucidated.[56] For it to be an effective modality, however, motor axons in the phrenic nerve and muscle fibers in the diaphragm need to remain functional, and these factors are very variable in patients with neuromuscular disorders in comparison with patients with high cervical spinal injury for whom such devices are mainly indicated. Nevertheless, studies suggest that even in SDB related to neuromuscular impairment, it may represent a means for delaying the need for mechanical ventilation.[57] No pharmacologic agents have been found to be beneficial in the treatment of SDB associated with neuromuscular disorders. Tracheostomy remains a definitive but invasive method of treating acute respiratory insufficiency, and its use in neuromuscular patients with SDB needs to be carefully considered on a case-by-case basis. Unfortunately, it may become necessary in patients unable to tolerate treatment with CPAP devices.

Box 8
Summary of AASM task force recommendations for titration of NIPPV settings

Recommendations for Titration

1. The recommended minimum starting inspiratory positive airway pressure (IPAP) and expiratory positive airway pressure (EPAP) should be 8 cm H_2O and 4 cm H_2O, respectively.

2. The recommended maximum IPAP should be 30 cm H_2O for patients $\geq$12 years and 20 cm H_2O for patients <12 years.

3. The recommended minimum and maximum levels of pressure support (PS) are 4 cm H_2O and 20 cm H_2O, respectively.

4. The minimum and maximum incremental changes in PS should be 1 and 2 cm H_2O, respectively.

Recommendations for Adjustment of IPAP, EPAP, and PS

1. IPAP and/or EPAP should be increased (as per AASM guidelines) until the following obstructive respiratory events are eliminated (no specific order): apneas, hypopneas, respiratory effort-related arousals, and snoring.

2. The PS should be increased every 5 minutes if the TV is low (<6–8 mL/kg).

3. The PS should be increased if the arterial Pco_2 remains 10 mm Hg or more above the Pco_2 goal at the current settings for 10 minutes or more. An acceptable goal for Pco_2 is a value less than or equal to the awake Pco_2.

4. The PS may be increased if respiratory muscle rest has not been achieved by NIPPV treatment at the current settings for 10 minutes of more.

5. The PS may be increased if the Spo_2 remains below 90% for 5 minutes or more and TV is low (<6–8 mL/kg).

Note:

- NIPPV treatment goals should be individualized, but typically include prevention of worsening of hypoventilation during sleep, improvement in sleep quality, relief of nocturnal dyspnea, and providing respiratory muscle rest.

- It is recommended by the task force that these titration studies be performed after careful mask fitting and a period of acclimatization at lower pressures, and that they be attended, in-laboratory studies.

- Transcutaneous or end-tidal CO_2 may be used to adjust NIPPV settings if adequately calibrated and ideally validated with arterial blood gas testing.

- Supplemental oxygen starting at 1 L/min and increased in increments of 1 L/min about every 5 minutes until an adequate Spo_2 is attained (>90%) is recommended in patients with an awake Spo_2 <88% or when the PS and respiratory rate have been optimized but the Spo_2 remains <90% for 5 minutes or more.

- A backup rate (ie, ST mode), starting at 10 breaths/min and increased in 1 to 2 breaths/min increments every 10 minutes, should be used in all patients with central hypoventilation, those with a significant number of central apneas or an inappropriately low respiratory rate, and those who unreliably trigger IPAP/EPAP cycles owing to muscle weakness. It may be used if adequate ventilation or adequate respiratory muscle rest is not achieved with the maximum (or maximum tolerated) PS in the spontaneous mode.

Data from Berry RB, Chediak A, Brown LK, et al. NPPV Titration Task Force of the American Academy of Sleep Medicine. Best clinical practices for the sleep center adjustment of noninvasive positive pressure ventilation (NPPV) in stable chronic alveolar hypoventilation syndromes. J Clin Sleep Med 2010;6(5):491–509.

The residual excessive daytime sleepiness that persists in some patients even with adequate titration and compliance with CPAP devices (and which may occur as a primary complaint in patients with myotonic dystrophy, see later discussion) may be treated with wakefulness-promoting agents such as modafanil and armodafanil, as well as stimulants such as methylphenidate and amphetamines. Restless legs syndrome (RLS, recently renamed Willis-Ekbom disease), seen in many neuromuscular disorders but particularly with postpolio syndrome (see later discussion), is treated with dopaminergic agents such as pramipexole, ropinirole, and rotigotine, in addition to iron supplementation in patients with serum ferritin levels lower than 50 ng/mL. Gabapentin and pregabalin have been used to treat RLS symptoms in patients with comorbid peripheral neuropathy, and several recent studies have confirmed the efficacy of a once-a-day dosing regimen of an extended-release form of gabapentin (gabapentin enacabril XR), which recently gained FDA approval for the treatment of RLS.[58]

SLEEP DYSFUNCTION IN INDIVIDUAL NEUROMUSCULAR DISEASES
Diseases of Motor Neurons

ALS, also known as motor neuron disease or Lou Gehrig disease, is a progressive neuromuscular disease characterized by degeneration of motor neurons in the cerebral cortex, brainstem, and anterior horn cells, leading to a combination of upper and lower motor neuron findings. Patients with ALS complain of excessive daytime somnolence and insomnia. In a recent study, 59% of patients with ALS had sleep complaints, compared with 36% of controls. ALS patients reported longer sleep latencies, poorer sleep efficiency, and increased sleep disturbances, as measured by the Pittsburgh Sleep Quality Index, compared with controls. The most common nocturnal complaints were nocturia (54%), sleep fragmentation (48%), and nocturnal cramps (45%).[59] Sleep fragmentation is often due to SDB, but many patients with ALS find compliance with CPAP challenging.[60]

Given that the course of this disease is a relentless loss of motor function, it is not surprising that SDB is a major concern and is a leading cause of morbidity and mortality. SDB in ALS is generally attributable to a combination of increased upper airway resistance and alveolar hypoventilation, as already described. In general, SDB and sleep complaints are late manifestations of ALS that occur when significant diaphragmatic weakness has begun, but there have been cases of sleep complaints being the presenting features of the disease.[61] However, a correlation between early-onset SDB and bulbar-onset ALS has not been found.[62]

There has been special interest in the PSG findings in patients with ALS. One study in particular looked at ALS patients without known respiratory dysfunction and found that the most common SDB was periodic mild oxygen desaturations that occurred independent of the sleep stage, possibly representing central drive dysfunction or respiratory muscle fatigue even in patients who do not demonstrate diaphragmatic involvement on diurnal studies.[63] Although studies have shown that a decreased PImax is associated with sleep dysfunction in patients complaining of orthopnea and excessive daytime sleepiness, daytime studies (FVC, PImax) tend to correlate poorly with any specific PSG findings.[64] PSG analysis in ALS patients confirms their complaints of decreased sleep efficiency and fragmented sleep architecture.[59]

The management of SDB in ALS has been described earlier, and basically consists of nocturnal upper airway bilevel positive-pressure pressurization. Several studies have shown that use of NIPPV prolongs survival in patients with ALS.[65] However, there have not been many large studies correlating improvement in sleep complaints with use of upper airway pressurization, which is clearly an area ripe for future research.

Spinal muscular atrophies (SMA) are a group of autosomally recessive inherited disorders caused by mutations of the survival motor neuron (SMN)-1 gene on chromosome 5 q11.2-13.3. There are several subtypes based on age of presentation, which in turn is dependent on the number of functioning copies of the SMN-2 gene. Symptoms are generally less severe and begin later in life in those with a greater number of copies of the SMN-2 gene. The most common types are acute infantile (SMA type 1 or Werdnig-Hoffman disease), chronic infantile (SMA type 2), chronic juvenile (SMA type 3 or Kugelberg-Welander disease), and adult-onset (SMA type 4) forms. SDB has been described in SMA. Testa and colleagues[66] found that infants and children affected by SMA types 1 and 2 had significantly higher AHI (mean 1.9/h) than controls (mean 0.3/h), and had paradoxic breathing in both quiet and active sleep. Studies have shown that nocturnal NIPPV eliminates SDB, normalizes sleep architecture, and improves subjective sleep quality and daytime alertness in children with SMA types 1 and 2.[67–69]

Poliomyelitis is a viral infection of the anterior horn cells (spinal poliomyelitis) and cranial motor neurons (bulbar poliomyelitis) caused by poliovirus, an RNA member of the enterovirus family, spread mainly by the feco-oral route. Patients with bulbar poliomyelitis may develop respiratory disturbances and sleep dysfunction in the acute and convalescent stages.[8] Postpolio syndrome refers to the development of new-onset weakness, pain, and fatigue several decades after the acute attack, affecting as many as half the patients with a history of poliomyelitis. The exact cause remains unclear but is thought to be secondary to degeneration of the distal terminal branches of enlarged motor units, perhaps as part of a normal aging process, in patients with already poor neuromuscular reserve.[70]

Studies have found that almost half of all patients with postpolio syndrome complain of sleep disturbances, specifically fatigue and excessive daytime sleepiness, headaches, and RLS.[71] Steljes and colleagues[72] studied the PSG findings in 13 postpolio patients and found respiratory abnormalities consisting of hypoventilation, apneas, and hypopneas associated with significant obstructions and desaturation. Recently, Silva and colleagues[73] similarly analyzed 60 PSGs of patients with postpolio syndrome and found poor sleep efficiency due to prolonged sleep latencies and high arousal indices. Araujo and colleagues[74] performed PSGs on 99 patients with postpolio syndrome, and found that 17% had significant PLMS (defined as a PLMS index of 5/h or greater); however, when compared with those patients with postpolio syndrome without significant PLMS, they found no significant difference in the AHI, awakening index, total sleep time, and sleep efficiency. However, there have not been many studies examining the relationship between postpolio syndrome and complaints of RLS. One study of 10 patients with postpolio syndrome who fulfilled the criteria for RLS found that there was a high correlation between the appearance of RLS symptoms and the onset of postpolio symptoms[75]; these patients responded positively to gabapentin and pramipexole.

Myopathies

Primary disorders of muscle often cause diaphragmatic weakness, generally late in the disease, leading to SDB. One important exception is acid-maltase deficiency, a form of inherited glycogen storage disease, in which there may be early diaphragmatic involvement causing nocturnal hypoventilation even before limb weakness becomes evident.[76] In the early stage of respiratory involvement in myopathies, SDB may manifest as REM-related alveolar hypoventilation, worsening to occur in NREM sleep and then in the wakeful state as the disease progresses. In addition, weakness of upper airway dilator muscles may cause superimposed OSA. In many patients with myopathies not affecting diaphragmatic function sufficiently enough to cause alveolar hypoventilation, REM-related hypopneas, apneas, and paradoxic breathing may occur (see **Fig. 6**).

Duchenne muscular dystrophy, an X-linked recessive mutation of the dystrophin gene causing instability of the sarcolemmal membrane, is characterized by a relentless progression of skeletal muscle weakness, initially beginning in the legs and pelvis, resulting in loss of ability to walk and stand. As the disease progresses, muscle is replaced by fibrous tissue, resulting in pseudohypertrophy of the calves. Muscle contractures and skeletal deformities (scoliosis) also occur late in the disease. The diagnosis can be made by family history, genetic testing, and muscle biopsy. Treatment is mostly supportive and average life expectancy is of the order of 25 years. Cardiomyopathy and subsequent arrhythmias are common, but respiratory failure and pneumonia late in the course of the disease are the leading causes of mortality. Although worst in REM sleep, alveolar hypoventilation in Duchenne muscular dystrophy occurs in all stages of sleep and is likely due to a combination of respiratory muscle weakness and scoliosis, causing a restrictive pulmonary deficit.[77] Severe sleep hypoxemia and hypercapnia often result. Obstructive apneas and hypopneas are also common, probably caused by poor upper airway muscle tone.[78] There have been contradictory reports regarding the benefit of NIPPV in Duchenne muscular dystrophy. One study found that preventive NIPPV did not improve respiratory handicap and reduced survival, and the investigators suggested that use of NIPPV for preventive purposes should be avoided in patients with FVC between 20% and 50% of predicted values[79] Other studies, however, found NIPPV useful in correcting nocturnal ABG abnormalities, improving daytime somnolence, and prolonging survival.[80,81] Clearly more studies are required in this population.

A large number of congenital myopathies (eg, nemaline rod myopathy, centrotubular and central core disease, merosin myopathies, and congenital muscular dystrophies) may also present with sleep complaints, respiratory insufficiency, and SDB. Although generally presenting in childhood, there have been case reports of these disorders having a delayed presentation in adulthood with respiratory failure.[82,83] Recently, investigators reported PSG findings in 12 children with congenital muscular dystrophies and found decreased total sleep time, decreased REM duration, and signs of upper airway resistance.[84] A study of 7 patients with a variety of neuromuscular diagnoses such as myasthenia gravis, limb-girdle muscular dystrophy, and 1 with Scotland myopathy showed that after 18 months of NIPPV therapy there was improvement in ABG and sleep quality, although there was no change in lung function.[85]

Myotonic dystrophy type 1 (DM1) is a multisystem disorder characterized by muscle weakness and myotonia, cataracts, cardiac conduction defects, frontal balding, and endocrine abnormalities. It is inherited in an autosomal dominant fashion. The main genetic defect is a triple nucleotide expansion mutation of the CTG sequence of the DMPK gene on the long arm of chromosome 19. Longer repeats lead to earlier and more severe manifestations of the disease. Sleep disturbances are very common and well documented in DM1, with more than 50% of these patients complaining of excessive daytime somnolence and up to two-thirds complaining of fatigue.[86] SDB is frequent in this population and may be due to a combination of OSA, central apneas, periodic breathing, and nocturnal hypoventilation. It is not predicted by daytime PFT.[87] Developmental orofacial structural abnormalities owing to poor muscle tone may further predispose this population to OSA.

Compared with controls, DM1 patients report longer sleep periods, less restorative sleep, more difficulty falling asleep, being less alert in the morning, and having more trouble staying awake after meals. Recent studies of the PSG characteristics of patients with adult-onset DM1 showed that compared with healthy controls, they had significantly reduced sleep efficiencies and higher PLMS indices,[88] increased REM densities ,and greater percentages of slow-wave sleep.[89]

The excessive daytime sleepiness of DM1 patients is often out of proportion to their degree of SDB, and persists despite adequate treatment of SDB. The degree of hypersomnolence has been found to weakly correlate with muscle-strength impairment, but not the number of CTG repeats.[90] DM1 patients have short sleep latencies on MSLT as well as short sleep-onset REM periods (SOREMPs), suggesting a narcoleptic phenotype. However, measurement of cerebrospinal fluid (CSF) hypocretin in these patients has provided inconsistent results; some studies found hypocretin levels to be comparable with those of controls,[91] whereas other reports found levels to be low[92]; no correlation has been made between the CSF hypocretin level and the degree of hypersomnolence.[93] Nevertheless, this along with the occurrence of periodic breathing has led some researchers to suggest a central mechanism, responsible for sleep dysfunction in DM1, as part of the multisystem involvement. A correlation has been found between the degree of corpus callosum atrophy and the severity of hypersomnolence detected on MSLT.[94]

Myotonic dystrophy type 2 (DM2 or proximal myotonic myopathy, PROMM), a more recently described myotonic disorder, is clinically and genetically distinct from DM1. It is caused by an autosomally dominant CCTG expansion mutation of intron 1 of zinc-finger 9 gene on chromosome 3. Given the rarity of this disorder, there have been fewer reports on sleep disturbances in DM2. Patients with DM2 seem to be less hypersomnolent, but more fatigued, than patients with DM1.[95] A recent analysis of the PSG findings in 6 DM2 patients[96] described increased arousals, decreased sleep efficiency, alpha-delta sleep, obstructive apneas, and paradoxic breathing in REM sleep. All of these patients had complained of excessive daytime sleepiness, snoring, or insomnia. MSLT performed in 4 of these patients showed reduced mean sleep latency without SOREMPs. A case of REM without atonia and dream-enacting behavior in a patient with DM2[97] was recently reported. As in DM1, an abnormality of central control of breathing and sleep-wakefulness related to a common generalized membrane abnormality of the brainstem may be responsible for sleep-wake and respiratory dysfunction.

Neuromuscular Junction Disorders

Myasthenia gravis, a postsynaptic neuromuscular junction disorder related to the production of antibodies against acetylcholine receptor antibodies, is characterized by prominent bulbar signs (dysarthria, dysphagia, and diplopia) and fatigable generalized muscle weakness. Respiratory muscle weakness is a common complication of myasthenic crises. There have been contradictory reports in the literature regarding the nature of SDB in myasthenia gravis. Some studies have suggested that OSA is more common in myasthenic patients than in controls,[98] with risk factors being age, presence of diaphragmatic weakness, and daytime alveolar hypoventilation. SDB was reported even in patients with controlled daytime myasthenic symptoms.[99] It has also been reported that most respiratory events are central apneas and hypopneas,[100,101] which were found to mainly occur in REM sleep in stable myasthenics.[102] Other investigators, however, found no causal relationship between stable myasthenia gravis and OSA, no correlation between pulmonary function and SDB in these patients, and no increased prevalence of central apneas.[103] Most published studies involved small numbers of patients, and the final verdict on the nature of SDB in myasthenia gravis awaits larger, controlled studies. Even fewer data exist on SDB in

Lambert-Eaton myasthenic syndrome, a presynaptic autoimmune disorder of the neuromuscular junction that may be complicated by respiratory failure.

Neuropathies

Polyneuropathies affect peripheral nerves in a symmetric fashion causing paresthesias, sensory loss, areflexia, and muscle weakness and wasting in a length-dependent manner, with symptoms being worse distally. Most neuropathies are acquired and are due to medical conditions such as diabetes mellitus, deficiencies of vitamin B12 or folic acid, hypothyroidism, or paraproteinemias. Respiratory involvement in neuropathies is rare; the most important exception is Guillian-Barré syndrome or acute inflammatory demyelinating polyradiculoneuropathy (AIDP), in which diaphragmatic involvement can cause respiratory insufficiency requiring mechanical ventilation. Sleep dysfunction appears to be most common in the acute phase of AIDP; a recent questionnaire-based study found that sleep disturbances were reported in more than half of such patients, and were most severe in the first week of hospitalization, improving thereafter. The most common findings included increased sleep latencies, sleep fragmentation, and reduced sleep periods.[104] Of interest, there have been reports of narcoleptic-type symptoms (sleep onset in REM sleep periods, REM sleep without atonia, hypnagogic hallucinations)[105] and low CSF hypocretin levels[106] in the acute phase of AIDP, suggesting possible central demyelination. On the other hand, long-term SDB was not found in a study of 34 patients recovering from AIDP despite the persistence of varying degrees of residual neurologic impairment.[107]

Charcot-Marie-Tooth (CMT) disease includes a large number of inherited, genetically heterogeneous neuropathies with both demyelinating and axonal forms. A small case-control study of 12 CMT type 1 patients who underwent PSG found significantly elevated AHI (mean 10.5/h) compared with controls (mean 1.5/h), correlating with neurologic disability.[108] Other investigators have reported similar findings.[109] Upper airway dysfunction and diaphragmatic weakness have been described in CMT type 2C, an axonal variant that is much rarer than CMT type 1, although large studies in this particular subtype are difficult. A recent Web-based survey among patients with various subtypes of CMT found that these patients reported significantly greater fatigue and daytime sleepiness; 79.3% of CMT patients complained of poor sleep quality compared with 17.2% of controls. Prevalence of RLS was 18.1% in CMT patients compared with 5.6% in controls. No significant differences were found among genetic subtypes.[110]

In addition, neuropathies and plexopathies involving the phrenic nerve have been reported, and may be a cause of respiratory insufficiency as well as SDB.[111] Phrenic nerve paralysis has been reported in patients with CMT complicated by diabetes mellitus,[112] and as a complication of various cardiac and thoracic surgeries.[113]

SUMMARY

Often overlooked and underdiagnosed, sleep dysfunction, particularly SDB, is common in many neuromuscular diseases. A high index of suspicion is crucial because patients are often unaware of the specific symptoms of SDB, attributing them to the underlying neurologic illness. A variety of diurnal and nocturnal tests, including blood gas analysis, pulmonary and sniff function testing, oximetry, and capnography are available to aid in making the diagnosis. However, there is still no consensus about the optimal daytime indicator in neuromuscular patients with suspected nocturnal hypoventilation. In-laboratory PSG and upper airway titration studies remain the gold standard for diagnosis and treatment. NIPPV is the mainstay of treatment of nocturnal respiratory failure

---

Illustrative Case

A 57-year-old man with a 2-year history of progressive limb weakness, atrophy, hyperreflexia, and fasciculations was diagnosed with ALS after nerve conduction studies and an EMG. Over the past 6 months he began to experience bulbar complaints, including dysarthria and dysphagia. He also began to complain of shortness of breath while lying down in bed at night, to the point where he needed to use 3 to 4 pillows to keep his body semi upright in order to fall asleep. He had a hard time falling asleep because of this, and his sleep was fitful, with frequent awakenings. He complained of always being tired and falling asleep watching television or at the movies. He had early-morning headaches and admitted to feeling depressed. He also snored loudly, and his wife noticed that he had pauses in his breathing during sleep. Real-time fluoroscopy of the chest showed no movement of the right hemidiaphragm and minimal movement of the left with inspiration.

He had an overnight diagnostic PSG that showed severe OSA with an AHI of 40/h and an Sao_2 nadir of 73%, with more than 85% of the night spent with an Sao_2 of less than 90%. He was titrated with a bilevel positive airway pressure device in the sleep laboratory. The highest pressure reached was 20/15 cm H_2O. At this pressure, his AHI was still moderately elevated (27/h).

Analysis of his overnight hypnogram (see **Fig. 3**) showed that at the highest bilevel pressure tried, the elevated AHI was mainly due to residual respiratory events in REM sleep; this pressure was sufficient to eliminate OSA in NREM supine sleep. However, low baseline Sao_2 persisted despite correction of OSA, even in NREM sleep. The Sao_2 remained persistently below 90% throughout the night, and cyclically worsened during cycles of REM sleep. This pattern was due to sleep hypoxemia, with superimposed event-related hypoxemia in REM sleep due to OSA. In patients with neuromuscular weakness, sleep hypoxemia is due to alveolar hypoventilation (see section on Pathophysiology of Sleep-Disordered Breathing in Neuromuscular Diseases), which may worsen in REM sleep. Patients with neuromuscular diseases may also experience OSA that is worse in REM sleep, resulting in the pattern seen in this patient. Addition of supplemental oxygen via nasal cannula at 2 L/min did not improve baseline Sao_2.

He subsequently returned for a repeat full-night titration study and was ultimately prescribed a bilevel device at a pressure of 26/20 cm H_2O, a pressure at which his AHI improved to 12/h including a long stretch of supine REM sleep. Addition of supplemental O_2 at 4 L/min to this pressure kept his Sao_2 above 90% for most of the night when overnight pulse oximetry was tested after 2 months of bilevel use. He reported better sleep continuity, a better mood, more energy during the day, and cessation of snoring.

---

in neuromuscular diseases, although the precise timing and indications for this therapy, as well as the long-term outcomes, especially on symptoms related to sleep dysfunction, remain to be elucidated with further research.

REFERENCES

1. Johns MW. A new method for measuring daytime sleepiness: the Epworth Sleepiness Scale. Sleep 1991;14(6):540–5.
2. Chervin RD, Aldrich MS, Pickett R, et al. Comparison of the results of the Epworth Sleepiness Scale and the Multiple Sleep Latency Test. J Psychosom Res 1997;42(2):145–55.
3. Benbadis SR, Mascha E, Perry MC, et al. Association between the Epworth Sleepiness Scale and the Multiple Sleep Latency Test in a clinical population. Ann Intern Med 1999;130(4 Pt 1):289–92.
4. Johns MW. Daytime sleepiness, snoring, and obstructive sleep apnea: the Epworth Sleepiness Scale. Chest 1993;103(1):30–6.
5. Furuta H, Kaneda R, Kosaka K, et al. Epworth Sleepiness Scale and sleep studies in patients with obstructive sleep apnea syndrome. Psychiatry Clin Neurosci 1999;53:301–2.

6. Steier J, Jolley CJ, Seymour J, et al. Screening for sleep-disordered breathing in neuromuscular disease using a questionnaire for symptoms associated with diaphragm paralysis. Eur Respir J 2011;37(2):400–5.

7. Mehta S. Neuromuscular disease causing acute respiratory failure. Respir Care 2006;51(9):1016–21.

8. Chokroverty S. Sleep and breathing in neuromuscular disorders. Handb Clin Neurol 2011;99:1087–108.

9. Mangera Z, Panesar G, Makker H. Practical approach to management of respiratory complications in neurological disorders. Int J Gen Med 2012;5: 255–63.

10. Culebras A. Sleep and neuromuscular disorders. Neurol Clin 2005;23(4): 1209–23.

11. Iber C, Ancoli-Israel S, Chesson AL, et al. The AASM manual for the scoring of sleep and associated events: rules, terminology, and technical specifications. Westchester (IL): American Academy of Sleep Medicine; 2007.

12. Mortimore IL, Bennett SP, Douglas NJ. Tongue protrusion strength and fatigu-ability: relationship to apnoea/hypopnoea index and age. J Sleep Res 2000; 9(4):389–93.

13. Eckert DJ, Sabiosky JP, Jordan AS, et al. Upper airway myopathy is not impor-tant in the pathophysiology of obstructive sleep apnea. J Clin Sleep Med 2007; 3(6):570–3.

14. Dhand UK, Dhand R. Sleep disorders in neuromuscular diseases. Curr Opin Pulm Med 2006;12(6):402–8.

15. Hutchinson D, Whyte K. Neuromuscular disease and respiratory failure. Pract Neurol 2008;8(4):229–37.

16. Hukins CA, Hillman DR. Daytime predictors of sleep hypoventilation in Duchenne muscular dystrophy. Am J Respir Crit Care Med 2000;161(1): 166–70.

17. Frankenstein L, Nelles M, Meyer FJ, et al. Validity, prognostic value and optimal cutoff of respiratory muscle strength in patients with chronic heart failure changes with beta-blocker treatment. Eur J Cardiovasc Prev Rehabil 2009;16:424.

18. Vilaró J, Ramirez-Sarmiento A, Martínez-Llorens JM, et al. Global muscle dysfunction as a risk factor of readmission to hospital due to COPD exacerba-tions. Respir Med 2010;104:1896.

19. Moore AJ, Soler RS, Cetti EJ, et al. Sniff nasal inspiratory pressure versus IC/TLC ratio as predictors of mortality in COPD. Respir Med 2010;104:1319.

20. Fiz JA, Carreres A, Rosell A, et al. Measurement of maximal expiratory pressure: effect of holding the lips. Thorax 1992;47:961.

21. Ragette R, Mellies U, Schwake C, et al. Patterns and predictors of sleep disor-dered breathing in primary myopathies. Thorax 2002;57(8):724–8.

22. Mellies U, Ragette R, Schwake C, et al. Daytime predictors of sleep disordered breathing in children and adolescents with neuromuscular disorders. Neuro-muscul Disord 2003;13(2):123–8.

23. Lechtzin N, Wiener CM, Shade DM, et al. Spirometry in the supine position improves the detection of diaphragmatic weakness in patients with amyotrophic lateral sclerosis. Chest 2002;121(2):436–42.

24. Varrato J, Siderowf A, Damiano P, et al. Postural change of forced vital capacity predicts some respiratory symptoms in ALS. Neurology 2001;57(2):357–9.

25. Bégin P, Mathieu J, Almirall J, et al. Relationship between chronic hypercapnia and inspiratory-muscle weakness in myotonic dystrophy. Am J Respir Crit Care Med 1997;156(1):133–9.

26. Kumar SP, Sword D, Petty RK, et al. Assessment of sleep studies in myotonic dystrophy. Chron Respir Dis 2007;4(1):15–8.

27. Winhammar JM, Joffe D, Simmul R, et al. Nocturnal hypoxia in motor neuron disease is not predicted by standard respiratory function tests. Intern Med J 2006;36(7):419–22.

28. Heritier F, Rahm F, Pasche P, et al. Sniff nasal inspiratory pressure; A noninvasive assessment of inspiratory muscle strength. Am J Respir Crit Care Med 1994; 150(6):1678–83.

29. Stefanutti D, Benoist MR, Sceinman P, et al. Usefulness of sniff nasal pressure in patients with neuromuscular or skeletal disorders. Am J Respir Crit Care Med 2000;162(4):1507–11.

30. Morgan RK, McNally S, Alexander M, et al. Use of sniff nasal-inspiratory force to predict survival in amyotrophic lateral sclerosis. Am J Respir Crit Care Med 2005;171(3):269–74.

31. Lyall RA, Donaldson N, Polkey MI, et al. Respiratory muscle strength and ventilatory failure in amyotrophic lateral sclerosis. Brain 2001;124(Pt 10):2000–13.

32. Carratù P, Cassano A, Gadaleta F, et al. Association between low sniff nasal-inspiratory pressure (SNIP) and sleep disordered breathing in amyotrophic lateral sclerosis: preliminary results. Amyotroph Lateral Scler 2001;12(6):458–63.

33. Anderson VB, McKenzie JA, Seton C, et al. Sniff nasal inspiratory pressure and sleep disordered breathing in childhood neuromuscular disorders. Neuromuscul Disord 2012;22(6):528–33.

34. Steier J, Kaul S, Seymour J, et al. The value of multiple tests of respiratory muscle strength. Thorax 2007;62:975–80.

35. Hart N, Plokey MI, Sharshar T, et al. Limitations of sniff nasal pressure in patients with severe neuromuscular weakness. J Neurol Neurosurg Psychiatry 2003;74: 1685–7.

36. de Carvalho M, Costa J, Pinto S, et al. Percutaneous nocturnal oximetry in amyotrophic lateral sclerosis: periodic desaturation. Amyotroph Lateral Scler 2009; 10(3):154–61.

37. Netzer N, Eliasson AH, Netzer C, et al. Overnight pulse oximetry for sleep-disordered breathing in adults: a review. Chest 2001;120(2):625–33.

38. Nardi J, Prigent H, Adala A, et al. Nocturnal oximetry and transcutaneous carbon dioxide in home-ventilated neuromuscular patients. Respir Care 2012; 57(9):1425–30.

39. Kim S, Park KS, Nam H, et al. Capnography for assessing nocturnal hypoventilation and predicting compliance with subsequent noninvasive ventilation in patients with ALS. PLoS One 2011;6(3):e17893.

40. Collop N, Anderson M, Boehlecke B, et al. Clinical guidelines for the use of unattended portable monitors in the diagnosis of obstructive sleep apnea in adult patients. Portable monitoring task force of the American Academy of Sleep Medicine. J Clin Sleep Med 2007;3(7):737–47.

41. Smith IE, King MA, Shneerson JM. Choosing a negative pressure ventilation pump: are there any important differences? Eur Respir J 1995;8:1792–5.

42. Shneerson JM, Simonds AK. Noninvasive ventilation for chest wall and neuromuscular disorders. Eur Respir J 2002;20(2):480–7.

43. Kleopa KA, Sherman M, Neal B, et al. BIPAP improves survival and rate of pulmonary function decline in patients with ALS. J Neurol Sci 1999;164(1):82–8.

44. Aboussouan LS, Khan SU, Meeker DP, et al. Effect of noninvasive positive-pressure ventilation on survival in amyotrophic lateral sclerosis. Ann Intern Med 1997;127:450–3.

45. Lo Coco D, Marchese S, Pesco MC, et al. Noninvasive positive-pressure venti-lation in ALS: predictors of tolerance and survival. Neurology 2006;67(5):761–5.
46. Lyall RA, Donaldson N, Fleming T, et al. A prospective study of quality of life in ALS patients treated with noninvasive ventilation. Neurology 2001;57(1): 153–6.
47. Newsom-Davis IC, Lyall RA, Leigh PN, et al. The effect of non-invasive positive pressure ventilation (NIPPV) on cognitive function in amyotrophic lateral scle-rosis (ALS): a prospective study. J Neurol Neurosurg Psychiatry 2001;71:482–7.
48. Boitano LJ, Jordan T, Benditt JO. Noninvasive ventilation allows gastrostomy tube placement in patients with advanced ALS. Neurology 2001;56(3):413–4.
49. Mustfa N, Walsh E, Bryant V, et al. The effect of noninvasive ventilation on ALS patients and their caregivers. Neurology 2006;66(8):1211–7.
50. Consensus conference report: clinical indications for noninvasive positive pres-sure ventilation in chronic respiratory failure due to restrictive lung disease, COPD, and nocturnal hypoventilation. Chest 1999;116(2):521–34.
51. Miller RG, Jackson CE, Kasarskis EJ, et al. Practice parameter update: the care of the patient with amyotrophic lateral sclerosis: drug, nutritional, and respiratory ther-apies (an evidence-based review). Report of the Quality Standards Subcommittee of the American Academy of Neurology. Neurology 2009;73(15):1218–26.
52. Jackson CE, Rosenfeld J, Moore DH, et al. A preliminary evaluation of a prospective study of pulmonary function studies and symptoms of hypoventi-lation in ALS/MND patients. J Neurol Sci 2001;191(1–2):75–8.
53. Berry RB, Chediak A, Brown LK, et al. NPPV titration task force of the American Academy of Sleep Medicine. Best clinical practices for the sleep center adjust-ment of noninvasive positive pressure ventilation (NPPV) in stable chronic alve-olar hypoventilation syndromes. J Clin Sleep Med 2010;6(5):491–509.
54. Gay PC, Edmonds LC. Severe hypercapnia after low-flow oxygen therapy in patients with neuromuscular disease and diaphragmatic dysfunction. Mayo Clin Proc 1995;70(4):327–30.
55. Scherer K, Bedlack RS. Diaphragm pacing in amyotrophic lateral sclerosis: a literature review. Muscle Nerve 2012;46(1):1–8.
56. Amirjani N, Kiernan MC, McKenzie DK, et al. Is there a case for diaphragm pacing for amyotrophic lateral sclerosis patients? Amyotroph Lateral Scler 2012;13(6):521–7.
57. Onders RP, Elmo M, Khansarinia S, et al. Complete worldwide operative expe-rience in laparoscopic diaphragm pacing: results and differences in spinal cord injured patients and amyotrophic lateral sclerosis patients. Surg Endosc 2009; 23(7):1433–40.
58. Lal R, Ellenbogen A, Chen D, et al. A randomized, double-blind, placebo-controlled, dose-response study to assess the pharmacokinetics, efficacy, and safety of gabapentin enacarbil in subjects with restless legs syndrome. Clin Neuropharmacol 2012;35(4):165–73.
59. Lo Coco D, Mattaliano P, Spataro R, et al. Sleep-wake disturbances in patients with amyotrophic lateral sclerosis. J Neurol Neurosurg Psychiatry 2011;82(8):839–42.
60. Barthlen GM, Lange DJ. Unexpectedly severe sleep and respiratory pathology in patients with amyotrophic lateral sclerosis. Eur J Neurol 2000;7(3):299–302.
61. Takekawa H, Kubo J, Miyamoto T, et al. Amyotrophic lateral sclerosis associated with insomnia and the aggravation of sleep-disordered breathing. Psychiatry Clin Neurosci 2001;55(3):263–4.
62. Kimura K, Tachibana N, Kimura J, et al. Sleep-disordered breathing at an early stage of amyotrophic lateral sclerosis. J Neurol Sci 1999;164(1):37–43.

63. Atalaia A, De Carvalho M, Evangelista T, et al. Sleep characteristics of amyotrophic lateral sclerosis in patients with preserved diaphragmatic function. Amyotroph Lateral Scler 2007;8(2):101–5.
64. David WS, Bundlie SR, Mahdavi Z. Polysomnographic studies in amyotrophic lateral sclerosis. J Neurol Sci 1997;152(Suppl 1):S29–35.
65. Carratù P, Spicuzza L, Cassano A, et al. Early treatment with noninvasive positive pressure ventilation prolongs survival in amyotrophic lateral sclerosis patients with nocturnal respiratory insufficiency. Orphanet J Rare Dis 2009;4:10.
66. Testa MB, Pavone M, Bertini E, et al. Sleep-disordered breathing in spinal muscular atrophy types 1 and 2. Am J Phys Med Rehabil 2005;84(9):666–70.
67. Mellies U, Dohna-Schwake C, Stehling F, et al. Sleep disordered breathing in spinal muscular atrophy. Neuromuscul Disord 2004;14(12):797–803.
68. Petrone A, Pavone M, Testa MB, et al. Noninvasive ventilation in children with spinal muscular atrophy types 1 and 2. Am J Phys Med Rehabil 2007;86(3):216–21.
69. Lemoine TJ, Swoboda KJ, Bratton SL, et al. Spinal muscular atrophy type 1: are proactive respiratory interventions associated with longer survival? Pediatr Crit Care Med 2012;13(3):e161–5.
70. Trojan DA, Cashman NR. Post-poliomyelitis syndrome. Muscle Nerve 2005;31:6–19.
71. van Kralingen KW, Ivanyi B, van Keimpema AR, et al. Sleep complaints in post-polio syndrome. Arch Phys Med Rehabil 1996;77(6):609–11.
72. Steljes DG, Kryger MH, Kirk BW, et al. Sleep in postpolio syndrome. Chest 1990; 98(1):133–40.
73. Silva TM, Moreira GA, Quadros AA, et al. Analysis of sleep characteristics in post-polio syndrome patients. Arq Neuropsiquiatr 2010;68(4):535–40.
74. Araujo MA, Silva TM, Moreira GA, et al. Sleep disorders frequency in post-polio syndrome patients caused by periodic limb movements. Arq Neuropsiquiatr 2010;68(1):35–8.
75. Marin LF, Carvalho LB, Prado LB, et al. Restless legs syndrome in post-polio syndrome: a series of 10 patients with demographic, clinical and laboratorial findings. Parkinsonism Relat Disord 2011;17(7):563–4.
76. Nabatame S, Taniike M, Sakai N, et al. Sleep disordered breathing in childhood-onset acid maltase deficiency. Brain Dev 2009;31(3):234–9.
77. Smith PE, Edwards RH, Calverley PM. Ventilation and breathing pattern during sleep in Duchenne muscular dystrophy. Chest 1989;96(6):1346–51.
78. Smith PE, Calverley PM, Edwards RH. Hypoxemia during sleep in Duchenne muscular dystrophy. Am Rev Respir Dis 1988;137(4):884–8.
79. Raphael J, Chevret S, Chastang C, et al. Randomised trial of preventive nasal ventilation in Duchenne muscular dystrophy. Lancet 1994;343(8913):1600–4.
80. Ishikawa Y, Ishikawa Y, Minami R. The effect of nasal IPPV on patients with respiratory failure during sleep due to Duchenne muscular dystrophy. Rinsho Shinkeigaku 1993;33(8):856–61 [in Japanese].
81. Vianello A, Bevilacqua M, Salvador V, et al. Long-term nasal intermittent positive pressure ventilation in advanced Duchenne's muscular dystrophy. Chest 1994; 105(2):445–8.
82. Kelly E, Farrell MA, McElvaney NG. Adult-onset nemaline myopathy presenting as respiratory failure. Respir Care 2008;53(11):1490–4.
83. Polat M, Tosun A, Ay Y, et al. Central core disease: atypical case with respiratory insufficiency in an intensive care unit. J Child Neurol 2006;21(2):173–4.
84. Pinard JM, Azabou E, Essid N, et al. Sleep-disordered breathing in children with congenital muscular dystrophies. Eur J Paediatr Neurol 2012. http://dx.doi.org/10.1016/j.ejpn.2012.02.009.

85. Barbe F, Quera-Salva MA, de Lattre J, et al. Long-term effects of nasal intermittent positive-pressure ventilation on pulmonary function and sleep architecture in patients with neuromuscular diseases. Chest 1996;110(5):1179–83.

86. Quera Salva MA, Blumen M, Jacquette A, et al. Sleep disorders in childhood-onset myotonic dystrophy type 1. Neuromuscul Disord 2006;16(9–10):564–70.

87. Pincherle A, Patruno V, Raimondi P, et al. Sleep breathing disorders in 40 Italian patients with Myotonic dystrophy type 1. Neuromuscul Disord 2012;22(3):219–24.

88. Romigi A, Izzi F, Pisani V, et al. Sleep disorders in adult-onset myotonic dystrophy type 1: a controlled polysomnographic study. Eur J Neurol 2011; 18(9):1139–45.

89. Yu H, Laberge L, Jaussent I, et al. Daytime sleepiness and REM sleep characteristics in myotonic dystrophy: a case-control study. Sleep 2011;34(2):165–70.

90. Laberge L, Bégin P, Montplaisir J, et al. Sleep complaints in patients with myotonic dystrophy. J Sleep Res 2004;13(1):95–100.

91. Ciafaloni E, Mignot E, Sansone V, et al. The hypocretin neurotransmission system in myotonic dystrophy type 1. Neurology 2008;70(3):226–30.

92. Iwata T, Suzuki N, Mizuno H, et al. A marked decrease of orexin in the cerebrospinal fluid in a patient with myotonic dystrophy type 1 showing an excessive daytime sleepiness. Rinsho Shinkeigaku 2009;49(7):437–9 [in Japanese].

93. Martínez-Rodríguez JE, Lin L, Iranzo A, et al. Decreased hypocretin-1 (Orexin-A) levels in the cerebrospinal fluid of patients with myotonic dystrophy and excessive daytime sleepiness. Sleep 2003;26(3):287–90.

94. Giubilei F, Antonini G, Bastianello S, et al. Excessive daytime sleepiness in myotonic dystrophy. J Neurol Sci 1999;164(1):60–3.

95. Tieleman AA, Knoop H, van de Logt AE, et al. Poor sleep quality and fatigue but no excessive daytime sleepiness in myotonic dystrophy type 2. J Neurol Neurosurg Psychiatry 2010;81(9):963–7.

96. Bhat S, Sander HW, Grewal RP, et al. Sleep disordered breathing and other sleep dysfunction in myotonic dystrophy type 2. Sleep Med, in press.

97. Chokroverty S, Bhat S, Rosen D, et al. REM behavior disorder in myotonic dystrophy type 2. Neurology 2012;78(24):2004.

98. Nicolle MW, Rask S, Koopman WJ, et al. Sleep apnea in patients with myasthenia gravis. Neurology 2006;67(1):140–2.

99. Shintani S, Shiozawa Z, Shindo K, et al. Sleep apnea in well-controlled myasthenia gravis. Rinsho Shinkeigaku 1989;29(5):547–53 [in Japanese].

100. Stepansky R, Weber G, Zeitlhofer J. Sleep apnea in myasthenia gravis. Wien Med Wochenschr 1996;146(9–10):209–10 [in German].

101. Gajdos P, Quera Salva MA. Respiratory disorders during sleep and myasthenia. Rev Neurol (Paris) 2001;157(11 Pt 2):S145–7 [in French].

102. Manni R, Piccolo G, Sartori I, et al. Breathing during sleep in myasthenia gravis. Ital J Neurol Sci 1995;16(9):589–94.

103. Prudlo J, Koenig J, Ermert S, et al. Sleep disordered breathing in medically stable patients with myasthenia gravis. Eur J Neurol 2007;14(3):321–6.

104. Karkare K, Sinha S, Taly AB, et al. Prevalence and profile of sleep disturbances in Guillain-Barré Syndrome: a prospective questionnaire-based study during 10 days of hospitalization. Acta Neurol Scand 2012. http://dx.doi.org/10.1111/j.1600-0404.2012.01688.

105. Cochen V, Arnulf I, Demeret S, et al. Vivid dreams, hallucinations, psychosis and REM sleep in Guillain-Barré syndrome. Brain 2005;128(Pt 11):2535–45.

106. Nishino S, Kanbayashi T, Fujiki N, et al. CSF hypocretin levels in Guillain-Barré syndrome and other inflammatory neuropathies. Neurology 2003;61(6):823–5.

107. Koeppen S, Kraywinkel K, Wessendorf TE, et al. Long-term outcome of Guillain-Barré syndrome. Neurocrit Care 2006;5(3):235–42.

108. Dziewas R, Waldmann N, Böntert M, et al. Increased prevalence of obstructive sleep apnoea in patients with Charcot-Marie-Tooth disease: a case control study. J Neurol Neurosurg Psychiatry 2008;7:829–31.

109. Dematteis M, Pépin JL, Jeanmart M, et al. Charcot-Marie-Tooth disease and sleep apnoea syndrome: a family study. Lancet 2001;357(9252):267–72.

110. Boentert M, Dziewas R, Heidbreder A, et al. Fatigue, reduced sleep quality and restless legs syndrome in Charcot-Marie-Tooth disease: a web-based survey. J Neurol 2010;257(4):646–52.

111. Barraclough A, Triplett J, Tuch P. Brachial neuritis with phrenic nerve involvement. J Clin Neurosci 2012;19(9):1301–2.

112. Chan CK, Mohsenin V, Loke J, et al. Diaphragmatic dysfunction in siblings with HMSN. Chest 1987;91:567–70.

113. Ostrowska M, de Carvalho M. Prognosis of phrenic nerve injury following thoracic interventions: four new cases and a review. Clin Neurol Neurosurg 2012;114(3):199–204.

Psychiatric Disorders and Sleep

Andrew D. Krystal, MD, MS

KEYWORDS

- Psychiatric disorders • Sleep • Insomnia • Depression • Anxiety
- Substance use disorders

KEY POINTS

- Psychiatric disorders can have a major impact on sleep.
- Sleep and sleep disorders can influence psychiatric conditions.
- Treatment of sleep disorders can improve psychiatric disorders.
- Sleep deprivation has a complex relationship with psychiatric disorders.

INTRODUCTION

It has long been appreciated that sleep problems are common among those with psychiatric disorders. The prevailing view has been that sleep problems are generally symptoms of the associated psychiatric conditions. Consistent with this point of view is that sleep problems are defining features of several psychiatric disorders and are included among the diagnostic criteria for these conditions.[1] However, there are several additional ways that psychiatric disorders and sleep are interrelated. The emerging view is that the relationships of psychiatric disorders with sleep are complex and are marked by bidirectional causality. For example, the long-standing view that treating some psychiatric conditions improves sleep is complemented by recent evidence suggesting that treating sleep disturbances can have important effects on the outcome of treatment of psychiatric conditions. Furthermore, contrary to the prevailing view, some sleep disorders increase the risks of developing episodes of psychiatric disorders. It is also the case that some treatments are used to treat both psychiatric disorders and sleep disorders.[2–6] Moreover, some treatments for psychiatric disorders may trigger disturbances of sleep, and some treatments for sleep

Disclosures: Grants/research support: NIH, Sanofi-Aventis, Cephalon, GlaxoSmithKline, Merck, Neurocrine, Pfizer, Sunovion/Sepracor, Somaxon, Takeda, Transcept, Phillips-Respironics, Neurogen, Evotec, Kingsdown Inc, Astellas, Abbott. Consultant: Abbott, Actelion, Arena, Astellas, Axiom, AstraZeneca, BMS, Cephalon, Eisai, Eli Lilly, GlaxoSmithKline, Jazz, Johnson and Johnson, King, Merck, Neurocrine, Neurogen, Novartis, Organon, Ortho-McNeil-Janssen, Pfizer, Respironics, Roche, Sanofi-Aventis, Somnus, Sunovion/Sepracor, Somaxon, Takeda, Transcept, Kingsdown Inc.
Sleep Research Laboratory and Insomnia Program, Department of Psychiatry, Duke University Medical Center, Box 3309, Durham, NC 27710, USA
E-mail address: kryst001@mc.duke.edu

disorders may increase the risks for psychiatric disorders.[7,8] A further complexity in the sleep–psychiatric disorders relationship is that sleep deprivation may have therapeutic effects for some psychiatric disorders but may aggravate others.[9] This article provides evidence that supports this point of view, reviewing data on sleep disturbances seen in patients with psychiatric disorders as well as data on the impact of sleep disturbances on psychiatric conditions. It is organized into 6 sections: (1) the sleep of patients with psychiatric disorders; (2) the risks of psychiatric disorders in those with sleep disturbances; (3) the impact of sleep disturbances on the course and treatment of psychiatric conditions; (4) the sleep effects of psychiatric treatments; (5) the impact of sleep deprivation on psychiatric disorders; and (6) a case report. This article is focused on the subset of psychiatric disorders that have the most important relationships with sleep: major depressive disorder (MDD; diagnostic criteria appear in **Box 1**); bipolar disorder (diagnostic criteria appear in **Box 2**); generalized anxiety disorder (GAD; diagnostic criteria appear in **Box 3**); posttraumatic stress disorder (PTSD) (diagnostic criteria appear in **Box 4**); schizophrenia (diagnostic criteria appear in **Box 5**); and alcoholism.[1]

THE SLEEP OF PATIENTS WITH PSYCHIATRIC DISORDERS
Major Depressive Disorder

Problems with sleep, which could include insomnia or hypersomnia, is one of the diagnostic criteria for MDD (see **Box 1**).[1] As such, it is not surprising that some type of sleep difficulty occurs in as many of 90% of MDD patients.[10] The type of sleep difficulty experienced by those with MDD can include difficulty falling asleep, difficulty staying asleep, insufficient sleep quality, nightmares, and daytime sleepiness. Troubles falling asleep and staying asleep have been documented polysomnographically; however, there are no studies finding objective evidence of daytime sleepiness with the multiple sleep latency test, the standard for clinical and research assessment of sleepiness.[11–14] Patients with MDD also appear to have alterations in their sleep stages that are evident with polysomnography, including: shortened latency to the

---

Box 1
Diagnostic criteria for MDD according to the *Diagnostic and Statistical Manual of Mental Disorders* (fourth edition, text revision) (DSM-IV TR)

The presence of 5 of the following 9 criteria symptoms over a period of at least 2 weeks whereby 1 of the 5 symptoms has to be either depressed mood or loss of interest or pleasure:

1. Depressed mood

2. Loss of interest or pleasure in activities

3. Change in appetite

4. Insomnia or hypersomnia

5. Psychomotor agitation or retardation

6. Fatigue

7. Feelings of worthlessness or guilt

8. Poor concentration and difficulty making decisions

9. Suicidal ideation

Data from American Psychiatric Association. Diagnostic and statistical manual of mental disorders. 4th edition. Text revision. Washington, DC: APA; 2000.

Box 2
DSM-IV TR diagnostic criteria for bipolar disorder

At least 1 manic episode that is defined by elevated or irritable mood accompanied by at least 3 associated symptoms, which could include:

1. Grandiosity

2. Decreased sleep need

3. Pressured speech

4. Flight of ideas

5. Easy distractibility

6. Increased goal-directed activity

7. Impulsivity

Data from American Psychiatric Association. Diagnostic and statistical manual of mental disorders. 4th edition. Text revision. Washington, DC: APA; 2000.

---

onset of rapid eye movement (REM) sleep (REM latency)[15–23]; increased number of eye movements per minute of REM sleep (REM density)[11,16,24,25]; increased percentage of the night that meets scoring criteria for REM sleep[11,14,23]; a longer duration of the first REM period[14,26,27]; and decreased amount of slow-wave sleep.[11,12,14,17,26,28]

The prolonged sleep onset and difficulties with sleep maintenance found in patients with MDD are established indicators of disturbance of sleep. However, the significance of the alterations in sleep stages seen in those with MDD is unknown. There is some evidence to suggest that shortened REM latency and diminished slow-wave sleep may be trait markers of MDD,[29–33] whereas the increased REM density and sleep disturbance appear to be state markers because they are most evident during episodes of depression.[30,34,35] However, these sleep-stage changes appear to be of limited clinical utility as they are not specific to those with MDD but are seen in those with other types of psychiatric disorders.[21]

Box 3
DSM-IV TR diagnostic criteria for GAD

Frequent excessive anxiety for at least 6 months that is accompanied by symptoms that may include:

Restlessness

Easy fatigability

Problems concentrating

Irritability

Muscle tension

Disturbed sleep

Data from American Psychiatric Association. Diagnostic and statistical manual of mental disorders. 4th edition. Text revision. Washington, DC: APA; 2000.

Box 4
DSM-IV TR diagnostic criteria for PTSD

A history of exposure to a traumatic event whereby the person has experienced, witnessed, or been confronted with an event or events that involve actual or threatened death or serious injury, or a threat to the physical integrity of oneself or others and the person's response involved intense fear, helplessness, or horror.

Duration is more than 1 month.

Is associated with clinically significant distress or impairment in social, occupational, or other important areas of functioning.

Symptoms from each of 3 symptom clusters below:

A. *Intrusive recollection*: The traumatic event is persistently re-experienced in at least one of the following ways:

  1. Recurrent and intrusive distressing recollections of the event, including images, thoughts, or perceptions. Note: in young children, repetitive play may occur in which themes or aspects of the trauma are expressed

  2. Recurrent distressing dreams of the event

  3. Acting or feeling as if the traumatic event were recurring (includes a sense of reliving the experience, illusions, hallucinations, and dissociative flashback episodes, including those that occur on awakening or when intoxicated). Note: in children, trauma-specific reenactment may occur

  4. Intense psychological distress at exposure to internal or external cues that symbolize or resemble an aspect of the traumatic event

  5. Physiologic reactivity on exposure to internal or external cues that symbolize or resemble an aspect of the traumatic event

B. *Avoidant/numbing*: Persistent avoidance of stimuli associated with the trauma and numbing of general responsiveness (not present before the trauma), as indicated by at least 3 of the following:

  1. Efforts to avoid thoughts, feelings, or conversations associated with the trauma

  2. Efforts to avoid activities, places, or people that arouse recollections of the trauma

  3. Inability to recall an important aspect of the trauma

  4. Markedly diminished interest or participation in significant activities

  5. Feeling of detachment or estrangement from others

  6. Restricted range of affect (eg, unable to have loving feelings)

  7. Sense of foreshortened future (eg, does not expect to have a career, marriage, children, or a normal life span)

C. *Hyperarousal*: Persistent symptoms of increasing arousal (not present before the trauma), indicated by at least 2 of the following:

  1. Difficulty falling or staying asleep

  2. Irritability or outbursts of anger

  3. Difficulty concentrating

  4. Hypervigilance

  5. Exaggerated startle response

Data from American Psychiatric Association. Diagnostic and statistical manual of mental disorders. 4th edition. Text revision. Washington, DC: APA; 2000.

Box 5
DSM-IV TR diagnostic criteria for schizophrenia

Social and/or occupational dysfunction occurring in the setting of at least 1 month whereby 2 or more of the following occur:

1. Delusions

2. Hallucinations

3. Disorganized speech

4. Disorganized behavior

5. Loss of motivation, flat affect, or alogia

Data from American Psychiatric Association. Diagnostic and statistical manual of mental disorders. 4th edition. Text revision. Washington, DC: APA; 2000.

Bipolar Disorder

For the manic phase of bipolar disorder, the diagnostic criteria include decreased need for sleep.[1] Therefore, as with MDD, it is not surprising that changes in sleep are nearly universal among those with bipolar mania.[36] However, the nature of the sleep problem in this condition, namely decreased need for sleep, is an alteration in sleep that is only seen in mania. Decreased need for sleep is not synonymous with insomnia. It is a condition whereby an individual can, and does, decrease one's sleep time, at least to some degree, without experiencing any impairment in function or quality of life. By contrast, insomnia is a condition whereby individuals experience impairments in function and/or quality of life caused by failing to experience sleep despite having the adequate opportunity to do so.[1] Diagnostic confusion might arise because those with mania may experience difficulties falling and staying asleep, much like insomnia patients. However, in the case of manic patients this problem arises because they are attempting to sleep more than the amount they need to be restored, whereas insomnia patients are unable to sleep enough to feel restored despite their efforts to do so.

During the depressed phase of bipolar disorder, the most common sleep complaint is hypersomnia, which reportedly occurs more frequently in those with bipolar depression than with unipolar depression.[37] The little research performed to determine if there is objective evidence of daytime sleepiness in patients with bipolar depression using the multiple sleep latency test has not found evidence of clinically significant sleepiness.[37]

The alterations in sleep seen with polysomnography in patients with bipolar mania are comparable with what has been observed in those with MDD.[38,39] This finding may indicate that there is a common pathophysiology in MDD and bipolar mania. However, it is important to keep in mind that these polysomnographic findings are also seen in those with other psychiatric conditions and, therefore, may not be reflective of specific pathophysiologic mechanisms.[21]

Generalized Anxiety Disorder

As with MDD and bipolar disorder, a change in sleep is among the core features of GAD. In this case the alteration is disturbance of sleep (difficulty falling or staying asleep), which affects over half of those with GAD.[1,40–42]

Few data exist on the polysomnographic features that characterize the sleep of patients with GAD. However, those that exist suggest that GAD patients have longer sleep onset latency, a greater number of arousals, and greater wake time during the night.[43,44] In contrast to bipolar disorder and MDD, GAD does not appear to be marked by any alterations in REM latency or percentage of the night comprising REM sleep. However, one study reported that compared with controls, GAD patients had a decreased percentage of the night spent in slow-wave sleep and a relative increase in the percentage of the night meeting criteria for stage 1 sleep.[43,44]

Posttraumatic Stress Disorder

Sleep problems are also among the diagnostic criteria for PTSD, although in this case the sleep difficulties include distressing dreams along with difficulties falling or staying asleep.[1] Accordingly, complaints of sleep difficulties are ubiquitous among those who have PTSD.[45]

Several studies including polysomnography have examined the sleep of patients with PTSD in an effort to explore the associated neurophysiologic changes.[46–50] The most consistent findings suggest disruption of sleep and include diminished total sleep time, which has been reported in 5 studies, and an elevation in the time spent awake after initially falling asleep (WASO), which has been noted in 3 reports.[46–50] In one additional study, there was an association between an increase in WASO and nightmares.[51] However, it should be noted that there are several studies that have not found evidence for sleep difficulties polysomnographically in PTSD patients.[52] This inconsistency may not be specific to PTSD, however. There is evidence that among patients with insomnia complaints occurring in other settings, there is often a weak relationship between polysomnographic and self-report measures of sleep.[53,54]

Another frequent polysomnographic finding in PTSD patients is an alteration in REM sleep, such as is seen in those with MDD and bipolar disorder. The most frequently reported REM sleep aberration has been an increase in REM density (eye movements per minute of REM sleep).[46,47,49] As already discussed, this measure of the "intensity" of REM sleep does not reflect a physiologic alteration specific to PTSD because it has also been reported to be elevated in those with MDD, which has a high-rate of comorbidity with PTSD.[55]

Schizophrenia

In contrast to the psychiatric disorders already discussed, sleep is not a core feature of schizophrenia. However, sleep problems, including difficulty falling and staying asleep and diminished sleep quality, are common in those suffering from schizophrenia, although systematic epidemiologic data on the prevalence of sleep disturbances in this population do not exist.[56–60] An additional type of sleep problem that has been reported to affect people with schizophrenia is shifts in circadian rhythm, which are reflected in a tendency to be awake at night and sleep during the day.[57,61] The reason for this is unknown; however, some have speculated that alcohol and illicit drug use or antipsychotic medications used to treat schizophrenia might play a role.

Several studies using polysomnography have attempted to characterize the neurophysiologic changes in sleep in persons with schizophrenia, and have identified the following differences from healthy controls: increased latency to sleep onset, increased wake time during the night, decreased total sleep time, decreased latency to the onset of REM sleep, decreased amount of slow-wave sleep, and a decrease in the amplitude of electroencephalogram (EEG) slow waves during non-REM sleep.[60,62–72]

In addition, those with schizophrenia have been identified to experience other sleep disorders at a relatively higher rate than the general population, including an increase in the prevalence of sleep-disordered breathing (15%) and periodic limb movements of sleep.[73]

Alcoholism

Two types of problems related to alcohol use can occur: dependence and abuse. Dependence is characterized by an adaptation occurring with repeated alcohol use that results in tolerance to the effects of alcohol and withdrawal symptoms occurring on discontinuation.[1] Abuse, on the other hand, is defined by problems arising in an individual's life as a result of adverse consequences deriving from the direct effects of alcohol.[1] Insomnia is extremely common among those who suffer from alcohol dependence and/or abuse, the prevalence of which is estimated to be 36% to 72%.[74–76] It is believed that the sleep disturbance stems from a rebound of wakefulness occurring as the effects of alcohol, which has sleep-promoting effects, wear off. In this regard, it has been reported that alcohol hastens sleep onset, suppresses REM sleep, and relatively increases the amount of non-REM sleep.[77] However, the effects are relatively short-lived and, as the sleep-enhancing effects dissipate through the night, a predisposition to sleep disruption and increased REM activity occur.[78] This problem is exacerbated as tolerance develops to the sleep-enhancing effects with repeated use.[1,21,79]

Like those with schizophrenia, those suffering from alcoholism may experience disruption of the usual circadian sleep-wake rhythm, which is also believed to derive from the sleep-enhancing effects of alcohol. It is hypothesized that regular daytime drinking may predispose to regular daytime sleeping, which tends to erode the usual circadian sleep rhythm.[78]

The sleep problems of those with alcohol-related problems are not restricted to periods when alcohol ingestion is occurring. The available evidence suggests that following periods of regular alcohol use, sleep disturbance may persist throughout several years of abstinence, during which a relative increase in REM sleep has been documented.[80]

THE RISKS OF PSYCHIATRIC DISORDERS IN THOSE WITH SLEEP DISTURBANCES

The risks of psychiatric disorders in those with sleep disturbances are less well appreciated than the sleep disturbances associated with psychiatric disorders. Nevertheless, the evidence that sleep disturbances are associated with an increased risk of developing psychiatric disorders has existed since the 1980s.

MDD

In terms of MDD, this evidence includes the suggestion that those with insomnia and those with hypersomnia are roughly 10 times as likely to have MDD as healthy controls without sleep disorders.[81–83] Also, a series of longitudinal studies indicate that having insomnia at one point in time significantly increases the risk for the subsequent development of new-onset MDD.[83–85]

GAD

There are also longitudinal data indicating that insomnia increases the risk for the subsequent development of anxiety disorders. Those with insomnia appear to have approximately double the risk of healthy controls.[81]

PTSD

To date there is no evidence suggesting that preexisting insomnia is a predisposing factor for the development of PTSD syndrome following an extreme event, although apparently no studies have specifically investigated this question. There is, however, one study suggesting that sleep complaints occurring at 1 month or longer after trauma were significant predictors of the presence of a diagnosis of PTSD at 1 year post trauma.[86] Though intriguing, this report is of uncertain significance.

Schizophrenia

Severe disturbance of sleep has been noted to occur before the development of episodes of acute psychotic decompensation in patients with schizophrenia.[59,87,88] However, it remains unknown whether this sleep disturbance is a harbinger of impending difficulties, or if it has any causal relationship.

Alcoholism

There is a body of evidence suggesting that sleep difficulties may increase the risks for alcoholism and may contribute to continued alcohol consumption among drinkers. Several longitudinal studies suggest that those with insomnia are at increased risk for the development of subsequent problems related to alcohol use in comparison with those without disturbed sleep.[81,89,90] Several studies suggest that those with alcoholism often use alcohol as a means to treat sleep difficulties. For instance, such individuals are more likely than those without alcoholism to choose alcohol as a way to improve sleep, and to report difficulty falling asleep if they do not drink alcohol before going to bed.[75,91,92]

THE IMPACT OF SLEEP DISTURBANCES ON THE COURSE AND TREATMENT OF PSYCHIATRIC CONDITIONS

There is a growing body of literature indicating that sleep disturbances affect the course and treatment of psychiatric conditions. Such reports include studies on the relationship between sleep disturbance and psychiatric symptoms as well as the relationship with treatment outcome and the risk of relapse in psychiatric conditions. Studies also document the impact of treating sleep disorders on the outcome of psychiatric conditions.

MDD

Though long thought of as a symptom of depression, insomnia appears to have an impact on the course and treatment response of MDD.[93] According to the symptom model, sleep disturbance would be expected to resolve with appropriate antidepressant therapy along with the other MDD symptoms. Although this certainly occurs to a degree, the available evidence suggests that in 20% to 44% of those with MDD, sleep difficulties fail to resolve despite the administration of standard antidepressant treatments.[90,94] This residual insomnia also appears to be associated with an increased risk of MDD relapse as well as several impairments including decreased concentration, sleepiness, and diminished performance capacity.[95,96]

Among those with MDD, there are several other ways that poor sleep appears to have an adverse impact on the course of MDD. Perhaps the most important and most concerning of these is that sleep disturbance appears to increase the risks of suicidal ideation, suicide attempts, and completed suicide. To date, at least 32 studies have identified that sleep disturbance is linked to suicidal ideation or completed suicide, including: 10 studies in children and adolescents; 22 studies in younger and older adults; and studies spanning multiple countries (United States, England, France, Canada, Turkey, Finland, Sweden, Brazil, China, and Japan).[97–112] Of note, these studies include 5 prospective studies, and in many the associations between sleep disturbance and suicidality remained after adjusting for depression severity.

However, despite all the evidence linking insomnia and suicidality, insomnia is generally overlooked as a suicide risk factor and as a means of preventing suicide in those with MDD.[113]

Sleep disturbance also has other adverse effects on the course of MDD. Those MDD patients with poor sleep have slower treatment response and lower remission rates than those without sleep disturbance.[114–117] Greater sleep disturbance is also independently correlated (independent of depression severity) with poorer quality of life in those with MDD.[118]

There is additional evidence to support the independent importance of disturbed sleep in MDD, and these data speak to the need to target treatment specifically to the sleep problems in those with MDD. Several studies indicate that targeting treatment to insomnia in addition to providing standard antidepressant therapy may not only improve sleep but also enhance the improvement in depression. In one such study, the hypnotics lormetazepam and flurazepam were compared with placebo as adjunctive insomnia therapies to antidepressant treatment with nortriptyline or maprotiline.[119] Those subjects randomized to lormetazepam had greater improvement in depression than subjects receiving placebo. In another study, coadministration of eszopiclone, 3 mg and fluoxetine led to greater improvement in sleep and a more rapid and greater improvement in depression (greater improvement in the Hamilton Depression Rating Scale with sleep items removed and greater percentage of responders and remitters) than fluoxetine plus placebo.[120,121] However, it should be noted that a study of identical design using zolpidem extended-release preparation 12.5 mg instead of eszopiclone found that insomnia therapy improved sleep and sleep-related daytime function but not depression outcome in comparison with placebo.[122] Lastly, a study was performed in which cognitive behavioral insomnia was compared with a behavioral control intervention in depressed patients treated with escitalopram.[123] In this study, those receiving the active insomnia therapy experienced a 62% remission rate compared with 33% for the control intervention.

Thus, 3 of 4 studies indicate that targeting treatment to insomnia improves not only sleep outcome but also response to depression treatment. In the one study where this was not the case, sleep and function were improved; however, it remains unclear as to why depression outcome did not improve.[122] Further studies will be needed to better understand the impact of insomnia therapy on MDD treatment outcomes. Nonetheless, multiple lines of research suggest that sleep disturbance has a substantial impact on MDD and the antidepressant response, and generally speak to the need to treat insomnia in those with MDD.

Bipolar Disorder

Relatively less research has been performed on the impact of sleep on the course of bipolar disorder. However, several studies indicate that preventing patients with bipolar disorder from sleeping predisposes them to the development of mania.[124–126] On this basis it has been hypothesized that sleep loss plays an etiologic role in the development of mania such that loss of sleep predisposes toward mania which, in turn, leads to further loss of sleep in a positive feedback cycle.[124]

Whether this is the case remains unclear, as are the mechanisms whereby sleep loss might predispose patients with bipolar disorder to develop mania. However, the clinical implications of this hypothesis are that management of bipolar patients should include interventions to prevent sleep loss and lengthen sleep time as a means of preventing and/or treating mania. Although this approach has yet to be systematically studied, it is probably no accident that all antimanic therapies have significant sleep-enhancing effects.

GAD

Relatively few data exist on the impact of sleep on the course of GAD. However, 2 placebo-controlled trials of adding insomnia cotherapy to the treatment of GAD with escitalopram have been performed.[127,128] These studies include a trial of eszopiclone, 3 mg plus escitalopram versus placebo plus escitalopram, and a trial of zolpidem extended-release, 12.5 mg plus escitalopram versus placebo plus escitalopram. Much like the results seen in nearly identical studies performed with MDD patients, eszopiclone significantly improved sleep and GAD response/remission compared with placebo, whereas zolpidem extended-release only improved sleep and sleep-associated daytime function compared with placebo. As with MDD, these studies support the utility and importance of targeted insomnia therapy in GAD patients. However, it remains unclear whether the treatment of insomnia might affect GAD outcome or whether there are specific characteristics of eszopiclone or zolpidem extended-release that may have affected their impact on GAD outcome.

PTSD

There are several placebo-controlled studies demonstrating that treatments aimed at improving sleep in patients with PTSD can improve daytime PTSD symptoms, including one study of eszopiclone, 3 mg administered at bedtime, 4 studies of prazosin administered at bedtime, and 1 study of a behavioral sleep intervention targeting insomnia and nightmares.[129–133] However, whether these sleep-targeted therapies have direct effects on daytime PTSD symptoms or whether daytime PTSD symptoms are improved because of improvements in sleep has not been definitively established. At least for prazosin, there is evidence that this agent improves daytime PTSD symptoms when administered during the day, so it is at least plausible that nighttime administration could directly improve daytime PTSD symptoms. While the half-life of this drug (2–4 hours) seems to preclude this possibility, it must be borne in mind that this medication has several active metabolites that could contribute to its therapeutic effect.[134] There are no data that indicate whether eszopiclone or behavioral sleep therapy might have direct effects on daytime PTSD symptoms.

Schizophrenia

Several studies suggest that disturbed sleep can adversely affect the symptoms and course of schizophrenia. In one study, self-ratings of sleep quality were significantly correlated with quality-of-life ratings.[57] As described earlier, sleep problems often occur before episodes with acute psychotic symptoms, although it is unclear whether sleep disturbance plays an etiologic role in these episodes or if it is simply the first symptom of decompensation.[59,72,88] A series of studies have also identified associations between polysomnographic sleep indices and the presence of subsets of schizophrenia symptoms, classified as either positive (delusions, hallucinations, and disorganized thought) or negative (affective flattening, avolition, alogia, attention problems). Greater positive-symptom severity has been found to be correlated with shorter REM latency, longer sleep-onset latency, and diminished sleep efficiency (total sleep time divided by time in bed).[65,71,87,135–137] At the same time greater negative-symptom severity has been found to be correlated with lower non-REM sleep EEG slow-wave amplitude and shorter REM-onset latency.[60,68,69,71,138] Furthermore, a greater likelihood of suicidal ideation has been found to be correlated with a greater percentage of the night spent in REM sleep and greater REM density (rapid eye movements per minute of REM sleep).[139,140] The clinical significance and pathophysiologic implications of these findings remain uncertain, as the polysomnographic alterations described are not specific to schizophrenia and the findings have not been consistently found across studies.

Alcoholism

Several studies suggest that sleep problems and polysomnographic alterations in sleep occurring after abstinence may play an important role in hastening relapse. The link between disturbed sleep during abstinence and relapse to drinking has been identified in several studies.[75,79,141] Polysomnographic sleep variables that have been found to be predictors of relapse include longer sleep-onset latency, decreased sleep efficiency, decreased percentage of the night spent in slow-wave sleep, shorter REM-onset latency, greater percentage of the night spent in REM sleep, and greater REM density.[142,143] The variable that best predicts relapse seems to vary with the duration of time since the abstinence period began, although this may not in fact be the case but may reflect that the findings are variable across studies that happened to focus on different time periods. Increased REM density immediately after stopping drinking has been reported to be the best predictor of relapse 3 to 4 months later. However, at 1 month after the onset of abstinence sleep-onset latency was found to be the best predictor of relapse, whereas at 5 months after the beginning of the abstinence period sleep-onset latency and sleep efficiency best predicted relapse at 1 year.[78,80,144]

Although these studies speak to the need to evaluate whether the treatment of sleep disturbances during abstinence might decrease the likelihood of relapse, only 2 placebo-controlled studies have been performed that address this question, both of which were small trials. One was a study of trazodone, 200 mg, which included only 16 subjects and found that this medication improved sleep compared with placebo but had no impact on relapse rate, although it could be reasonably argued that the study was underpowered to assess this outcome.[145] The other study evaluated gabapentin, 1500 mg in only 21 subjects and, although there was a decrease in relapse rate, there was no difference between drug and placebo groups regarding sleep parameters.[146]

Based on the limited amount of work performed, it remains unclear whether treating sleep problems during abstinence decreases the rate of subsequent relapse to drinking, and studies addressing this issue are clearly needed.

THE SLEEP EFFECTS OF PSYCHIATRIC TREATMENTS
MDD

Many antidepressant medications have been documented to have effects on polysomnographic sleep variables. Some are used to treat sleep disturbance, some have a tendency to disturb sleep, and some have a tendency to cause or exacerbate periodic leg movements of sleep (PLMS) and/or restless legs syndrome. In terms of the effects of antidepressant on polysomnographic sleep indices, several studies have documented that antidepressant treatments including monoamine oxidase inhibitors, tricyclic antidepressants electroconvulsive therapy, selective serotonin reuptake inhibitors, and serotonin-norepinephrine reuptake inhibitors, suppress REM sleep.[21,147–153] These findings have served as the basis for the hypothesis that suppression of REM sleep is an important part of the mechanism of action of antidepressant therapies. However, evidence to the contrary is provided by several effective antidepressant agents, bupropion, nefazodone, mirtazapine, and trazodone, which do not suppress REM sleep,[154] although these medications appear to have other polysomnographic effects including increasing the amount of slow-wave sleep and increasing the amplitude of EEG slow-waves in non-REM sleep.[155–160]

Several antidepressants are also used to treat problems falling and/or staying asleep and are used for the treatment of insomnia, although few have been demonstrated to have therapeutic effects in placebo-controlled studies. The antidepressants most commonly used for this purpose are trazodone, mirtazapine, amitriptyline, and doxepin, which, other than mirtazapine are prescribed in lower dosages than typically used to treat depression when administered to treat insomnia.[2] Data from placebo-controlled trials supporting a sleep onset and/or maintenance exist only for doxepin and trimipramine, although studies performed in depressed patients or healthy controls suggest that amitriptyline and mirtazapine might have therapeutic effects in this setting.[157,161–171]

Another sleep-related effect of antidepressant medications is that some can disturb sleep. The norepinephrine and dopamine reuptake inhibitor bupropion, selective serotonin reuptake inhibitors, and serotonin norepinephrine reuptake inhibitors all have an adverse effect rate of insomnia/sleep disturbance that is in the range of 1.5 to 3 times that of placebo.[154]

Many antidepressants also have the potential to cause or exacerbate PLMS and restless legs syndrome.[172] Agents most often associated with this are selective serotonin reuptake inhibitors, serotonin norepinephrine reuptake inhibitors, and mirtazapine.[172,173]

Bipolar Disorder

Few studies document the sleep effects of agents used to treat bipolar disorder. Most of the available relevant data relate to antipsychotic medications that are often used to treat mania. The sleep effects of these agents are discussed in the next section. Otherwise, data exist only for lithium, long a mainstay of the treatment of patients with bipolar disorder. This agent has been found to increase slow-wave sleep, suppress REM sleep, and increase REM latency.[174] Like many of the antidepressant medications, lithium has also been reported to cause or exacerbate restless legs syndrome.[175]

Schizophrenia

Several publications document the sleep effects of antipsychotic medications, the most common pharmacologic therapies administered to patients with schizophrenia. The sleep-related effect of these medications that is of most clinical importance is their tendency to enhance sleep. This effect may be responsible for daytime sedation, which may further impair the already limited daytime functional capacity of many patients with schizophrenia, although for patients with disturbed sleep this type of effect may be beneficial.[176] Systematic studies of the effects of antipsychotic medications have been performed in patients with mood disorders, those with schizophrenia, and healthy controls. Both quetiapine (25 and 100 mg) and ziprasidone (40 mg) were evaluated in trials in healthy controls where sleep during a night with noise disturbance was compared with a night during which no disturbance took place.[177,178] Quetiapine was found to shorten sleep-onset latency and to improve total sleep time, sleep efficiency, and sleep quality, and also suppressed REM sleep.[177] Ziprasidone increased total sleep time, sleep efficiency, and sleep quality, and decreased the number of awakenings, but also decreased the percentage of REM and increased REM density and the percentage of slow-wave sleep.[178] Several relatively small studies document the sleep effects of olanzapine. These studies were performed in those with schizophrenia and those with mood disorders, and indicate that this medication decreases sleep-onset latency and wake time after sleep onset and increases sleep efficiency, sleep-quality ratings, and the amount and percentage of slow-wave sleep.[179–186] Small studies also document that clozapine decreases awakenings and wake time after sleep onset, and increases total sleep time and amount of slow-wave sleep,[187,188] and that risperidone, 0.5 to 1 mg decreases wake time after sleep onset as well as the amount of REM sleep.[189]

Because so few data exist on the sleep effects of these agents that derive from placebo-controlled trials, it is helpful to consider the rates of reported daytime sedation adverse effects in placebo-controlled trials with these medications, although in some cases daytime sedation may not be accompanied by nighttime sleep enhancement because of slow absorption, and in the case of agents with short half-lives, daytime somnolence rates will substantially underestimate their nighttime sleep enhancement. Based on these data the agents with the highest rates of sedation are clozapine, chlorpromazine, and thioridazine (33%–60%), followed by risperidone and olanzapine (approximately 30%) and haloperidol (23%), whereas the agents with the least associated sedation are quetiapine and ziprasidone (16%) and aripiprazole (12%).[176]

Because of their dopamine antagonism, antipsychotic medications may also cause or exacerbate PLMS and restless legs syndrome and, owing to the potential for weight gain, these agents may increase the risks of developing sleep-disordered breathing.[176]

Alcoholism

Only one study has been performed regarding the sleep effects of a treatment for alcoholism. This study evaluated acamprosate in 24 subjects before and 2 weeks after discontinuation of alcohol consumption, and found that it decreased wake time after sleep onset and shortened REM latency.[190]

THE IMPACT OF SLEEP DEPRIVATION ON PSYCHIATRIC DISORDERS

A notable, and perhaps surprising, aspect of the relationship of sleep and psychiatric disorders is that sleep deprivation can have a profound effect on individuals with mood disorders.

MDD

A night of sleep deprivation has been reported to have robust antidepressant effects. Studies evaluating this phenomenon suggest that at least 50% of those with MDD meet response criteria following a single night of sleep deprivation.[191–193] However, the clinical utility of sleep deprivation as an antidepressant treatment is limited by the fact that the benefits generally disappear when the treated patient sleeps, even if the period of sleep is short.[193,194] Attempts to prolong the benefits of sleep deprivation with medications and other interventions have met with limited success,[195,196] such that sleep deprivation is not implemented as a treatment for depression in clinical practice to any significant extent. However, it continues to attract attention as a window into the pathophysiology of MDD and the mechanisms of action of antidepressant treatments.

There is also limited literature related to attempts to treat MDD with chronic (3 weeks), in-laboratory, REM sleep deprivation, which is based on the evidence that many effective antidepressant therapies suppress REM sleep.[197] Unlike a night of total sleep deprivation, one study found that chronic REM deprivation leads to gradual and persistent improvement in depression,[197] although attempts to replicate this finding have not succeeded in doing so.

Bipolar Disorder

In contrast to MDD, sleep deprivation tends to exacerbate symptoms in those with bipolar disorder, predisposing individuals with this condition to develop mania. A series of studies whereby patients with bipolar disorder underwent experimental sleep deprivation provide the basis for this conclusion.[36,124–126] The mechanism by which sleep deprivation predisposes patients with bipolar disorder to mania remains unknown. Furthermore, sleep deprivation has never been demonstrated to trigger or exacerbate mania in naturalistic studies in patients with bipolar disorder. However, it is generally assumed that this occurs; therefore, prudent clinical care should include taking steps to prevent sleep loss in those with bipolar disorder when depressed and/or euthymic, and to increase sleep in bipolar patients when manic.

SUMMARY

Psychiatric disorders and sleep are related in important ways. In contrast to the long-standing view of this relationship that viewed sleep problems as symptoms of psychiatric disorders,[93] there is growing experimental evidence that the relationship between psychiatric disorders and sleep is complex and includes bidirectional causation. Although much has been learned about the psychiatric disorders–sleep relationship, much remains unknown. For example, further studies are needed to determine whether improvement of sleep improves MDD outcome and why some treatments for sleep problems appear to differentially affect the antidepressant response. In some cases correlations have been identified between alterations in sleep and the course and/or outcome of psychiatric conditions, and further work will be needed to determine if these are causal links.

From a clinical point of view, the available research on the psychiatric disorder–sleep relationship speaks to the need to direct treatment toward sleep disorders and not simply to treat what is assumed to be an underlying psychiatric condition. There is some reason to believe that this has the potential to improve the course and treatment response of some psychiatric conditions. This work also speaks to the need to be aware of the sleep effects of psychiatric interventions, which may in turn affect the course and treatment response of the psychiatric condition being treated.

There are also research implications of the body of literature elucidating the psychiatric disorder–sleep relationship. This literature suggests that the boundaries between sleep disorders and some psychiatric disorders may be indistinct and that in many cases the causal relationships between them are unclear. Nonetheless, the work in this field has increased over time and our understanding of these causal relationships has significantly evolved from the long-held symptom model of sleep disturbance.[93] Although much additional research is needed to address the limitations of the current body of literature and to help us better understand the relationships between psychiatric disorders and sleep, the advances made to date suggest that this work promises to improve our understanding of both sleep and psychiatric conditions, and to provide better clinical care for patients with psychiatric disorders and sleep disorders.

Case study

Ms B. is a 39-year-old woman with 2 children who had no history of sleep problems until approximately 1 year ago when she lost her job. At that point she developed problems falling asleep and staying asleep, which were associated with fatigue, anxiety, irritability, and difficulty with concentration. Four months after she lost her job she got a new job, which she liked, but her sleep problems did not improve. As a result, she made an appointment to see her primary care provider and was given a handout that listed good sleep hygiene practices and was told that she should get diphenhydramine from the drug store and take 25 to 50 mg at bedtime. She followed the sleep hygiene rules on the handout and began taking the diphenhydramine, but it caused her to be "fuzzy-headed" during the day so she stopped using it after only 2 nights. Her sleep problems subsequently worsened so she returned to her primary care provider, who referred her to the Sleep Clinic for an evaluation.

At the Sleep Clinic a careful evaluation was performed. Ms B. reported that she was currently taking no medications, had no medical illnesses, and no prior history of psychiatric disorder. She denied daytime sleepiness and had no symptoms suggestive of a breathing-related sleep disorder, restless legs syndrome, or periodic movements of sleep. She had impeccable sleep hygiene. She had no family history of sleep problems but she did have a positive family history of major depression (mother and sister). She had no history of substance-use disorders, did not drink alcohol, and had no history of mania, psychosis, or anxiety problems other than anxiety about her sleep. However, 2 months before the evaluation she: began to stay at home more; lost interest in her book club and stopped enjoying spending time with friends; had to struggle to get herself to do her usual childcare activities that she had always enjoyed; developed crying spells; lost her appetite, losing 12 lb in the last 2 months without intending to lose weight; felt hopeless about sleeping better or feeling better; and increasingly worried about her worsening sleep problem.

She was diagnosed with major depression and comorbid insomnia. Treatment with a sedating antidepressant such as mirtazapine or a tricyclic antidepressant was suggested as a means to treat both the depression and the sleep difficulty. However, she did not want to take these medications because of the risks of weight gain and sexual dysfunction. As a result, she was treated with a nonsedating antidepressant, bupropion XL, 150 mg every day along with a sleep-targeted therapy, eszopiclone (3 mg). After she began treatment with this regimen her sleep immediately improved. Other symptoms of depression were somewhat improved at a 3-week follow-up visit. At that point her bupropion XL was increased to 300 mg daily. At a 6-week follow-up appointment her sleep and depression symptoms were absent. At 12 weeks after initiating treatment an attempt was made to taper the eszopiclone; however, her sleep difficulties returned. As a result, the eszopiclone was restarted and her sleep difficulties again improved. After 6 months of treatment an attempt to taper the eszopiclone was successfully made without return of sleep difficulties. Her bupropion XL was continued for another 6 months and subsequently discontinued. She remained free of depression and sleep difficulties through her last follow-up visit, which took place 1 year later.

REFERENCES

1. American Psychiatric Association. Diagnostic and statistical manual of mental disorders, 4th edition, text revision. Washington, DC: APA; 2000.
2. Krystal AD. A compendium of placebo-controlled trials of the risks/benefits of pharmacological treatments for insomnia: the empirical basis for U.S. clinical practice. Sleep Med Rev 2009;13(4):265–74.
3. Walsh JK, Schweitzer PK. Ten-year trends in pharmacologic treatment of insomnia. Sleep 1999;22:371–5.
4. Thorpy M. Current concepts in the etiology, diagnosis and treatment of narcolepsy. Sleep Med 2001;2:5–17.
5. Santosh PJ, Taylor E. Stimulant drugs. Eur Child Adolesc Psychiatry 2000; 9(Suppl 1):127–43.

6. Nierenberg AA, Dougherty D, Rosenbaum JF. Dopaminergic agents and stimulants as antidepressant augmentation strategies. J Clin Psychiatry 1998; 59(Suppl 5):60–3.
7. Bakshi R. Fluoxetine and restless legs syndrome. J Neurol Sci 1996;142(1–2): 151–2.
8. Baran AS, Richert AC. Obstructive sleep apnea and depression. CNS Spectr 2003;8:128–34.
9. Giedke H, Schwarzler F. Therapeutic use of sleep deprivation in depression. Sleep Med Rev 2002;6:361–77.
10. Thase ME. Antidepressant treatment of the depressed patient with insomnia. J Clin Psychiatry 1999;60(Suppl 17):28–31.
11. Waller DA, Hardy BW, Pole R, et al. Sleep EEG in bulemic, depressed and normal subjects. Biol Psychiatry 1989;25:661–4.
12. Kupfer DJ, Ulrich RF, Coble PA, et al. Electroencephalographic sleep of younger depressives. Arch Gen Psychiatry 1985;42:806–10.
13. Gillin JC, Duncan WC, Pettigrew KD, et al. Successful separation of depressed, normal and insomniac subjects by EEG sleep data. Arch Gen Psychiatry 1979; 36:85–90.
14. Berger M, Doerr P, Lund RD, et al. Neuroendocrinological and neurophysiological studies in major depressive disorders: are there biological markers for the endogenous subtype? Biol Psychiatry 1982;17:1217–42.
15. Kupfer DJ, Foster FG. Interval between onset of sleep and rapid-eye-movement sleep as an indicator of depression. Lancet 1972;2:684–6.
16. Kupfer DJ, Reynolds CF III, Ehlers CL. Comparison of EEG sleep measures among depressive subtypes and controls in older individuals. Psychiatry Res 1989;27:13–21.
17. Kupfer DJ, Ulrich RF, Coble PA, et al. Application of automated REM and slow-wave sleep analysis, II: testing the assumptions of the two-process model of sleep regulation in normal and depressed subjects. Psychiatry Res 1985;13: 335–43.
18. Snyder F. Dynamic aspects of sleep disturbance in relation to mental illness. Biol Psychiatry 1969;1:119–30.
19. Hartmann E, Verdone P, Snyder F. Longitudinal studies of sleep and dreaming patterns in psychiatric patients. J Nerv Ment Dis 1966;142:117–26.
20. Mendels J, Hawkins DR. Sleep and depression: a controlled EEG study. Arch Gen Psychiatry 1967;16:344–54.
21. Benca RM, Obermeyer WH, Thisted RA, et al. Sleep and psychiatric disorders: a meta-analysis. Arch Gen Psychiatry 1992;49:651–68.
22. Quitkin FM, Rabkin JG, Stewart JW, et al. Sleep of atypical depressives. J Affect Disord 1985;8:61–7.
23. Emslie GJ, Rush AJ, Weinberg WA, et al. Children with major depression show reduced rapid eye movement latencies. Arch Gen Psychiatry 1990;47:119–24.
24. Jones DA, Kelwala S, Bell J, et al. Cholinergic REM sleep induction response correlation with endogenous depressive subtype. Psychiatry Res 1985;14: 99–110.
25. Foster FG, Kupfer DJ, Coble PA, et al. Rapid eye movement sleep density. An objective indicator in severe medial-depressive syndromes. Arch Gen Psychiatry 1976;33:1119–23.
26. Borbely AA, Tobler I, Loepfe M, et al. All night spectral analysis of the sleep EEG in untreated depressives and normal controls. Psychiatry Res 1984;12: 27–33.

27. Feinberg M, Gillin JC, Carroll BJ, et al. EEG studies of sleep in the diagnosis of depression. Biol Psychiatry 1982;17:305–16.
28. Kupfer DJ, Reynolds CF III, Ulrich RF, et al. Comparison of automated REM and slow wave sleep analysis in young and middle-aged depressed subjects. Biol Psychiatry 1986;21:189–200.
29. Giles DE, Etzel BA, Reynolds CF III, et al. Stability of polysomnographic parameters in unipolar depression: a cross-sectional report. Biol Psychiatry 1989;25:807–10.
30. Thase ME, Fasiczka AL, Berman SR, et al. Electroencephalographic sleep profiles before and after cognitive behavioral therapy of depression. Arch Gen Psychiatry 1998;55:138–44.
31. Hauri PJ, Chernic D, Hawkins DR, et al. Sleep of depressed patients in remission. Arch Gen Psychiatry 1974;31:386–91.
32. Rush AJ, Erman MK, Giles DE, et al. Polysomnographic findings in recently drug-free and clinically remitted depressed patients. Arch Gen Psychiatry 1986;43:878–84.
33. Lee JH, Reynolds CF III, Hoch CC, et al. Electroencephalographic sleep in recently remitted, elderly depressed patients in double-blind placebo maintenance therapy. Neuropsychopharmacology 1993;8:143–50.
34. Schulz H, Lund RD, Cording C, et al. Bimodal distribution of REM sleep latencies in depression. Biol Psychiatry 1979;14:595–600.
35. Kerkhofs M, Hoffman G, De Martelaere V, et al. Sleep EEG recordings in depressive disorders. J Affect Disord 1985;9:47–53.
36. Wehr TA, Sack DA, Rosenthal NE. Sleep reduction as a final common pathway in the genesis of mania. Am J Psychiatry 1987;144:201–4.
37. Nofzinger EA, Thase ME, Reynolds CF III, et al. Hypersomnia in bipolar depression: a comparison with narcolepsy using the multiple sleep latency test. Am J Psychiatry 1991;148:1177–81.
38. Hudson JI, Lipinski JF, Frankenburg FR, et al. Electroencephalographic sleep in mania. Arch Gen Psychiatry 1988;45:267–73.
39. Linkowski P, Kerkhofs M, Rielaert C, et al. Sleep during mania in manic-depressive males. Eur Arch Psychiatry Neurol Sci 1986;235:339–41.
40. Monti JM, Monti D. Sleep disturbance in generalized anxiety disorder and its treatment. Sleep Med Rev 2000;4:263–76.
41. Reynolds CF 3rd, Shaw DH, Newton TF, et al. EEG sleep in outpatients with generalized anxiety: as preliminary comparison with depressed outpatients. Psychiatry Res 1983;8:81–9.
42. Uhde TW. Anxiety disorders. In: Kryger MH, Roth T, Dement WC, editors. Principles and practice of sleep medicine. 3rd edition. W.B. Saunders; 2000. p. 1123–39.
43. Saletu B, Anderer P, Brandstätter N, et al. Insomnia in generalized anxiety disorder: polysomnographic, psychometric and clinical investigations before, during and after therapy with a long- versus a short-half-life benzodiazepine (quazepam versus triazolam). Neuropsychobiology 1994;29(2):69–90.
44. Fuller KH, Waters WF, Binks PG, et al. Generalized anxiety and sleep architecture: a polysomnographic investigation. Sleep 1997 May;20(5):370–6.
45. Ross RJ, Ball WA, Sullivan KA, et al. Sleep disturbance as the hallmark of post-traumatic stress disorder. Am J Psychiatry 1989;146:697–707.
46. Mellman TA, Kulick-Bell R, Ashlock LE, et al. Sleep events among veterans with combat-related posttraumatic stress disorder. Am J Psychiatry 1995;152:110–5.

47. Mellman T, Kumar A, Kulick-Bell R, et al. Nocturnal/daytime urine noradrenergic measures and sleep in combat-related PTSD. Biol Psychiatry 1995;38:174–9.

48. Mellman TA, Nolan B, Hebding J, et al. A polysomnographic comparison of veterans with combat-related PTSD, Depressed men, and non-ill controls. Sleep 1997;20:46–51.

49. Dow BM, Kelsoe JR Jr, Gillin JC. Sleep and dreams in Vietnam PTSD and depression. Biol Psychiatry 1996;39:42–50.

50. Kobayashi I, Huntley E, Lavela J, et al. Subjectively and objectively measured sleep with and without posttraumatic stress disorder and trauma exposure. Sleep 2012;35(7):957–65.

51. Woodward SH, Arsenault NJ, Murray C, et al. Laboratory sleep correlates of nightmare complaint in PSTD inpatients. Biol Psychiatry 2000;48:1081–7.

52. Hurwitz TD, Mahowald MW, Kuskowski M, et al. Polysomnographic sleep is not clinically impaired in Vietnam combat veterans with chronic posttraumatic stress disorder. Biol Psychiatry 1998;44:1066–73.

53. Krystal AD, Edinger JD, Wohlgemuth WK, et al. NREM sleep EEG frequency spectral correlates of sleep complaints in primary insomnia subtypes. Sleep 2002;25(6):630–40.

54. Krystal AD, Edinger JD. Sleep EEG predictors and correlates of the response to cognitive behavioral therapy for insomnia. Sleep 2010;33(5):669–77.

55. Breslau N. The epidemiology of posttraumatic stress disorder: what is the extent of the Problem? J Clin Psychiatry 2001;62(Suppl 17):16–22.

56. Doi Y, Minowa M, Uchiyama M, et al. Psychometric assessment of subjective sleep quality using the Japanese version of the Pittsburgh Sleep Quality Index (PSQI-J) in psychiatric disordered and control subjects. Psychiatry Res 2000;97(2–3):165–72.

57. Hofstetter JR, Mayeda AR, Happel CG, et al. Sleep and daily activity preferences in schizophrenia: associations with neurocognition and symptoms. J Nerv Ment Dis 2003;191(6):408–10.

58. Hofstetter JR, Lysaker PH, Mayeda AR. Quality of sleep in patients with schizophrenia is associated with quality of life and coping. BMC Psychiatry 2005;5(13):1–5.

59. Van Kammen DP, Van Kammen WB, Peters JL, et al. CSF MHPG, sleep and psychosis in schizophrenia. Clin Neuropharmacol 1986;9(Suppl 4):575–7.

60. Van Kammen DP, Van Kammen WM, Peters J, et al. Decreased slow-wave sleep and enlarged lateral ventricles in schizophrenia. Neuropsychopharmacology 1988;1:265–71.

61. Martin JL, Jeste DV, Ancoli-Israel S. Older schizophrenia patients have more disrupted sleep and circadian rhythms than age-matched comparison subjects. J Psychiatr Res 2005;39(3):251–9.

62. Chouinard S, Poulin J, Stip E, et al. Sleep in untreated patients with schizophrenia: a meta-analysis. Schizophr Bull 2004;30(4):957–67.

63. Caldwell DF, Domino EF. Electroencephalographic and eye movement patterns during sleep in chronic schizophrenia patients. Electroencephalogr Clin Neurophysiol 1967;22:414–20.

64. Poulin J, Daoust AM, Forest G, et al. Sleep architecture and its clinical correlates in first episode and neuroleptic-naive patients with schizophrenia. Schizophr Res 2003;62(1–2):147–53.

65. Feinberg I, Braum N, Koresko RL, et al. Stage 4 sleep in schizophrenia. Arch Gen Psychiatry 1969;21:262–6.

66. Hiatt JF, Floyd TC, Katz PH, et al. Further evidence of abnormal non-rapid-eye-movement sleep in schizophrenia. Arch Gen Psychiatry 1985;42:797–802.

67. Jus K, Bouchard M, Jus AK, et al. Sleep EEG studies in untreated long-term schizophrenic patients. Arch Gen Psychiatry 1973;29:386–90.

68. Keshaven MS, Reynolds CF 3rd, Miewald J, et al. Slow-wave sleep deficits and outcome in schizophrenia and schizoaffective disorder. Acta Psychiatr Scand 1995;91(5):289–92.

69. Keshavan MS, Miewald J, Haas G, et al. Slow-wave sleep and symptomatology in schizophrenia and related psychotic disorders. J Psychiatr Res 1995;29:303–14.

70. Stern M, Fram D, Wyatt R, et al. All night sleep studies of acute schizophrenics. Arch Gen Psychiatry 1969;20:470–7.

71. Tandon R, Shipley JE, Taylor S, et al. Electroencephalographic sleep abnormalities in schizophrenia. Relationship to positive/negative symptoms and prior neuroleptic treatment. Arch Gen Psychiatry 1992;49(3):185–94.

72. Zarcone VP, Benson KL, Berger PA. Abnormal rapid eye movement latencies in schizophrenia. Arch Gen Psychiatry 1987;44:45–8.

73. Benson KL, Zarcone VP. Sleep abnormalities in schizophrenia and other psychotic disorders. In: Oldham JM, Riba MS, editors. Review of psychiatry, vol. 13. Washington, DC: American Psychiatric Press; 1994. p. 677–705.

74. Baekeland F, Lundwall L, Shanahan TJ, et al. Clinical correlates of reported sleep disturbance in alcoholics. Q J Stud Alcohol 1974;35:1230–41.

75. Brower KJ, Aldrich MS, Robinson EA, et al. Insomnia, self-medication, and relapse to alcoholism. Am J Psychiatry 2001;158:399–404.

76. Brower KJ. Insomnia, alcoholism and relapse. Sleep Med Rev 2003;7(6):523–39.

77. Lobo LL, Tufik S. Effects of alcohol on sleep parameters of sleep-deprived healthy volunteers. Sleep 1997;20:52–9.

78. Gillin JC, Drummond SP. Medication and substance abuse. In: Kryger MH, Roth T, Dement WC, editors. Principles and practice of sleep medicine. 3rd edition. W.B. Saunders; 2000. p. 1176–95.

79. Adamson J, Burdick JA. Sleep of dry alcoholics. Arch Gen Psychiatry 1973;28: 146–9.

80. Drummond SP, Gillin JC, Smith TL, et al. The sleep of abstinent pure primary alcoholic patients: natural course and relationship to relapse. Alcohol Clin Exp Res 1998;22:1796–802.

81. Breslau N, Roth T, Rosenthal L, et al. Sleep disturbance and psychiatric disorders: a longitudinal epidemiologic study of young adults. Biol Psychiatry 1996;39:411–8.

82. Mellinger GD, Balter MB, Uhlenhuth EH. Insomnia and its treatment. Prevalence and correlates. Arch Gen Psychiatry 1985;42:225–32.

83. Ford DE, Kamerow DB. Epidemiologic study of sleep disturbance and psychiatric disorders: an opportunity for prevention? JAMA 1989;262:1479–84.

84. Livingston G, Blizard B, Mann A. Does sleep disturbance predict depression in elderly people? A study in inner London. Br J Gen Pract 1993;43:445–8.

85. Chang PP, Ford DE, Mead LA, et al. Insomnia in young men and subsequent depression. Am J Epidemiol 1997;146:105–14.

86. Koren D, Arnon I, Lavie P, et al. Sleep complaints as early predictors of posttraumatic stress disorder: a 1-year prospective study of injured survivors of motor vehicle accidents. Am J Psychiatry 2002;159(5):855–7.

87. Zarcone VP, Benson KL. BPRS symptom factors and sleep variables in schizophrenia. Psychiatry Res 1997;66:111–20.

88. Chemerinski E, Ho BC, Flaum M, et al. Insomnia as a predictor for symptom worsening following antipsychotic withdrawal in schizophrenia. Compr Psychiatry 2002;43(5):393–6.

89. Weissman MM, Greenwald S, Nino-Murcia G, et al. The morbidity of insomnia uncomplicated by psychiatric disorders. Gen Hosp Psychiatry 1997;19(4): 245–50.

90. Nierenberg AA, Keefe BR, Leslie VC, et al. Residual symptoms in depressed patients who respond acutely to fluoxetine. J Clin Psychiatry 1999;60:221–5.

91. Roehrs T, Papineau K, Rosenthal L, et al. Ethanol as a hypnotic in insomniacs: self administration and effects on sleep and mood. Neuropsychopharmacology 1999;20(3):279–86.

92. Skoloda TE, Alterman AI, Gottheil E. Sleep quality reported by drinking and non-drinking alcoholics. In: Gottheil EL, Elmsford NY, editors. Addiction research and treatment. New York: Pergamon Press; 1979. p. 102–12.

93. NIH. Consensus conference. Drugs and insomnia. The use of medications to promote sleep. JAMA 1984;11(251):2410–4.

94. Carney CE, Segal ZV, Edinger JD, et al. A comparison of rates of residual insomnia symptoms following pharmacotherapy or cognitive-behavioral therapy for major depressive disorder. J Clin Psychiatry 2007;68(2):254–60.

95. Reynolds CF III, Frank E, Houck PR, et al. Which elderly patients with remitted depression remain well with continued interpersonal psychotherapy after discontinuation of antidepressant medication? Am J Psychiatry 1997;154: 958–62.

96. Asnis GM, Chakraburtty A, DuBoff EA, et al. Zolpidem for persistent insomnia in SSRI-treated depressed patients. J Clin Psychiatry 1999;60:668–76.

97. Agargun MY, Kara H, Solmaz M. Sleep disturbances and suicidal behavior in patients with major depression. J Clin Psychiatry 1997;58:249–51.

98. Agargun M, Kara H, Solmaz M. Subjective sleep quality and suicidality in patients with major depression. J Psychiatr Res 1997;31(3):377–81.

99. Agargun M, Cilli A, Kara H, et al. Repetitive and frightening dreams and suicidal behavior in patients with major depression. Compr Psychiatry 1998;39(4): 198–202.

100. Agargun MY, Besiroglu L, Cilli AS, et al. Nightmares, suicide attempts, and melancholic features in patients with unipolar major depression. J Affect Disord 2007;98:267–70.

101. Choquet M, Menke H. Suicidal thoughts during early adolescence: prevalence, associated troubles and help-seeking behavior. Acta Psychiatr Scand 1989;81: 170–7.

102. Choquet M, Kovess V. Suicidal thoughts among adolescents: an intercultural approach. Adolescence 1993;28(111):649–61.

103. McCall WV, Blocker JN, D'Agostino R Jr, et al. Insomnia severity is an indicator of suicidal ideation during a depression clinical trial. Sleep Med 2010;11(9): 822–7.

104. Bernert R, Joiner T, Cukrowicz K, et al. Suicidality and sleep disturbances. Sleep 2005;28(9):1135–41.

105. Chellappa SL, Araújo JF. Sleep disorders and suicidal ideation in patients with depressive disorder. Psychiatry Res 2007;153:131–6.

106. Fawcett J, Scheftner WA, Fogg L, et al. Time-related predictors of suicide in major affective disorder. Am J Psychiatry 1990;147:1189–94.

107. Vignau J, Bailly D, Duhamel A, et al. Epidemiologic study of sleep quality and troubles in French secondary school adolescents. J Adolesc Health 1997;21: 343–50.

108. Sjöström N, Waern M, Hetta J. Nightmares and sleep disturbances in relation to suicidality in suicide attempters. Sleep 2007;30:91–5.

109. Smith M, Perlis M, Haythornthwaite J. Suicidal ideation in outpatients with chronic musculoskeletal pain. Clin J Pain 2004;20(2):111–8.
110. Roberts R, Roberts C, Chen I. Functioning of adolescents with symptoms of disturbed sleep. J Youth Adolesc 2001;30(1):1–18.
111. Tanskanen A, Tuomilehto J, Vinamaki H, et al. Nightmares are predictors of suicide. Sleep 2001;24(7):844–7.
112. Turvey CL, Conwell Y, Jones MP, et al. Risk factors for late-life suicide: a prospective, community-based study. Am J Geriatr Psychiatry 2002;10:398–406.
113. Oquendo MA, Mann JJ. Intervention research for suicidal behaviour. Lancet 2003;362(9387):844–5.
114. Buysse D, Reynolds CF, Houck PR, et al. Does lorazepam impair the antidepressant response to nortriptyline and psychotherapy? J Clin Psychiatry 1997; 58(10):426–32.
115. Dew M, Reynolds CF, Houck PR, et al. Temporal profiles of the course of depression during treatment. Predictors of pathways toward recovery in the elderly. Arch Gen Psychiatry 1997;54(11):1016–24.
116. Thase M, Buysse DJ, Frank E, et al. Which depressed patients will respond to interpersonal psychotherapy? The role of abnormal EEG sleep profiles. Am J Psychiatry 1997;154(4):502–9.
117. Winokur A, Reynolds CF. The effects of antidepressants and anxiolytics on sleep physiology. Prim Psychiatr 1994;1:22–7.
118. McCall WV, Reboussin BA, Cohen W. Subjective measurement of insomnia and quality of life in depressed inpatients. J Sleep Res 2000;9:43–8.
119. Nolen WA, Haffmans PM, Bouvy PF, et al. Hypnotics as concurrent medication in depression. A placebo-controlled, double-blind comparison of flunitrazepam and lormetazepam in patients with major depression, treated with a (tri)cyclic antidepressant. J Affect Disord 1993;28:179–88.
120. Fava M, McCall WV, Krystal A, et al. Eszopiclone co-administered with fluoxetine in patients with insomnia coexisting with major depressive disorder. Biol Psychiatry 2006;59(11):1052–60.
121. Krystal A, Fava M, Rubens R, et al. Evaluation of eszopiclone discontinuation after cotherapy with fluoxetine for insomnia with coexisting depression. J Clin Sleep Med 2007;3(1):48–55.
122. Fava M, Asnis GM, Shrivastava RK, et al. Improved insomnia symptoms and sleep-related next-day functioning in patients with comorbid major depressive disorder and insomnia following concomitant zolpidem extended-release 12.5 mg and escitalopram treatment: a randomized controlled trial. J Clin Psychiatry 2011;72(7):914–28.
123. Manber R, Edinger JD, Gress JL, et al. Cognitive behavioral therapy for insomnia enhances depression outcome in patients with comorbid major depressive disorder and insomnia. Sleep 2008;31(4):489–95.
124. Wehr TA. Sleep loss as a possible mediator of diverse causes of mania. Br J Psychiatry 1991;159:576–8.
125. Wehr TA, Goodwin FK, Wirz-Justice A, et al. 48-hour sleep-wake cycles in manic-depressive illness: naturalistic observations and sleep deprivation experiments. Arch Gen Psychiatry 1982;39:559–65.
126. Zimanova J, Vojtechovsky M. Sleep deprivation as a potentiation of antidepressant pharmacotherapy. Act Nerv Super (Praha) 1974;16:188–9.
127. Fava M, Asnis GM, Shrivastava R, et al. Zolpidem extended-release improves sleep and next-day symptoms in comorbid insomnia and generalized anxiety disorder. J Clin Psychopharmacol 2009;29(3):222–30.

128. Pollack M, Kinrys G, Krystal A, et al. Eszopiclone coadministered with escitalopram in patients with insomnia and comorbid generalized anxiety disorder. Arch Gen Psychiatry 2008;65(5):551–62.
129. Germain A, Richardson R, Moul DE, et al. Placebo-controlled comparison of prazosin and cognitive-behavioral treatments for sleep disturbances in US Military Veterans. J Psychosom Res 2012;72(2):89–96.
130. Pollack MH, Hoge EA, Worthington JJ, et al. Eszopiclone for the treatment of posttraumatic stress disorder and associated insomnia: a randomized, double-blind, placebo-controlled trial. J Clin Psychiatry 2011;72(7):892–7.
131. Raskind MA, Peskind ER, Kanter ED, et al. Reduction of nightmares and other PTSD symptoms in combat veterans by prazosin: a placebo-controlled study. Am J Psychiatry 2003;160(2):371–3.
132. Taylor FB, Martin P, Thompson C, et al. Prazosin effects on objective sleep measures and clinical symptoms in civilian trauma posttraumatic stress disorder: a placebo-controlled study. Biol Psychiatry 2008;63(6):629–32.
133. Raskind MA, Peskind ER, Hoff DJ, et al. A parallel group placebo controlled study of prazosin for trauma nightmares and sleep disturbance in combat veterans with post-traumatic stress disorder. Biol Psychiatry 2007;61(8):928–34.
134. Taylor FB, Lowe K, Thompson C, et al. Daytime prazosin reduces psychological distress to trauma specific cues in civilian trauma posttraumatic stress disorder. Biol Psychiatry 2006;59(7):577–81.
135. Lauer CJ, Schreiber W, Pollmacher T, et al. Sleep in schizophrenia: a polysomnographic study on drug-naïve patients. Neuropsychopharmacology 1997;16:51–60.
136. Neylan TC, Van Kammen DP, Kelley ME, et al. Sleep in schizophrenic patients on and off haloperidol therapy. Arch Gen Psychiatry 1992;49:643–9.
137. Benson KL, Zarcone VP. REM sleep eye movement activity in schizophrenia and depression. Arch Gen Psychiatry 1993;50:474–82.
138. Taylor SF, Tandon R, Shipley JE, et al. Sleep-onset REM periods in schizophrenic patients. Biol Psychiatry 1991;30:205–9.
139. Keshavan MS, Reynolds CF, Montrose D, et al. Sleep and suicidality in psychotic patients. Acta Psychiatr Scand 1994;89:122–5.
140. Lewis CF, Tandon R, Shipley JE, et al. Biological predictors of suicidality in schizophrenia. Acta Psychiatr Scand 1996;94:416–20.
141. Foster JH, Peters TJ. Impaired sleep in alcohol misusers and dependent alcoholics and the impact upon outcome. Alcohol Clin Exp Res 1999;23(6):1044–51.
142. Allen RP, Wagman AM, Funderburk FR, et al. Slow wave sleep: a predictor of individual differences in response to drinking? Biol Psychiatry 1980;15:345–8.
143. Gillin JC, Smith TL, Irwin M, et al. Increased pressure for rapid eye movement sleep at time of hospital admission predicts relapse in nondepressed patients with primary alcoholism at 3-month follow-up. Arch Gen Psychiatry 1994;51:189–97.
144. Brower KJ, Aldrich MS, Hall JM. Polysomnographic and subjective sleep predictors of alcoholic relapse. Alcohol Clin Exp Res 1998;22:1864–71.
145. Le Bon O, Murphy JR, Staner L, et al. Double-blind, placebo-controlled study of the efficacy of trazodone in alcohol post-withdrawal syndrome: polysomnographic and clinical evaluations. J Clin Psychopharmacol 2003;23(4):377–83.
146. Brower KJ, Myra Kim H, Strobbe S, et al. Randomized double-blind pilot trial of gabapentin versus placebo to treat alcohol dependence and comorbid insomnia. Alcohol Clin Exp Res 2008;32(8):1429–38.
147. Bowers M, Kupfer DJ. Central monoamine oxidase inhibition and REM sleep. Brain Res 1971;35:561–4.

148. Wyatt RJ, Fram DH, Buchbinder R, et al. Treatment of intractable narcolepsy with a monoamine oxidase inhibitor. N Engl J Med 1971;285:987–91.

149. Wyatt RJ, Fram DH, Kupfer DJ, et al. Total prolonged drug-induced REM sleep suppression in anxious-depressed patients. Arch Gen Psychiatry 1971;24: 145–55.

150. Gillin JC, Wyatt RJ, Fram D, et al. The relationship between changes in REM sleep and clinical improvement in depressed patients treated with amitriptyline. Psychopharmacology (Berl) 1978;59:267–72.

151. Kupfer DJ, Spiker DG, Coble PA, et al. Sleep and treatment prediction in endogenous depression. Am J Psychiatry 1981;138:429–34.

152. Thase ME. Depression and sleep: pathophysiology and treatment. Dialogues Clin Neurosci 2006;8:217–26.

153. Mayers AG, Baldwin DS. Antidepressants and their effect on sleep. Hum Psychopharmacol 2005;20:533–59.

154. Krystal AD, Thase ME, Tucker VL, et al. Bupropion HCL and sleep in patients with depression. Clin Psych Rev Current Psychiatry Reviews 2007;3:123–8.

155. Scharf MB, Sachais BA. Sleep laboratory evaluation of the effects and efficacy of trazodone in depressed insomniac patients. J Clin Psychiatry 1990;51:13–7.

156. Mouret J, Lemoine P, Minuit MP, et al. Effects of trazodone on the sleep of depressed subjects—a polygraphic study. Psychopharmacology 1988;95:37–43.

157. Winokur A, Sateia MJ, Hayes JB, et al. Acute effects of mirtazapine on sleep continuity and sleep architecture in depressed patients: a pilot study. Biol Psychiatry 2000;48(1):75–8.

158. Winokur A, DeMartinis NA 3rd, McNally DP. Comparative effects of mirtazapine and fluoxetine on sleep physiology measures in patients with major depression and insomnia. J Clin Psychiatry 2003;64(10):1224–9.

159. Parrino L, Spaggiari MC, Boselli M, et al. Clinical and polysomnographic effects of trazodone CR in chronic insomnia associated with dysthymia. Psychopharmacology 1994;116:389–95.

160. Ware JC, Pittard JT. Increased deep sleep after trazodone use: a double-blind placebo- controlled study in healthy young adults. J Clin Psychiatry 1990; 51(Suppl):18–22.

161. Krystal AD, Lankford A, Durrence HH, et al. Efficacy and safety of doxepin 3 and 6 mg in a 35-day sleep laboratory trial in adults with chronic primary insomnia. Sleep 2011;34(10):1433–42.

162. Krystal AD, Durrence HH, Scharf M, et al. Efficacy and safety of doxepin 1 mg and 3 mg in a 12-week sleep laboratory and outpatient trial of elderly subjects with chronic primary insomnia. Sleep 2010;33(11):1553–61.

163. Scharf M, Rogowski R, Hull S, et al. Efficacy and safety of doxepin 1 mg, 3 mg, and 6 mg in elderly patients with primary insomnia: a randomized, double-blind, placebo-controlled crossover study. J Clin Psychiatry 2008;69(10):1557–64.

164. Roth T, Rogowski R, Hull S, et al. Efficacy and safety of doxepin 1 mg, 3 mg, and 6 mg in adults with primary insomnia. Sleep 2007;30(11):1555–61.

165. Roth T, Zorick F, Wittig R, et al. The effects of doxepin HCl on sleep and depression. J Clin Psychiatry 1982;43(9):366–8.

166. Feuillade P, Pringuey D, Belugou JL, et al. Trimipramine: acute and lasting effects on sleep in healthy and major depressive subjects. J Affect Disord 1992;24:135–45.

167. Hajak G, Rodenbeck A, Voderholzer U, et al. Doxepin in the treatment of primary insomnia: a placebo-controlled, double-blind, polysomnographic study. J Clin Psychiatry 2001;62(6):453–63.

168. Hohagen F, Montero RF, Weiss E. Treatment of primary insomnia with trimipramine: an alternative to benzodiazepine hypnotics? Eur Arch Psychiatry Clin Neurosci 1994;244(2):65–72.

169. Riemann D, Voderholzer U, Cohrs S, et al. Trimipramine in primary insomnia: results of a polysomnographic double-blind controlled study. Pharmacopsychiatry 2002;35(5):165–74.

170. Hartmann E, Cravens J. The effects of long term administration of psychotropic drugs on human sleep, IV: the effects of chlorpromazine. Psychopharmacology (Berl) 1973;33:203–18.

171. Ruigt GS, Kemp B, Groenhout CM, et al. Effect of the antidepressant Org 3770 on human sleep. Eur J Clin Pharmacol 1990;38:551–4.

172. Hoque R, Chesson AL Jr. Pharmacologically induced/exacerbated restless legs syndrome, periodic limb movements of sleep, and REM behavior disorder/REM sleep without atonia: literature review, qualitative scoring, and comparative analysis. J Clin Sleep Med 2010;6(1):79–83.

173. Yang C, White DP, Winkelman JW. Antidepressants and periodic leg movements of sleep. Biol Psychiatry 2005;58:510–4.

174. Kupfer DJ, Reynolds CF III, Weiss BL, et al. Lithium carbonate and sleep in affective disorders: further considerations. Arch Gen Psychiatry 1974;30:79–84.

175. Terao T, Terao M, Yoshimura R, et al. Restless legs syndrome induced by lithium. Biol Psychiatry 1991;30:1167–70.

176. Krystal AD, Goforth H, Roth T. Effects of antipsychotic medications on sleep in schizophrenia. Int Clin Psychopharmacol 2008;23:150–60.

177. Cohrs S, Rodenbeck A, Guan Z, et al. Sleep-promoting properties of quetiapine in healthy subjects. Psychopharmacology 2004;174:421–9.

178. Cohrs S, Meier A, Neumann AC, et al. Improved sleep continuity and increased slow wave sleep and REM latency during ziprasidone treatment: a randomized, controlled, crossover trial of 12 healthy male subjects. J Clin Psychiatry 2005;66:989–96.

179. Salin-Pascual RJ, Herrera-Estrella M, Galicia-Polo L, et al. Olanzapine acute administration in schizophrenic patients increases delta sleep and sleep efficiency. Biol Psychiatry 1999;46(1):141–3.

180. Salin-Pascual RJ, Herrera-Estrella M, Galicia-Polo L, et al. Low delta sleep predicted a good clinical response to olanzapine administration in schizophrenic patients. Rev Invest Clin 2004;56:345–50.

181. Sharpley AL, Vassallo CM, Cowen PJ. Olanzapine increases slow-wave sleep: evidence for blockade of central 5-HT2C receptors in vivo. Biol Psychiatry 2000;47(5):468–70.

182. Sharpley AL, Vassallo CM, Pooley EC. Allelic variation in the 5-HT2C receptor (HT2RC) and the increase in slow wave sleep produced by olanzapine. Psychopathology 2001;153:271–2.

183. Sharpley AL, Attenburrow ME, Hafizi S, et al. Olanzapine increases slow wave sleep and sleep continuity in SSRI-resistant depressed patients. J Clin Psychiatry 2005;66(4):450–4.

184. Gimenez S, Clos S, Romero S, et al. Effects of olanzapine, risperidone and haloperidol on sleep after a single oral morning dose in healthy volunteers. Psychopharmacology 2007;190(4):507–16.

185. Lindberg N, Virkkunen M, Tani P, et al. Effect of a single-dose of olanzapine on sleep in healthy females and males. Int Clin Psychopharmacol 2002;17(4):177–84.

186. Moreno RA, Hanna MM, Tavares SM, et al. A double-blind comparison of the effect of the antipsychotics haloperidol and olanzapine on sleep in mania. Braz J Med Biol Res 2007;40(3):357–66.
187. Hinze-Selch D, Mullington J, Orth A, et al. Effects of clozapine on sleep: a longitudinal study. Biol Psychiatry 1997;42:260–6.
188. Lee JH, Woo JI, Meltzer HY. Effects of clozapine on sleep measures and sleep-associated changes in growth hormone and cortisol in patients with schizophrenia. Psychiatry Res 2001;103:157–66.
189. Sharpley AL, Bhagwagar Z, Hafizi S, et al. Risperidone augmentation decreases rapid eye movement sleep and decreases wake in treatment-resistant depressed patients. J Clin Psychiatry 2003;64:192–6.
190. Staner L, Boeijinga P, Danel T, et al. Effects of acamprosate on sleep during alcohol withdrawal: a double-blind placebo-controlled polysomnographic study in alcohol-dependent subjects. Alcohol Clin Exp Res 2006;30(9):1492–9.
191. Pflug B, Tolle R. Disturbance of the 24-hour rhythm in endogenous depression by sleep deprivation. Int Pharmacopsychiatry 1971;6:187–96.
192. Post RM, Kotin J, Goodwin FK. Effects of sleep deprivation on mood and central amine metabolism in depressed patients. Arch Gen Psychiatry 1976;33:627–32.
193. Van den Burg W, Van den Hoofdakker RH. Total sleep deprivation on endogenous depression. Arch Gen Psychiatry 1975;32:1121–5.
194. Weigand M, Berger M, Zulley J, et al. The influence of daytime naps on the therapeutic effect of sleep deprivation. Biol Psychiatry 1987;22:386–9.
195. Sack DA, Dancan W, Rosenthal NE, et al. The timing and duration of sleep in partial sleep deprivation therapy of depression. Acta Psychiatr Scand 1988; 77:219–24.
196. Berger M, Vollmann J, Hohagen F, et al. Sleep deprivation combined with consecutive sleep phase advance as a fast-acting therapy in depression: an open pilot trial in medicated and unmedicated patients. Am J Psychiatry 1997;154:870–2.
197. Vogel GW, Thurmond A, Gibbons P, et al. REM sleep reduction effects on depressive syndromes. Arch Gen Psychiatry 1975;32:765–77.

Index

Note: Page numbers of article titles are in **boldface** type.

A

ABGs. *See* Arterial blood gases (ABGs)
Acetylcholine
    in alertness, 969
Acromegaly
    CSA and, 1118
Actigraphy
    in sleep assessment, 1003
Adenosine
    in sleep promotion, 972–973
ADHD. *See* Attention-deficit/hyperactivity disorder (ADHD)
ADNFLE. *See* Autosomal dominant nocturnal frontal lobe epilepsy (ADNFLE)
Advanced sleep phase disorder (ASPD), 1175–1177
Advanced sleep phase syndrome, 1175–1177
Age
    as factor in OSA, 1101
Alcohol avoidance
    in OSA management, 1109
Alcohol use
    as factor in OSA, 1102
Alcoholism
    in persons with sleep disturbances
        risk factors for, 1396
    sleep problems associated with, 1395
    treatment of
        sleep effects of, 1401
        sleep problems impact on, 1399
Alertness
    acetylcholine in, 969
Antidepressants
    for insomnia, 1059
Antiepileptics
    for insomnia, 1059
Antipsychotics
    atypical
        for insomnia, 1059
Anxiety
    sleep disorders and, 1017
Anxiety disorders
    in children
        sleep disorders related to, 1206

Neurol Clin 30 (2012) 1415–1433
http://dx.doi.org/10.1016/S0733-8619(12)00083-7
0733-8619/12/$ – see front matter © 2012 Elsevier Inc. All rights reserved.

neurologic.theclinics.com

United States Postal Service

Statement of Ownership, Management, and Circulation
(All Periodicals Publications Except Requestor Publications)

1. Publication Title										2. Publication Number									3. Filing Date
Neurologic Clinics										0	0	0	-	7	1	2			9/14/12

4. Issue Frequency	5. Number of Issues Published Annually	6. Annual Subscription Price
Feb, May, Aug, Nov	4	$285.00

7. Complete Mailing Address of Known Office of Publication (Not printer) (Street, city, county, state, and ZIP+4®)	Contact Person
Elsevier Inc. 360 Park Avenue South New York, NY 10010-1710	Stephen R. Bushing Telephone (Include area code) 215-239-3688

8. Complete Mailing Address of Headquarters or General Business Office of Publisher (Not printer)

Elsevier Inc., 360 Park Avenue South, New York, NY 10010-1710

9. Full Names and Complete Mailing Addresses of Publisher, Editor, and Managing Editor (Do not leave blank)

Publisher (Name and complete mailing address)

Kim Murphy, Elsevier, Inc., 1600 John F. Kennedy Blvd. Suite 1800, Philadelphia, PA 19103-2899

Editor (Name and complete mailing address)

Donald Mumford, Elsevier, Inc., 1600 John F. Kennedy Blvd. Suite 1800, Philadelphia, PA 19103-2899

Managing Editor (Name and complete mailing address)

Sarah Barth, Elsevier, Inc., 1600 John F. Kennedy Blvd. Suite 1800, Philadelphia, PA 19103-2899

10. Owner (Do not leave blank. If the publication is owned by a corporation, give the name and address of the corporation immediately followed by the names and addresses of all stockholders owning or holding 1 percent or more of the total amount of stock. If not owned by a corporation, give the names and addresses of the individual owners. If owned by a partnership or other unincorporated firm, give its name and address as well as those of each individual owner. If the publication is published by a nonprofit organization, give its name and address.)

Full Name	Complete Mailing Address
Wholly owned subsidiary of	1600 John F. Kennedy Blvd., Ste. 1800
Reed/Elsevier, US holdings	Philadelphia, PA 19103-2899

11. Known Bondholders, Mortgagees, and Other Security Holders Owning or Holding 1 Percent or More of Total Amount of Bonds, Mortgages, or Other Securities. If none, check box ☐ None

Full Name	Complete Mailing Address
N/A	

12. Tax Status (For completion by nonprofit organizations authorized to mail at nonprofit rates) (Check one)
The purpose, function, and nonprofit status of this organization and the exempt status for federal income tax purposes:
☐ Has Not Changed During Preceding 12 Months
☐ Has Changed During Preceding 12 Months (Publisher must submit explanation of change with this statement)

PS Form 3526, September 2007 (Page 1 of 3 (Instructions Page 3)) PSN 7530-01-000-9931 PRIVACY NOTICE: See our Privacy policy in www.usps.com

13. Publication Title		14. Issue Date for Circulation Data Below
Neurologic Clinics		August 2012

15. Extent and Nature of Circulation			Average No. Copies Each Issue During Preceding 12 Months	No. Copies of Single Issue Published Nearest to Filing Date
a. Total Number of Copies (Net press run)			1101	840
b. Paid Circulation (By Mail and Outside the Mail)	(1)	Mailed Outside-County Paid Subscriptions Stated on PS Form 3541 (Include paid distribution above nominal rate, advertiser's proof copies, and exchange copies)	520	479
	(2)	Mailed In-County Paid Subscriptions Stated on PS Form 3541 (Include paid distribution above nominal rate, advertiser's proof copies, and exchange copies)		
	(3)	Paid Distribution Outside the Mails Including Sales Through Dealers and Carriers, Street Vendors, Counter Sales, and Other Paid Distribution Outside USPS®	249	255
	(4)	Paid Distribution by Other Classes Mailed Through the USPS (e.g. First-Class Mail®)		
c. Total Paid Distribution (Sum of 15b (1), (2), (3), and (4))		▶	769	734
d. Free or Nominal Rate Distribution (By Mail and Outside the Mail)	(1)	Free or Nominal Rate Outside-County Copies Included on PS Form 3541	78	84
	(2)	Free or Nominal Rate In-County Copies Included on PS Form 3541		
	(3)	Free or Nominal Rate Copies Mailed at Other Classes Through the USPS (e.g. First-Class Mail)		
	(4)	Free or Nominal Rate Distribution Outside the Mail (Carriers or other means)		
e. Total Free or Nominal Rate Distribution (Sum of 15d (1), (2), (3) and (4))		▶	78	84
f. Total Distribution (Sum of 15c and 15e)		▶	847	818
g. Copies not Distributed (See instructions to publishers #4 (page #3))		▶	254	22
h. Total (Sum of 15f and g)		▶	1101	840
i. Percent Paid (15c divided by 15f times 100)			90.79%	89.73%

16. Publication of Statement of Ownership

☐ If the publication is a general publication, publication of this statement is required. Will be printed in the November 2012 issue of this publication.   ☐ Publication not required

17. Signature and Title of Editor, Publisher, Business Manager, or Owner

Stephen R. Bushing – Inventory Distribution Coordinator   Date September 14, 2012

I certify that all information furnished on this form is true and complete. I understand that anyone who furnishes false or misleading information on this form or who omits material or information requested on the form may be subject to criminal sanctions (including fines and imprisonment) and/or civil sanctions (including civil penalties).

PS Form 3526, September 2007 (Page 2 of 3)

Moving?

Make sure your subscription moves with you!

To notify us of your new address, find your **Clinics Account Number** (located on your mailing label above your name), and contact customer service at:

Email: journalscustomerservice-usa@elsevier.com

800-654-2452 (subscribers in the U.S. & Canada)
314-447-8871 (subscribers outside of the U.S. & Canada)

Fax number: 314-447-8029

Elsevier Health Sciences Division
Subscription Customer Service
3251 Riverport Lane
Maryland Heights, MO 63043

*To ensure uninterrupted delivery of your subscription, please notify us at least 4 weeks in advance of move.

Printed and bound by CPI Group (UK) Ltd, Croydon, CR0 4YY

08/06/2025

01896875-0007